Essential Evidence

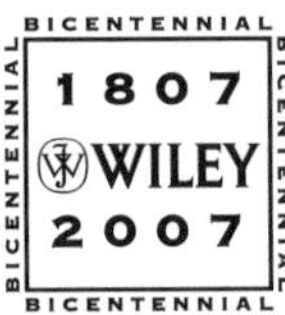

The Wiley Bicentennial–Knowledge for Generations

Each generation has its unique needs and aspirations. When Charles Wiley first opened his small printing shop in lower Manhattan in 1807, it was a generation of boundless potential searching for an identity. And we were there, helping to define a new American literary tradition. Over half a century later, in the midst of the Second Industrial Revolution, it was a generation focused on building the future. Once again, we were there, supplying the critical scientific, technical, and engineering knowledge that helped frame the world. Throughout the 20th Century, and into the new millennium, nations began to reach out beyond their own borders and a new international community was born. Wiley was there, expanding its operations around the world to enable a global exchange of ideas, opinions, and know-how.

For 200 years, Wiley has been an integral part of each generation's journey, enabling the flow of information and understanding necessary to meet their needs and fulfill their aspirations. Today, bold new technologies are changing the way we live and learn. Wiley will be there, providing you the must-have knowledge you need to imagine new worlds, new possibilities, and new opportunities.

Generations come and go, but you can always count on Wiley to provide you the knowledge you need, when and where you need it!

William J. Pesce
President and Chief Executive Officer

Peter Booth Wiley
Chairman of the Board

Essential Evidence

Medicine that Matters

David Slawson
University of Virginia

Allen Shaughnessy
Tufts University

Mark Ebell
Medical College of Georgia

Henry Barry
Michigan State University

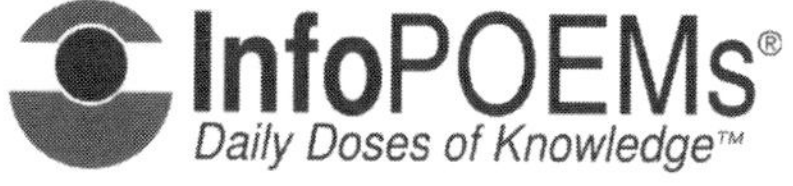

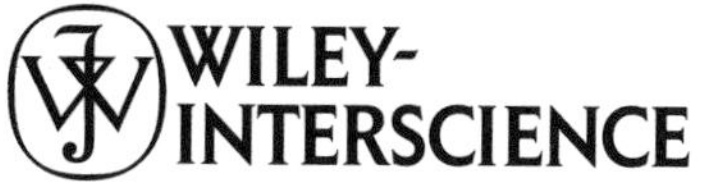

A JOHN WILEY & SONS, INC., PUBLICATION

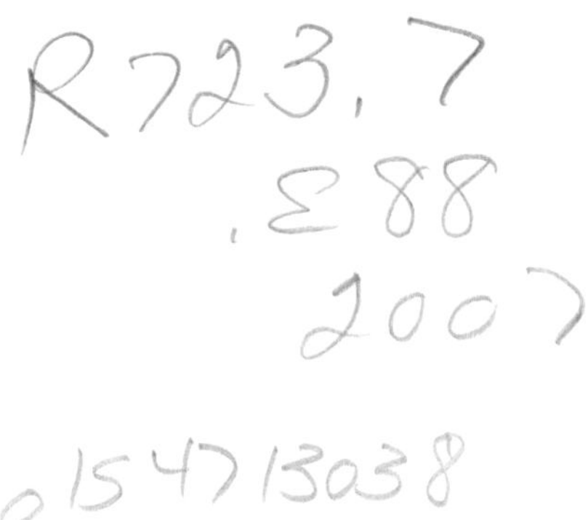

Published by John Wiley & Sons, Inc., Hoboken, New Jersey
Published simultaneously in Canada

For general information on our other products and services or for technical support, please contact our Customer Care Department within the United States at (800) 762-2974, outside the United States at (317) 572-3993 or fax (317) 572-4002.

Wiley also publishes its books in a variety of electronic formats. Some content that appears in print may not be available in electronic formats. For more information about Wiley products, visit our web site at www.wiley.com.

Library of Congress Cataloging-in-Publication Data:
ISBN 978-0-470-17890-4

Printed in the United States of America

10 9 8 7 6 5 4 3 2 1

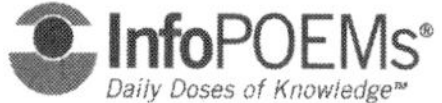

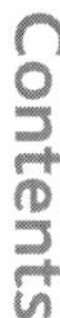

Contents

Contents

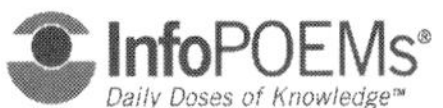

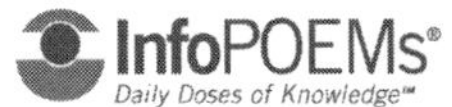
InfoPOEMs®
Daily Doses of Knowledge℠

Contents

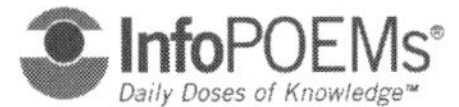
InfoPOEMs®
Daily Doses of Knowledge™

Contents

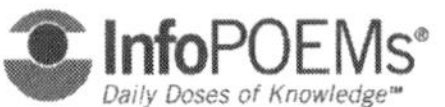
InfoPOEMs®
Daily Doses of Knowledge™

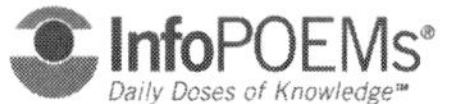

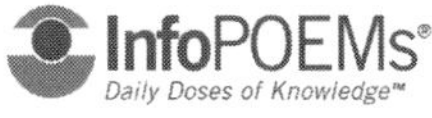

Contents

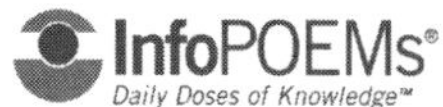
InfoPOEMs
Daily Doses of Knowledge

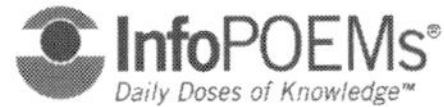
InfoPOEMs
Daily Doses of Knowledge

Contents

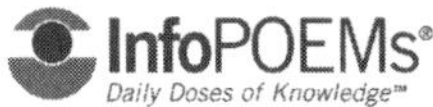

Preface

As you read this preface, tens of thousands of medical researchers from around the world are conducting studies. Thousands of editors are evaluating papers to determine whether the researchers' hard work will see the light of day on their journal pages. Countless journalists, newsletter writers, bloggers, and web masters are summarizing the results of published research for their readers. And, no doubt, several of your own patients are, at this very moment, printing or copying research findings to bring to you for your opinion.

Although almost all of it is good, and some of it is interesting, most of this research is not ready for "prime time." Our goal for writing *Essential Evidence* is to sort, evaluate, and summarize recent research findings most helpful for physicians striving to provide the best care for their patients. We have filtered through the mountain of research recently published to find the study results that can – and should – change your practice.

How do we do it? Each month, five editors survey 118 journals – almost 200 individual issues – looking for valid research that focuses on outcomes patients care about. From over 2000 articles published in these journals every month, we are able to find about 25 articles that meet these criteria. We translate the 2500 words of research-speak into short, structured, unbiased 250 word synopses written for busy clinicians. The editorial board members savage these synopses, we rewrite them, and the finished product is proofread, translated into languages other than English, and then made into what has become known as an InfoPOEM (Patient-Oriented Evidence that Matters). This manual is a collection of the best, relevant InfoPOEMs from the past several years.

Essential Evidence begins with two chapters providing a brief synopsis of some of the key concepts of evidence-based medicine and some tips on keeping up and on finding information when you need it. Do not skip these chapters – they will help you understand the rest of the book.

The remaining chapters, organized by disease category, provide InfoPOEMs, or rather one-page synopses of recent research studies of importance to everyday clinical practice. Some of the information may be well known to you; much of it, however, will be new and will change your practice for the better. The book ends with a short glossary of common terms.

One of the best characteristics of medicine is that knowledge continuously changes; it is also one of its worst characteristics. It is our hope that this book provides some new knowledge to you that will, ultimately, benefit your patients.

 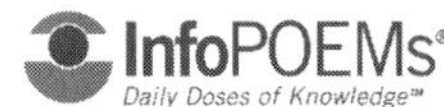

Taking an Evidence-Based Approach to the Care of Patients

We have always used evidence in the practice of medicine. This evidence has come from many sources. So, what is evidence-based medicine (EBM)?

EBM is simply the recognition that there is a hierarchy of evidence in medicine. It says that evidence derived from controlled clinical research has a better likelihood of being correct than evidence derived from other sources. What is so hard about that?

The Problem

The problem with EBM is when the "evidence-based" answer conflicts with what seems to make sense or with what we have always done. Yet there are numerous examples in the recent history of medicine in which controlled clinical research did not prove that what we have always done was best.

The most recent example is the finding that estrogen replacement therapy in postmenopausal women does not protect against heart disease. It is well known that the incidence of heart disease increases following the onset of menopause. We also knew, from *uncontrolled* studies, that women taking estrogen also seemed to have less heart disease.

And then the controlled studies were done. Some women received estrogen, while others did not. When studied in this way, it was shown that the incidence of heart disease was the same whether or not the women received estrogen.

The Language of EBM

Another problem is the language used in presenting research findings. Here are some common terms used in EBM:

- **p-value:**
  - P stands for "probability," the likelihood that the difference observed between two groups could have arisen by chance.
  - The usual p-value is arbitrarily set at 0.05; it means that there is a 5% probability that the difference is actually due to chance.
  - It does not tell you the *importance* of the difference.
  - In the phrase, "51.7% of warfarin recipients developed a DVT as compared with 36.9% of enoxaparin recipients (p = 0.003)," the probability of this difference being due to chance is 0.003 or 0.3%.

- **Confidence Interval (CI)**
  - Sort of a statistic of a statistic. Although studies present a specific number, the confidence interval gives us the range of likely possibilities with a given degree of certainty.
  - A 95% CI tells us that we can be fairly (95%) certain that the true value will fall within this range.

- For example, a difference between treatment A and treatment B might be 42% (95% CI 22%–66%). The difference could only be 22% or could be as high as 66%.

- **Number Needed to Treat (NNT)**
  - When we treat patients, we do so because all have the potential to benefit. Not all patients actually *will* benefit. The NNT is the number of patients that need to be treated for one to receive benefit.
  - NNTs often are very large for prevention. For example, the NNT for treatment of mild hypertension is 700: one stroke, heart attack, or death will be prevented in 700 people receiving treatment for 1 year. Why so high? Most people with mild hypertension will not have a stroke or a heart attack or die. So, even though they received treatment, most patients will not see the benefit, because they were unlikely to have a bad outcome in the first place.
  - For treatment, NNTs are much lower. *Helicobacter pylori* eradication treatment has an NNT of 1.2 – that is because almost everyone is successfully treated.
  - NNTs are best used to get a "feel" for a benefit or to compare one treatment with another.

- **Concealed Allocation**
  - When subjects begin a study, they are allocated to a group, frequently a treatment or a placebo group. There is a risk that researchers performing the study enroll some patients into the study based on what group they will be in. Concealing allocation from the investigator will prevent this from happening.
  - It is not, however, the same as blinding, which occurs *after* the study is started.
  - For example, in many of the studies evaluating the effectiveness of breast cancer screening, researchers knew whether an individual patient would be allocated to the screening (with mammography) or to the no-screening group before enrolling them. If they did not want the particular patient in the group to which they would be assigned, they simply did not enroll them into the study.
  - As a result, the patients in these studies who received mammography were, on average, 6 months older, better educated, and economically better off, three factors that are associated with decreased mortality.

- **Blinding**
  - Preventing people involved in the study from knowing the treatment a subject is receiving.
  - "Double-blinding" means that neither the researcher nor the subject knew what treatment was used.
  - Also called "masking."

Too Much Information, Too Few Answers

We live in the information age. Through various electronic sources, we have unprecedented access to medical information.

So do our patients. The sheer amount of information can quickly overwhelm them – and us.

Along with its volume, much of this information is preliminary, speculative, or will turn out to be just plain wrong. Knowledge develops in medicine in a tedious process of exploratory research followed, only rarely, by well-done confirmatory research.

Taking an Evidence-Based Approach

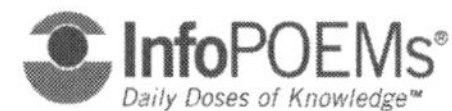

We realized about 15 years ago, just as the EBM movement was just getting started, that most doctors and other health professionals do not have time to read and understand even a small fraction of the medical literature. It occurred to us that busy clinicians need a service that scrutinizes the medical information for them and identifies and presents the information to them that they can really use.

POEMs – Patient-Oriented Evidence that Matters

But how could we separate the useful medical information from the "not ready for prime time" information? For this we turned to patient-oriented evidence that matters – *POEMs* – a concept we first identified in the early 1990s.

A POEM in clinical medicine is valid, new research information that meets three criteria:

- The research evaluates the effect of a test, drug, procedure, or intervention on an outcome that *patients* care about.
- The problem studied is common to practice and the intervention is feasible.
- The information has the potential to cause clinicians to change their practice.

Determining whether the research studies an outcome that patients care about is not as obvious as it should be. Much research, however, does not directly study whether subjects lived longer or better; it is simply too difficult to study.

Instead, much medical research evaluates intermediate, or surrogate outcomes, such as blood levels or effects of drugs on receptors. Other research may find a relationship between a treatment and outcome but the research design is not strong enough to decide whether it is a *cause-and-effect* relationship.

Relevant and Valid Information

POEMs summarize research that is of high enough quality to demonstrate a cause-and-effect relationship and that focus on outcomes that matter to people rather than on intermediate or surrogate outcomes. A POEM, in other words, presents relevant and valid information.

Relevant information that matters to us also involves diseases or health problems that we see and interventions that are available to us to use in practice. Information, for example, about a new treatment for shistosomiasis is going to be useful to only a small group of clinicians and will not rise to the level of POEM-hood for most.

The final requirement for POEM status is that the information has the potential to induce us to change our practice. Information that confirms that what we currently do is correct may be gratifying but it is not that useful.

The POEMs Process

To identify POEMs in the medical literature, each month we review over 120 journals, looking for articles that meet our criteria for relevance and validity. The articles are critically appraised for relevance and validity and the most important aspects of the research – including an interpretation of the results – are summarized in a 300-word POEM written in a style readable by non-researchers.

The **Clinical Question** poses the question the study seeks to answer.

The **Level of Evidence (LOE)** is a rating from 1a (best) to 5 (worst) of how well the study is designed to show bias.

The **Bottom Line** summarizes the findings of the research and is designed to help clinicians understand how best to apply the results.

Vitamin A may promote osteoporosis

Clinical Question:

Can excessive vitamin A intake increase the risk of osteoporotic hip fractures?

Bottom Line:

Long-term intake of a diet high in vitamin A, especially retinol (from vitamin supplements), may increase the risk of osteoporotic hip fractures in women. Postmenopausal estrogen reduced the risk of fractures in women who took excessive amounts of vitamin A. Too much of a good thing is not always good! (LOE = 1b)

Reference:

Feskanich D, Singh V, Willett WC, Colditz GA. Vitamin A intake and hip fractures among postmenopausal women. JAMA 2002;287:47-54.

Study Design:

Cohort (prospective)

Setting:

Population-based

The **Synopsis** provides a concise overview of the study design and results. Although concise like an abstract, InfoPOEM synopses adhere to our criteria for validity evaluation and only contain the most significant and applicable details, written in an easy-to-understand style with minimal "research-speak."

The **Setting** identifies the environment in which the study took place (outpatient, inpatient, emergency department, etc.)

Synopsis:

Excessive dietary intake of vitamin A antagonizes the ability of vitamin D to maintain calcium levels, may contribute to accelerated bone resorbtion, and thus may increase the risk of clinical fractures. Using data from our old friend, the Nurses' Health Study, the authors examined the relationship between vitamin A intake from foods and supplements and the risk of hip fracture among postmenopausal women. After controlling for confounding factors (smoking, alcohol use, hormone use, body weight), women in the group with the highest vitamin A intake had a 48% higher risk of hip fracture (RR = 1.48; 95% CI, 1.05 - 2.07; P = 0.003) compared with women with the lowest vitamin A intake. Most of the risk was attributable primarily to retinol intake (from multivitamins). This risk was reduced by postmenopausal estrogen use. Beta carotene intake, primarily from carrots, did not contribute significantly to fracture risk.

Using POEMs to Improve Practice

The editors chose the POEMs in this compilation because they present valid information relevant to the practice of medicine. All of the research has been published in the past several years.

The POEMs are organized into general categories. They can be read in order or the book can be opened and browsed. The index provides a quick look-up to use this book as a reference.

What happens when you find a POEM that suggests to you a new way of practice? Be sure to read the complete synopsis to read and understand what the POEM is telling you and to understand the magnitude of the benefit of the new treatment or study. Check the level of evidence to determine the strength of the study.

Taking an Evidence-Based Approach

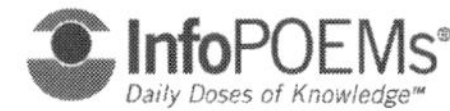

Changing with Confidence

Think about the effect the change will have on your practice. Will you be able to confirm the results in your own practice? It is likely you will not if the new practice is a preventive treatment that might take years before you will see a difference.

Remember that these POEMs have been carefully screened for validity and the results will be similar in your own practice. You can change with confidence based on much of this information.

How to Become an Information Master: Feeling Good about NOT Knowing Everything

Buried under Information

Most of us have a loose system of staying up to date with new findings. Colleagues, local experts, consultants, pharmaceutical representatives, perhaps a yearly CME meeting, the stolen few minutes to read a journal, and even the local newspaper story on medicine serve to keep us aware of innovations in medicine.

When we have questions, we turn again to colleagues, save the question for later, punch a few keys on the computer, or tap our PDA screen. Yet few clinicians, when they admit it to themselves, are really confident in their knowledge of current best practices.

Becoming a Master of Information

Information Mastery is a set of skills that can help clinicians feel confident in their knowledge. More important, it allows us to feel confident that what we *do not* know is not that important.

It involves finding the most valid and relevant information in the least amount of time. Information is valid if it is based on sound clinical science. Information is relevant if it demonstrates that what we do for patients helps them live long, functional, symptom-free lives.

Patients First

The most important component of Information Mastery is that the patient – not pathophysiologic reasoning, schools of thought, specialty-specific approaches, or effective marketing – is the center of all care decisions. Patient outcomes that matter – decreased pain, better quality of life, lower mortality, and even cost – supersede the need to adhere to tradition, defend turf, bow to authority, engage in mental gymnastics, or other lapses that continue to plague the practice of medicine.

Looking for Answers to Questions

Rather than get caught up in the swirl of information and non-information, many practicing clinicians turn to textbooks – both printed and electronic – colleagues, newsletters, e-mail lists, and experts for answers. These answers are seductive because they are so easy to use and believable.

However, they all have limitations. Printed textbooks cannot keep up with the speed of change in medicine. The validity is often uncertain of recommendations in both printed and electronic textbooks, along with many review articles in journals. Experts who write these chapters and articles often selectively present the evidence.

Lost in the Information

On the other hand, studies evaluating the effect of medical research have shown that study results that should influence medical care fail to do so because the results are lost among all of

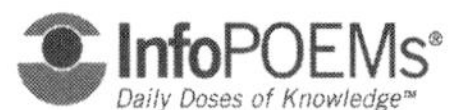

the other clinically important information. We are so overwhelmed by information that we fail to identify the truly important stuff.

No matter what source of information to which we turn, we would like to spend the least amount of time and energy to find the best. Ideally, we would like information that is readily applicable to everyday practice, accurate, and easy to obtain.

What Makes Information *Useful?*

These three factors can be represented by what we call the *Information Mastery Usefulness Equation*:

$$\text{Usefulness of information source} = \frac{\text{relevance} * \text{validity}}{\text{work}}$$

For an information source to be useful, it must present information that is valid, relevant – patient-oriented – and takes little time, effort, or money to obtain.

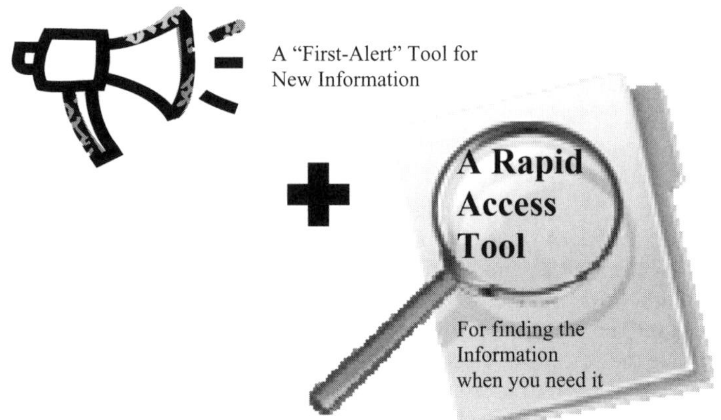
A "First-Alert" Tool for New Information
A Rapid Access Tool
For finding the Information when you need it

Two Tools Needed

So, how do we find information that is relevant? Two tools are needed to manage information.

- The first tool is a "First-Alert" system that tells us of new relevant and valid findings from the best research. *Daily InfoPOEMs* is such a service, delivering POEMs such as those in this book to your desktop every day.

Criteria for a high-quality foraging tool. A transparent process that:

- Filters out disease-oriented research and presents only patient-oriented research outcomes
- Demonstrates that a validity assessment has been performed using appropriate criteria
- Assigns levels of evidence, based on appropriate validity criteria, to individual studies
- Provides specific recommendations, when feasible, on how to apply the information, placing it into clinical context
- Comprehensively reviews the literature for a specific specialty or discipline
- Coordinates with a high-quality hunting tool

Reprinted by permission from: Slawson DC, Shaughnessy AF. Teaching evidence-based medicine: Should we be teaching information management instead? Acad Med 2005;80:685–89.

- The second tool helps you find the information when you need to use it. InfoRetriever is one such tool, allowing you quick access to all POEMs along with other information sources.

Criteria for a high-quality hunting tool. A transparent process that:

- Uses a specific, explicit method for comprehensively searching the literature to find relevant *and* valid information
- Provides key recommendations supported by patient-oriented outcomes when possible and, when not, specified as preliminary when supported only by disease-oriented outcomes
- Assigns levels of evidence[i] or strength of recommendation[ii] to key recommendation using appropriate criteria
- Coordinates with a high quality foraging tool

Reprinted by permission from: Slawson DC, Shaughnessy AF. Teaching evidence-based medicine: Should we be teaching information management instead? Acad Med 2005;80:685–89.

Becoming an Information Master

We are fortunate to live in a time in which the technology allows us access to an overabundance of information. Some of this information is useful; the rest is either not useful or is misleading.

The two tools outlined above separate out the useful information from the "not ready for prime time" non-information. Every clinician needs to develop a system for keeping up with changes in medicine, and for finding this new information again when needed.

---

[i] Oxford Center for Evidence-Based Medicine. Levels of evidence and grades of recommendation. http://www.cebm.net/levels_of_evidence.asp. Accessed December 13, 2004.

[ii] Ebell MH, Siwek J, Weiss BD, Woolf SH, Susman J, Ewigman B, Bowman, M. Strength of recommendation taxonomy (SORT): a patient-centered approach to grading evidence in the medical literature. J Am Board Fam Pract 2004;17:59–67.

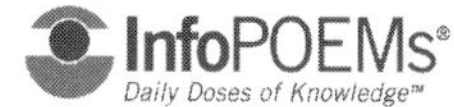

Both tools are necessary. Without both, either you will not know that new information is available or you will not know where to find it when you need it.

Busy clinicians wishing to deliver high-quality health care must rapidly identify and use high-quality information in the course of their practice. Clinicians armed with high-quality tools at the point of care are the true Information Masters of the information age.

Checklist

- Develop "First-Alert" system. Use services that evaluate information for validity and relevance rather than just presenting the information.
- Find a rapid-access tool to find the information again when you need it. You should be able to find the answer to your question in less than 30 seconds.
- Improve your practice. Once you find the information, change your practice to improve the care of your patients.

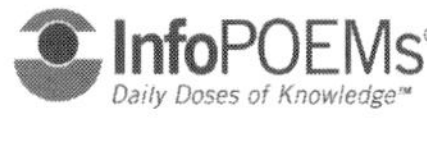

InfoPOEMs (Patient-Oriented Evidence that Matters)

Most women with breast cancer have no risk factors

Clinical question

How important is family history as a risk factor for developing breast cancer?

Bottom line

Although family history is an important risk factor for the development of breast cancer, the magnitude of risk is dependent on the age at diagnosis and the age of the woman concerned. Having said this, about 90% of women who develop breast cancer have no family history, and 90% of women with a first-degree relative with breast cancer do not develop breast cancer. (LOE = 1a)

Reference

Collaborative Group on Hormonal Factors in Breast Cancer. Familial breast cancer: collaborative reanalysis of individual data from 52 epidemiological studies including 58,209 women with breast cancer and 101,986 women without the disease. Lancet 2001;358:1389–1399.

Study Design

Meta-analysis (non-RCT)

Setting

Population-based

Synopsis

These authors collected data on over 150,000 individual patients (58,209 with breast cancer) included in 52 cohort studies of risk factors for developing breast cancer. The data confirm that having a first-degree relative with breast cancer increases a woman's risk: 1.8, 2.9 and 3.6 for one, two or three affected relatives, respectively. The risk appears greatest for first-degree relatives diagnosed earlier in life and is a greater burden for younger women. Childbearing history had no influence on risk in women with a family history of breast cancer. Compared with nulliparous women, the more babies a woman had, the lower the risk. Compared with nulliparous women, the younger age at first childbirth, the lower the risk (age over 30 appears to have about the same risk as being nulliparous). Reflecting hormonal exposure, women with earlier menopause were at lower risk, women who hadn't been on oral contraceptives for more than 10 years, and women who had never been on hormone replacement therapy were at the lowest risk. Most women with breast cancer had no identifiable risk factors.

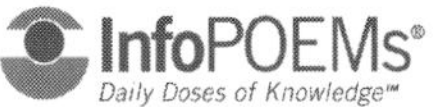

Raloxifene reduces breast cancer risk (CORE)

Clinical question

Does raloxifene (Evista) prevent breast cancer?

Bottom line

Previous research has shown that raloxifene can protect against breast cancer after 4 years of use. In this 4-year extension of the original study, this protection continued. (LOE = 1b)

Reference

Martino S, Cauley JA, Barrett-Connor E, et al. Continuing outcomes relevant to Evista: breast cancer incidence in postmenopausal osteoporotic women in a randomized trial of raloxifene. J Natl Cancer Inst 2004;96:1751–1761.

Study Design

Randomized controlled trial (double-blinded)

Funding

Industry

Allocation

Uncertain

Setting

Outpatient (any)

Synopsis

This is a continuation of the Multiple Outcomes of Raloxifene Evaluation (MORE) trial that found that raloxifene (Evista) decreased the incidence of invasive breast cancer among postmenopausal women with osteoporosis (number needed to treat [NNT] = 93 for 4 years; 95% CI, 61–161; Breast Cancer Res Treat 2001; 65:125–34 and 2001; 67:191[erratum]). This study is a continuation designed to assess raloxifene's longer term safety and efficacy. Of the 6511 patients in the MORE trial, 4011 chose to continue in this trial (Continuing Outcomes Relevant to Evista; CORE). This drop off between the 2 studies is likely to introduce bias in favor of the treatment group. In the CORE trial, the researchers didn't re-randomize patients; they merely continued the same allocation (1286 took placebo, 2725 took raloxifene) and maintained the double blinding of the original trial. To be eligible, women had to be 80 years or younger, have osteoporosis by bone density measurement, and had to be at least 2 years beyond menopause. Finally, the researchers evaluated the outcomes by intention to treat. During the 4 years of the CORE trial, significantly more patients taking placebo developed breast cancer (2.3% vs 1.1%; NNT = 84; 95% CI, 45–282). There was no significant difference in total mortality, total adverse events, serious adverse events, or drug discontinuations. However, there was a significant increase in pulmonary emboli when all 8 years of data were combined (absolute risk reduction = 0.46%; number needed to treat to harm = 214; 95% CI, 117–10,000).

Essential Evidence: Medicine that Matters, Edited by David Slawson, Allen Shaughnessy, Mark Ebell, and Henry Barry.

Raloxifene and tamoxifen equally effective in reducing breast cancer risk

Clinical question

What are the relative effects of raloxifene and tamoxifen on reducing the risk of developing invasive breast cancer?

Bottom line

Tamoxifen (Nolvadex, Tamofen) and raloxifene (Evista) are similarly effective for reducing the risk of invasive breast cancer in postmenopausal women. Although women taking tamoxifen are at an increased risk of thromboembolic events and cataracts, they report improved sexual function compared with women taking raloxifene. All-cause mortality and overall quality-of-life were similar in both treatment groups. (LOE = 1b–)

Reference

Vogel VG, Costantino JP, Wickerham DL, et al, for the National Surgical Adjuvant Breast and Bowel Project (NSABP). Effect of tamoxifen vs raloxifene on the risk of developing invasive breast cancer and other disease outcomes. The NSABP study of tamoxifen and raloxifene (STAR) P-2 trial. JAMA 2006;295:2727–2741.

Study Design

Randomized controlled trial (double-blinded)

Funding

Industry + govt

Allocation

Concealed

Setting

Outpatient (any)

Synopsis

These investigators identified postmenopausal women, 35 years or older, with at least a 5-year predicted breast cancer risk of 1.66% on the Gail model. A total of 19,747 consenting women (mean age = 58.5 years) met inclusion criteria. More than 93% of participants were white. Eligible women randomly received (concealed allocation assignment) tamoxifen (20 mg/d) or raloxifene (60 mg/d) for a maximum of 5 years. Follow-up occurred for more than 94% of women for a mean of 3.9 years. The authors do not specifically state whether individuals assessing outcomes remained blinded to treatment group assignment. Using intention-to-treat analysis, there were no significant differences between the 2 groups in the risk of either invasive or noninvasive breast cancer, uterine cancer, other invasive cancers, ischemic heart disease events, stroke, osteoporotic fractures, or all-cause mortality. Thromboembolic events and cataracts occurred significantly less often in the raloxifene group. A related study in the same issue (JAMA 2006;295) reported no significant differences between the treatment groups in physical health, mental health, or depression, but the tamoxifen group reported better sexual function.

Essential Evidence: Medicine that Matters, Edited by David Slawson, Allen Shaughnessy, Mark Ebell, and Henry Barry.

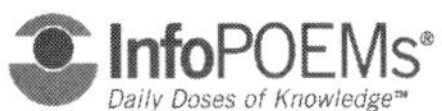

Raloxifene decreases breast cancer risk, no effect on cardiovascular disease risk (RUTH)

Clinical question

What is the effect of raloxifene on the risks of cardiovascular disease and breast cancer?

Bottom line

For every 1000 women who take raloxifene for 5 years, we can expect 4 to 5 additional strokes, 6 additional episodes of venous thromboembolism (VTE), 6 fewer invasive breast cancers, and 6 to 7 fewer clinical vertebral fractures. The cost for this mixed bag of benefits and harms would be approximately $1000 per woman per year, for a total cost of $5,000,000 at current drug prices. (LOE = 1b)

Reference

Barrett-Connor E, Mosca L, Collins P, et al, for the Raloxifene Use for The Heart (RUTH) Trial Investigators. Effects of raloxifene on cardiovascular events and breast cancer in postmenopausal women. N Engl J Med 2006;355:125–137.

Study Design	Funding	Allocation
Randomized controlled trial (double-blinded)	Industry	Concealed

Setting

Outpatient (any)

Synopsis

Previous studies have shown that raloxifene appears to reduce the risk of breast cancer and may also have beneficial cardiovascular effects. In the current Raloxifene Use for The Heart (RUTH) trial, 10,101 postmenopausal women 55 years or older with known cardiovascular disease (or at high risk for it) were randomly assigned to raloxifene 60 mg per day or placebo. Patients with recent myocardial infarction, bypass surgery, or percutaneous coronary intervention were excluded, as were women who had a history of cancer or VTE, recent unexplained uterine bleeding, heart failure, liver or renal disease, or who had recently used estrogen or other sex hormones. The mean age of participants was 67 years, 84% were white, 10% had a family history of breast cancer, and approximately 40% had a 5-year risk of breast cancer greater than 1.66% (the usual cutoff for considering prophylactic therapy). Approximately half had a history of coronary artery disease and 45% were diabetic. Groups were balanced at the start of the study except for a statistically significant difference in the cardiovascular risk score (7.9 in the raloxifene group vs 7.8 in the placebo group). However, it is unlikely that this small difference was clinically meaningful. Women were followed up for a mean of 5.6 years, and outcomes were adjudicated by a committee blinded to treatment assigned. There was no difference between groups in the risk of "all bad cardiovascular things," death from coronary disease, or nonfatal myocardial infarction. Among women taking raloxifene, there was a trend toward more strokes (0.95% vs 0.86% per year; P = .07) and a greater risk of VTE (0.39% vs 0.27% per year; P = .02; number needed to treat to harm = 833/year). However, the risk of invasive breast cancer was lower in the raloxifene group (0.15% vs 0.27% per year; P = .003; number needed to treat [NNT] = 833/year), as was the risk of clinical vertebral fracture (0.24% vs 0.37% per year; P = .007; NNT = 769). There was no difference in the risk of clinical nonvertebral fracture or all-cause mortality.

Essential Evidence: Medicine that Matters, Edited by David Slawson, Allen Shaughnessy, Mark Ebell, and Henry Barry.

MRI more accurate than mammogram in high-risk patients

Clinical question

Is magnetic resonance imaging more accurate than mammography in women at high risk of breast cancer?

Bottom line

Magnetic resonance imaging is better at ruling out breast cancer (i.e., more sensitive) than mammography, but is also more likely to produce false-positive results (less specific). It is also more expensive and leads to more unnecessary biopsies and follow-up studies. This makes it inappropriate for an average-risk or low-risk group, but it may be a good option for high-risk women who understand these limitations. (LOE = 2b)

Reference

Kriege M, Brekelmans CT, Boetes C, et al. Efficacy of MRI and mammography for breast-cancer screening in women with a familial or genetic predisposition. N Engl J Med 2004;351:427–437.

Study Design	Funding	Setting
Cohort (prospective)	Government	Outpatient (any)

Synopsis

Magnetic resonance imaging (MRI) is an expensive test, but it may be more sensitive than mammography. The authors identified 1909 Dutch women aged 25 years to 70 years with at least a 15% or more lifetime risk of breast cancer. This group included 358 mutation carriers, 1052 with a 30% to 49% risk, and 499 with a 15% to 29% risk. Of this group, 4.6% were lost to follow-up, largely because they underwent prophylactic mastectomy. Another 4.7% refused MRI, usually because of claustrophobia. The mean age was 40 years, only 15% had never had breast cancer screening, and approximately 75% were premenopausal. Women underwent a clinical breast examination every 6 months, as well as annual MRI and mammography, which were interpreted independently by radiologists blinded to the results of the other study. The women were followed up for a median of 2.9 years. A Breast Imaging Reporting and Data System (BI-RADS) classification of 0 ("need additional imaging"), 3, 4 or 5 was considered a positive screening test result (a classification of 1 or 2 indicates normal or nearly normal). The reference standard was histologic examination, and sensitivity and specificity were calculated by comparing the number of cancers detected by each method plus any interval cancers. In addition to sensitivity and specificity, the ability to detect earlier cancers was also evaluated by comparison with an unscreened control group who had a similar risk of breast cancer. MRI was more than twice as sensitive as mammography regardless of the cutoff used to define an abnormal test result (79% vs 33%), although it was somewhat less specific (89.8% for BI-RADS of 0, 3, 4, or 5 as abnormal compared with 95% for mammography). The area under the receiver operating characteristic curve, a measure of overall diagnostic accuracy, was significantly greater for MRI (0.83 vs 0.69). However, the lower specificity means that women underwent more unnecessary additional follow-up exams (420 vs 207) and had more unnecessary biopsies (24 vs 7) because of the addition of MRI screening. The comparison with unscreened control groups, although imperfect, found that fewer women screened with both MRI and mammography were node-positive.

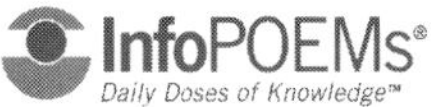

MRI more sensitive than mammography in high-risk women (MARIBS)

Clinical question

In women at high risk of breast cancer, is MRI alone or in combination with mammography better at detecting cancers than mammography alone?

Bottom line

Among women at high risk for breast cancer, MRI detects more cancers than mammography. The combination of both, however is most accurate. But please be careful with this information: This study doesn't tell us if high-risk patients have better outcomes with MRI, mammography, or both. (LOE = 2b–)

Reference

Leach MO, Boggis CR, Dixon AK, et al, for the MARIBS study group. Screening with magnetic resonance imaging and mammography of a UK population at high familial risk of breast cancer: a prospective multicentre cohort study (MARIBS). Lancet 2005;365:1769–1778.

Study Design	Funding	Setting
Cohort (prospective)	Government	Outpatient (any)

Synopsis

Women were eligible to participate in this study if they were asymptomatic, aged between 35 years and 49 years, known carriers of genetic mutations linked with breast cancer (BRCA1, BRCA2, or TP53), first-degree relatives of someone with one of these genetic mutations, or if they had a strong family history of breast or ovarian cancer. The women had annual mammography and contrast-enhanced breast magnetic resonance imaging (MRI), each of which were read independently by 2 pairs of radiologists. Each pair was unaware of the results of the other test. The gold standard for this study was based on histopathology or the absence of a new cancer in the year following the test. The absence of cancer at 1 year is the commonly accepted definition of a true negative. Of 649 women screened, 13% had a mutation of BRCA1 and 6% of BRCA2. By the end of the seventh year of the study, 35 cancers were found. It is important to point out that not all women got both the MRI and mammogram, so the authors only report data on those who had both. This has the potential for introducing biases into the study, especially if the order of MRI and mammography wasn't random. For all women in the study, MRI was slightly better at ruling out cancers than mammography (negative likelihood ratio [LR–] for MRI = 0.28; 95% CI, 0.12–0.5; LR– for mammogram = 0.65; 0.44–0.83), and mammography was slightly better at ruling in cancers (positive likelihood ratio [LR+] for MRI = 4.1; 3–5.3; LR+ for mammogram = 5.7; 3–11.6). The overall sensitivity was 77% for MRI and 40% for mammography and the specificities were 81% and 93%, respectively. MRI was much better at detecting cancers than mammography among women with BRCA mutations or with first-degree relatives with BRCA mutations (sensitivity = 92% vs 23%), but was less specific (79% vs 92%). This means that MRI produces more false-positives, as well. In this study, the combination of MRI and mammography was much better than either alone.

Essential Evidence: Medicine that Matters, Edited by David Slawson, Allen Shaughnessy, Mark Ebell, and Henry Barry.

Digital mammography more sensitive for younger women

Clinical question

Is digital mammography more accurate than traditional film mammography?

Bottom line

Digital mammography is more sensitive than film mammography for women younger than 50, premenopausal and perimenopausal women, and women with dense breasts. It does not result in more unnecessary biopsies, but is between 1.5 times and 4 times as costly as film mammography. The survival benefit is almost certainly less impressive than the difference in accuracy. For example, if 10 in 10,000 pre- or peri-menopausal women have cancer, using digital mammography will detect 2 additional cancers (72% vs 51% sensitivity). If the digital mammogram costs $100 more then we will have spent $500,000 (10,000 × $100/2) to detect 1 additional cancer. A formal cost effectiveness analysis is underway and widespread adoption of this technology should await its completion. (LOE = 1b)

Reference

Pisano ED, Gatsonis C, Hendrick E, et al, for the Digital Mammographic Imaging Screening Trial (DMIST) Investigators Group. Diagnostic performance of digital versus film mammography for breast-cancer screening. N Engl J Med 2005;353:1846–1847.

Study Design

Diagnostic test evaluation

Funding

Government

Setting

Outpatient (any)

Synopsis

The authors enrolled 49,528 women, of whom 42,760 followed the protocol and had adequate follow-up information. The mean age of participants was 55 years, 84% were white, 28% were premenopausal, and 47% had dense breasts. All underwent both digital and film mammography (in random order), and each mammogram was independently and blindly interpreted by a different radiologist. Breast density was also rated, and patients had biopsy or aspiration of all suspicious-appearing lesions. Patients had a follow-up mammogram after 1 year. The reference standard was a pathologic diagnosis of breast cancer within 455 days of the initial mammogram. Patients were considered to be free of cancer if they had a negative biopsy result or if their 1-year follow-up mammogram was negative. Overall, this was a well-designed diagnostic comparison. A total of 335 cancers were diagnosed, 231 invasive and 103 ductal carcinoma in situ (DCIS). The area under the receiver operating characteristic curve (AUROCC) was used to compare the accuracy of digital and film mammography overall and for different subgroups (a higher AUROCC is better, with 1.0 being a perfect test). There was no significant difference in overall accuracy between digital and film mammography for the entire study population. However, digital mammograms were significantly more accurate than film mammograms for women younger than 50 years (AUROCC = 0.84 vs 0.69), for women with heterogeneously dense or extremely dense breasts (AUROCC = 0.78 vs 0.68) and for premenopausal or perimenopausal women (AUROCC = 0.82 vs 0.67). The difference in accuracy as measured by the AUROCC was primarily due to increased sensitivity: after 1 year, 78% vs 51% for women younger than 50 years, 72% vs 51% for pre- and perimenopausal women, and 70% vs 55% for women with dense breasts. (The sensitivities are lower than those usually reported because the authors used a longer follow-up interval than usual, resulting in more false-negative results).

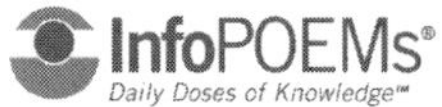

Mammography results in overdiagnosis

Clinical question

Does screening mammography result in the identification and treatment of breast cancers that would never be clinically apparent?

Bottom line

Approximately 10% of women (95% CI, 1%–18%) who have confirmed breast cancer and who receive treatment, never would have had clinically apparent symptoms without a screening mammogram. So, in addition to the possibility of having a false-positive mammogram result sometime in their lives, 1 in 10 women who have a real diagnosis of breast cancer undergo treatment that, although seemingly curative, ultimately has no beneficial effect on them because they would never have developed clinically apparent breast cancer. (LOE = 2b–)

Reference

Zackrisson S, Andersson I, Janzon L, Manjer J, Garne JP. Rate of over-diagnosis of breast cancer 15 years after end of Malmo mammographic screening trial: follow-up study. BMJ 2006;332:689–692.

Study Design

Randomized controlled trial (nonblinded)

Funding

Self-funded or unfunded

Allocation

Concealed

Setting

Population-based

Synopsis

There are 2 possible harmful outcomes of screening for breast cancer. The first is a false-positive result, telling a woman she may have breast cancer only to find out on biopsy that she doesn't. A more subtle negative outcome is the risk of overdiagnosis, in which breast cancer is detected by mammography in a woman who would otherwise have lived her life never knowing that she had breast cancer. The authors conducting this analysis used the results of the Malmo mammogram screening trial. These authors enrolled 42,283 women and randomized them to receive mammography or no mammography. They enrolled women over a 10-year period and then followed up for another 15 years. As would be expected, significantly more women receiving mammography were identified as having breast cancer than were nonscreened women. However, there continued to be more diagnoses of breast cancer in the screened group than in the nonscreened group, even though during the follow-up period women in both groups had regular mammograms. Since any woman who was identified as having breast cancer was no longer part of the screening group, the initially unscreened women should have caught up and had more breast cancers identified when they started regular mammograms. That they didn't indicates that overdiagnosis occurred in the woman initially assigned to screening mammogram. Overall, approximately 10% (95% CI, 1%–18%) of the woman who had mammograms and were given a diagnosis of breast cancer were overdiagnosed, meaning they would have never have known they had breast cancer – or have received treatment – except for the screening program.

Essential Evidence: Medicine that Matters, Edited by David Slawson, Allen Shaughnessy, Mark Ebell, and Henry Barry.

Annual mammography starting at 40 doesn't lower breast cancer mortality

Clinical question
Does starting annual mammography at age 40 decrease breast cancer mortality?

Bottom line
This study found that 10 years of annual mammography starting at age 40 produced no statistically significant reduction in breast cancer mortality. The screening of women in this age group is controversial and the limitations of these data won't settle the arguments. (LOE = 1b)

Reference
Moss SM, Cuckle H, Evans A, et al, for the Trial Management Group. Effect of mammographic screening from age 40 years on breast cancer mortality at 10 years' follow-up: a randomised controlled trial. Lancet 2006;368:2053–2060.

Study Design
Randomized controlled trial (nonblinded)

Funding
Government

Allocation
Concealed

Setting
Population-based

Synopsis
Women in England, Scotland, and Wales aged between 39 years and 41 years were randomly assigned to annual mammography (n = 53,884) or usual care (n = 106,956). The research team evaluated the women until they were 48 years of age (mean follow-up = 10.7 years; more than 99% accounted for). The main outcomes, breast cancer mortality and all-cause mortality, came from the National Health Service Central Register and were analyzed via intention to treat. Overall, 81% of the women had at least 1 mammogram and those screened women had, on average, 5.6 mammograms during the study period. The authors state, but give no data, that their evidence indicates that the extent of screening in the control group is small. During the study, the cost of screening in this age group was not covered by the National Health Service and would therefore be borne at personal expense. At the end of the study, the differences between groups in all-cause mortality (1.66 vs 1.72 per 1000 person-years) and breast cancer mortality (0.18 vs 0.22 per 1000 person years) were not statistically significant. However, the study was originally designed to have 80% power to detect a 20% relative reduction in breast cancer mortality. But the study group ran out of money and didn't recruit as many women as they had planned. The final study had 72% power. In other words, although this was a well-conducted study, the statistical aspects are limited. For example, compared with usual care, we would need to screen 2512 (95% CI, 1149–13,544) to prevent 1 breast cancer death over 10 years.

Essential Evidence: Medicine that Matters, Edited by David Slawson, Allen Shaughnessy, Mark Ebell, and Henry Barry.

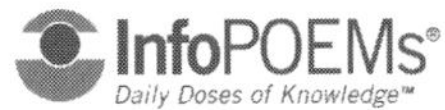

Many unnecessary Pap smears are performed after hysterectomy

Clinical question

How often are women undergoing Pap smear screening even though they are not at risk of cervical cancer?

Bottom line

Many American women who have had a hysterectomy with removal of the cervix for benign disease continue to undergo routine Papanicolaou (Pap) test despite a lack of supporting evidence and a clear recommendation from the United States Preventive Services Task Force against routine screening. Conversely, the vast majority of American women who die from cervical cancer were either underscreened or never screened for cervical disease, most likely as a result of real or perceived cost barriers. The money saved by not inappropriately performing Pap tests on low-risk women would pay for the cost of screening the 17 million women in the United States who are currently underscreened for cervical cancer (J Womens Health and Gender Based Med 2002; 11:103–9.). (LOE = 2b)

Reference

Sirovich BE, Welch HG. Cervical cancer screening among women without a cervix. JAMA 2004;291:2990–2993

Study Design

Cross-sectional

Setting

Population-based

Synopsis

Since 1996, the United States Preventive Services Task Force has suggested that routine Pap tests are unnecessary for women who have undergone hysterectomy with removal of the cervix for benign disease, placing them no longer at risk of cervical cancer. Many clinicians still perform Pap tests on these women, purportedly to screen for vaginal cancer. Since the risk of vaginal cancer is so low, however, women currently screened for cervical cancer with an intact cervix are not routinely screened for vaginal cancer. To determine the frequency of inappropriate screening, the authors used data from a survey conducted by the Centers for Disease Control and Prevention from 1992 to 2002 reporting the proportion of women with a hysterectomy who had a subsequent Pap test within 3 years. During this 10-year period, 22 million US women 18 years of age and older underwent hysterectomy, representing 21% of the population. The proportion of these women reporting a subsequent Pap test within 3 years before (68.5%) and 3 years after (69.1%) the Task Force recommendations in 1996 did not change. The authors estimate that half these women had hysterectomies that spared the cervix or were performed for cervical neoplasia, resulting in almost 10 million women being screened unnecessarily.

Essential Evidence: Medicine that Matters, Edited by David Slawson, Allen Shaughnessy, Mark Ebell, and Henry Barry.

Specific HPV strains are associated with cervical cancer risk

Clinical question

Do some oncogenic strains of HPV confer more risk of severe dysplasia or cancer than others?

Bottom line

Human papillomavirus (HPV) testing results that are positive for types 16 or 18 are associated with a 14% to 17% risk of cervical intraepithelial neoplasia 3 (CIN3) or greater over the following 10 years. Other oncogenic types are associated with a much lower risk (approximately 3%), and for women who test negative for HPV the risk is less than 1%. (LOE = 1b)

Reference

Khan MJ, Castle PE, Lorincz AT, et al. The elevated 10-year risk of cervical precancer and cancer in women with human papillomavirus (HPV) type 16 or 18 and the possible utility of type-specific HPV testing in clinical practice. J Natl Cancer Inst 2005;97:1072–1079.

Study Design

Cohort (prospective)

Funding

Unknown/not stated

Allocation

Concealed

Setting

Outpatient (any)

Synopsis

Essentially all cervical cancers are associated with HPV infection. HPV testing by Hybrid Capture 2 was performed in this cohort study of almost 21,000 women, and outcomes of CIN3 or greater within the next 10 years were determined. Women were categorized as positive for HPV16 (n = 455), positive for HPV18 (n = 154), positive for 1 of 11 other HPV oncogenic subtypes (n = 2211), or negative. Seventeen percent of women with HPV16 were given a diagnosis of CIN3 or greater over the next 10 years; 14% of those with HPV18; 3% of those with other oncogenic types; and 0.8% of those who were HPV negative. For the almost 13,000 women older than 30 years with negative cytology at baseline and a negative HPV result, only 0.5% had CIN3 or greater over the following 10 years.

Essential Evidence: Medicine that Matters, Edited by David Slawson, Allen Shaughnessy, Mark Ebell, and Henry Barry.

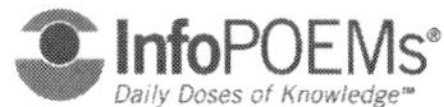

Vaccine effective against HPV

Clinical question

Is a vaccine effective against human papillomavirus strains associated with cervical cancer?

Bottom line

A bivalent vaccine against human papillomavirus (HPV) types 16 and 18 is well-tolerated and effective in reducing HPV infection and HPV-associated cytologic abnormalities. What we need now is a larger, longer-termed, adequately powered study to look at the effect of this vaccine on the development of cervical cancer. (LOE = 1b)

Reference

Harper DM, Franco EL, Wheeler C, et al. Efficacy of a bivalent L1 virus-like particle vaccine in prevention of infection with human papillomavirus types 16 and 18 in young women: a randomised controlled trial. Lancet 2004;364:1757–1765.

Study Design

Randomized controlled trial (double-blinded)

Funding

Industry

Allocation

Concealed

Setting

Population-based

Synopsis

This team of researchers randomly assigned healthy women aged 15 to 25 years with no more than 6 sexual partners and no history of condyloma or cervical cancer to receive a bivalent vaccine active against HPV serotypes 16 and 18 or placebo. They administered the vaccine or placebo at 0, 1, and 6 months. They evaluated the patients after 27 months to determine the presence of HPV infection or cytologic abnormalities. Using an intention-to-treat approach to these outcomes, the vaccine was 95% effective against persistent HPV infection and 93% effective against cytologic abnormalities associated with HPV. In the intention-to-treat analysis, the absolute reduction in new HPV infections was 6.4% (number needed to treat [NNT] = 16) and 3.5% for persistent infections (NNT = 29). Other than local injection site symptoms, there were no differences in side effects between the active and placebo vaccines.

Essential Evidence: Medicine that Matters, Edited by David Slawson, Allen Shaughnessy, Mark Ebell, and Henry Barry.

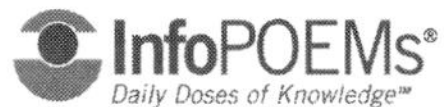

Bivalent vaccine against HPV effective for 4.5 years

Clinical question

Does a vaccine confer long-term protection against human papillomavirus strains associated with cervical cancer?

Bottom line

A bivalent vaccine against human papillomavirus (HPV) types 16 and 18 is well-tolerated and effective in reducing HPV infection and HPV-associated cytologic abnormalities for 4.5 years. (LOE = 1b)

Reference

Harper DM, Franco EL, Wheeler CM, et al, for the HPV Vaccine Study group. Sustained efficacy up to 4.5 years of a bivalent L1 virus-like particle vaccine against human papillomavirus types 16 and 18: follow-up from a randomised control trial. Lancet 2006;367:1247–1255.

Study Design	Funding	Allocation
Randomized controlled trial (double-blinded)	Industry	Concealed

Setting

Population-based

Synopsis

We previously reviewed the initial report from this study (Lancet 2004;364:1757–65) that demonstrated after 27 months that a bivalent vaccine active against HPV serotypes 16 and 18 was more effective than placebo in reducing HPV infection and HPV-associated cytologic abnormalities. In this study, the investigators provide additional follow-up on 776 of 1113 women from the original study who received all 3 doses of vaccine or placebo, and for whom treatment allocation remained double blinded. In the original study, women were eligible if they were 15 to 25 years old, had no more than 6 sexual partners and had no history of condyloma or cervical cancer. They administered the vaccine or placebo at 0, 1, and 6 months. In the intention-to-treat analysis for the subsequent follow-up period, the absolute reduction in new HPV infections was 7.4% (number needed to treat [NNT] = 14; 95% CI, 10–23). If you combine the results for events occurring during the initial study period with the results from this follow-up period, the absolute reduction is 13.7% (NNT = 8; 6–10). Furthermore, no vaccinated woman developed HPV 16/18-associated CIN1 or worse (and only 2 developed HPV 16/18-associated ASCUS) compared with 1.7% of those receiving placebo (NNT = 59; 30–182). Interestingly, this vaccine also appeared to have some cross-protection against HPV 45 and HPV 31. Additional data and analyses are needed to understand the mechanisms of cross-protection and its importance to lesion development. Finally, the vaccine was well-tolerated. A total of 14% of those vaccinated reported at least one adverse side effect compared with 22% of those receiving placebo; 3% reported at least one new onset chronic disease compared with 5% taking placebo; and 4% reported at least one serious adverse event compared with 5% taking placebo.

Essential Evidence: Medicine that Matters, Edited by David Slawson, Allen Shaughnessy, Mark Ebell, and Henry Barry.

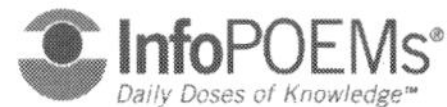

Liquid-based not better than conventional Pap

Clinical question

Is liquid-based cytology better than conventional cytology in detecting high-grade cervical disease?

Bottom line

High-quality studies fail to demonstrate that liquid-based cervical cytology is more reliable or more accurate at detecting high-grade abnormalities than conventional cytology. (LOE = 2a)

Reference

Davey E, Barratt A, Irwig L, et al. Effect of study design and quality on unsatisfactory rates, cytology classifications, and accuracy in liquid-based versus conventional cervical cytology: a systematic review. Lancet 2006;367:122–132.

Study Design

Systematic review

Funding

Government

Setting

Outpatient (any)

Synopsis

These authors searched MEDLINE and EMBASE to find studies that directly assessed liquid-based cytology and conventional cytology in cervical cancer screening. The studies had to have used a manual review of the slides rather than automated screening systems. The team also reviewed the bibliographies of included studies to find additional candidates. They didn't look for unpublished studies. Since positive results of novel technologies and interventions are more likely to be published, this raises the possibility of bias in favor of liquid-based cytology. Two reviewers independently assessed study eligibility with discrepancies resolved by consensus. Additionally, 2 reviewers independently assessed the methodologic validity of the studies. These reviewers were blinded to the study results. The 56 eligible studies included more than 1.2 million slides. The quality of the studies was generally poor and only two thirds used a gold standard. None of the studies were ideal and only 5 were considered high quality. There was no significant difference in the rate of unsatisfactory smears, especially in larger studies. Overall, the rates of cytologic abnormalities were similar; in the high-quality studies, however, conventional cytology was more likely to detect high-grade cervical lesions. If there was significant publication bias, it is more likely that this systematic review would make liquid-based cytology would look better.

Essential Evidence: Medicine that Matters, Edited by David Slawson, Allen Shaughnessy, Mark Ebell, and Henry Barry.

Endometrial sampling adequate for diagnosing endometrial cancer

Clinical question

Is endometrial sampling a suitable substitute for D & C for the diagnosis of endometrial cancer in postmenopausal women?

Bottom line

Outpatient endometrial sampling is a highly accurate diagnostic test for endometrial cancer when compared with D & C. In the hands of the clinicians participating in the studies included in this meta-analysis, an inadequate sample could be considered a negative test result. It is uncertain whether that conclusion is generalizable to other clinicians. (LOE = 1a)

Reference

Clark TJ, Mann CH, Shah N, Khan KS, Song F, Gupta JK. Accuracy of outpatient endometrial biopsy in the diagnosis of endometrial cancer: a systematic quantitative review. Br J Obstet Gynecol 2002;109:313–321.

Study Design

Meta-analysis (other)

Setting

Various (meta-analysis)

Synopsis

This was a meta-analysis of 11 studies of endometrial sampling as diagnostic test for endometrial cancer. The methodology was top notch. Summary likelihood ratios were calculated as measures of diagnostic accuracy. Six brands of devices were represented, of which the most common was the Pipelle device (n = 7 studies). Postmenopausal women represented 79% of the populations studied. The reference (gold) standard was most often dilatation and curettage (D & C), though hysterectomy and directed biopsy were accepted in some studies. In all included studies the reference standard procedure was performed regardless of endometrial biopsy results. The biggest weakness of the group of studies was lack of reporting of blinding (9 of the 11). For adequate endometrial samples, the pooled likelihood ratios for endometrial cancer were 66.48 (95% CI, 30.04–147.13) for a positive test result and 0.14 (95% CI, 0.08–0.27) for a negative test result. The pretest probability of endometrial cancer was 6.3%. It increased to 81.7% with a positive test result, and decreased to 0.9% with a negative test result. If inadequate samples were considered as negative test results, the results were even more accurate.

Essential Evidence: Medicine that Matters, Edited by David Slawson, Allen Shaughnessy, Mark Ebell, and Henry Barry.

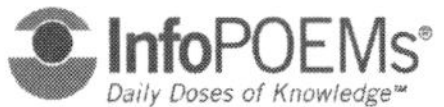

Melanoma incidence really not rising

Clinical question

Has the incidence of skin melanoma increased?

Bottom line

This study provides preliminary evidence that the incidence of melanoma is increasing not because of factors such as skin burns and ozone layer holes, but simply because more dermatologists are biopsying more lesions. In a 5-year period the incidence of melanoma increased 2.4-fold, whereas the biopsy rate over this same period increased a similar 2.5 times. (LOE = 2c)

Reference

Welch HG, Woloshin S, Schwartz LM. Skin biopsy rates and incidence of melanoma: population based ecological study. BMJ 2005;33:481–484.

Study Design

Ecologic

Funding

Government

Setting

Population-based

Synopsis

The incidence of skin melanoma is now 6 times higher than in 1950. The researchers conducting this study attempted to determine whether the true incidence is rising or whether the increase is simply due to an increased biopsy rate. Histologic diagnosis of melanoma is difficult, and several studies have shown that pathologists cannot agree on which samples are really melanoma (see: Pathology as art appreciation: melanoma diagnosis. http://www.jr2.ox.ac.uk/bandolier/band37/b37-2.html). This study compared skin biopsy rates for people older than 65 years with the incidence of melanoma over 5 years in 9 geographical areas in the United States. Over this period the number of biopsies in this age group increased 2.5-fold, from 1 in 35 people to 1 in 14 people. The incidence of melanoma increased 2.4-fold, from 1 in every 2222 people to 1 in every 925 people. Despite this increase in diagnoses, mortality due to melanoma changed little. Although these data don't prove it, they suggest that the increase in melanoma diagnoses is simply because more lesions are being biopsied that wouldn't have been biopsied in the past.

Essential Evidence: Medicine that Matters, Edited by David Slawson, Allen Shaughnessy, Mark Ebell, and Henry Barry.

Lifetime risk of mole transforming to melanoma very low

Clinical question

What is the risk that any given mole will become a melanoma?

Bottom line

Using a theoretical model and existing sources of data, the authors estimate that the lifetime risk that a mole will become melanoma in a 50-year-old man is 1 in 2000 and in a 50-year-old woman is 1 in 9000. These findings call into question the cost-effectiveness of surveillance programs and frequent excisions, especially for young or low-risk patients. (LOE = 2c)

Reference

Tsao H, Bevona C, Goggins W, Quinn T. The transformation rate of moles (melanocytic nevi) into cutaneous melanoma. Arch Dermatol 2003;139:282–288.

Study Design

Decision analysis

Setting

Population-based

Synopsis

This is an interesting question, and may be helpful as we talk to our patients about moles and melanoma. The authors took data from a variety of sources, including surveys of the number per adult of melanocytic nevi at least 2 to 3 mm in diameter and a community-based pathology database of skin biopsies. They created a theoretical model to determine the transformation rate, and stratified their findings by age. The risk that any single mole on a 30 year old will become a melanoma by age 80 was 38 in 100,000 in men and 11 in 100,000 in women. The lifetime risk of transformation to melanoma gradually increases in men from 31.6 in 100,000 in 20 year olds to 50.1 in 100,000 in 50 year olds (that is, 1 in 3000 to 1 in 2000).

Essential Evidence: Medicine that Matters, Edited by David Slawson, Allen Shaughnessy, Mark Ebell, and Henry Barry.

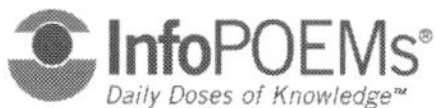

0.7% of congenital melanocytic nevi become malignant

Clinical question

What is the risk that a congenital melanocytic nevus will undergo malignant transformation?

Bottom line

Less than 1% of congenital melanocytic nevi (CMN) reported in the medical literature underwent malignant transformation, although the heterogeneous nature of the studies permits only a broad estimate of risk. The true rate of malignant transformation may be lower because of selection bias inherent in smaller studies. (LOE = 2a)

Reference

Krengel S, Hauschild A, Schafer T. Melanoma risk in congenital melanocytic naevi: a systematic review. Br J Dermatol 2006;155:1–8.

Study Design

Meta-analysis (other)

Funding

Unknown/not stated

Setting

Outpatient (any)

Synopsis

Congenital melanocytic nevi (CMN) are pigmented lesions of varying size that are present at or shortly after birth. They occur in between 0.2% and 2.1% of infants, and range in size from less than 1 square centimeter to hundreds of square centimeters. Previous case series and cohort studies have provided varying estimates of the risk of malignant transformation. This systematic review identified 14 relevant articles after a comprehensive literature search. Studies with fewer than 20 patients or those with fewer than 3 years of follow-up were appropriately excluded. Eight studies were retrospective and 6 were prospective, and the mean follow-up ranged from 3.4 to nearly 24 years. Six studies had fewer than 100 patients; 2 studies were quite large, with 1008 and 3922 patients. The proportion of patients with melanoma ranged from 0% to 10.7% (6 of 56 patients in 1 small retrospective study). The age at diagnosis of melanoma ranged from birth to 57 years, with a mean age of 15 years. Overall, 49 melanomas were reported in 46 of 6571 patients (0.7%). Most (75%) arose in so-called "garment nevi," which are greater than 40 cm in diameter. Because of the higher rate in small studies, suggesting selection bias, this figure of 0.7% probably represents an upper bound. The largest, and perhaps best, population-based study found that 0.2% of all newborns were registered as having CMN, of whom only 2 (0.05%) underwent malignant transformation after a median follow-up of 10 years.

Essential Evidence: Medicine that Matters, Edited by David Slawson, Allen Shaughnessy, Mark Ebell, and Henry Barry.

Dermoscopy with validated criteria more sensitive than unaided eye

Clinical question

Does use of a dermoscope improve the accuracy of diagnosis of melanoma?

Bottom line

Dermoscopy, especially when used in conjunction with the Menzies method, is more sensitive than the unaided eye in diagnosing melanoma. This technique is not widely used in the United States and deserves further study. We don't know whether it was the validated criteria or the use of dermoscopy that made the intervention more sensitive. (LOE = 2b)

Reference

Dolianitis C, Kelly J, Wolfe R, Simpson P. Comparative performance of 4 dermoscopic algorithms by nonexperts for the diagnosis of melanocytic lesions. Arch Dermatol 2005;141:1008–1014.

Study Design

Diagnostic test evaluation

Funding

Foundation

Setting

Outpatient (any)

Synopsis

Dermoscopy, also called dermatoscopy, involves use of a low-power handheld microscope (typically 10×) used with or without oil immersion to view suspicious skin lesions (http://www.dermoscopy.org/default.asp). Previous studies have shown that in expert hands it increases the accuracy of diagnosis. In this study, 60 physicians (35 general practitioners, 10 dermatologists, and 16 dermatology trainees) were presented with unaided photos of 40 lesions and asked to use their standard clinical judgment to make a diagnosis of melanoma or nonmelanoma. They were then presented with dermascopic images of the same lesions 4 times in succession and asked to apply 4 different set of standard, validated criteria for diagnosing melanoma (the ABCD rule, the Menzies method, a 7-point checklist, and pattern analysis). They were instructed in each of these methods using a CD-ROM. Interrater reliability for key melanoma diagnostic features was fair, with kappas in the range from 0.21 to 0.56. The unaided eye using a standard photo of the lesion was 61% sensitive and 85% specific with a 73% diagnostic accuracy. The dermoscopic photo used in conjunction with each of the 4 sets of criteria were more sensitive (68% for pattern analysis, 77% for the ABCD rule, 81% for the 7-point checklist, and 85% for the Menzies method). The specificity of pattern analysis is similar to the clinical examination (85%). The specificity of all other methods ranged from 73% to 80%. In this situation, sensitivity is more important than specificity; you don't want to miss any cancers, and the biopsy is an even more specific test that will hopefully sort out the nonmalignant tumors. Note that this study does not tell us that patients diagnosed with dermoscopy live longer or better lives: it's not a POEM. Rather, it's a SMORE (Surrogate Marker Of Relevant Outcomes), if one assumes that more accurate diagnosis of melanoma leads to better outcomes.

Essential Evidence: Medicine that Matters, Edited by David Slawson, Allen Shaughnessy, Mark Ebell, and Henry Barry.

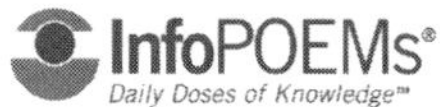

Larger margins better in melanoma >2mm thick

Clinical question

What is the optimal margin for excision of melanomas at least 2-mm thick?

Bottom line

There is a greater likelihood of local or regional recurrence of melanoma in patients who have a 1-cm margin compared with those who have excision with a 3-cm margin. However, the benefit in terms of disease-specific mortality is only marginally significant, and is nonsignificant for all-cause mortality. (LOE = 1b)

Reference

Thomas JM, Newton-Bishop J, A'Hern R, et al. Excision margins in high-risk malignant melanoma. N Engl J Med 2004;350:757–766.

Study Design

Randomized controlled trial (single-blinded)

Setting

Outpatient (specialty)

Synopsis

A previous study found no difference in outcomes for patients with melanoma who had excisions with 2-cm or 4-cm margins. This larger study randomized 900 patients (allocation concealed) with a melanoma at least 2-mm thick to either 1-cm or 3-cm margins. These are relatively high-risk lesions. The mean age of included patients was 57 years, and approximately half were women. Most had an initial 1-mm biopsy margin followed by later 1-cm or 3-cm excision. Patients were followed up for a median of 60 months, although no details are given on how often or in what way patients were evaluated. Outcomes were adjudicated by a central group blinded to treatment group. Groups were similar at baseline and analysis was by intention to treat. Patients with a 1-cm margin were more likely to have a locoregional recurrence at 3 years (168 vs 142; hazard ratio [HR] = 1.26; 95% CI, 1.0–1.59). There was also a trend toward a greater likelihood of death from melanoma (128 vs 105; HR = 1.24; 95% CI, 0.96–1.61). However, there was no significant difference in the likelihood of death from any cause (144 vs 137; HR = 1.07; 95% CI, 0.85–1.36).

Antioxidants don't prevent GI cancers, and may increase overall mortality

Clinical question
Do antioxidants prevent gastrointestinal cancers?

Bottom line
Antioxidants do not prevent gastrointestinal cancers. In fact, in pooled results of high-quality studies, antioxidants increased overall mortality. (LOE = 1a)

Reference
Bjelakovic G, Nikolova D, Simonetti RG, Gluud C. Antioxidant supplements for prevention of gastrointestinal cancers: a systematic review and meta-analysis. Lancet 2004;364:1219–1228.

Study Design
Meta-analysis (randomized controlled trials)

Funding
Foundation

Setting
Various (meta-analysis)

Synopsis
This is a Cochrane Review that follows their usual rigorous methods of searching, identification of unpublished data, and data extraction. The authors included all trials that randomized participants to supplementation with antioxidants (beta-carotene, vitamins A, C, and E, and selenium, as different combinations or separately) versus placebo, and that reported the incidence of gastrointestinal cancers. The authors assessed the methodological quality of trials and calculated whether the findings were consistent across trials. A total of 14 randomized controlled trials with 170,525 patients were evaluated. The number of patients in each trial ranged from 226 to nearly 40,000. Half the studies of cancer incidence were of good quality; 7 of the 9 that also reported mortality were of good quality. None of the supplements protected against esophageal cancer, gastric cancer, colorectal cancer, or pancreatic cancer. In the high-quality studies, antioxidants increased overall mortality (8.0% vs 6.6%). This translates to a number needed to treat to harm of 69 for 1 additional death (95% CI, 58–85). It is interesting to note that 4 trials of selenium (3 with unclear or poor methodology) reduced the incidence of gastrointestinal cancer (odds ratio = 0.49; 95% CI, 0.36–0.67). Selenium should be evaluated in randomized trials with sound methods.

Essential Evidence: Medicine that Matters, Edited by David Slawson, Allen Shaughnessy, Mark Ebell, and Henry Barry.

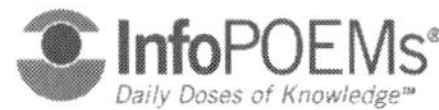

Vitamin E doesn't lower women's risk of cardiovascular disease or cancer

Clinical question

Is vitamin E effective in reducing the risk of cardiovascular disease and cancer among healthy women?

Bottom line

Vitamin E does not reduce the risk of cardiovascular disease, cancer, or total mortality among healthy women 45 years or older. (LOE = 1b)

Reference

Lee IM, Cook NR, Gaziano JM, et al. Vitamin E in the primary prevention of cardiovascular disease and cancer. The Women's Health Study: A randomized controlled trial. JAMA 2005;294:56–65.

Study Design

Randomized controlled trial (double-blinded)

Funding

Industry + govt

Allocation

Concealed

Setting

Population-based

Synopsis

Evidence from observational trials suggests that vitamin E may be effective in preventing cardiovascular disease and cancer in women. In the Women's Health Study, the investigators randomized (concealed allocation assignment) 39,876 healthy women, 45 years or older, to receive either (1) 600 IU natural-source vitamin E every other day, (2) placebo and 100 mg aspirin every other day, or (3) placebo only in a 2 × 2 factorial design. Individuals blinded to treatment group assignment assessed outcomes. Follow-up occurred for an average of 10.1 years for more than 97% of the subjects. Using intention-to-treat analysis, vitamin E did not significantly reduce the risk of major cardiovascular events, including myocardial infarction, ischemic stroke, or hemorrhagic stroke. Although vitamin E slightly reduced the risk of cardiovascular death (number needed to treat for 10.1 years = 586; 95% CI, 306–6058), all-cause mortality was not significantly reduced. Vitamin E did not significantly reduce the risk of any cancer, including breast, lung, and colorectal cancers. Cancer mortality was not significantly lower in any group.

Essential Evidence: Medicine that Matters, Edited by David Slawson, Allen Shaughnessy, Mark Ebell, and Henry Barry.

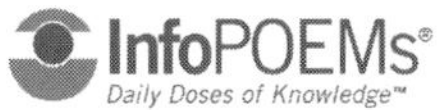

Antioxidants don't prevent colorectal cancer

Clinical question

Can colorectal cancer risk be decreased with antioxidant supplements?

Bottom line

Antioxidant supplementation for up to 6 years does not decrease the risk of colorectal adenomatous polyps and thus, by extension, does not reduce the risk of colorectal cancer. Vitamin E may increase the risk of colorectal adenoma. (LOE = 1a–)

Reference

Bjelakovic G, Nagorni A, Nikolova D, Simonetti RG, Bjelakovic M, Gluud C. Meta-analysis: antioxidant supplements for primary and secondary prevention of colorectal adenoma. Aliment Pharmacol Ther 2006;24:281–291.

Study Design

Meta-analysis (randomized controlled trials)

Funding

Self-funded or unfunded

Setting

Outpatient (any)

Synopsis

The researchers conducted this analysis using standard methodology and searched 5 databases for all randomized trials comparing beta-carotene, vitamin A, vitamin C, vitamin E, or selenium with no treatment or placebo on the development of colorectal adenoma, a cancer precursor. They also searched for unpublished studies. They report that they used The Cochrane Collaboration methodology for conducting the meta-analysis but they don't give details of how they chose studies for inclusion or how they abstracted the data. They assessed the research for quality, identifying the studies as high quality or low quality according to study design. There was no publication bias. The 8 trials used in this analysis included a total of 17,260 participants, though most of the patients (88%) were in a single high-quality study. This study enrolled patients without previous adenoma; the rest of the studies enrolled participants with previously removed colorectal adenomas (6 studies) or previous colorectal cancer (1 study). Overall, there was no benefit of antioxidant supplementation on the development of colorectal adenoma. High-quality studies showed no effect or a slight increase of risk of adenoma with antioxidants; the small, low-quality studies found a benefit with antioxidants. When analyzed separately, none of the individual antioxidants had a beneficial effect on adenoma rates. Vitamin E, used in the largest study, produced a statistically significant increase in the risk of colorectal adenoma (relative risk = 1.7; 95% CI, 1.1–2.8).

Essential Evidence: Medicine that Matters, Edited by David Slawson, Allen Shaughnessy, Mark Ebell, and Henry Barry.

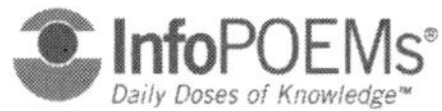

Mammography, FOBT and CXR don't reduce all-cause mortality

Clinical question

Do commonly used cancer screening tests actually reduce all-cause mortality?

Bottom line

Randomized trials of screening that report only cancer-specific mortality present more biased data than when all-cause mortality is reported. This goes back to basics. When we measure death, we all get a score of one. Patients die; doctors can't change that. Although we have some interventions that maximize survival (aspirin for primary prevention, immunizations, and so forth), it is unclear if screening for colon, lung, or breast cancer are among those successful interventions. (LOE = 2c)

Reference

Black WC, Haggstrom DA, Welch HG. All-cause mortality in randomized trials of cancer screening. J Natl Cancer Inst 2002;94:167–173.

Study Design

Other

Setting

Outpatient (any)

Synopsis

All-cause mortality is the least biased way of reporting the mortality benefit attributed to therapy or screening. These authors explore this in a semi-systematic way. They took the references from "an authoritative text," supplemented it with a PubMed search and identified 12 trials that reported both disease-specific mortality (what most authors report) and all-cause mortality: 7 trials of of mammography, 3 of fecal occult blood testing (FOBT), and 2 of chest radiography (CXR). In the mammography studies, four reported improved breast cancer mortality. When all-cause mortality is used, only 1 demonstrated a benefit (and the methods of this particular study have been criticized). In the 3 studies of FOBT, all demonstrated reductions in cancer-specific mortality, but none demonstrated significant effect on all-cause mortality. The two studies of CXR showed that patients had increased cancer-specific mortality. When all-cause mortality is considered, the patients receiving CXR were still worse off, but the magnitude of harm was different in one of the studies.

Essential Evidence: Medicine that Matters, Edited by David Slawson, Allen Shaughnessy, Mark Ebell, and Henry Barry.

Spiral CT detects early lung cancer, but screening use is premature

Clinical question

Can spiral computed tomography screening detect small lung cancers that are potentially curable?

Bottom line

The authors point to this study as evidence to support widespread use of spiral computed tomography (CT) scans to screen for lung cancer in high-risk patients. However, there are important problems with this recommendation. The unintended negative consequences of screening are of particular concern with a disease like lung cancer. A patient's continued tobacco use because he is reassured by negative screening increases his risk of heart disease and other malignancies. Two randomized controlled trials that look at all-cause mortality are underway. Also, while the authors point to the low cost ($200) of a scan, this does not include the cost of positron-emission tomography (PET) scans, follow-up CT scans, and biopsies. Finally, the radiation associated with repeated CT scans (even "low-dose" scans) is not trivial and will cause some cancers even as it detects others early. (LOE = 2b)

Reference

The International Early Lung Cancer Action Program Investigators, Henschke CI, Yankelevitz DF, et al. Survival of patients with stage I lung cancer detected on CT screening. N Engl J Med 2006;355:1763–1771.

Study Design	Funding	Setting
Cohort (prospective)	Government	Outpatient (any)

Synopsis

Screening programs are thought to be most effective for tumors that grow at an intermedate speed. Those that grow too fast are often untreatable by the time they are detected, while those that grow very slowly may never require treatment. Lung cancers are thought to fall into the former category, and studies have shown that sputum cytology and chest x-ray are not effective screening tools for this disease. In this study, patients at high risk for lung cancer because of current or previous tobacco use (83%), occupational exposure (5%), or exposure to second-hand smoke (12%) were recruited. The 31,567 participants underwent a baseline spiral CT scan between 1993 and 2005. The 4186 patients who had at least one suspicious nodule went through a management algorithm that could involve antibiotics for suspected infection, repeat CT in 3 months, or immediate PET scan followed by biopsy if the lesion remained suspicious. A total of 405 patients from this group of 4186 had lung cancer diagnosed. The remaining patients had a second screening between 7 months and 18 months later. Of this group, 1460 had newly identified noncalcified nodules and 74 had lung cancer. Five patients had an interim diagnosis of lung cancer before completing their second screening examination. Of the 484 patients with a diagnosis of lung cancer, 412 had clinical stage I lung cancer, defined as: no nodal involvement; no metastases; and if there was more than one adenocarcinoma, they were all 30 mm or less in diameter. The estimated 10-year survival for all patients with screening-detected lung cancer was 80%; 92% for those with stage I disease. Eight patients chose not to be treated, and all died within 5 years after diagnosis. Unfortunately, we are not given any information about these patients, who may well have chosen to forego treatment because of other major comorbidities.

Essential Evidence: Medicine that Matters, Edited by David Slawson, Allen Shaughnessy, Mark Ebell, and Henry Barry.

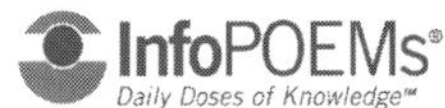

Cancer linked to some diabetes treatments

Clinical question

Is there a relationship between cancer-related mortality and treatments for type 2 diabetes mellitus?

Bottom line

Death due to cancer seems to be more prevalent in patients with type 2 diabetes treated with either insulin or a sulfonylurea than in patients treated with metformin (Glucophage). It may be that hyperinsulinemia increases cancer risk, or that metformin is protective. Another explanation could be that, although cancer is related to certain medication use, it is not caused by their use. We need a controlled study to answer these questions. (LOE = 2b)

Reference

Bowker SL, Majumdar SR, Veugelers P, Johnson JA. Increased cancer-related mortality for patients with type 2 diabetes who use sulfonylureas or insulin. Diabetes Care 2006;29:254–258.

Study Design	Funding	Setting
Cohort (retrospective)	Foundation	Population-based

Synopsis

Insulin resistance and the resulting hyperinsulinemia has been linked to a number of disorders, especially, of course, to type 2 diabetes mellitus. The sequela of the metabolic syndrome are also a consequence, and there is some evidence that cancer is related. Insulin and insulin-like growth factor are required at all stages of cell growth, cancerous or not. Data from the United Kingdom Prospective Diabetes Study (UKPDS) suggest the possibility of an increase in all-cause mortality for patients with type 2 diabetes treated with insulin. The researchers conducting this provocative study identified 10,309 new users of metformin or sulfonylureas in Canada using a drug plan database. They monitored the patients for an average 5.4 years using a computerized vital statistics file. All patients were followed up. The patients were an average 63.4 years old, and 55% were men. In this type of study, no intervention particular to the study was performed; the patients were treated by their individual physicians as they saw fit and the outcomes of the patients were determined over time. Since the patients were not specifically assigned to therapy, imbalances could have (and did) occur. The average age of the patients who were started on a sulfonylurea was 5 years older than the metformin-treated patients (66.9 years vs 61.8 years; $P < .0001$). A greater proportion of men were in the sulfonylurea group (58.6% vs 53.5%; $P < .0001$) and more patients initially started on metformin eventually were given insulin (16.3% vs 9.2%; $P < .0001$). All of these imbalances can be adjusted statistically, though an ideal study would randomly assign patients to prevent such imbalances. A total of 407 cancer-related deaths (3.9%) occurred in the whole group. Before statistical adjustment, 3.5% of patients receiving metformin died of a cancer-related illness compared with 4.9% patients in the sulfonylurea-treated group ($P = .001$). After statistical adjustment, deaths were still 30% higher in the group treated with a sulfonylurea than in the group taking metformin (hazard ratio [HR] = 1.3; 95% CI, 1.1–1.6; $P = .012$). In addition, cancer-related mortality was almost twice as high in patients treated with insulin, regardless of other treatment (HR = 1.9; 1.5–2.4).

Essential Evidence: Medicine that Matters, Edited by David Slawson, Allen Shaughnessy, Mark Ebell, and Henry Barry.

Finasteride of mixed benefit in preventing prostate cancer

Clinical question

Does finasteride reduce the risk of prostate cancer?

Bottom line

Finasteride 5 mg daily reduces the overall risk of prostate cancer from 24.4% to 18.4%, but increases the risk of high-grade disease from 5.1% to 6.4%. Since the latter is the cancer that matters in terms of mortality, and because the drug is associated with significant cost and adverse effects, it is not recommended for the prevention of prostate cancer. Patients starting finasteride for the prevention of urinary retention should be informed of these risks. (LOE = 1b)

Reference

Thompson IM, Goodman PJ, Tangen CM, et al. The influence of finasteride on the development of prostate cancer. N Engl J Med 2003;349:215–224.

Study Design

Randomized controlled trial (double-blinded)

Setting

Outpatient (any)

Synopsis

Finasteride (Proscar) inhibits the conversion of testosterone to dihydrotestosterone; it is thought that having less of this potent androgen may reduce the risk of prostate cancer. However, this theory has never been tested. In the current trial, men older than 55 years with, at most, moderate symptoms of benign prostatic hypertrophy (BPH), a normal digital rectal examination (DRE) result, and a prostate specific antigen (PSA) level of less than or equal to 3.0 ng/mL were recruited from 221 sites and randomized to oral finasteride 5 mg each day or placebo. We aren't told whether they were recruited from primary care or specialty clinics (although I suspect the latter), and 20% had a first-degree relative with prostate cancer. The allocation method was not described, but groups were balanced at baseline. Although the analysis is described as intention to treat, only men with a tissue biopsy at the end of the study were actually included. The participants had annual DRE and PSA testing, and underwent prostate biopsy if they had an abnormal DRE result or a PSA level greater than 4.0 ng/mL. All patients were supposed to undergo prostate biopsy at the end of the study, although approximately 1 in 4 refused in each group. The plan was to follow each man for 7 years, but it was stopped early by the monitoring committee, meaning that approximately 20% were followed up for less than 7 years. The overall likelihood of prostate cancer was lower in the finasteride group (18.4% vs 24.4%; $P < .001$; number needed to treat [NNT] = 16). However, there were more high-grade cancers (Gleason score 7 to 10) in the finasteride group (6.4% vs 5.1%; $P = .005$; number needed to treat to harm [NNTH] = 77). There was no difference in overall mortality over the 7-year follow-up period, although the study was too small and too short to be able to detect such a difference if it did exist. Patients taking finasteride had a greater risk of erectile dysfunction (NNTH = 16), loss of libido (NNTH = 17), and reduced volume of ejaculate (NNTH = 8), and a lower risk of benign prostatic hypertrophy (NNT = 29), incontinence (NNT = 333), and urinary retention (NNT = 48). It is interesting that more than 40% of patients had a prostate biopsy during the follow-up period because of symptoms, abnormal DRE result, or elevated PSA level. That illustrates part of the harm associated with prostate cancer screening, which must be balanced against any potential benefits.

Essential Evidence: Medicine that Matters, Edited by David Slawson, Allen Shaughnessy, Mark Ebell, and Henry Barry.

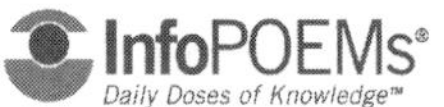

Prostate cancer screening every 4 years as good as annually

Clinical question

Is a 4-year screening interval as effective as annual screening for prostate cancer?

Bottom line

The 4-year rate of developing prostate cancer in screened men between the ages of 55 years and 75 years is pretty low. Although this study can't tell us whether men are better or worse off as a result of screening, it suggests that for those men who choose to be screened, annual screening isn't necessary. Other, smaller studies have similarly found that men with low prostate-specific antigen (PSA) levels don't need annual screening. (LOE = 2b)

Reference

van der Cruijsen-Koeter IW, van der Kwast TH, Schröder FH. Interval carcinomas in the European Randomized Study of Screening for Prostate Cancer (ERSPC)-Rotterdam. J Natl Cancer Inst 2003;95:1462–1466.

Study Design

Randomized controlled trial (nonblinded)

Setting

Population-based

Synopsis

This team studied more than 17,000 men between the ages of 55 years and 74 years randomized to screening or no screening. This study reports on the cohort of men being screened with rectal examinations, PSA, and ultrasound (n = 8350). After the first 4 years of follow-up, they report on the incidence of prostate cancer as confirmed by a review of the cancer registry. This could underestimate the true incidence of cancer. During the first screening, 412 men were given a diagnosis of prostate cancer; only 25 more cases were detected after enrollment. This translates to an incidence of 21 cases per 1000 person-years among men in the screened arm. Since the intervention group had ultrasound, these data may not reflect what one might find if PSA were used alone.

False-positive PSA associated with increased worry, fears

Clinical question

Do men who receive a positive prostate specific antigen (PSA) test result subsequently shown to be wrong worry more about prostate cancer than men who receive a negative result?

Bottom line

False positive results of screening tests are not benign but carry with them a psychological cost. As with women receiving false-positive mammogram results, men receiving false-positive prostate specific antigen (PSA) test results report having thought and worried more about prostate cancer despite receiving a negative follow-up test (prostate biopsy) result. They also think, like women, that the false-positive result makes them more likely to develop prostate cancer. Screening can be bad for our patients' mental health. (LOE = 1b)

Reference

McNaughton-Collins M, Fowler FJ, Caubet JF, et al. Psychological effects of a suspicious prostate cancer screening test followed by a benign biopsy result. Am J Med 2004;117:719–725.

Study Design

Cohort (prospective)

Funding

Foundation

Setting

Outpatient (primary care)

Synopsis

The investigators identified 167 men from a group of consecutive men who had a negative biopsy following a suspicious PSA test. In other words, these men had a false positive PSA result. For comparison, they also identified 233 men who had a normal PSA test. The men were mailed a brief questionnaire about 6 weeks after their biopsy or normal PSA test result. Overall, 85% of the men responded by returning the survey, which is a very good response for a survey. Of the men who had a false positive PSA, 49% reported having thought about prostate cancer either "a lot" or "some of the time" compared with 18% of controls ($P < .001$). As compared with 8% in the control group, 40% of the men in the false positive group also worried "a lot" (7%) or "some of the time" (33%) about the possibility of developing prostate cancer. The false positive group did not worry more than the control group about dying soon. Sixty-two percent of the men with a negative biopsy reported being "a lot" reassured by the result, despite the 10% false negative rate associated with biopsy. As with women undergoing mammogram, instead of being angry at the erroneous PSA, men with a false positive PSA but a normal biopsy felt they "dodged a bullet": Significantly more men in this group reported their lives changed for the better (31% vs. 13%, $P < .001$). And, similar to women experiencing a false positive mammogram, the men in the false positive group were more likely to think their chance of getting prostate cancer was "much more" or "a little more than average" (36% vs. 18% in the control group, $P < .001$).

Essential Evidence: Medicine that Matters, Edited by David Slawson, Allen Shaughnessy, Mark Ebell, and Henry Barry.

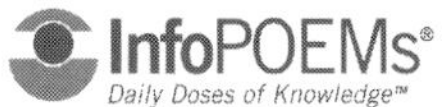

Elevated PSA should be confirmed before biopsy

Clinical question

How often does an elevated PSA level return to normal?

Bottom line

Isolated elevations of serum prostate-specific antigen (PSA) frequently return to normal. Clinicians and their patients with an elevated PSA have 3 choices: (1) immediate referral for biopsy; (2) immediate repeat of the PSA test; or (3) wait 4 to 6 weeks and repeat the test. The repeat testing interval of 4 to 6 weeks is based on studies reporting the time needed for an elevated PSA to return to normal after biopsy or surgery for noncancerous conditions. Studies of prostate cancer progression conclude that a delay of several months from diagnosis to surgery does not affect outcomes. Thus, choice #3 is likely the best one for most patients before proceeding with further testing or referral. (LOE = 2b)

Reference

Eastham JA, Riedel E, Scardino PT, et al. Variation of serum prostate-specific antigen levels. An evaluation of year-to-year fluctuations. JAMA 2003;289:2695–2700.

Study Design

Cohort (prospective)

Setting

Outpatient (specialty)

Synopsis

Routine use of the PSA as a screening tool has been questioned because of its lack of specificity – meaning that many men with elevated levels do not have prostate cancer and thus undergo unnecessary and potentially harmful treatment or further testing. A variety of different methods have been studied to improve the specificity of the PSA, including age-specific reference levels, PSA velocity of change, and percentage-free PSA. Given that natural biological variations in PSA levels occur, the authors used blood samples obtained during the Polyp Prevention Trial from 1351 men aged 35 years or older with 1 or more colonic adenomas. Samples were obtained at least yearly for up to 4 years and were stored between 1 and 9 years prior to their analysis. Participants with a history of prostate cancer, those developing prostate cancer during the study period, and those with fewer than 2 blood samples were excluded from the final analysis. Most of the participants (n = 972; 79%) had PSA measurements at baseline and yearly for 4 years. Using any of the PSA thresholds, 37% of the men would have met at least 1 of the criteria for an abnormal test result. Nearly half these men subsequently had a normal PSA level on 1 or more subsequent follow-ups, including 44% with a PSA level greater than 4 ng/mL; 40% with a level greater than 2.5 ng/mL; 55% with a level above the age-specific cutoff; and 53% with level 4 ng/mL to 10 ng/mL and a free-to-total ratio of less than 0.25 ng/mL.

Essential Evidence: Medicine that Matters, Edited by David Slawson, Allen Shaughnessy, Mark Ebell, and Henry Barry.

Radical prostatectomy improves outcomes in symptom-detected prostate cancer

Clinical question

What is the best treatment for moderately differentiated or well-differentiated prostate cancer?

Bottom line

Radical prostatectomy is better than watchful waiting for men with moderately differentiated or well-differentiated prostate cancer, especially (and perhaps only) in men younger than 65 years. Although these are the best data on treatment in this group to date, only 5% of the men in this study had their cancer detected by screening. Whether these data generalize to men with screening-detected prostate cancer is unclear but will likely be assumed by most clinicians and their patients. (LOE = 1b)

Reference

Bill-Axelson A, Holmberg L, Ruutu M, et al, for the Scandinavian Prostate Cancer Group Study No. 4. Radical prostatectomy versus watchful waiting in early prostate cancer. N Engl J Med 2005;352:1977–1984.

Study Design

Randomized controlled trial (single-blinded)

Funding

Government

Allocation

Concealed

Setting

Outpatient (specialty)

Synopsis

This is a 3-year follow-up study to one originally reported in 2002. The researchers randomized men with localized, well-differentiated, or moderately differentiated prostate cancer according to World Health Organization grading to either radical prostatectomy or watchful waiting. Gleason scores were 2 to 4 for 13% of the men, 5 or 6 for 48%, 7 for 23%, and 8 to 10 for 5%. The Gleason score was unknown for 11% of patients. Only 5% of cancers were detected by screening, although more than 85% had a prostate-specific antigen (PSA) level higher than 4.0 ng/mL. Allocation was concealed, outcomes were blindly assessed, and analysis was by intention to treat. The vast majority of patients, however, stayed in the group to which they were assigned. The median duration of follow-up was 8.2 years, and 10-year follow-up data were available for 222 patients. The researchers prespecified several subgroup analyses by age, Gleason score, and PSA. Overall, results became more favorable for radical prostatectomy with an increased duration of follow-up. All-cause mortality was lower in the radical prostatectomy group (27% vs 32%; P = .04; number needed to treat [NNT] = 20), as was disease-specific mortality (9.6% vs 14.9%; P = .01; NNT = 19). The likelihood of local progression and distant metastases was also lower in the treated group. Radical prostatectomy was especially beneficial in men younger than 65 years; there was little difference between watchful waiting and surgery in patients older than 65. Although there was no association between the benefit of surgery and the Gleason score, more than 70% had a Gleason score of 5 to 7. Therefore, there were too few patients with lower or higher Gleason scores to confidently assess the benefit of surgery in those groups or in men with screening-detected prostate cancer.

Essential Evidence: Medicine that Matters, Edited by David Slawson, Allen Shaughnessy, Mark Ebell, and Henry Barry.

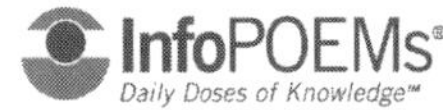

Early metoprolol in acute MI: no benefit, possible harm (COMMIT; CCS-2)

Clinical question

Does the early use of metoprolol improve outcomes in patients with acute myocardial infarction?

Bottom line

The early use of metoprolol in patients with acute myocardial infarction who are also receiving thrombolytics and aspirin provides no short-term benefit compared with placebo. Since the early use, however, increases the risk of cardiogenic shock, it may be wise to delay starting metoprolol until the patient is hemodynamically stable. (LOE = 1b)

Reference

Chen ZM, Pan HC, Chen YP, et al, for the COMMIT (ClOpidogrel and Metoprolol in Myocardial Infarction Trial) Collaborative Group. Early intravenous then oral metoprolol in 45,852 patients with acute myocardial infarction: randomised placebo-controlled trial. Lancet 2005;366:1622–1632.

Study Design	Funding	Allocation	Setting
Randomized controlled trial (double-blinded)	Industry + govt	Concealed	Inpatient (any location)

Synopsis

Studies of beta-blockers for secondary prevention of acute myocardial infarction were generally performed in the years before the widespread use of thrombolytics. This study had 2 key components. One component evaluated whether adding clopidogrel to aspirin was beneficial for patients with acute myocardial infarction. The second part of the study, presented here, assessed whether adding metoprolol to current standard practice (aspirin and thrombolytics) is of any value to those patients. More than 45,000 patients presenting to Chinese hospitals with suspected acute myocardial infarction within 24 hours of the onset of the symptoms were randomly assigned to receive metoprolol or placebo. The research team excluded patients scheduled for primary percutaneous intervention and patients with "a small likelihood of benefit and high risk of adverse effects" from the study medications, a fairly subjective exclusion. The treating physicians were encouraged to prescribe beta-blockers and aspirin after discharge. The first 3 doses (5 mg or placebo) were given intravenously every 5 minutes as long as the heart rate remained near 50 beats per minute and the systolic blood pressure remained above 90 mm Hg. After these 3 doses, the patient received 50 mg metoprolol or placebo every 6 hours for the first day. From the second day on, the patients received 200 mg sustained-release metoprolol or placebo once daily for up to 4 weeks or until discharge from the hospital. The main outcomes, assessed via intention to treat, were all-cause mortality and the composite of death, reinfarction, and cardiac arrest assessed during the first 28 days or until hospital discharge. Only one patient in each group was lost to follow-up. There was no difference between the 2 groups in total mortality (~8%) or in the composite outcome (9.4% on metoprolol and 9.9% on placebo). The study was powerful enough to detect a 10% difference in event rates. More patients taking metoprolol developed cardiogenic shock during the first 24 hours than those taking placebo (5% vs 3.9%). One would need to treat 90 patients with metoprolol to harm one (95% CI, 67–136).

Essential Evidence: Medicine that Matters, Edited by David Slawson, Allen Shaughnessy, Mark Ebell, and Henry Barry.

Insulin/dextrose infusion ineffective in AMI (HI-5)

Clinical question

Does intensive control of blood glucose in patients with acute myocardial infarction decrease mortality?

Bottom line

Intensive control of blood glucose in patients with known diabetes or in patients with hyperglycemia at the time of admission for acute myocardial infarction (AMI) does not decrease either short-term or long-term mortality. (LOE = 1b–)

Reference

Cheung NW, Wong VW, McLean M. The hyperglycemia: intensive insulin infusion in infarction (HI-5) study. Diabetes Care 2006;29:765–770.

Study Design

Randomized controlled trial (nonblinded)

Funding

Industry + govt

Allocation

Uncertain

Setting

Inpatient (ICU only)

Synopsis

Previous studies have produced conflicting results regarding the benefit of insulin and glucose infusions as an adjunct treatment of AMI. These investigators enrolled 240 patients with evidence of AMI and either known diabetes mellitus or a blood glucose level of at least 140 mg/dL (8.8 mmol/L) on admission. They randomly assigned the patients, allocation concealment uncertain, to receive either their usual care for diabetes or to an intensive treatment group. Metformin was temporarily discontinued. The intensive treatment group were given insulin at 2 units per hour and 5% dextrose at 80 mL per hour for at least 24 hours, with the insulin titrated to maintain blood glucose between 72 mg/dL and 180 mg/dL (4–10 mmol/l). Patients also underwent standard AMI treatment. The insulin/dextrose treatment did not reduced mortality during the hospital stay or at 3 or 6 months. The door is not completely shut, however, on this treatment: Mortality was lower in patients for whom a mean blood glucose level of less than 144 mg/dL (8.1 mmol/L) was achieved (2% vs 11% at 6 months; P = .02). However, these patients also were more likely to have received percutaneous angioplasty instead of thrombolytic treatment. These results echo the findings in the DIGAMI-2 study (Eur Heart J 2005;26:650–651).

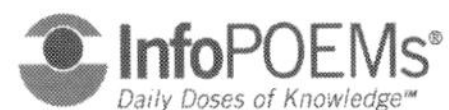

Early initiation of statins following ACS does not improve outcomes

Clinical question

Does early initiation of statin therapy following the onset of acute coronary syndromes reduce the short-term risk of death, recurrent myocardial infarction, or stroke?

Bottom line

Early initiation of statin therapy within 14 days of the onset of acute coronary syndromes (ACS) does not reduce the risk of death, recurrent myocardial infarction (MI), or stroke up to 4 months. (LOE = 1a)

Reference

Briel M, Schwartz GG, Thompson PL, et al. Effects of early treatment with statins on short-term clinical outcomes in acute coronary syndromes. A meta-analysis of randomized controlled trials. JAMA 2006;295:2046–2056.

Study Design

Meta-analysis (randomized controlled trials)

Funding

Industry

Setting

Various (meta-analysis)

Synopsis

During the initial period following the onset of ACS the risk is high for recurrent events and death due to vessel occlusions from vulnerable coronary plaques. To study the efficacy of statins in reducing the short-term risk of adverse clinical outcomes, these investigators thoroughly searched (without any language restrictions) electronic databases including the Cochrane Registry, reference lists of identified articles, recently published editorials, topical reviews, and they contacted authors of significant publications. Eligible trials fulfilled the following criteria: Randomized trial design comparing statin treatment with usual care; initiation of treatment within 14 days of onset of ACS; and follow-up for at least 30 days. Two authors independently assessed trial eligibility and quality. Twelve studies, comprising 13,024 individuals with a mean age ranging from 53 to 69 years, met inclusion criteria. Early statin therapy did not significantly reduce the risk of death, MI, or stroke at either 1 or 4 months following ACS. In addition, there were no significant risk reductions for secondary outcomes including total death, total MI, total stroke, cardiovascular death, fatal or nonfatal MI, or revascularization procedures. The authors found no evidence for heterogeneity among the studies (ie, the results were basically similar among all the trials). A formal analysis found little evidence for publication bias.

Essential Evidence: Medicine that Matters, Edited by David Slawson, Allen Shaughnessy, Mark Ebell, and Henry Barry.

Antibiotics not effective in acute coronary syndromes

Clinical question

Are antibiotics effective in the treatment of acute coronary syndromes?

Bottom line

Antibiotic therapy is no more effective than placebo in reducing the morbidity or mortality in patients with acute coronary syndromes. (LOE = 1a–)

Reference

Andraws R, Berger JS, Brown DL. Effects of antibiotic therapy on outcomes of patients with coronary artery disease. A meta-analysis of randomized controlled trials. JAMA 2005;293:2641–2647.

Study Design

Meta-analysis (randomized controlled trials)

Funding

Self-funded or unfunded

Setting

Various (meta-analysis)

Synopsis

Chlamydia pneumoniae infection is associated with the initiation and progression of atherosclerosis. Clinical trials investigating the effect of antibiotic therapy aimed at eradicating infection with Chlamydia on the outcomes of acute coronary syndromes are mixed. The investigators comprehensively searched multiple databases, including MEDLINE, the Cochrane Central Register for Controlled Trials, bibliographies of retrieved articles, and abstracts from major scientific meetings for potential clinical trials. Only English-language randomized placebo-controlled trials were included. From an initial total of 110 reports, only 11 enrolling 19,217 patients met inclusion criteria. The most common treatment was a single antibiotic such as roxithromycin, azithromycin, clarithromycin, or gatifloxacin. Overall, antibiotic therapy had no significant effect compared with placebo on reducing all-cause mortality or on the combined end point of myocardial infarction and unstable angina. The results were minimally heterogeneous, but exclusion of any single trial from the analysis did not alter the overall findings. There was no evidence of significant publication bias.

Essential Evidence: Medicine that Matters, Edited by David Slawson, Allen Shaughnessy, Mark Ebell, and Henry Barry.

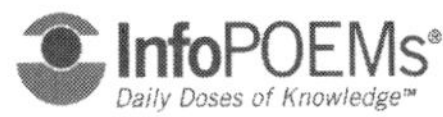

ABCDE approach to non-ST-segment elevation ACS

Clinical question

What is the optimal management of non-ST-segment elevation acute coronary syndrome?

Bottom line

The "ABCDE" approach can serve as a simplified guide for applying the best evidence in the care of patients with non-ST-segment elevation acute coronary syndrome. ABCDE stands for Antiplatelet, Anticoagulation, and ACE inhibition, Beta-blockade and Blood pressure control, Cholesterol treatment and Cigarette smoking cessation, Diabetes management and Diet, and Exercise. (LOE = 1a)

Reference

Gluckman TJ, Sachdev M, Schulman SP, Blumenthal RS. A simplified approach to the management of non-ST-segment elevation acute coronary syndromes. JAMA 2005;293:349–357.

Study Design

Practice guideline

Funding

Foundation

Setting

Various (meta-analysis)

Synopsis

Although practice guidelines abound on the best treatment of acute coronary syndromes (ACS), a simplified method for applying the best evidence would likely be beneficial for many busy clinicians. The authors searched standard evidence-based sources, including the Cochrane database and MEDLINE for controlled studies on the treatment of non-ST-segment elevation ACS (NSTE-ACS). No information is given on an independent assessment of review and evaluation or the potential for publication bias. The authors do discuss the strength of evidence for their individual recommendations. To simplify recommendations, they summarize them through an "ABCDE" approach as follows: A: "Antiplatelet therapy, including aspirin for all patients indefinitely, initially with 162–325 mg followed by 75–160 mg daily thereafter, clopidogrel for all patients unless anticipated need for urgent CABG surgery for up to 1 year, and Gp IIb/IIIa inhibitor therapy for all patients with continuing ischemia, an elevated troponin level, a TIMI risk score greater than 4, or anticipated PCI; "Anticoagulation", including preferably low molecular weight heparin or unfractionated heparin unless creatinine clearance is less than 60 mL/min or CABG surgery within 24 hours; "ACE inhibition or AT1 receptor blockade for all patients with left ventricular dysfunction (EF less than 40%); heart failure, or hypertension.B: "Beta-blockade" for all patients and "Blood pressure control", with goal of blood pressure at least 130/85 mmHg or lower. C: "Cholesterol treatment" for all patients with the goal of a LDL-C level less than 70 mg/dL; and "Cigarette smoking cessation". D: "Diabetes management: and "Diet", in particular with the Mediterranean diet. E: "Exercise", preferably with a cardiac rehabilitation program.

Essential Evidence: Medicine that Matters, Edited by David Slawson, Allen Shaughnessy, Mark Ebell, and Henry Barry.

Door-to-balloon time important in STEMI

Clinical question
Does time to reperfusion using coronary angioplasty ("door-to-balloon time") affect mortality rates?

Bottom line
Mortality resulting from ST-segment elevation myocardial infarction (STEMI) is independently related to the time it takes to administer percutaneous coronary intervention (PCI) following presentation to the emergency department. The relationship is still seen in patients who present several hours after symptoms begin. If you have a choice of hospitals, find out their door-to-balloon times and send patients to the faster one. (LOE = 2b)

Reference
McNamara RL, Wang Y, Herrin J, et al, for the NRMI Investigators. Effect of door-to-balloon time on mortality in patients with ST-segment elevation myocardial infarction. J Am Coll Cardiol 2006;47:2180–2186.

Study Design
Cohort (retrospective)

Funding
Government

Setting
Emergency department

Synopsis
Faster use of thrombolytic therapy in the treatment of STEMI is associated with better outcomes, though this relationship is not as solid for PCI. The investigators conducting this study evaluated the role of speed of reperfusion therapy in a US registry. The registry contained data on 29,222 patients treated at 395 hospitals with PCI within 6 hours of presentation. The investigators excluded data from hospitals performing fewer than 20 PCIs over the 4 years of data collection. In-hospital mortality was associated with delays in treatment in a linear fashion with rates of 3.0%, 4.2%, 5.7%, and 7.4% at less than 91 minutes, 91 to 120 minutes, 121 to 150 minutes, and greater than 150 minutes, respectively ($P < .01$). In other words, 1 additional death is avoided for every 23 patients treated within 90 minutes rather than after 150 minutes. This trend was seen regardless of the time between symptom onset and presentation to the hospital. Faster administration of PCI was associated with improved outcomes in patients with at least one risk factor for STEMI, but not for patients with no risk factors.

Essential Evidence: Medicine that Matters, Edited by David Slawson, Allen Shaughnessy, Mark Ebell, and Henry Barry.

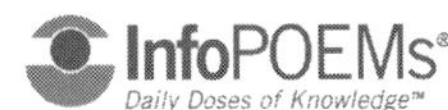

Routine invasive strategy may be preferred for ACS

Clinical question

Is a routine or selective invasive strategy more effective in the treatment of acute coronary syndrome?

Bottom line

High-risk patients with unstable angina or non-ST-segment elevation myocardial infarction (NSTEMI) and positive cardiac biomarkers benefit from immediate coronary angiography and revascularization when appropriate. Similar patients with negative cardiac biomarkers appear to do as well with initial pharmacologic treatment, reserving angiography and revascularization for those with evidence of ongoing ischemia. (LOE = 1a–)

Reference

Mehta SR, Cannon CP, Fox KA, et al. Routine vs selective invasive strategies in patients with acute coronary syndrome. A collaborative meta-analysis of randomized trials. JAMA 2005;293:2908–2917.

Study Design	Funding	Setting
Meta-analysis (randomized controlled trials)	Government	Various (meta-analysis)

Synopsis

Optimal treatment for patients with unstable angina or NSTEMI remains controversial. The investigators comprehensively searched MEDLINE, the Cochrane Registry of Controlled Trials, abstracts from major cardiology meetings, and cross-references from original articles and reviews for relevant trials comparing benefits and risks of routine versus selective invasive treatment strategies. A routine invasive strategy was defined as all patients with unstable angina or NSTEMI undergoing immediate coronary angiography followed by revascularization when appropriate. A selective invasive strategy was defined as all patients being initially treated pharmacologically, followed by angiography and revascularization only for those with persistent symptoms or evidence of ongoing ischemia. Only randomized trials with adequate concealment and follow-up were included in the review. Two individuals independently assessed the individual trials and extracted pertinent data. Of 84 initially identified articles, only 7 involving 9208 patients met inclusion criteria. Follow-up occurred for a mean of 17 months. Mortality was significantly increased during the initial hospitalization in the routine invasive strategy group (1.8% vs 1.1% in the selective invasive strategy group), but after discharge the routine strategy was associated with a significantly lower mortality (3.8% vs 4.9%). Overall, the composite outcome of death or recurrent myocardial infarction was lower in patients in the routine group than in the selective group (12.2% vs 14.4%; number needed to treat = 45; 95% CI, 28–119). Higher risk patients with elevated cardiac biomarkers (eg, troponin and creatine kinase levels) at baseline benefited the most from the routine invasive strategy, but there was no benefit to the routine strategy for patients with negative biomarkers. There was some heterogeneity in the outcomes of the various trials, but the authors speculate that it's related to the concurrent use of other medications in some, but not all, trials. Trials published after 1999 demonstrated the most benefit to routine invasive strategy, suggesting a positive impact of improved treatment protocols.

Essential Evidence: Medicine that Matters, Edited by David Slawson, Allen Shaughnessy, Mark Ebell, and Henry Barry.

Intensive medical tx + selective PCI preferred for non-ST ACS

Clinical question

What is the best way to manage patients with non-ST-segment acute coronary syndrome?

Bottom line

An intensive medical program with selective use of angiography and percutaneous coronary interventions is at least as good as a more aggressive strategy of catheterizing everyone. (LOE = 1b)

Reference

de Winter RJ, Windhausen F, Cornel JH, et al, for the Invasive versus Conservative Treatment in Unstable Coronary Syndromes (ICTUS) Investigators. Early invasive versus selectively invasive management for acute coronary syndromes. N Engl J Med 2005;353:1095–1104.

Study Design	Funding	Allocation
Randomized controlled trial (single-blinded)	Industry + govt	Concealed

Setting

Inpatient (any location) with outpatient follow-up

Synopsis

Although previous studies of an early invasive strategy in patients with non-ST-segment elevation acute coronary syndrome (ACS) have found a reduction in combined end points, reduction in mortality was much less impressive or absent, and new developments in conservative treatment of ACS such as clopidogrel and intensive lipid lowering may make the latter a more attractive option. In this Dutch study, 1200 patients with ACS and no ST-segment elevation at 42 hospitals were randomly assigned (allocation concealed) to selective invasive management or early invasive management with coronary angiography within 48 hours and percutaneous coronary intervention when indicated. The former group underwent coronary angiography only if they developed refractory angina, hemodynamic or rhythmic instability, or had ischemia on a predischarge stress test. Physicians were encouraged to give all patients intensive medical therapy including aspirin on arrival, enoxaparin for at least 48 hours, clopidogrel (Plavix), and atorvastatin (Lipitor) 80 mg per day. Patients were followed up for 1 year, outcomes were blindly assessed, and analysis was by intention to treat. The median age was 62 years, 74% were men, 25% had a history of previous myocardial infarction, and 14% were diabetic. Not surprisingly, patients in the early invasive group were much more likely to undergo revascularization after 1 year (79% vs 54%), usually involving placement of a stent. After 1 year, the composite end point of death, nonfatal myocardial infarction, or rehospitalization for angina was similar between the 2 groups (22.7% for the early invasive group vs 21.2% for the selectively invasive group). Patients in the early invasive group had more myocardial infarctions (15% vs 10%; P = .005; number needed to treat = 20), but fewer rehospitalizations (7.4% vs 10.9%; P = .04; NNT = 29). Most important, mortality was identical between groups. The study was adequately powered to find a 25% relative risk reduction in the primary outcome.

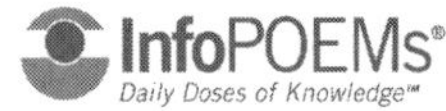

Invasive tx slightly better in non-ST-elevation ACS (RITA3)

Clinical question

Do patients with non-ST-elevation acute coronary syndromes have better long-term outcomes if managed conservatively or on the basis of arteriography?

Bottom line

In this study, patients with acute coronary syndromes when managed according to arteriography experience slightly better 5-year mortality rates (P = .054) than those managed conservatively. (LOE = 2b)

Reference

Fox KA, Poole-Wilson P, Clayton TC, et al. 5-year outcome of an interventional strategy in non-ST-elevation acute coronary syndrome: the British Heart Foundation RITA 3 randomised trial. Lancet 2005;366:914–920.

Study Design

Randomized controlled trial (nonblinded)

Funding

Industry + govt

Allocation

Uncertain

Setting

Inpatient (any location) with outpatient follow-up

Synopsis

The clinicians in this study were uncertain about the best way to initially manage 1810 patients with cardiac pain associated with electrocardiographic evidence of coronary artery disease (CAD) or evidence of previous CAD, or an elevated serum cardiac marker. The patients were randomized to conservative medical management (n = 915) or coronary angiography within 72 hours (n = 895). Medical treatment included beta-blockers and aspirin plus enoxaparin, unless contraindicated. For patients assigned to angiography, the subsequent management was left entirely to the discretion of the physician. The main outcome, 5-year mortality, was assessed by personnel unaware of treatment allocation via intention to treat. Although there were no significant differences after 1 year, at the end of 5 years, 14% of patients treated conservatively died compared with 11% of patients treated according to arteriography (P = .054). In a planned exploratory analysis on the basis of risk levels, patients at highest risk derived the greatest benefit from invasive management.

Essential Evidence: Medicine that Matters, Edited by David Slawson, Allen Shaughnessy, Mark Ebell, and Henry Barry.

In ACS, 5 years of invasive tx decreases MI but not all cause mortality (FRISC-II)

Clinical question

Are the long-term outcomes of invasive intervention better than those for medical management in the face of acute coronary syndromes?

Bottom line

In this study of patients with non-ST-elevation acute coronary syndromes, patients treated invasively had fewer subsequent myocardial infarctions after 5 years than patients treated medically. The benefits are seen mainly in men, nonsmokers, and patients with at least 2 risk factors. (LOE = 1b)

Reference

Lagerqvist B, Husted S, Kontny F, et al, for the Fast Revascularisation during InStability in Coronary artery disease (FRISC-II) Investigators. 5-year outcomes in the FRISC-II randomised trial of an invasive versus a non-invasive strategy in non-ST-elevation acute coronary syndrome: a follow-up study. Lancet 2006;368:998–1004.

Study Design

Randomized controlled trial (nonblinded)

Funding

Industry + govt

Allocation

Concealed

Setting

Inpatient (any location) with outpatient follow-up

Synopsis

The FRISC-II was a randomized trial designed to study the effects of invasive intervention or medical management of patients with acute coronary syndromes. This study reports the 5-year follow up on more than 99% of the original participants. The patients were eligible if they had less than 48 hours of chest pain with signs of myocardial ischemia or non-ST-elevation myocardial infarction. All patients received aspirin and dalteparin for at least 5 days. Those in the intervention group received aspirin and dalteparin every day until their revascularization; their last dose was the evening before the procedure. Patients also received beta-blockers unless contraindicated. During the first 24 months, the study team directly contacted patients. After this, the data for vital status were obtained from national population registries and the national registries of cause of death. The researchers used intention-to-treat analysis to analyze the outcomes. At the end of 5 years, there was no difference in all-cause morality (9.7% in the group managed invasively; 10.1% in the group managed medically). However, the patients managed invasively had fewer myocardial infarctions (12.9% vs 17.7%; number needed to treat = 21; 95% CI, 13–56). The benefit was seen mainly in men, nonsmokers, and patients with 2 or more risk factors.

Essential Evidence: Medicine that Matters, Edited by David Slawson, Allen Shaughnessy, Mark Ebell, and Henry Barry.

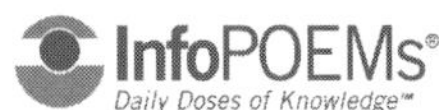

Captopril = losartan for reducing all-cause mortality after MI

Clinical question
Is losartan more effective than captopril after acute myocardial infarction?

Bottom line
Previous studies have demonstrated that, compared with placebo, ACE inhibitors improve outcomes after acute myocardial infarction. This adequately-powered study shows that losartan (Cozaar) is no more effective than captopril (Capoten) in reducing all-cause mortality or cardiovascular mortality in patients with left ventricular dysfunction after acute myocardial infarction. Since the losartan was better tolerated, it may be a reasonable alternative for those unable to tolerate captopril. (LOE = 1b)

Reference
Dickstein K, Kjekshus J. Effects of losartan and captopril on mortality and morbidity in high-risk patients after acute myocardial infarction: the OPTIMAAL randomised trial. Lancet 2002;360:752–760.

Study Design
Randomized controlled trial (double-blinded)

Setting
Inpatient (any location) with outpatient follow-up

Synopsis
This study, the OPTIMAAL trial, was designed to see if losartan (Cozaar) was superior to captopril (Capoten) in treating high-risk patients after acute myocardial infarction. They studied patients over 50 years of age with an acute myocardial infarction who also had signs or symptoms of heart failure in the acute phase, with an ejection fraction under 35% or other physiologic markers of left ventricular dysfunction. They excluded patients with systolic BP < 100 mm Hg, those already on an ACE inhibitor or angiotensin II antagonist, unstable angina, those with planned revascularization and those with hemodynamically unstable valvular disease and arrhythmias. The researchers randomly assigned (masked allocation) to receive captopril (6.25 mg three times daily titrated to 50 mg three times daily; n = 2733) or losartan (12.5 mg daily titrated to 50 mg daily; n = 2744). They followed the patients for an average of 2.7 years. The main outcome was all-cause mortality. All study end-points were assessed by researchers blinded to allocation and analyzed by intention to treat. To ensure adequate power, the researchers designed the study to continue until 937 patients died. At the end of the study, the overall mortality was similar between the groups. Four hundred forty-seven (16.4%) of the patients on captopril died compared to 499 (18.2%) on losartan. Of all the secondary outcomes, the only significant difference was for cardiovascular mortality (13.3% for captopril versus 15.3% on losartan). Since they looked at multiple endpoints, it is possible this may have been a chance occurrence. On the other hand, the pooled drop out rate was less for losartan (17% versus 23%).

Essential Evidence: Medicine that Matters, Edited by David Slawson, Allen Shaughnessy, Mark Ebell, and Henry Barry.

Captopril better than valsartan or combination post-MI

Clinical question

Does valsartan or the combination of valsartan and captopril offer benefits over captopril alone after myocardial infarction?

Bottom line

Captopril and valsartan are similarly effective when given to patients with acute myocardial infarction (AMI) and left ventricular dysfunction (LVD). The combination of both is no more effective, and is associated with more adverse effects. Captopril is less expensive and causes less hypotension and renal problems, although it causes slightly more cough. (LOE = 1b)

Reference

Pfeffer MA, McMurray JJ, Velazquez EJ, et al. Valsartan, captopril, or both in myocardial infarction complicated by heart failure, left ventricular dysfunction, or both. N Engl J Med 2003;349:1893–1906.

Study Design

Randomized controlled trial (double-blinded)

Setting

Inpatient (any location) with outpatient follow-up

Synopsis

This study included adults with an AMI in the previous 10 days, evidence of LVD, serum creatinine level less than 2.5 mg/dL, and a systolic blood pressure at least 100 mm Hg. Allocation was concealed and outcomes were adjudicated by a group unaware of treatment assignment. Patients were randomized to valsartan (Diovan, n = 4909), captopril (Capoten, n = 4909), or both (n = 4885) and followed up for a mean of 24.7 months. Valsartan was initially dosed at 20 mg orally once a day and the dose advanced with a goal of 80 mg orally twice a day in the hospital and 160 mg orally twice a day by 3 months. Similarly, captopril was started at 6.25 orally once a day and advanced to 25 mg orally 3 times daily in the hospital and 50 mg orally 3 times daily at 3 months. Finally, the group receiving both medications started at valsartan 20 mg plus captopril 6.25 mg orally once a day, advanced to valsartan 40 mg orally twice a day plus captopril 25 mg orally 3 times daily during hospitalization, and valsartan 80 mg orally twice a day plus captopril 50 mg orally 3 times a day at 3 months. Analysis was by intention to treat for the primary outcome of all-cause mortality. There was no difference between groups in all-cause mortality (19.9% for valsartan, 19.5% for captopril, and 19.3% for both) or in the likelihood of the "all bad cardiovascular things" outcome (32.8% for valsartan, 33.4% for captopril, and 32.3% for both). After 1 year, more patients stopped taking valsartan plus captopril than those taking only 1 of the medications (19.8% for both, 15.3% for valsartan, 16.8% for captopril). Adverse events were most likely in the valsartan plus captopril group (28.9% vs 22.8% and 21.8%; $P < .05$). Hypotension (15.1% vs 11.9%; $P < .05$; NNTH = 30) and renal problems (4.9% vs 3.0%; $P < .05$; NNTH = 54) were more common in the valsartan group than the captopril group. Cough (1.7% vs 5.0%; $P < .05$; NNTH = 30) was less common in the valsartan group. Angioedema occurred no more than 0.5% in any group and never required intubation.

Essential Evidence: Medicine that Matters, Edited by David Slawson, Allen Shaughnessy, Mark Ebell, and Henry Barry.

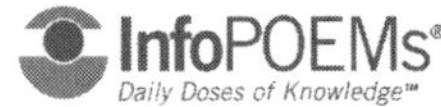

Implantable defibrillators are not effective post-MI

Clinical question

Do implantable cardioverter-defibrillators improve outcomes in at-risk patients after myocardial infarction?

Bottom line

Implantable cardioverter-defibrillators do not reduce mortality in patients with myocardial infarction who are at high risk for ventricular arrhythmia. (LOE = 1b)

Reference

Hohnloser SH, Kuck KH, Dorian P, et al. Prophylactic use of an implantable cardioverter-defibrillator after acute myocardial infarction. N Engl J Med 2004;351:2481–2488.

Study Design

Randomized controlled trial (single-blinded)

Funding

Industry

Allocation

Concealed

Setting

Inpatient (any location) with outpatient follow-up

Synopsis

Implantable cardioverter-defibrillators (ICDs) can reduce mortality in selected patients. In this industry-sponsored study, adults with a recent myocardial infarction, a left ventricular ejection fraction less than or equal to 0.35, and either relative tachycardia (>80 beats per minute) or decreased heart rate variability were randomized to either ICD or usual care. This was an open-label trial with no attempt at sham surgery or sham ICD implantation. The primary outcomes of all-cause mortality or death due to cardiac arrhythmia were blindly assessed and analysis was by intention to treat. The groups were balanced at the beginning of the study, with 332 in the ICD group and 342 in the control group. Patients were followed up for a mean of 30 months, with a maximum follow-up of 48 months. On the bright side, patients in the ICD group experienced significantly fewer arrhythmic deaths (1.5% vs 3.5%; number needed to treat = 50; 95% CI, 27–209). On the not-so-bright side, they also experienced more nonarrhythmic deaths (6.1% vs 3.5%; number needed to treat to harm = 38; 20–150). There was no significant difference between groups regarding the most important patient-oriented outcome: all-cause mortality (7.5% for the ICD group vs 6.9% for the control group). The difference in nonarrhythmic deaths was largely caused by more cardiac nonarrhythmic deaths. The authors speculate that a group of patients with severe heart disease are "saved" from an arrhythmic death only to die from pump failure without any clinically important increase in the overall lifespan. Implantable defibrillators have been shown to be effective in patients with non-ischemic cardiomyopathy (JAMA 2004;292:2874–79).

Essential Evidence: Medicine that Matters, Edited by David Slawson, Allen Shaughnessy, Mark Ebell, and Henry Barry.

Start warfarin at 10 mg faster for outpatient anticoagulation

Clinical question

Is starting warfarin with 10 mg better than 5 mg better in outpatients?

Bottom line

A nomogram for warfarin dosing, starting with 10 mg daily for the first 2 days, results in quicker achievement of therapeutic oral anticoagulation, allowing shorter therapy with low-molecular-weight heparin in outpatients treated for venous thromboembolism. (LOE = 1b)

Reference

Kovacs MJ, Rodger M, Anderson DR, et al. Comparison of 10-mg and 5-mg warfain initiation nomograms together with low-molecular-weight heparin for outpatient treatment of acute venous thromboembolism. Ann Intern Med 2003;138:714–719.

Study Design

Randomized controlled trial (double-blinded)

Setting

Outpatient (specialty)

Synopsis

For many outpatients started on warfarin for venous thromboembolism, a dosing nomogram, starting with 5 mg daily with adjustments based on international normalized ratios (INRs) collected at 3, 4, 5, and 6 days after initiation, is a quick and easy way to achieve anticoagulation. This study evaluated a nomogram starting with 10 mg for the first 2 days, checking the INR only on the third and fifth days. The 201 patients ranged in age from 18 to 98 years, with 16% older than 75 years. They were randomly assigned (allocation was concealed) to receive warfarin using either a previously developed (Ann Intern Med 1997;12:333) nomogram starting with 5 mg or a new algorithm based on 2 daily doses of 10 mg. The 5-mg algorithm was based on inpatient therapy. Warfarin was started on the first day along with at least 5 days of low-molecular-weight heparin. Analysis was by intention to treat. Patients started on 10 mg daily achieved a therapeutic INR 1.4 days earlier than the 5-mg group (4.2 days vs 5.6 days). Rates of recurrent thromboembolism and major bleeding episodes over 90 days were not different between the 2 groups, although the study may not have been large enough to find a difference if one exists.

Essential Evidence: Medicine that Matters, Edited by David Slawson, Allen Shaughnessy, Mark Ebell, and Henry Barry.

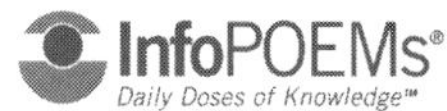

Use an algorithm to start warfarin in older patients

Clinical question

Can an algorithm predict the final warfarin dose in elderly hospitalized patients?

Bottom line

This algorithm, which starts with a lower dose than other algorithms, is effective in predicting the final dose of warfarin required by patients older than 70 years. (LOE = 2b)

Reference

Siguret V, Gouin I, Debray M, et al. Initiation of warfarin therapy in elderly medical inpatients: A safe and accurate regimen. Am J Med 2005;118:137–142.

Study Design

Cohort (prospective)

Funding

Unknown/not stated

Setting

Inpatient (any location)

Synopsis

We have several algorithms available for when initiating warfarin (Coumadin), elderly patients present a unique challenge because of their use of multiple medications, their higher risk of bleeding from overanticoagulation, and because their usual dose is lower than that of younger patients. This study evaluated a new algorithm designed for patients at least 70 years of age who are hospitalized and require initiation of oral anticoagulation. The authors derived their algorithm in one set of patients and then evaluated its effectiveness in a second group of consecutive patients drawn from 9 study centers. The average age of this confirmation group of 96 patients was 84.6 years. Fifteen patients could not be analyzed, primarily because they were discharged before reaching a maintenance dose. The algorithm starts with warfarin 4 mg given daily for 3 days at dinnertime. An international normalized ratio (INR) was obtained on the morning of the fourth day and the dose was adjusted according to the algorithm. Doses were adjusted until the maintenance dose was reached, which was defined as the dose required to yield an INR of between 2.0–3.0 on 2 consecutive samples drawn at least 2 days apart and after at least 4 days of the same dose. The dose predicted by the algorithm on day 4 was equal to the actual maintenance dose in 73% of the patients (95% CI, 64%–81%). The average time needed to achieve a therapeutic INR was 6.7 days. No patients had an INR greater than 4.0 during the study, although one patient died as the result of an intracranial hemorrhage with an INR in the therapeutic range (the patient also received heparin). Here is the nomogram: Days 1, 2, 3 – Give warfarin 4 mg. On Day 4 – Check INR in the morning; according to the result, give the following dose (daily): 1.0 to <1.3 = 5 mg; 1.3 to <1.5 = 4 mg; 1.5 to <1.7 = 3 mg; 1.7 to <1.9 = 2 mg; 1.9 to <2.5 = 1 mg. If the INR is 2.5 or higher, measure INR daily and hold warfarin until INR drops to <2.5, then resume at 1 mg.

Essential Evidence: Medicine that Matters, Edited by David Slawson, Allen Shaughnessy, Mark Ebell, and Henry Barry.

Self-monitoring of anticoagulation safe, effective

Clinical question

Can patients taking warfarin monitor and adjust their doses safely and effectively?

Bottom line

Although many patients will not wish to do so, home monitoring of anticoagulation status and subsequent self-adjustment of dosing is safe and effective. Self-monitoring of anticoagulation is a bit trickier than home blood glucose monitoring, and approximately 30% of patients dropped out during the training period. The testing equipment is expensive ($1300 US), a cost-effectiveness analysis has not been done, and there is no evidence that it leads to better clinical outcomes (ie, less bleeding and less recurrent embolic events). (LOE = 2b)

Reference

Fitzmaurice DA, Murray ET, McCahon D, et al. Self management of oral anticoagulation: randomised trial. BMJ 2005;331:1057–1062.

Study Design

Randomized controlled trial (nonblinded)

Funding

Government

Allocation

Concealed

Setting

Outpatient (primary care)

Synopsis

The marketing of simple point-of-care tools for determining anticoagulation opens up the possibility of patients self-monitoring and adjusting their own warfarin doses. These UK researchers tested this possibility in patients taking warfarin chronically for a variety of reasons. Starting by identifying 2530 patients who might be eligible, they ended up recruiting 617 adults (25%) with a long-term indication for anticoagulation who had taken warfarin for at least 6 months. All patients were considered capable of self management. Using concealed allocation, the researchers randomly assigned patients to continue either routine care or to self-monitoring. Following 2 training sessions, the patients were given testing equipment (Coaguchek S) and a dose-adjustment algorithm. The patients checked their coagulation status every 2 weeks, or weekly following a dosing change. The percentage of time the international normalized ratio (INR) was in the therapeutic range was similar between the patients who continued self-management (~70%) and the patients in routine care (72% vs 68%). Patients with a target INR of 2.5 were in the therapeutic range 74% of the time. Of patients with a higher target INR of 3.5, they were in their therapeutic range only 55% of the 12-month study period, but this percentage was significantly higher than before the study was started (45%). The rate of adverse effects was low in the routine care and self-management groups: 2.8 vs. 2.7 events per 100 patients per year. Serious bleeding rates and serious thrombosis rates were similar in both groups. These results are slightly better than a recent study conducted in Italy (Ann Intern Med 2005;142:1–10).

Essential Evidence: Medicine that Matters, Edited by David Slawson, Allen Shaughnessy, Mark Ebell, and Henry Barry.

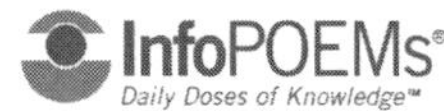

Self-monitoring anticoagulation superior at preventing venous thromboembolics events

Clinical question

Do patients monitor and manage their oral anticoagulation at least as well as professionals?

Bottom line

Patients who self-monitor oral anticoagulation had fewer thromboembolic events than those using standard approaches to monitoring. However, self-monitoring should only be offered to literate and motivated patients. Additionally, the machines are costly and not universally covered by insurance. (LOE = 1a)

Reference

Heneghan C, Alonso-Coello P, Garcia-Alamino JM, Perera R, Meats E, Glasziou P. Self-monitoring of oral anticoagulation: a systematic review and meta-analysis. Lancet 2006;367:404–411.

Study Design

Meta-analysis (randomized controlled trials)

Funding

Self-funded or unfunded

Setting

Outpatient (any)

Synopsis

These investigators searched multiple databases for randomized controlled trials comparing self-monitoring of oral anticoagulation with standard monitoring. Additionally, they sought ongoing trials and data from equipment manufacturers in an attempt to find unpublished data. Three reviewers independently assessed each study for inclusion with discrepancies resolved by consensus. Additionally, they assessed each study's methodologic quality. Ultimately, the authors identified 14 studies including 1309 patients. These were generally small studies with an average of 94 patients. In all studies, the self-monitored patients maintained their international normalization ratio within target at least as well as those with standard monitoring. More important, only 2.2% of self-monitored patients had thromboembolic events compared with 4.6% receiving standard care (number needed to treat = 43; 95% CI, 27–92). In the studies that directly measured them, outcomes of major hemorrhage and overall death were also significantly better in the self-monitoring groups. A word of caution: A high proportion of patients (31%–88%) didn't enroll or dropped out because of the complexity of self-management.

Essential Evidence: Medicine that Matters, Edited by David Slawson, Allen Shaughnessy, Mark Ebell, and Henry Barry.

INR 1.5–1.9 less effective than 2.0–3.0 for idiopathic DVT

Clinical question

Is low-intensity warfarin as effective as conventional anticoagulation to prevent recurrent venous thromboembolism?

Bottom line

Low-intensity anticoagulation with a target international normalized ratio (INR) of 1.5 to 1.9 results in more episodes of recurrent venous thromboembolism (VTE) than conventional warfarin therapy (number needed to treat = 100) for patients with idiopathic VTE. The rate of major bleeding was similar between groups, so low-intensity therapy did not appear to be safer. Low-intensity therapy works better than placebo, but existing trials are not large enough to demonstrate a benefit in the risk of major bleeds. (LOE = 1b)

Reference

Kearon C, Ginsberg JS, Kovacs MJ, et al. Comparison of low-intensity warfarin therapy with conventional-intensity warfarin therapy for long-term prevention of recurrent venous thromboembolism. N Engl J Med 2003;349:631–639.

Study Design

Randomized controlled trial (double-blinded)

Setting

Outpatient (any)

Synopsis

A recent study showed that a lower intensity target for anticoagulation (INR 1.5–1.9) in patients 6 months after an initial episode of idiopathic VTE reduced the risk of recurrent VTE more than placebo (N Engl J Med 2003; 348:1425–34). That study found a low risk of major bleeding in patients on the low-intensity warfarin of 0.9 episodes/100 patient years. This study takes the next step of comparing low-intensity warfarin therapy with conventional warfarin therapy (INR 2.0–3.0). Patients (n = 738) were randomized with concealed allocation to either low-intensity or conventional warfarin therapy. A series of fake reports were generated to adjust the warfarin dose for low-intensity patients, so their physician would think they were keeping the INR between 2 and 3 when in reality it was between 1.5 and 1.9. Patients were assessed every 6 months, told to come in if they had symptoms of VTE, and followed up for a mean of 2.4 years. Only symptomatic recurrences were considered, and bleeding was considered major if it required transfusion with 2 or more units of blood, was associated with a drop of 2 points of hemoglobin, or was in the wrong place (for example, the brain). The groups were balanced at the start of the study, and similar numbers of patients left the study in each group. Patients in the low-intensity group had more recurrent VTE than those in the conventional therapy group (1.9 vs 0.9 per 100 person-years; P = .03). There was a trend toward more deaths in the low-intensity group (P = .09) and no significant difference in major bleeding episodes (1.1 vs 0.9 per 100 person-years). This was surprising; The authors themselves had estimated 3 major bleeding episodes per 100 person-years when planning their study, on the basis of the rate found in their previous smaller study of long-term anticoagulation (N Engl J Med 1999; 340:901).

Essential Evidence: Medicine that Matters, Edited by David Slawson, Allen Shaughnessy, Mark Ebell, and Henry Barry.

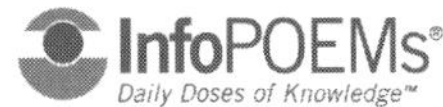

Oral vitamin K works faster than subcutaneous

Clinical question

In patients overdosed on warfarin, is oral vitamin K any better than subcutaneous administration?

Bottom line

Patients with excessive INRs while on warfarin will respond more rapidly to oral administration of vitamin K 1 mg than if the drug is given subcutaneously. (LOE = 1b–)

Reference

Crowther MA, Douketis JD, Schnurr T, et al. Oral vitamin K lowers the international normalized ratio more rapidly than subcutaneous vitamin K in the treatment of warfarin-associated coagulopathy. A randomized, controlled trial. Ann Intern Med 2002;137:251–254.

Study Design

Randomized controlled trial (non-blinded)

Setting

Various

Synopsis

Occasionally patients on warfarin will have excessive anticoagulation requiring rapid reversal with vitamin K. This study compared vitamin K 1 mg given either orally or subcutaneously to asymptomatic patients with an international normalized ratio (INR) between 4.5 and 10. This randomized study of 51 patients used concealed allocation to enroll patients (increasing the likelihood of similar groups) but neither patients nor their treating physician was blinded to the treatment. One day following administration of vitamin K, 58% of patients receiving oral dosing and 24% of patients receiving subcutaneous therapy had INRs of 1.8 to 3.2 (P = 0.015; NNT = 3). No patient receiving oral vitamin K and two patients receiving subcutaneous vitamin K had an increase in INR the following day. No bleeding or thrombotic event occurred in any of the patients. This dose of vitamin K is lower than the 2.5–5 mg often used. Higher doses do not work any better yet will depress the INR for several days after administration. The lower dose comes with a catch – it is not available in the U.S. (as phytonadione) and has to be prepared by a pharmacist from the injectable form. Another option is to one-quarter for the 5 mg tablet.

Essential Evidence: Medicine that Matters, Edited by David Slawson, Allen Shaughnessy, Mark Ebell, and Henry Barry.

Oral vitamin K effective for warfarin overdose

Clinical question

Is oral vitamin K as effective as intravenous vitamin K in patients with warfarin overdose?

Bottom line

Low doses of oral vitamin K are as effective as intravenous (IV) vitamin K in patients with an elevated international normalized ratio (INR) due to excessive warfarin action. At an INR of greater than 10, the 2 routes of administration produce equivalent results. At lower elevations of INR (6 to 10), IV administration produces a greater lowering within the first 12 hours, but by 24 hours the average INR is the same. Note that IV vitamin K is not recommended because of the risk of anaphylaxis and that previous research has shown oral vitamin K to be superior to subcutaneous administration (Crowther MA. Ann Intern Med 2002; 137:251–54). (LOE = 1b–)

Reference

Lubetsky A, Yonath H, Olchovsky D, et al. Comparison of oral vs intravenous phytonadione (vitamin K) in patients with excessive anticoagulation. Arch Intern Med. 2003;163:2469–2473.

Study Design

Randomized controlled trial (nonblinded)

Setting

Outpatient (any)

Synopsis

The researchers enrolled 61 consecutive patients receiving warfarin who presented with an INR of 6.0 or more but had no major bleeding. Patients were randomly allocated (allocation strategy was concealed from the enrolling physician) to receive treatment with either IV or oral vitamin K. Patients receiving oral therapy were given either 2.5 mg if their INR was between 6 and 10 (71% of patients) or 5 mg if their INR was greater than 10. Patients in the IV group were treated with low-dose IV phytonadione, 0.5 mg if their INR was between 6 and 10 and 1 mg if their INR was greater than 10. This IV dose is lower than is typically used, but higher doses have not been shown to hasten reversal of anticoagulation but simply to extend the time the patient is refractory to warfarin. In patients with an INR of 6 to 10, the response was faster with IV admininistration, with the average INR declining to between 2 and 4 within 6 hours, compared with 24 hours for the same response with oral administration. At 12 hours, approximately twice as many patients were reversed with IV use. At 24 hours there was no difference in the number of patients who had reversal. This difference in response rate may not be clinically relevant because patients at this level of anticoagulation do not generally need rapid reversal. For patients with an INR of 10 or more, there was no difference between IV and oral responses at any time. However, the power of the study is probably not large enough to find a small difference if one exists. There were no bleeding or thrombotic episodes in any of the patients over the following 28 days of follow-up.

Essential Evidence: Medicine that Matters, Edited by David Slawson, Allen Shaughnessy, Mark Ebell, and Henry Barry.

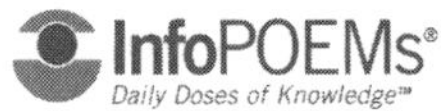

Clinical decision rules accurately predict stroke risk in atrial fibrillation

Clinical question

Which patients with atrial fibrillation would benefit from anticoagulation?

Bottom line

Clinical decision rules, especially the well validated SPAF score, can help identify groups of patients with atrial fibrillation that are likely and unlikely to benefit from anticoagulation. (LOE = 1a)

Reference

Gage BF, van Walraven C, Pearce L, et al. Selecting patients with atrial fibrillation for anticoagulation: Stroke risk stratification in patients taking aspirin. Circulation 2004;110:2287–2292.

Study Design	Funding	Setting
Decision rule (validation)	Government	Various (meta-analysis)

Synopsis

We sometimes choose to anticoagulate patients with atrial fibrillation to prevent stroke. If the risk of stroke is low (<2%) the harms of anticoagulation generally outweigh the benefits. If the risk of stroke is high (>4%), the benefits of anticoagulation outweigh the risks for most patients. In between we have to look carefully at their risk for hemorrhage. This article tested the ability of five clinical decision rules to accurately identify low risk patients who don't need anticoagulation and high risk patients who do. The validation population consisted of pooled data from 2580 patients in the aspirin arm (75 to 325 mg daily) in six randomized controlled trials. The mean age was 72, 37% were women, 46% were hypertensive, and 22% had a prior stroke or transient ischemic attack. All five rules were able to divide patients into low, moderate, and high risk groups. However, the number of patients in the low risk group varied from 175 to 983 and in the high risk group from 223 to 1543. Clearly, identifying a greater percentage of patients in the low and high risk groups is better than having a lot in the intermediate group where no definitive advice can be made. A score that did this well was the Stroke Prevention in Atrial Fibrillation (SPAF) rule. Patients who had any of the following were considered high risk by the SPAF rule: systolic blood pressure >160 mm Hg, prior ischemia, women over age 75, recent heart failure, or left ventricular ejection fraction <=25%. Patients who were high risk had a 3.6% risk of stroke (95% CI 2.7 to 4.7, n = 884). Patients who had none of the high risk factors but carried a diagnosis of hypertension were moderate risk and had a 2.7% risk of stroke (95% CI 1.8 to 4.0, n = 462). Finally, low risk patients were those who were not moderate or high risk and had a 1.1% risk of stroke (95% CI 0.7 to 1.8, n = 668). The authors like the CHADS2 rule, named for the elements in the score (Congestive heart failure, Hypertension, Age, Diabetes, and prior Stroke or transient ischemic attack). However, this score placed the majority of patients in the intermediate group, which is less helpful for clinical decision-making.

Essential Evidence: Medicine that Matters, Edited by David Slawson, Allen Shaughnessy, Mark Ebell, and Henry Barry.

Thromboembolism just as likely with atrial flutter

Clinical question

Is the presence of atrial flutter a risk factor for developing thromboembolism?

Bottom line

In this small study, lone atrial flutter resulted in a stroke risk higher than that of lone atrial fibrillation. These patients are also more likely than the general population to develop atrial fibrillation. (LOE = 1b)

Reference

Halligan SC, Gersh BJ, Brown RD, et al. The natural history of lone atrial flutter. Ann Intern Med 2004;140:265–268.

Study Design

Cohort (prospective)

Setting

Outpatient (any)

Synopsis

The authors started with 567 patients who were seen with atrial flutter (over a 30-year period). After excluding patients with concomittant illness, they ended up with 59 patients who had a regular rhythm with an atrial rate between 240 and 350 beats per minute. Those patients' average age was 70 years and most (75%) developed recurrent episodes or chronic flutter. Most were treated with rate-controlling therapy, and approximately half (n = 31) received aspirin or warfarin to prevent embolic events. Atrial fibrillation subsequently developed in 33 patients within an average of 5 years. Nineteen patients (32%) experienced at least 1 cerebrovascular ischemic event. Six of these 19 patients developed atrial fibrillation before the subsequent ischemic event. The mean time to development of the ischemic event was 4.3 years. In comparison with a second group of 145 patients with lone atrial fibrillation, patients with atrial flutter were more likely to be women and to be older. Patients with atrial flutter had a higher incidence of ischemic stroke or transient ischemic attack than patients with atrial fibrillation (hazard ratio = 2.6, 95% CI, 1.2–5.3).

Essential Evidence: Medicine that Matters, Edited by David Slawson, Allen Shaughnessy, Mark Ebell, and Henry Barry.

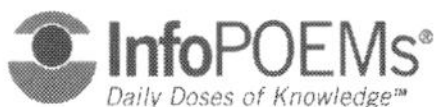

Warfarin prevents more strokes than clopidorel + ASA in atrial fibrillation (ACTIVE)

Clinical question

Is warfarin better than clopidogrel plus aspirin in preventing strokes in patients with atrial fibrillation?

Bottom line

Warfarin is superior to the combination of clopidogrel (Plavix) plus aspirin in preventing strokes and systemic emboli in high-risk patients with atrial fibrillation. (LOE = 2b)

Reference

ACTIVE Writing Group on behalf of the ACTIVE Investigators; Connolly S, Pogue J, Hart R, et al. Clopidogrel plus aspirin versus oral anticoagulation for atrial fibrillation in the Atrial fibrillation Clopidogrel Trial with Irbesartan for prevention of Vascular Events (ACTIVE W): a randomised controlled trial. Lancet 2006;367:1903–1912.

Study Design

Randomized controlled trial (nonblinded)

Funding

Industry

Allocation

Concealed

Setting

Outpatient (any)

Synopsis

In this study, more than 6700 patients with atrial fibrillation eligible for – and willing to take – oral anticoagulation were included if they had at least one of the following characteristics: more than 75 years of age; treated for hypertension; a previous stroke, transient ischemic attack, or non-CNS systemic embolism; left ventricular ejection fraction less than 45%; or peripheral artery disease. They also included younger patients if they had diabetes or coronary artery disease. Eligible patients were randomly assigned to once-daily clopidogrel (75 mg) plus aspirin (75 to 100 mg daily) or warfarin titrated to a target international normalized ratio of between 2.0 and 3.0. The primary study outcomes (stroke, non-CNS systemic embolism, myocardial infarction, or vascular death), assessed by researchers masked to treatment assignment, were evaluated by intention to treat. The study was terminated early because of the clear superiority of oral anticoagulation. After 1.3 years of follow-up, bad outcomes occurred in 4.9% of patients taking oral anticoagulation compared with 7.0% in those treated with clopidogrel plus aspirin (number needed to treat = 48; 95% CI, 31–101). They found minimal differences in all individual events, except stroke and non-CNS embolism. The rate of major bleeding complications was comparable in patients taking clopidogrel plus aspirin (2.42% per year) and patients taking warfarin (2.21% per year). However, the rate of minor bleeding was lower in patients treated with warfarin (11.4% vs 13.6%).

Essential Evidence: Medicine that Matters, Edited by David Slawson, Allen Shaughnessy, Mark Ebell, and Henry Barry.

Ximelagatran effective in preventing stroke in atrial fibrillation

Clinical question

Is ximelagatran as effective as warfarin in preventing stroke in patients with nonvalvular atrial fibrillation?

Bottom line

In this manufacturer-sponsored, open-label study, patients with atrial fibrillation and at increased risk for stroke treated with either ximelagatran or warfarin have comparable outcomes. If these results are confirmed independently, ximelagatran may become the preferred treatment, since it doesn't require monitoring and may cause fewer bleeding complications. (LOE = 2b)

Reference

Executive Steering Committee on behalf of the SPORTIF III Investigators. Stroke prevention with the oral direct thrombin inhibitor ximelagatran compared with warfarin in patients with non-valvular atrial fibrillation (SPORTIF III): randomised controlled trial. Lancet 2003;362:1691–1698.

Study Design

Randomized controlled trial (nonblinded)

Setting

Other

Synopsis

Patients with atrial fibrillation were recruited from hospitals, doctor's offices, and health-care clinics to participate in this manufacturer-sponsored open-label study comparing fixed doses of ximelagatran (n = 1704) with warfarin dosed to maintain an international normalized ratio (INR) between 2.0 and 3.0 (n = 1703). Patients also needed to have at least one additional stroke risk factor to be included: hypertension, older than 75 years, previous thromboembolic phenomena, left ventricular ejection fraction less than 40%, symptomatic congestive heart failure, or older than 65 years with coronary artery disease or diabetes mellitus. There were a large number of exclusion criteria, including: recent stroke, transient ischemic attack, acute coronary syndrome, conditions associated with increased bleeding risk, endocarditis, planned major surgery, or cardioversion. Allocation to treatment group was masked. The primary outcome, all stroke (ischemic or hemorrhagic) and systemic embolic events, was assessed via intention to treat. The secondary end points, also assessed by intention to treat, included bleeding; treatment discontinuation; ischemic stroke, transient ischemic attack, systemic embolism; and death, stroke, systemic embolism, and acute myocardial infarction. The study was designed to have 90% power, a minimum of 12 months of follow-up per patient, and an aggregate of 80 primary events. The main outcomes were assessed by local study-affiliated neurologists or stroke specialists, masked to treatment. The authors had data on all but 10 patients who never took the study drug. Slightly more patients taking warfarin completed the study (86% vs 82% taking ximelagatran). The total mortality was approximatley the same in each group (4.6%). The mean length of follow-up was 17 months. In the group treated with warfarin, 56 patients had primary events during 2440 patient-years (yearly rate = 2.3%) compared with 40 patients in the ximelagatran group during 2446 patient-years (yearly rate = 1.6%). This difference was not significant. The rate of secondary events in each group was similar, with the exception of bleeding complications. These occurred less often in the ximelagatran group (26% per year) than in the warfarin group (30% per year).

Essential Evidence: Medicine that Matters, Edited by David Slawson, Allen Shaughnessy, Mark Ebell, and Henry Barry.

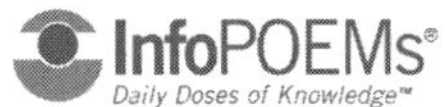

Quality of life with rate or rhythm control in atrial fibrillation (AFFIRM)

Clinical question

In patients with atrial fibrillation does rhythm control offer a quality of life benefit over controlling heart rate?

Bottom line

Attempting to maintain sinus rhythm in patients with atrial fibrillation, in addition to having no effect on mortality, does not improve the patients' quality of life as measured by a number of different scales. Patients who were profoundly symptomatic were not enrolled in this study and the results may not apply to them. (LOE = 1b−)

Reference

The AFFIRM Investigators. Quality of life in atrial fibrillation: The atrial fibrillation follow-up investigation of rhythm management (AFFIRM) study. Am Heart J 2005;149:112–120.

Study Design	Funding	Allocation
Randomized controlled trial (double-blinded)	Government	Uncertain

Setting

Outpatient (specialty)

Synopsis

The AFFIRM study showed that stable patients with atrial fibrillation had similar survival whether they received rate or rhythm control. This predefined substudy evaluated the effect of the two therapies on quality of life. The investigators randomly selected 25% of the sites participating in the AFFIRM study to enroll patients into this quality of life study as well. The 716 patients were similar demographically to the other patients in the study: an average age of 70 years, 62% male, 93% white, with 62% of the patients experiencing recurrent atrial fibrillation at the time of entry. The patients were treated to control either their heart rate during atrial fibrillation or were treated with the goal of maintaining normal cardiac rhythm. They were observed for up to 6 years and were asked annually to complete several quality of life questionnaires. To the question, "In general, would you say your health is . . ." a similar proportion, about 20% of patients in each group perceived their health to be excellent or very good. Using the Ladder of Life questionnaire, which asks patients to rate their life at present, 5 years ago and 5 years from now. In both groups the present life satisfaction score improved significantly from baseline in both groups and remained improved over 4 years ($P < .05$) Health status using the Medical Outcomes Study SF-36 questionnaire, were similar in both groups and dropped from baseline, although the scores in both groups were lower than the general US population for the age group. The cardiac version of the QoL Index and the Symptom Checklist scores were similar between the two groups at all times. The researchers went the next step and analyzed patients by actual response to therapy (atrial fibrillation or not) and found no difference in quality of life scores. The study had sufficient power to detect a 10% difference in scores if one was truly present.

Essential Evidence: Medicine that Matters, Edited by David Slawson, Allen Shaughnessy, Mark Ebell, and Henry Barry.

Rate control better than rhythm control in atrial fibrillation (AFFIRM)

Clinical question

Is rate control or rhythm control the preferred strategy in high-risk patients with atrial fibrillation?

Bottom line

Rhythm control is no better and probably worse than rate control for high-risk patients with atrial fibrillation. These results may not apply to younger, healthier patients. (LOE = 1b)

Reference

AFFIRM Investigators. A comparison of rate control and rhythm control in patients with atrial fibrillation. N Engl J Med 2002;347:1825–1833.

Study Design

Randomized controlled trial (nonblinded)

Setting

Outpatient (any)

Synopsis

We have traditionally tried to be fairly aggressive, at least initially, in the management of atrial fibrillation, with the goal of keeping patients in normal sinus rhythm. To do so often requires multiple episodes of cardioversion and potentially toxic antiarrhythmic drugs. Many patients are managed with rate control and anticoagulation alone, though. This study was designed to compare these strategies. This was a federally funded study. Patients were included if they were over age 65 years or if they had "other risk factors for stroke or death." Unfortunately, we aren't told what qualifies as a risk factor for death, which, technically, could include having a pulse. Patients were only included if atrial fibrillation was likely to be recurrent and cause problems if it persisted, and if they were candidates for anticoagulation. The 4060 enrolled patients were randomized to receive rate or rhythm control and followed for a mean of 3.5 years. The rate control group could be given a beta-blocker, calcium-channel blocker, digoxin, or a combination of these drugs. Digoxin and beta-blockers were most widely used, followed by diltiazem and then verapamil. Adequate rate control was achieved in 80% of patients in this group, and about a third were in sinus rhythm after 5 years. The rhythm-control strategy involved use of a wide range of antiarrhythmic drugs (most often amiodarone, provided free by the manufacturer, followed by sotalol and propafenone), and 368 of 2033 (18.1%) underwent at least one attempt at cardioversion. More patients crossed over from rhythm to rate control than vice versa (27.3% vs 11.6% after 3 years, and 37.5% vs 14.9% after 5 years). The percentage in the rhythm control group who were actually in sinus rhythm was 82.4% at 1 year, 73.3% at 3 years, and 62.6% after 5 years. More patients in the rate control group were taking warfarin (85% vs approximately 70%); anticoagulation was mandated in the rate control group but only encouraged in the rhythm control group. We are not given any information on concealment of allocation or masking of the outcome assessors. There was a trend, although not statistically significant ($p = .08$) toward increased mortality in the rhythm control group. These patients also had more hospitalizations (80.1% vs 73.0%, $p < .001$) than those in the rate control group, and more pulmonary, gastrointestinal, or arrhythmic adverse events prompting discontinuation of a drug. The number of strokes was similar between groups, and most occurred in the minority of patients who either were not taking warfarin or had an INR < 2.0.

Essential Evidence: Medicine that Matters, Edited by David Slawson, Allen Shaughnessy, Mark Ebell, and Henry Barry.

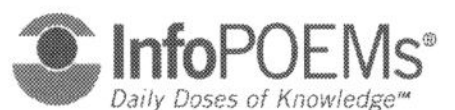

Amiodarone > sotalol > placebo for maintaining NSR in atrial fibrillation (SAFE-T)

Clinical question

What drug nest maintains normal sinus rhythm in patients with atrial fibrillation?

Bottom line

Amiodarone was more effective than sotalol at maintaining normal sinus rhythm in patients with chronic atrial fibrillation. However, there was a worrisome trend toward increased mortality in the active treatment groups, and other studies have not found a benefit of rhythm therapy over rate control with anticoagulation. (LOE = 1b)

Reference

Singh BN, Singh SN, Reda DJ, and the Sotalol Amiodarone Atrial Fibrillation Efficacy Trial (SAFE-T) Investigators. Amiodarone versus sotalol for atrial fibrillation. N Engl J Med 2005;352:1861–1872.

Study Design	Funding	Allocation	Setting
Randomized controlled trial (double-blinded)	Industry + govt	Concealed	Outpatient (specialty)

Synopsis

Rhythm control is no better than rate control as long as patients with chronic atrial fibrillation (AF) are properly anticoagulated (AFFIRM trial, N Engl J Med 2002;347:1825–33). However, some researchers question these results, arguing that rhythm control is still the optimal regimen. In this study, 665 patients with nonparoxysmal AF and no significant heart failure, renal failure, or long QT syndrome were randomized to receive amiodarone, sotalol, or placebo in a 2:2:1 ratio. All patients were anticoagulated. Amiodarone treatment began at 800 mg per day for 2 weeks, then decreased to 600 mg per day for 2 weeks, then to 300 mg per day for the rest of the first year and 200 mg per day after that. Sotalol was initiated at 80 mg twice daily for the first week and then advanced to 160 mg twice daily. If patients had not converted to sinus rhythm at 28 days, they underwent cardioversion. Patients in whom AF recurred underwent cardioversion. If AF still recurred, the study drug was withdrawn and patients were followed up for 1 year. Otherwise, they were followed up for up to 4.5 years. Approximately 1 in 4 patients in the sotalol and amiodarone groups converted to normal spontaneous rhythm during the first month, compared with only 1 of 100 in the placebo group. The total rate of conversion after cardioversion was 79.8% in the amiodarone group, 79.9% in the sotalol group, and 68.2% in the placebo group. The time to recurrence of AF was 487 days for amiodarone, 74 days for sotalol, and 6 days for placebo (P = .001). At 1 year the recurrence rate was 48% for amiodarone, 68% for sotalol, and 87% for placebo (number needed to treat = 2.5 for amiodarone vs placebo, and 5 for sotalol vs placebo). There was no difference between amiodarone and sotalol for patients with ischemic heart disease, though. There were 13 deaths in the amiodarone group, 15 in the sotalol group, and only 3 in the placebo group. Although the placebo group was smaller, there was still a trend toward increased mortality in the active treatment groups (4.4 vs 2.8 per 100 person-years follow-up; P = .13). The only significant adverse effect was an increase in minor bleeding with amiodarone compared with sotalol and placebo.

Essential Evidence: Medicine that Matters, Edited by David Slawson, Allen Shaughnessy, Mark Ebell, and Henry Barry.

Mediterranean diet associated with lower all cause mortality

Clinical question

Does a Mediterranean diet reduce mortality?

Bottom line

This excellent study lends further strength to the association between a Mediterranean diet (rich in vegetables, legumes, fruits, nuts, cereals, olive oil, fish, and alcohol and low in meat) and a reduction in all-cause mortality. Salut! (LOE = 2b)

Reference

Trichopoulou A, Costacou T, Bamia C, Trichopoulos D. Adherence to a Mediterranean diet and survival in a Greek population. N Engl J Med 2003;348:2599–2608.

Study Design

Cohort (prospective)

Setting

Population-based

Synopsis

It's hard to go wrong with a diet containing pasta, olive oil, and red wine, and it may even make you live longer! There have been numerous ecologic studies suggesting that a Mediterranean diet high in vegetables, legumes, fruits, nuts, cereals, olive oil, fish, and alcohol; moderate in cheese and yogurt; and low in saturated lipids, meat, and poultry is associated with greater longevity. This is the largest prospective study to date of this hypothesis. The researchers identified 25,917 community-dwelling Greeks, and excluded 3874 with coronary heart disease, diabetes mellitus, or cancer at enrollment. They did a detailed assessment of diet and lifestyle, and rated the participants adherence to the Mediterranean diet on a scale from 0 (not at all) to 9 (perfect adherence – lots of veggies, seafood, wine, and pasta!) The median follow-up was 3.7 years. This was not a randomized trial, so the outcomes were adjusted for age, sex, smoking status, body mass index, and energy expenditure. The mean body mass index was 28.1 for men and 28.8 for women, making them a slightly pudgy group; 60% were women and more than half of all participants had never smoked. Other than the ratio of monounsaturated lipids to saturated lipids, individual dietary factors were not associated with mortality. However, every 2-point increase in the Mediterranean diet score was associated with a 25% reduction in the risk of death from any cause, a 33% reduction in the risk of death from coronary heart disease, and a 24% reduction in the risk of death from cancer. The benefit was greater in women, in persons older than 55 years, in never-smokers, in heavier folks, and in sedentary persons.

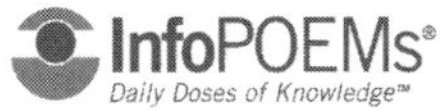

Coffee does not increase risk of developing CAD

Clinical question

Does coffee consumption increase the risk of heart disease?

Bottom line

There is no evidence that coffee consumption increases the likelihood that someone will develop heart disease. (LOE = 2b)

Reference

Lopez-Garcia E, van Dam RM, Willett WC, et al. Coffee consumption and coronary heart disease in men and women: a prospective cohort study. Circulation 2006;113:2045–2053.

Study Design

Cohort (prospective)

Funding

Government

Setting

Population-based

Synopsis

Many patients avoid coffee, often on the advice of their physicians, because of concerns that it may increase the risk of heart disease. The current study is the largest and longest to date on the subject and combines data from the Health Professionals Follow-up Study (N = 44,005) and the Nurses' Health Study (N = 84,488). These studies began in 1986 and 1976, respectively, and provide 14 years and 20 years of follow-up. None of the participants had coronary artery disease (CAD) at the beginning of the study. Participants reported their typical daily caffeine consumption via surveys every 4 years. The primary outcome was nonfatal myocardial infarction or fatal CAD before June 1, 2000. Perhaps the most remarkable thing about the study was that approximately one third of the male health professionals and one fourth of the nurses drank no coffee at all! After adjusting for age, smoking, and other risk factors, the relative risks for the primary outcome among men were all between 0.72 and 1.07, and none were statistically significant. Results were similar for women. No association was found for total caffeine intake, decaffeinated coffee, or tea either.

Essential Evidence: Medicine that Matters, Edited by David Slawson, Allen Shaughnessy, Mark Ebell, and Henry Barry.

Vitamin E has no effect on cardiovascular disease

Clinical question

Does vitamin E have a role in the treatment or prevention of heart disease?

Bottom line

Vitamin E has no effect on the cardiovascular system. It is not useful for the prevention or treatment of heart disease. (LOE = 1a)

Reference

Shekelle PG, Morton SC, Jungvig LK, et al. Effect of supplemental vitamin E for the prevention and treatment of cardiovascular disease. J Gen Intern Med 2004;19:380–389.

Study Design

Meta-analysis (randomized controlled trials)

Setting

Various (meta-analysis)

Synopsis

This systematic review started with a search of 11 databases to find research on vitamin E or its relatives. The authors did a nice job of locating the 8173 studies in any language, and of narrowing this number to 84 controlled trials of vitamin E that evaluated clinical outcomes. In 6 studies ranging from 2 years to 7 years of follow-up, vitamin E supplementation did not affect mortality when used as either secondary or primary prevention. Cardiovascular death rates were not different when the 5 large studies were combined. Vitamin E therapy also had no effect on rates of fatal or nonfatal myocardial infarction. Vitamin E also did not increase the risk of any outcomes, which is reassuring. These studies evaluated thousands of patients. However, most of the studies were of low quality (Jadad score =< 3 of a possible 5).

Essential Evidence: Medicine that Matters, Edited by David Slawson, Allen Shaughnessy, Mark Ebell, and Henry Barry.

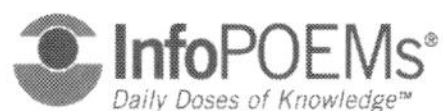

Lowering homocysteine does not reduce cardiovascular disease (HOPE 2)

Clinical question

Is supplementation to lower homocysteine levels an effective treatment for cardiovascular disease or disease prevention?

Bottom line

Supplementation with folic acid and B vitamins is ineffective for adults 55 years and older with known cardiovascular disease (CVD) or diabetes. A second report in the same issue found that similar supplementation in patients with a recent acute myocardial infarction was not helpful and may actually increase the risk of a bad cardiovascular outcome (relative risk = 1.22; 95% CI, 1.0–1.5). (LOE = 1b)

Reference

Lonn E, Yusuf S, Arnold MJ, et al, for the Heart Outcomes Prevention Evaluation (HOPE) 2 Investigators. Homocysteine lowering with folic acid and B vitamins in vascular disease. N Engl J Med 2006;354:1567–1577.

Study Design	Funding	Allocation
Randomized controlled trial (double-blinded)	Government	Concealed

Setting

Outpatient (any)

Synopsis

An elevated level of homocysteine is an independent predictor of the risk of developing CVD. The leap that many physicians and patients have made (unsubstantiated by any evidence) is that lowering homocysteine levels through the use of B vitamins and folic acid supplements will therefore prevent or treat CVD. The current study is the first to evaluate this hypothesis in a prospective, randomized trial. The authors enrolled 5522 patients older than 54 years with known coronary, cerebrovascular, or peripheral vascular disease, or diabetes plus one additional risk factor for CVD. They then randomized the patients (allocation concealed) to receive either 2.5 mg folic acid, 50 mg vitamin B6, and 1 mg vitamin B12 or matching placebo daily. Patients came from countries in which folate fortification of food is mandatory (United States and Canada) and not mandatory (Brazil, Western Europe, and Slovakia). Compliance with treatment was good: More than 90% and patients were followed up for a mean of 5 years. Groups were balanced at the start of the study and analysis was by intention to treat. As expected, homocysteine levels dropped and vitamin levels increased in the active treatment group. However, there was no difference between groups in the combined risk of cardiovascular death, myocardial infarction, or stroke (18.8% vs 19.8%; relative risk = 0.95; 95% CI, 0.84–1.07). There was also no difference regarding this combination of outcomes in patients in the top tertile of homocysteine levels (23.9% vs 24%). There was no difference in outcomes between countries that did or did not fortify foods with folate. Regarding individual outcomes, there were slightly fewer strokes (4.0% vs 5.3%), but more hospitalizations for unstable angina (9.7% vs 7.9%) with supplementation. The study was powered to detect a 17% to 20% relative reduction in the risk of the primary outcome. A second report in the same issue of the journal also failed to find any benefit for secondary prevention of cardiovascular events in patients with a recent acute myocardial infarction (N Engl J Med 2006;345:1578–1588). In fact, they found evidence of possible harm from B vitamin supplementation in this group of high-risk patients.

Omega 3 fatty acids do not affect mortality

Clinical question

Does supplementation with omega 3 fatty acids decrease mortality, cardiovascular disease, or cancer in adults?

Bottom line

Overall, omega 3 fatty acid supplementation does not decrease mortality or cardiovascular disease as compared with placebo. This study combined both primary and secondary prevention; that is, it included people with and without coronary heart disease. (LOE = 1a)

Reference

Hooper L, Thompson RL, Harrison RA, et al. Risks and benefits of omega 3 fats for mortality, cardiovascular disease, and cancer: systematic review. BMJ 2006;332:752–760.

Study Design

Systematic review

Funding

Government

Setting

Various (meta-analysis)

Synopsis

The authors of this review, which is an update of a previous Cochrane review, identified 48 randomized controlled trials and 41 cohort studies evaluating the effect of fish oil supplementation on overall mortality, cardiovascular disease, and cancer in adults. They identified these studies using the usual rigorous Cochrane methodology and analyzed the results from randomized trials separately from cohort data. The studies included patients with and without pre-existing coronary heart disease. As a result, the authors of this study combined both primary and secondary prevention research. Omega 3 fatty acids were given either as supplements or as a recommendation to eat more oily fish. In randomized trials enrolling more than 30,000 patients, omega 3 supplementation did not significantly reduce mortality (relative risk [RR] = 0.87; 95% CI, 0.73–1.03) or the likelihood of a cardiovascular event (RR = 1.09; 0.87–1.37). Long-chain omega 3 fatty acids did not produce different results than short-chain fats. Cancer was neither increased nor decreased in either clinical trials or cohort studies. The lack of benefit demonstrated in this study conflicts with the results of an earlier meta-analysis of the effect in patients with coronary heart disease (Am J Med 2002;112:298–304). However, this is the second study published after that meta-analysis that did not find a benefit overall.

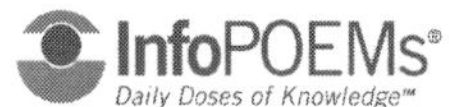

Folic acid supplementation does not reduce cardiovascular disease risk nor mortality

Clinical question

Does folic acid supplementation decrease morbidity or mortality from cardiovascular diseases?

Bottom line

The available evidence does not support the use of folic acid supplementation as secondary prevention of cardiovascular disease events, stroke, or all-cause mortality among patients with preexisting vascular diseases. (LOE = 1a)

Reference

Bazzano LA, Reynolds K, Holder KN, He J. Effect of folic acid supplementation on risk of cardiovascular diseases. A meta-analysis of randomized controlled trials. JAMA 2006;296:2720–2726.

Study Design

Meta-analysis (randomized controlled trials)

Funding

Government

Setting

Various (meta-analysis)

Synopsis

These investigators searched MEDLINE, reference lists from relevant studies, and contacted experts in the field to identify trials investigating the effect of folic acid supplementation on cardiovascular disease risk. No language restrictions were applied. Inclusion criteria included randomized controlled trials of folic acid supplementation with a duration of at least 6 months. Two investigators independently performed the search and identified reports meeting inclusion criteria. Discrepancies were resolved by consensus discussion with a third investigator. From an initial pool of 165 potentially relevant studies, the authors included a total of 12 trials representing data from 16,958 patients with preexisting cardiovascular or renal disease. The dosage of folic acid in the intervention groups ranged from 0.5 mg per day to 15 mg per day. All trials reported a reduction in homocysteine levels. However, compared with control patients, there was no significant reduction in the risk of total cardiovascular disease events, stroke, or all-cause mortality among patients using folic acid supplementation. A formal analysis found no evidence for publication bias or significant heterogeneity among the various trials (no significant differences in reported outcomes among the various individual trials). The longest follow-up period for any of the individual trials was 5 years, so it is possible that a benefit could occur with more prolonged use. Multiple large trials are currently underway addressing this issue.

Essential Evidence: Medicine that Matters, Edited by David Slawson, Allen Shaughnessy, Mark Ebell, and Henry Barry.

Fenofibrate doesn't prevent coronary events in DM (FIELD)

Clinical question

In patients with type 2 diabetes, does fenofibrate prevent coronary events?

Bottom line

In this study, patients with type 2 diabetes treated with fenofibrate (Antara, Lofibra, Tricor) had no significant reduction in coronary events compared with patients treated with placebo. There was a small reduction, however, in nonfatal myocardial infarctions, total cardiovascular disease, and revascularization. (LOE = 1b)

Reference

Keech A, Simes RJ, Barter P, et al, for the FIELD study investigators. Effects of long-term fenofibrate therapy on cardiovascular events in 9795 people with type 2 diabetes mellitus (the FIELD study): randomised controlled trial. Lancet 2005;366:1849–1861.

Study Design

Randomized controlled trial (double-blinded)

Funding

Industry + govt

Allocation

Concealed

Setting

Outpatient (any)

Synopsis

In this study, nearly 10,000 patients between the ages of 50 and 75 years with type 2 diabetes mellitus were randomly assigned to receive 200 mg micronized fenofibrate every day or a matching placebo. The patients all had a total cholesterol level between 3.0 mmol/L and 6.5 mmol/L (115 and 250 mg/dL), plus either a total cholesterol/HDL cholesterol ratio of 4.0 or higher, or a triglyceride level between 1.0 mmol/L and 5.0 mmol/L (88 and 440 mg/dL), with no clear indication for, or treatment with, lipid-modifying therapy at the start of the study. After randomization, the patients were seen every 4 to 6 months for up to 5 years. Subsequent decisions about adding other medications were left to the discretion of the treating physician. The study was designed to have enough power to detect modest differences in the rate of events. The outcomes for this study were analyzed by intention to treat and were assessed by evaluators unaware of the treatment group. The median follow up was 5 years and the researchers were able to account for more than 99% of the patients. The patients treated with placebo were more likely to receive subsequent nonstudy lipid-lowering medications (17% vs 8%). There was no significant difference in coronary events (6% vs 5%) between groups, although patients treated with placebo had more nonfatal myocardial infarctions (8.4% vs 6.4%; number needed to treat [NNT] = 100; 95% CI, 58–406). Patients taking fenofibrate also were less likely to have a cardiovascular event (NNT = 69; 95% CI, 36–1060) or revascularization (NNT = 67; 95% CI, 40–194). A systematic review* of fibrates has shown a significant increase in all-cause mortality (number needed to treat to harm = 132 for 4.4 years). In this study, there was also a nonsignificant increase in all-cause mortality (14.2/1000 vs 12.9/1000; P = .18). *Studer M, Briel M, Leimenstoll B, Glass TR, Bucher HC. Effect of different antilipidemic agents and diets on mortality. A systematic review. Arch Intern Med 2005;165:725–30

Essential Evidence: Medicine that Matters, Edited by David Slawson, Allen Shaughnessy, Mark Ebell, and Henry Barry.

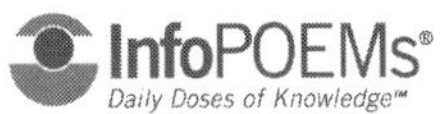

Optimal oral antiplatelet therapy for vascular disease

Clinical question

Which antiplatelet agents, used alone or in combination, are effective in preventing recurrent vascular events?

Bottom line

Aspirin is the recommended oral first-line antiplatelet therapy for patients with ST-segment elevation myocardial infarction. Aspirin or clopidogrel is recommended for those with initial transient ischemic attack (TIA)/ischemic stroke, chronic stable angina, or peripheral arterial disease, and aspirin plus clopidogrel should be used for those with non-ST-segment elevation acute coronary syndrome. For second-line therapy, the combination of aspirin and clopidogrel is recommended for recurrent acute coronary syndrome. The combination of aspirin and extended-release dipyridamole is recommended for patients with recurrent TIA/ischemic stroke in the absence of known coronary artery disease. Further studies are needed before making firm recommendations on the management of patients with recurrent TIA/ischemic stroke and known coronary artery disease. (LOE = 1a–)

Reference

Tran H, Anand SS. Oral antiplatelet therapy in cerebrovascular disease, coronary artery disease, and peripheral arterial disease. JAMA 2004;292:1867–1874.

Study Design	Funding	Setting
Systematic review	Industry	Various (meta-analysis)

Synopsis

Aspirin prevents recurrent vascular events in a wide range of high-risk patients, but it is unknown if other antiplatelet agents, alone or in combination with aspirin, are more effective. The investigators searched multiple databases, and reference lists of trials, review articles, and scientific statements and guidelines of official societies. They included randomized trials comparing an antiplatelet regimen to either placebo or another antiplatelet regimen assessing outcomes for at least 10 days. They identified 111 trials enrolling nearly 100,000 patients. No formal assessment of publication bias was done, nor was any specific analysis done to determine homogeneity of the results. Recommended oral first-line antiplatelet therapy is aspirin for patients with ST-segment elevation myocardial infarction; aspirin or clopidogrel for those with initial transient ischemic attack (TIA)/ischemic stroke, chronic stable angina, or peripheral arterial disease (since aspirin is less expensive, clopidogrel should be reserved only for aspirin-intolerant patients); and aspirin plus clopidogrel for those with non-ST-segment elevation acute coronary syndrome. For second-line therapy, the combination of aspirin and clopidogrel is recommended for recurrent acute coronary syndrome. The combination of aspirin and clopidogrel does not lower the incidence of recurrent vascular events in patients with recurrent TIAs/ischemic stroke, but does increase the risk of major and life-threatening bleeding. The combination of aspirin and extended-release dipyridamole is recommended for patients with recurrent TIA/ischemic stroke in the absence of known coronary artery disease. Ticlopidine is beneficial for various vascular conditions, but frequent side effects – some serious – limit its usefulness.

Essential Evidence: Medicine that Matters, Edited by David Slawson, Allen Shaughnessy, Mark Ebell, and Henry Barry.

Clopidogrel + ASA no better than ASA alone for high-risk patients

Clinical question

Is the combination of clopidogrel and aspirin better than aspirin alone for patients with, or at high risk for, vascular disease?

Bottom line

The use of the combination of clopidogrel (Plavix) and aspirin should be limited to carefully defined groups of patients with acute coronary syndromes. It is not recommended for the broader group of patients with coronary disease, cerebrovascular disease, or multiple risk factors such as diabetes, hyperlipidemia, and hypertension. (LOE = 1b)

Reference

Bhatt DL, Fox KA, Hacke W, et al, for the CHARISMA Investigators. Clopidogrel and aspirin versus aspirin alone for the prevention of atherothrombotic events. N Engl J Med 2006;354:1706–1717.

Study Design	Funding	Allocation
Randomized controlled trial (double-blinded)	Industry	Concealed

Setting

Outpatient (any)

Synopsis

The combination of aspirin and clopidogrel has been recommended for selected patients with acute coronary syndromes (ACS), such as those with non-ST elevation myocardial infarction (MI) or those with recurrent ACS. (Tran H, Anand SS. JAMA 2004;292:1867–74.) These investigators asked whether a broader group of patients would benefit from the combination. The authors enrolled patients 45 years or older who had documented coronary artery disease, cerebrovascular disease, or peripheral vascular disease, or if they had multiple risk factors for vascular disease. The most common risk factors in the latter group were diabetes (82%), hypertension (49%), hyperlipidemia (60%), or advanced age (51%). The patients' median age was 64 years and 30% were women. Participants were randomly assigned (allocation concealed) to either 75 mg clopidogrel plus 75 mg to 162 mg aspirin each given once daily or low-dose aspirin plus placebo. The primary outcome was a composite of MI, stroke, or death and was adjudicated by a panel blinded to treatment assignment. A total of 15,603 patients were enrolled and followed up for a median of 28 months. Analysis was by intention to treat. There was no difference between groups regarding the primary composite outcome and no difference for any of the individual elements (MI, stroke, or death). A predefined secondary composite end point added hospitalization for ischemic events, such as transient ischemic attack or revascularization, to the primary outcome. There was a very small benefit (16.7% vs 17.9%; $P = .04$; number needed to treat = 194 per year) of combination therapy for this secondary composite end point. However, there was also a trend toward more severe bleeding and a significant increase in moderate bleeding in the group given both clopidogrel and aspirin (2.1% vs 1.3%; $P < .001$; number needed to treat to harm = 291 per year). Severe bleeding was defined as intracranial hemorrhage, fatal bleeding, or bleeding that required significant clinical intervention, such as surgery, transfusion, or the use of intotropic agents.

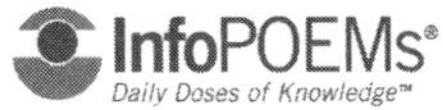

Clopidogrel beneficial added to ASA, fibrinolytic in STEMI

Clinical question

Does clopidogrel (Plavix) improve outcomes in patients with ST-segment elevation myocardial infarction when added to thrombolytic therapy and aspirin?

Bottom line

Adding clopidogrel to aspirin and fibrinolytic therapy during the first week in patients with ST-segment elevation myocardial infarction reduces the likelihood of recurrent myocardial infarction and ischemia leading to revascularization over a 30-day period (number needed to treat = 15). The short-term risk of major bleeding was low. This trial does not address how long patients should continue to take clopidogrel after the first week of treatment. (LOE = 1b)

Reference

Sabatine MS, Cannon CP, Gibson CM, et al. Addition of clopidogrel to aspirin and fibrinolytic therapy for myocardial infarction with ST-segment elevation. N Engl J Med 2005;352:1179–1189.

Study Design

Randomized controlled trial (double-blinded)

Funding

Industry

Allocation

Concealed

Setting

Inpatient (any location) with outpatient follow-up

Synopsis

Adults younger than 75 years presenting within 12 hours of the onset of an ST-elevation myocardial infarction (STEMI) were all given a thrombolytic, heparin (if indicated with that particular thrombolytic), and aspirin. Their mean age was 57 years, 80% were men, 50% were smokers, and 9% had a previous myocardial infarction [MI]. They were also randomized (allocation concealed) to receive an initial bolus of 300 mg clopidogrel (Plavix) followed by 75 mg daily or matching placebo until angiography, and followed up for 30 days. Almost all (94%) underwent angiography at 48 to 192 hours to assess vessel patency; those that didn't undergo angiography received the study drug for 8 days. Exclusions included those already taking clopidogrel, those with cerebrovascular disease or previous bypass surgery, those who were clinically unstable, and those who received too large a dose of heparin. There were 1752 in the clopidogrel group and 1739 in the placebo group, and these groups were balanced at the start of the study. The primary outcome was a mix of disease-oriented (infarct artery occlusion) and patient-oriented (death or recurrent MI) outcomes and analysis was by intention to treat. The primary outcome was less likely in patients receiving clopidogrel (15% vs 21.7%; $P < .05$; number needed to treat [NNT] = 15; 95% CI, 11–24), particularly in patients younger than 65 years. Most of this benefit was due to a reduction in recurrent ischemia or recurrent MI. There was no difference between groups in death from cardiovascular causes. The risk of major bleeding was similar between groups at 30 days and there was no significant difference in the risk of minor bleeding.

Essential Evidence: Medicine that Matters, Edited by David Slawson, Allen Shaughnessy, Mark Ebell, and Henry Barry.

Aspirin reduces risk of CV events, increases risk of bleeding

Clinical question

Is aspirin beneficial in the primary prevention of adverse cardiovascular events in both women and men?

Bottom line

Primary prevention with aspirin reduces the risk of adverse cardiovascular events in both women and men. In particular, aspirin reduces the risk of stroke in women and the risk of myocardial infarction (MI) in men. The risk of major bleeding is significantly increased with regular aspirin therapy in both sexes and overall mortality is unchanged. Patients and their clinicians should weigh their independent risks and benefits before deciding on regular aspirin use. (LOE = 1a)

Reference

Berger JS, Roncaglioni MC, Avanzini F, Pangrazzi I, Tognoni G, Brown DL. Aspirin for the primary prevention of cardiovascular events in women and men. A sex-specific meta-analysis of randomized controlled trials. JAMA 2006;295:306–313.

Study Design

Meta-analysis (randomized controlled trials)

Funding

Unknown/not stated

Setting

Various (meta-analysis)

Synopsis

Although aspirin reduces the risk of adverse cardiovascular events in high-risk adults, it is uncertain if women derive the same benefit as men. The investigators thoroughly searched MEDLINE, the Cochrane Central Registry of Controlled Trials, bibliographies of retrieved trials, and reports presented at major scientific meetings for randomized trials evaluating the risks and benefits of aspirin treatment for the primary prevention of cardiovascular events. Six randomized trials with a total of 95,456 individuals, including 51,342 women, were identified. Follow-up occurred for an average of 6.4 years among the various studies. In women, aspirin therapy was associated with a significant 12% reduction in cardiovascular events (odds ratio [OR] = 0.88; 95% CI, 0.70–0.97; number needed to treat [NNT] = 316, 180–3805) and 17% reduction in stroke (OR = 0.83; 95% CI, 0.70–0.97; NNT = 457, 259–2597). There was no significant beneficial effect of aspirin in reducing the risk of MI or cardiovascular mortality. In men, there was a similar 14% reduction in cardiovascular events (OR = 0.86; 95% CI, 0.78–0.94; NNT = 155, 98–364) and a 32% reduction in MI risk (OR = 0.68; 95% CI, 0.54–0.86; NNT = 114, 79–261). There was no significant beneficial effect of aspirin in reducing the risk of stroke or cardiovascular mortality. Aspirin treatment significantly increased the risk of major bleeding in both men and women and all-cause mortality was unchanged. There was no evidence of publication bias and the outcomes of the various trials were homogenous.

Essential Evidence: Medicine that Matters, Edited by David Slawson, Allen Shaughnessy, Mark Ebell, and Henry Barry.

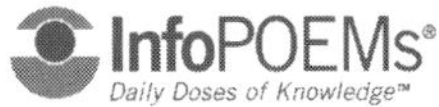

Aspirin + PPI safer than clopidogrel if history of GI bleed

Clinical question

What is the best antithrombotic for patients with a history of upper gastrointestinal bleeding?

Bottom line

For patients with a history of bleeding peptic ulcer, the combination of aspirin and a proton pump inhibitor twice a day was safer in terms of bleeding side effects than clopidogrel. While esomeprazole was used in this study, generic omeprazole 20 mg given twice a day provides the same degree of acid suppression at a much lower cost. This study calls into question the overall safety of clopidogrel, which has been promoted as not increasing the risk of bleeding significantly. (LOE = 1b)

Reference

Chan FK, Ching JY, Hung LC, et al. Clopidogrel versus aspirin and esomeprazole to prevent recurrent ulcer bleeding. N Engl J Med 2005;352:238–244.

Study Design

Randomized controlled trial (double-blinded)

Funding

Government

Allocation

Concealed

Setting

Inpatient (any location) with outpatient follow-up

Synopsis

Clopidogrel (Plavix) has been recommended by the American College of Cardiology as the preferred drug for patients who require an antithrombotic agent to prevent heart disease but who also have a history of bleeding peptic ulcer. This study compared clopidogrel with the combination of aspirin and esomeprazole in this setting. Patients with a source of upper gastrointestinal bleeding (52% gastric ulcer, 34% duodenal ulcer, 8% both, 6% other erosions) who had healing confirmed endoscopically were randomized to clopidogrel 75 mg daily plus esomepraozle placebo twice daily or aspirin 80 mg daily plus esomeprazole 20 mg twice daily. Groups were fairly well balanced at the outset, allocation was concealed, and analysis was by intention-to-treat. Patients were treated for 12 months. The primary outcome (hematemesis, melena, or a decrease in hemoglobin of at least 2 gm/dl accompanied by endoscopic evidence of ulcer or erosion) was seen in 8.6% of the clopidogrel group and 0.7% of the aspirin plus esomeprazole group ($p = 0.001$, number needed to treat [NNT] = 13). Three patients in the clopidogrel group had severe bleeding complications not related to the gastrointestinal tract compared with none in the aspirin group, including two intraventricular hemorrhages, one of which was fatal. There were more deaths in the clopidogrel group (8 vs 4) but this difference was not statistically significant. There was no difference between groups in the likelihood of adverse cardiovascular events (9 vs 11).

Electron beam tomography not helpful

Clinical question

Is electron beam tomography a useful motivational tool to change behavior and improve cardiovascular risk?

Bottom line

Results of electron beam tomography provided to asymptomatic patients at average risk of coronary artery disease and their clinicians had no effect on creating behavior change aimed at lowering cardiovascular risk. Interestingly, the use of a "stages of change" case management program aimed at individual participants did have a positive effect on lowering risk. We should be skeptical of any new test purported to motivate patients to change their behavior – including checking cholesterol and blood sugar – until it has been subjected to the rigors of a randomized controlled trial. (LOE = 1b)

Reference

O'Malley PG, Feuerstein IM, Taylor AJ. Impact of electron beam tomography, with or without case management, on motivation, behavioral change, and cardiovascular risk profile. A randomized controlled trial. JAMA 2003;289:2215–2223.

Study Design

Randomized controlled trial (nonblinded)

Setting

Outpatient (any)

Synopsis

Laboratory tests, such as bone mineral density measurement, carotid artery intimal thickness measurement, C-reactive protein, pulmonary function tests, and fasting blood sugar, are frequently used to assess risks and motivate patients to adopt more healthy behaviors. Minimal, if any, evidence supports this contention. Electron beam tomography (EBT), the new kid on the block, is being similarly used for the detection of subclinical coronary artery disease (CAD). To assess the motivational effect of EBT on behavioral change, 450 asymptomatic consenting active-duty US Army personnel aged 39 to 45 years were randomly assigned (concealed allocation assignment) to 1 of 4 intervention arms: (1) EBT results given to patients and their physicians who provided usual care; (2) EBT results given to both patients and their physicians who provided intensive case management (ICM) – a team approach of doctors, nurses, and dietitians with frequent contact tailored to individual patients' "stages of behavioral change"; (3) EBT results withheld from both patients and their usual care physicians; and (4) EBT results withheld from both patients and their ICM physicians. A total of 90% of the subjects were available at the 1-year follow-up evaluation. Baseline and follow-up cardiovascular risk was assessed using the 10-year Framingham Risk Score (FRS) by individuals blind to clinical status and intervention group. Data were analyzed by an intention-to-treat approach. The average risk at baseline was 5.85%. There was no significant risk change between the groups who received EBT results with those who did not. Comparing the groups who received ICM with those receiving usual care, the mean absolute risk change in the 10-year FRS was −0.06% vs +0.74% (P = .003).

Essential Evidence: Medicine that Matters, Edited by David Slawson, Allen Shaughnessy, Mark Ebell, and Henry Barry.

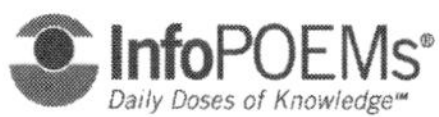

Chest pain relief by NTG doesn't predict active CAD

Clinical question

Does relief of chest pain by nitroglycerin predict active coronary artery disease?

Bottom line

A response – or lack of a response – to nitroglycerin does not predict active coronary artery disease (CAD) in patients presenting to an emergency department with chest pain. A coin flip would yield similar results. (LOE = 2b)

Reference

Henrikson CA, Howell EE, Bush DE et al. Chest pain relief by nitroglycerin does not predict active coronary artery disease. Ann Intern Med 2003;139:979–986.

Study Design

Cohort (prospective)

Setting

Emergency department

Synopsis

The researchers of this study enrolled 459 patients admitted to an emergency department with a diagnosis of "rule out myocardial infarction" or "chest pain" who also received one dose of sublingual or spray nitroglycerin. The goal was to determine whether a 50% reduction in the patients' chest pain predicted what was termed "active coronary artery disease." Active CAD was defined as one of the following: elevated serum troponin T level, 70% or greater stenosis on angiography, positive exercise test result, or clinical diagnosis of active CAD made by the attending physician and confirmed by a study cardiologist unaware of the response to nitroglycerin. The researchers even used results of testing performed up to 6 months before the hospitalization to characterize a patient as having active CAD. Of all the patients receiving nitroglycerin, 39% had at least 50% relief of their symptoms of chest pain and 61% did not. A total of 141 patients (31%) received a diagnosis of active CAD. Only one third of these patients (35%) had pain relief. In contrast, 41% of patients without active CAD experienced relief. At 4 months, clinical outcomes were similar in patients with and without chest pain with nitroglycerin.

Essential Evidence: Medicine that Matters, Edited by David Slawson, Allen Shaughnessy, Mark Ebell, and Henry Barry.

Ranolazine adds little to maximum antianginal therapy (ERICA)

Clinical question

In patients with frequent angina symptoms, does the addition of ranolazine to maximum therapy with amlodipine and nitroglycerin improve symptoms?

Bottom line

Ranolazine (Ranexa), added to maximum dosing of amlodipine, decreases angina episodes and nitroglycerin doses slightly more than placebo does; patients taking ranolazine experienced approximately 1 fewer episode, on average, every 2 weeks. These results occurred in patients with frequent symptoms – at least 4 anginal episodes per week – and its effect is likely to be less pronounced in patients with less frequent symptoms. (LOE = 1b)

Reference

Stone PH, Gratsiansky NA, Blokhin A, Huang IZ, Meng L; ERICA Investigators. Antianginal efficacy of ranolazine when added to treatment with amlodipine: the ERICA (Efficacy of Ranolazine in Chronic Angina) trial. J Am Coll Cardiol 2006;48:566–575.

Study Design

Randomized controlled trial (double-blinded)

Funding

Industry

Allocation

Concealed

Setting

Outpatient (any)

Synopsis

Ranolazine is thought to allow more energy to be produced for every molecule of oxygen delivered to the cells of the heart. The mainly eastern European investigators conducting this study enrolled 565 patients with pronounced symptomatic coronary artery disease and at least 3 episodes of angina weekly despite treatment with 10 mg amlodipine (Norvasc) daily. This is a fairly select group, since patients could not be taking any other antianginal drugs, except long-acting or sublingual nitroglycerin. Almost all patients were white; their average age was 62 years. The participants were randomized, using concealed allocation, to receive either placebo or extended-release ranolazine at a dose of 500 mg twice daily for 1 week, then 1000 mg twice daily for 6 weeks. The addition of either placebo or ranolazine to maximum doses of amlodipine resulted in a pronounced drop in the number of weekly angina episodes, from an average baseline rate of 5.6 episodes per week to an average of 3.3 in the placebo group and 2.9 in the treated group. The difference in rates between placebo and ranolazine, a treatment effect of 0.43 episodes per week, was statistically significant (P = .028). Weekly sublingual nitroglycerin use similarly decreased in both groups and was more pronounced in the treatment group (2.03 vs 2.68 doses per week; P = .014).

Essential Evidence: Medicine that Matters, Edited by David Slawson, Allen Shaughnessy, Mark Ebell, and Henry Barry.

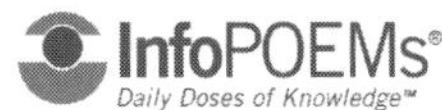

Better outcomes with CABG than PCI with stent for 2,3 vessel disease

Clinical question

Which is the better treatment for multivessel coronary disease: bypass surgery or stenting?

Bottom line

Coronary artery bypass grafting (CABG) is associated with lower long-term mortality than percutaneous coronary interventions (PCI) with stenting for most anatomic groups in patients with multivessel disease, and a lower risk of requiring revascularization in the 3 years following intervention. Of course, this was an observational study and the groups were quite different at baseline, so we must be cautious about drawing firm treatment conclusions, even with appropriate statistical adjustments. Stenting is less invasive and is associated with lower unadjusted in-hospital mortality, so it remains a good option for many patients. (LOE = 2b)

Reference

Hannan EL, Racz MJ, Walford G, et al. Long-term outcomes of coronary-artery bypass grafting versus stent implantation. N Engl J Med 2005;352:2174–2183.

Study Design	Funding	Setting
Cohort (prospective)	Unknown/not stated	Inpatient (any location) with outpatient follow-up

Synopsis

Randomized trials comparing PCI with CABG were done before stenting was widely used. This analysis used data from 2 New York cardiac registries, 1 for PCI and 1 for CABG. Data were collected for all patients undergoing CABG or PCI with stent placement for at least 1 lesion between 1997 and 2000. All patients had at least a 70% stenosis in 2 of the main coronary arteries. Patients with left main disease or myocardial infarction within 24 hours of the procedure were excluded. The groups were quite different: Patients in the CABG group were older (67 vs 65 years), more likely to be male (70.9% vs 68.6%), more likely to be white (89.2% vs 87%), and more likely to have a decreased ejection fraction. The researchers were unable to determine how many patients were lost to follow-up. The analysis first identified factors that were associated with the risk of death and adjusted for these factors in a multivariate analysis. Separate analyses were done for the different anatomical combinations of 2-vessel and 3-vessel disease. Patients were followed up for a mean of 706 days in the CABG group and 585 days in the stent group. The adjusted hazard ratio for death after CABG compared with the risk for stent was between 0.64 and 0.76 for the 5 different types of 2- and 3-vessel disease. The benefit was generally greater for patients with diabetes (hazard ratio = 0.59–0.71). There was no difference between outcomes for CABG or stent for patients with 2-vessel disease not including the proximal left anterior descending (LAD) artery and decreased ejection fraction. The benefit was greatest for patients with 3-vessel disease involving the LAD artery. Patients undergoing stent were much more likely to require revascularization with CABG (7.8% vs 0.3%) or subsequent PCI (27.3% vs 4.6%). Not surprisingly, unadjusted inpatient mortality was higher in the CABG group (1.75% vs 0.68%).

Essential Evidence: Medicine that Matters, Edited by David Slawson, Allen Shaughnessy, Mark Ebell, and Henry Barry.

Adding ACEI doesn't improve outcomes in stable angina w/nl LVEF (PEACE)

Clinical question

Does adding an angiotensin-converting enzyme inhibitor improve outcomes among patients with stable angina and no evidence of heart failure?

Bottom line

Adding the angiotensin-converting enzyme inhibitor trandolapril (Mavik) to standard medical treatment of patients with stable angina and normal left ventricular function did not reduce their risk of adverse cardiovascular outcomes. Although higher risk patients and those with less well controlled risk factors may still benefit from this intervention, this study didn't assess those groups. (LOE = 1b)

Reference

PEACE Trial Investigators. Angiotensin-converting-enzyme inhibition in stable coronary artery disease. N Engl J Med 2004;351:2058–2068.

Study Design	Funding	Allocation	Setting
Randomized controlled trial (double-blinded)	Industry + govt	Concealed	Outpatient (any)

Synopsis

The HOPE and EUROPA trials found that angiotensin-converting enzyme inhibitors (ACE) inhibitors improve cardiovascular outcomes in patients with vascular disease but with no evidence of overt heart failure. This study attempted to extend these findings to an even lower risk group using the ACE inhibitor trandolapril (Mavik). The researchers recrutied patients older than 50 years with documented coronary artery disease and a left ventricular ejection fraction of greater than 40%, excluding patients in poor health, with renal failure, recent unstable angina, or who had recently used an ACE inhibitor. Only patients who tolerated the active drug during a run-in phase were allowed into the study, a step that increases the likelihood of finding a benefit for the drug. The mean age of participants was 65 years, 18% were women, 55% had had a myocardial infarction (MI), 92% were white, and 17% were diabetic. Patients were randomized (allocation concealed) to trandolapril 2 mg per day, increased to 4 mg per day if tolerated, or matching placebo. Outcomes were blindly assessed and analysis was by intention to treat. The primary outcome began as death or nonfatal MI, but was expanded to include coronary revascularization as a way to reduce sample size and save money halfway through the study. The final sample included 4158 in the trandolapril group and 4132 in the placebo group; patients were followed for a median of 4.8 years. During the study, the safety monitoring committee recommended that all diabetic patients with microalbuminuria be given an ACE inhibitor, effectively removing them from the study. Removing data for these patients did not affect the overall study results. Much to the investigators' surprise, there was no difference between groups regarding the primary outcome (21.9% in the trandolapril group vs 22.5% in the placebo group) at the end of the study. They hypothesize that this is due to the lower overall risk of the patients in the PEACE study compared with those in the HOPE and EUROPA trials. Certainly, when patients are at greater risk of bad outcomes, they tend to benefit more from interventions, so this argument may have merit. Another explanation is that trandolapril is less effective than ramipril (HOPE) or perindopril (EUROPA), although the extent of blood pressure lowering (3 mm) was similar to that in the HOPE and EUROPA studies.

Essential Evidence: Medicine that Matters, Edited by David Slawson, Allen Shaughnessy, Mark Ebell, and Henry Barry.

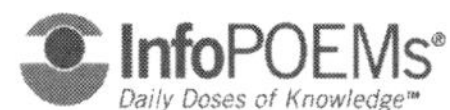

Rofecoxib increases risk of cardiovascular events

Clinical question

Does rofecoxib (Vioxx) increase the risk of cardiovascular events?

Bottom line

For every 62 patients who take rofecoxib instead of placebo for 3 years, 1 additional patient will experience a serious cardiovascular event. Remember, there is no greater symptomatic relief with COX-2 inhibitors than with older drugs; acetaminophen is a very safe alternative. The decrease in risk of serious gastrointestinal complications is marginal with COX-2 inhibitors and the cost is high. (LOE = 1b)

Reference

Bresalier RS, Sandler RS, Quan H, et al, for the Adenomatous Polyp Prevention on Vioxx (APPROVe) Trial Investigators. Cardiovascular events associated with rofecoxib in a colorectal adenoma chemoprevention trial. N Engl J Med 2005;352:1092–1102.

Study Design

Randomized controlled trial (double-blinded)

Funding

Industry

Allocation

Concealed

Setting

Outpatient (any)

Synopsis

The manufacturer of rofecoxib (Vioxx) designed this study to help include the prevention of colon polyps as an indication for the drug. Because of concerns about the safety of rofecoxib raised by earlier the studies, the Food and Drug Administration asked the researchers to also monitor cardiovascular outcomes. The authors identified 2,586 adults older than 40 years who had a history of colon polyps; some patients taking aspirin were allowed into the study (ultimately, 1 in 6). After a placebo run-in period to assure that patients would be compliant, they were randomized (allocation concealed) to receive rofecoxib 25 mg or placebo once daily for up to 3 years. Groups were balanced at the start of the study, but more patients in the rofecoxib group withdrew because of adverse clinical events (16% vs 11%). Outcomes were assessed blindly and analysis was by intention to treat. The likelihood of any cardiovascular event was higher in the rofecoxib group (3.6% vs 2.0%). One additional cardiovascular event would occur in every 62 patients treated with rofecoxib for three years (95% CI 35–330). This increased was largely the result of more myocardial infarction and other cardiac events. The number of strokes was also greater in the rofecoxib group, but this difference was not statistically significant (15 vs 7). The risk of adverse events was as high or higher during the second 18-month period compared with the first. There were 10 deaths in each group.

Essential Evidence: Medicine that Matters, Edited by David Slawson, Allen Shaughnessy, Mark Ebell, and Henry Barry.

Celecoxib increases risk of cardiovascular complications

Clinical question

Does celecoxib (Celebrex) increase the risk of cardiovascular events?

Bottom line

One additional cardiovascular event or cardiovascular death occurs for every 126 patients treated for 1 year with celecoxib. There appears to be a dose response relationship. It is difficult to justify continued use of this and other coxibs, except in the most exceptional circumstances. (LOE = 1b)

Reference

Solomon SD, McMurray JJ, Pfeffer MA, et al, for the Adenoma Prevention with Celecoxib (APC) Study Investigators. Cardiovascular risk associated with celecoxib in a clinical trial for colorectal adenoma prevention. N Engl J Med 2005;352:1071–1080.

Study Design

Randomized controlled trial (double-blinded)

Funding

Industry

Allocation

Concealed

Setting

Outpatient (specialty)

Synopsis

This study was an attempt to broaden the indication of this widely used drug even further by seeing if celecoxib (Celebrex) can prevent recurrent colon polyps. When the results of a similar study of rofecoxib (Vioxx) were released to the media, the authors of this study decided to similarly analyze their existing data to look for cardiovascular complications. In this study, 2035 patients aged 32 to 88 years with a history of a single large colon adenoma or multiple adenomas were randomized (allocation concealed) to placebo, celecoxib 200 mg twice daily, or celecoxib 400 mg twice daily. Groups were balanced at the start of the study, analysis was by intention to treat, and patients were followed up for 3 years. Cardiovascular endpoints were blindly assessed and mortality data were available for all patients. Although 41% of patients were hypertensive, only 4% had a history of myocardial infarction (MI); 2% had a history of stroke; 7%, angina; and 2%, heart failure. After 2.8 to 3.1 years of follow-up, the likelihood of cardiovascular death, MI, stroke, or heart failure was 1.0% in the placebo group, 2.3% in the 200 mg group, and 3.4% in the 400 mg group. The increase in this group of outcomes between the 400 mg and placebo groups was statistically significant, with a 95% confidence interval of 1.4% to 7.8%. The difference between the 200 mg and placebo groups just missed being statistically higher with celecoxib (95% CI 0.9 to 5.5). The number needed to treat to harm for treating with 400 mg per day for 3 years is 42, or 126 per year of use.

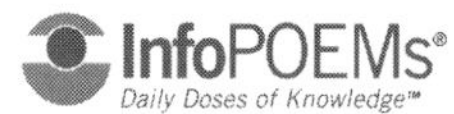

Rofecoxib, diclofenac and indomethacin increase risk of CVD

Clinical question

Which NSAIDs increase the risk of cardiovascular disease (CVD)?

Bottom line

Rofecoxib (Vioxx), diclofenac (Voltaren, Cataflam), and indomethacin (Indocin) are associated with a significant increased risk of CVD. It is likely that all NSAIDs carry some risk, but the risks may vary between medicines. Current evidence does not point to an increased risk for low dose (over the counter) ibuprofen and this remains safe to use at recommended doses. (LOE = 2a−)

Reference

McGettigan P, Henry D. Cardiovascular risk and inhibition of cyclooxygenase. A systematic review of the observational studies of selective and nonselective inhibitors of cyclooxygenase 2. JAMA 2006;296:1633–1644.

Study Design

Systematic review

Funding

Foundation

Setting

Various (meta-analysis)

Synopsis

Recent evidence that rofecoxib (Vioxx) increases the risk of CVD has raised concern about other nonsteroidal anti-inflammatory drugs (NSAIDs). These investigators searched multiple databases including MEDLINE, EMBASE, the Cochrane Library, abstracts of scientific meetings and bibliographies of relevant studies for reports on cardiovascular events and NSAID use. Of 7086 potentially eligible titles, 17 case-control including 86,193 cases and 6 cohort studies including 75, 520 users met study criteria. Most exclusions were a result of reports not providing sufficient information on study outcomes or the drugs of interest. The mean age of study participants was rarely less than 55 years, and in most cases was grater than 60 years. Two individuals independently extracted data and assessed study quality with disagreements resolved by consensus. Individual studies underwent assessment using a standardized instrument. All studies scored well (7–8 points in total from a possible 9). As expected, rofecoxib use significantly increased the risk of CVD, with risk being highest with doses in excess of 25 mg/day. Diclofenac (Voltaren, Cataflam) and indomethacin (Indocin) were also associated with a significantly increased risk of CVD. Data on meloxicam (Mobic) came from 3 trials, only one of which showed a statistically significant elevated risk. Authors of the article state that these data do not allow definite conclusions about the risk of meloxicam. Celecoxib (Celebrex), naproxen, piroxicam and inbuprofen exposure did not increase CVD risk. Stay tuned, however, as more studies are forthcoming shortly. In a related study in the same journal (Zhang J, Ding E, Song Y. JAMA; 296:1619–32), only rofecoxib was associated with a significant increased risk of renal events and heart arrhythmia. Celecoxib (Celebrex) was significantly associated with a reduced risk of renal dysfunction.

Essential Evidence: Medicine that Matters, Edited by David Slawson, Allen Shaughnessy, Mark Ebell, and Henry Barry.

BNP improves outcomes in evaluation of dyspnea

Clinical question

Does use of the B-type natriuretic peptide test in the diagnosis of acute dyspnea improve patient outcomes?

Bottom line

Knowledge of the B-type natriuretic peptide level during initial evaluation in the emergency department is associated with more rapid initiation of appropriate treatment, less need for hospitalization and intensive care, a shorter length of stay, and lower costs. The next question is whether the BNP can replace other tests like the chest x-ray or echocardiogram for some patients. (LOE = 1b)

Reference

Mueller C, Scholer A, Laule-Kilian K, et al. Use of B-type natriuretic peptide in the evaluation and management of acute dyspnea. N Engl J Med 2004;350:647–654.

Study Design

Randomized controlled trial (single-blinded)

Setting

Emergency department

Synopsis

New tests are often introduced without a careful examination of their effect on patient-oriented outcomes. Accuracy alone is not reason enough to adopt a test. More important reasons are that its use helps patients live better or longer lives or that it adds or reduces cost. B-type natriuretic peptide [BNP] is accurate in diagnosing heart failure (HF) in patients presenting with acute dyspnea (N Engl J Med 2002; 106: 416–22). This study looks at the larger impact of this test's use in clinical practice. Of 665 consecutive adults presenting to a Swiss emergency department with acute dyspnea, 452 met the inclusion criteria. Patients with an obvious traumatic cause, serum creatinine levels greater than 2.8 mg/dL, cardiogenic shock, or who requested transfer to another hospital were excluded. The mean age of patients was 71 years and half were women. Patients were randomly assigned (allocation concealed) to usual care supplemented by a rapid BNP level, or the usual diagnostic protocol without knowledge of BNP level. Clinicians were advised that a BNP level less than 100 pg/mL made HF unlikely, a result greater than 500 pg/mL made HF very likely, and that intermediate values required additional information and clinical judgment to make the diagnosis. The BNP was not measured during any subsequent hospitalization. All patients underwent a careful history and physical examination, electrocardiogram, chest x-ray, and blood tests other than BNP. Echocardiography and pulmonary function testing were strongly recommended for all patients, although the percentage actually having the tests was not reported. Outcomes were assessed by a group blinded to treatment assignment. The rate of admission to the hospital was lower in the BNP group (75% vs 85%; absolute risk reduction = 10%; number needed to treat [NNT] = 10), as was the rate of admission to the intensive care unit (15% vs 24%; NNT = 11). Patients in the BNP group were treated more quickly (63 vs 90 mins), spent less time in the hospital (8 vs 11 days), and their care cost less money ($5410 vs $7264) than those whose physicians did not have that test result. There was no difference in either in-hospital or 30-day mortality and no difference in 30-day readmission rates.

Essential Evidence: Medicine that Matters, Edited by David Slawson, Allen Shaughnessy, Mark Ebell, and Henry Barry.

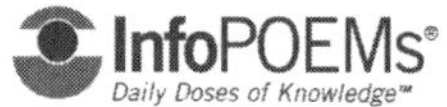

BNP testing beneficial with CHF + pulmonary dx

Clinical question

In patients with pulmonary disease, can B-type natriuretic peptide testing effectively guide therapy?

Bottom line

In patients with pre-existing pulmonary disease, B-type natriuretic peptide (BNP) testing in the emergency department is effective at distinguishing an exacerbation due to heart failure (HF) from that caused by pulmonary disease. As a result, hospitalizations are fewer, probably because of initiation of more appropriate therapy in the emergency department. Also, the duration of the hospital stay is shorter and the cost is less. (LOE = 1b)

Reference

Mueller C, Laule-Kilian K, Frana B, et al. Use of B-type natriuretic peptide in the management of acute dyspnea in patients with pulmonary disease. Am Heart J 2006;151:471–477.

Study Design

Randomized controlled trial (single-blinded)

Funding

Foundation

Allocation

Concealed

Setting

Emergency department

Synopsis

This report is a subgroup analysis of the BASEL study (N Engl J Med 2004;350:647–54), which showed the effectiveness of BNP testing in the management of patients with HF who present with acute decompensation to an emergency department. In this analysis, 226 patients had a history of pulmonary disease: 72% had a history of chronic obstructive pulmonary disease or asthma. Other pulmonary diseases included a history of pneumonia, pulmonary embolism, and interstitial lung disease. Patients were randomly assigned (allocation concealed) to usual care supplemented by a rapid BNP test, or the usual diagnostic protocol without knowledge of BNP level. Clinicians were advised that a BNP level less than 100 pg/mL made HF unlikely, a result greater than 500 pg/mL made HF very likely, and that intermediate values required additional information and clinical judgment to make the diagnosis. The BNP was not measured during any subsequent hospitalization. Outcomes were assessed by a group blinded to treatment assignment. HF was the major cause of acute dyspnea in 39% of patients, closely followed by an exacerbation of obstructive pulmonary disease (33%), and pneumonia (16%). Patients in the BNP group were less likely to be admitted (81% vs 91%; P = .034) and spent less time in the hospital (9 days vs 12 days; P = .001). The median cost of care was lower in the BNP group ($4841 US vs $5671 US; P = .008). In-hospital mortality was similar in both groups. These results parallel the results demonstrated in the complete BASEL study.

Essential Evidence: Medicine that Matters, Edited by David Slawson, Allen Shaughnessy, Mark Ebell, and Henry Barry.

Serial BNP levels predict risk of death and CHF after ACS

Clinical question

Are serial assessments of B-type natriuretic peptide levels useful in the prognosis of patients with unstable coronary artery disease?

Bottom line

Serial determination of B-type natriuretic peptide (BNP) during follow-up of patients after an acute coronary syndrome (ACS) helps predict the risk of subsequent death or congestive heart failure (CHF). It remains uncertain whether having this information will lead to a change in clinical management that improves patient-oriented outcomes or simply increases costs without any added benefit. (LOE = 1b)

Reference

Morrow DA, de Lemos JA, Blazing MA, et al. Prognostic value of serial B-type natriuretic peptide testing during follow-up of patients with unstable coronary artery disease. JAMA 2005;294:2866–2871.

Study Design

Cohort (prospective)

Funding

Industry

Setting

Inpatient (any location) with outpatient follow-up

Synopsis

BNP is released from cardiac muscle in response to ischemic stress. Elevated base-line levels in patients with ACS are associated with both short-term and long-term mortality. To determine the value of serial measurements after an ACS, the investigators prospectively followed up 4497 patients with non-ST elevation or ST-elevation ACS enrolled in a clinical trial evaluating early intensive versus less aggressive statin treatment. Follow-up occurred for 3618 (85%) and 2966 (70%) of patients at 4 months and 12 months, respectively. Individuals performing tests were blinded to clinical outcomes and treatment allocation. A total of 230 deaths and 163 incident cases of CHF occurred during follow-up. After adjustment for other risk factors, elevated levels of BNP (greater than 80 pg/mL) at 4 months and 12 months were significantly associated with an increased risk of subsequent death or new CHF (hazard ratio [HR] = 3.9; 95% CI, 2.6–6.0; and HR = 4.7; 95% CI, 2.5–8.9, respectively) . Patients with elevated levels of BNP at study entry and with follow-up BNP levels of less than 80 pg/mL had a nonsignificantly increased risk compared with patients with BNP levels of less than 80 pg/mL at both visits. Patients with elevated BNP levels at baseline and at 4 months had the highest risk of death or new CHF.

Essential Evidence: Medicine that Matters, Edited by David Slawson, Allen Shaughnessy, Mark Ebell, and Henry Barry.

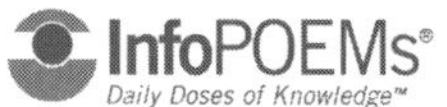

Higher BNP and N-ANP predict CV events

Clinical question

Does an elevated B-natriuretic peptide in an asymptomatic patient predict adverse cardiovascular events?

Bottom line

B-natriuretic peptide and N-terminal atrial natriuretic peptide are independent predictors of adverse cardiovascular events. However, it is not at all clear what to do with this information, or whether having this information leads to improved clinical outcomes. Use of these tests for prognosis should therefore await further clinical trials that examine the benefit or harm or intervening in patients with an elevated BNP level. (LOE = 1b)

Reference

Wang TJ, Larson MG, Levy D, et al. Plasma natriuretic peptide levels and the risk of cardiovascular events and death. N Engl J Med 2004;350:655–663.

Study Design

Cohort (prospective)

Setting

Population-based

Synopsis

B-natriuretic peptide (BNP) and N-terminal atrial natriuretic peptide (N-ANP) are released in response to atrial or ventricular wall stretch and are widely used in the diagnosis of heart failure. Their role as predictors of cardiovascular mortality has not been well studied. The authors identified 3346 Framingham Offspring Study participants with no known heart failure (all underwent baseline echocardiography) or renal failure. Their mean age was 58 years, 47% were men, 10% had diabetes, 15% smoked, and only a small percentage had a previous myocardial infarction (7% of men, 1% of women). Patients were followed up prospectively for a mean of 5.2 years, and outcomes were adjudicated by a central group blinded to the BNP or N-ANP levels. Results were adjusted for risk factors such as age, sex, hypertension, diabetes, lipids, body mass index, serum creatinine, and tobacco use. The authors found that the risk of death increased by 27% for each 1 standard deviation increase in BNP and by 41% for a similar increase in N-ANP. The risk of individual end points, such as first major cardiovascular event, diagnosis of heart failure, atrial fibrillation, or stroke or transient ischemic attack, were all increased for patients with a BNP level greater than the 80th percentile (20 pg/mL for men and 23.3 pg/mL for women). However, there was no association with coronary heart disease events.

Essential Evidence: Medicine that Matters, Edited by David Slawson, Allen Shaughnessy, Mark Ebell, and Henry Barry.

ARBs = ACEIs for all-cause mortality in heart failure

Clinical question

Do angiotensin receptor blockers offer advantages over ACE inhibitors in patients with heart failure?

Bottom line

ARBs are no better than ACE inhibitors in preventing all cause mortality in patients with heart failure. Treating 23 patients for 2 years with an ARB and an ACE inhibitor, instead of an ACE inhibitor alone, may prevent 1 hospitalization, although this finding is largely from a single study of valsartan and further studies are needed to confirm this benefit given the greatly increased cost of such a regimen. (LOE = 1a)

Reference

Jong P, Demers C, McKelvie RS, Liu PP. Angiotensin receptor blockers in heart failure: meta-analysis of randomized controlled trials. J Am Coll Cardiol 2002;39:463–470.

Study Design

Meta-analysis of randomized controlled trials

Setting

Various (meta-analysis)

Synopsis

This is an excellent meta-analysis. The authors did a careful search using the Cochrane Collaboration strategy. They included 17 randomized, blinded clinical trials of at least 4 weeks' duration that compared an angiotensin receptor blocker (ARB) with an angiotensin converting enzyme (ACE) inhibitor in patients with New York Heart Association grade II–IV heart failure. Abstracts and non-peer-reviewed studies were excluded, as were studies that did not report death or hospitalization as an end point. Analyses used the intention-to-treat principle, and heterogeneity of studies was tested. There were 4 main comparisons: ARB vs control (either placebo or ACE inhibitor), ARB vs placebo, ARB vs ACE inhibitor, and ARB plus ACE inhibitor vs ACE inhibitor alone. For all cause mortality, there was no benefit to ARB in any of these comparisons. Regarding the risk of hospitalization, there was a small benefit for the combination of ARB plus ACE inhibitor over ACE inhibitor alone (odds ratio = 0.74; 95% CI, 0.64–0.86; number needed to treat = 23 for approximately 2 years).

Essential Evidence: Medicine that Matters, Edited by David Slawson, Allen Shaughnessy, Mark Ebell, and Henry Barry.

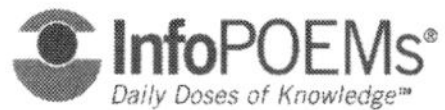

Optimal digoxin range for men 0.5 to 0.8 ng/ml

Clinical question

What is the optimal serum digoxin concentration for men with heart failure?

Bottom line

The optimal serum digoxin concentration at 1 month in men with stable heart failure in sinus rhythm is 0.5 to 0.8 ng/mL. Higher levels are associated with either no reduction or an increase in mortality. (LOE = 1b−)

Reference

Rathore SS, Curtis JP, Want Y, Bristow MR, Krumholz HM. Association of serum digoxin concentration and outcomes in patients with heart failure. JAMA 2003;289:871–878.

Study Design

Randomized controlled trial (double-blinded)

Setting

Outpatient (any)

Synopsis

Recent findings from the Digitalis Investigation Group (DIG) trial suggest strongly that only men with heart failure benefit from treatment with digoxin. In this post hoc analysis of data from the original 3-year randomized controlled trial, the authors assessed variations in serum digoxin concentration (SDC) and their associations with mortality. Findings from other studies have suggested that lower SDCs may lead to a reduction in mortality. Men were clinically stable with a left ventricular ejection fraction of 45% or less and were in sinus rhythm. Blood samples were drawn at least 6 hours after their previous digoxin dose. Men assigned to digoxin therapy were divided into 3 groups based on their SDC. Outcomes were assessed by individuals blinded to treatment group assignment. Of the 1171 men with SDCs assessed at 1 month, 572 (49%) had an SDC of 0.5 to 0.8 ng/mL, 322 (27%) had an SDC of 0.9 to 1.1 ng/mL, and 277 (24%) had an SDC of 1.2 ng/mL or higher. Men with an SDC of 0.5 to 0.8 ng/mL had a 6.3% lower mortality rate compared with men taking placebo. There was no associated reduction in mortality among men with SDCs of 0.9 to 1.1 ng/mL. However, men with SDCs of 1.2 ng/mL and higher had an 11.8% increased mortality rate compared with men in the placebo group. The association between higher SDC levels and increased mortality persisted after adjustment for potentially confounding variables.

Essential Evidence: Medicine that Matters, Edited by David Slawson, Allen Shaughnessy, Mark Ebell, and Henry Barry.

Digoxin increases mortality in women with heart failure

Clinical question

Does digoxin have a different effect in women than in men?

Bottom line

As compared with its use in men, digoxin increases mortality in women with CHF, and, given the small benefit of digoxin (only a possible reduction in hospitalization rates for women) it should be avoided. While careful attention to digoxin levels may avoid bad outcomes in women, we have no proof of this. (LOE = 1b–)

Reference

Rathore SS, Wang Y, and Krumholz HM. Sex-based differences in the effect of digoxin for the treatment of heart failure. N Engl J Med 2002;347:1403–1411.

Study Design

Randomized controlled trial (double-blinded)

Setting

Outpatient (any)

Synopsis

The Digitalis Investigation Group (DIG) trial randomized 5281 men and 1519 women with congestive heart failure (CHF) to either digoxin or placebo. After 3 years of follow-up, they found a reduction in hospitalization but no change in mortality. This reanalysis of the DIG data looked at the outcomes separately for men and women. While post-hoc analyses like these can be accused of data-dredging, in this case they had a valid hypothesis based on data from other studies suggesting a differential outcome for women and men with CHF. Women in the DIG study were very different from the men: older, higher median ejection fraction, shorter duration of CHF, and greater severity of disease by NYHA class. In the analysis, the authors looked at the interaction between sex and digoxin use. They found that women, but not men, had a higher all-cause mortality on digoxin (absolute risk increase 5.8%). Thus, for every 17.8 women who took digoxin for 3 years, there was one additional death. An obvious question is whether women received too much digoxin, and therefore had more toxicity. While men and women received similar doses per unit of body mass index (0.0093 mg vs 0.0084 mg), the median serum digoxin level was a bit higher for women at 1 month (0.9 vs 0.8 ng/ml, p = 0.007). At 12 months, the levels were the same, though (0.6 ng/ml) and there was no significant difference in the percentage with a level over 2.0 ng/ml at 1 and 12 months. Also, there was no difference in hospitalizations for digoxin toxicity.

Essential Evidence: Medicine that Matters, Edited by David Slawson, Allen Shaughnessy, Mark Ebell, and Henry Barry.

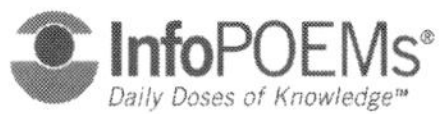

Nesiritide for CHF may increase mortality risk

Clinical question

Is nesiritide (Natrecor) effective in the treatment of patients with congestive heart failure?

Bottom line

Although it improves short-term symptoms, nesiritide (Natrecor) may increase the risk of death at 30 days when used in the treatment of acute decompensated heart failure. This review should mandate a large-scale, adequately powered, randomized trial to definitively evaluate this treatment. (LOE = 1a–)

Reference

Sackner-Bernstein JD, Kowalski M, Fox M, Aaronson K. Short-term risk of death after treatment with nesiritide for decompensated heart failure. A pooled analysis of randomized controlled trials. JAMA 2005;293:1900–1905.

Study Design

Meta-analysis (randomized controlled trials)

Funding

Unknown/not stated

Setting

Various (meta-analysis)

Synopsis

Nesiritide (Natrecor) improves symptoms in patients with acute congestive heart failure but long-term safety and efficacy is uncertain. The investigators obtained all registered controlled trials on file from the US Food and Drug Administration and searched PubMed and abstracts from annual meetings of various cardiology and heart association meetings for additional studies. Included studies were randomized double-blind group studies of nesiritide administered as a single infusion versus placebo reporting 30-day mortality. Only 3 trials with a total of 862 subjects met all inclusion criteria. Although not statistically significant, 30-day mortality was higher among patients in the nesiritide group (7.2% vs 4.0%; P = .059). There was no evidence for heterogeneity among the 3 trials. The authors did not analyze the potential for publication bias to affect the results.

Implantable defibrillators reduces mortality in NYHA Class II heart failure

Clinical question

For patients with moderate or severe heart failure, is amiodarone or an implanatable defibrillator the best way to reduce mortality?

Bottom line

Patients with moderate to severe heart failure benefit from an implantable ICD (NNT = 14 for 4 year mortality). However, the benefit was confined to the subgroup with NYHA Class II disease in this study. Those with NYHA Class III HF did not benefit from ICD, and amiodarone actually increased mortality in that subgroup. (LOE = 1b)

Reference

Bardy GH, Kerry LL, Mark DB, et al. Amiodarone or an implantable cardioverter-defibrillator for congestive heart failure. N Engl J Med 2005;352:225–237.

Study Design	Funding	Allocation
Randomized controlled trial (nonblinded)	Industry + govt	Uncertain

Setting

Outpatient (specialty)

Synopsis

Patients with heart failure are at increased of sudden death. Could these patients benefit from an implantable cardioverter-defibrillator (ICD)? The researchers in this study recruited patients with moderate systolic heart failure (HF) defined as an ejection fraction of less than 35%. Patients were identified as having ischemic HF if they had at least one coronary artery with 75% stenosis or a history of acute myocardial infarction (AMI). Patients were randomly assigned (allocation concealment uncertain) to receive either amiodarone (median dose 300 mg daily, n = 845), placebo pill (n = 847), or a single lead ICD programmed to treat only sustained ventricular tachycardia or ventricular fibrillation (n = 829). Groups were balanced at the beginning of the study, with an average age of 60 years, 23% being women, and an average ejection fraction of 25%. Patients were followed for a mean of 45 months and the vital status (i.e. whether they were alive or dead) was known for each of the 2521 patients at the end of the study. About one-third of patients with an ICD were shocked at some point during follow-up. All-cause mortality was lower in the ICD group than in the amiodarone or placebo groups (22% vs 28% vs 29%, p = 0.007, number need to treat compared with amiodarone = 17 over four years). Patients with NYHA Class II HF had a clear benefit, while those with NYHA Class III HF did not. The authors argue that we should embrace the results for patients with NYHA Class II HF but ignore those for patients with more severe disease, since other studies in studies with different inclusion criteria showed greater absolute benefit with greater disease. The alternate view is that in patients with more severe disease, the episode of VT or VF is an indicator of worsening death and the ICD merely prolongs the inevitable for a few days or weeks. It is also noteworthy that amiodarone did not improve survival compared with placebo in patients with NYHA Class II heart failure and actually increased mortality in those with Class III HF (hazard ratio 1.44, 95% CI 1.05 to 1.97), and that there was no difference overall between patients with ischemic and non-ischemic causes of HF.

Essential Evidence: Medicine that Matters, Edited by David Slawson, Allen Shaughnessy, Mark Ebell, and Henry Barry.

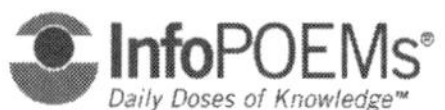

Herbs may reduce cholesterol, no data on clinical outcomes

Clinical question
Can herbal supplements reduce cholesterol?

Bottom line
The herbal supplements fenugreek, red yeast rice, artichoke, and guggul may reduce cholesterol, although the quality and consistency of studies is poor. There is no evidence that using these herbs improves clinical outcomes, although they do appear to be safe. (LOE = 1b–)

Reference
Coon JST, Ernst E. Herbs for serum cholesterol reduction: a systematic review. J Fam Pract 2003;52:468–478.

Study Design
Systematic review

Setting
Various (meta-analysis)

Synopsis
There is reasonably good evidence that garlic modestly lowers cholesterol, but we have no reason to believe it improves patient-oriented outcomes. This thorough review of the literature looked at other herbs, such as fenugreek, red yeast rice, artichoke, and guggul (whatever that is; it sounds like a character from the Lord of the Rings to me). They found 25 studies, but 13 had a Jadad score of 2 or lower on a scale from 0 to 5, and all but a few were quite small. Results were mixed, and in many cases the herb lowered cholesterol levels, but no more than placebo. None of the studies measured patient-oriented outcomes.

Essential Evidence: Medicine that Matters, Edited by David Slawson, Allen Shaughnessy, Mark Ebell, and Henry Barry.

Statins prevent CAD

Clinical question

Are statins effective in preventing coronary artery disease?

Bottom line

Statins reduce 5-year overall mortality, and specifically decrease cardiovascular mortality and morbidity. The patients at highest baseline risk derive the greatest benefit. (LOE = 1a)

Reference

Baigent C, Keech A, Kearney PM, et al, for the Cholesterol Treatment Trialists' (CTT) Collaborators. Efficacy and safety of cholesterol-lowering treatment: prospective meta-analysis of data from 90,056 participants in 14 randomised trials of statins. Lancet 2005;366:1267–1278.

Study Design

Meta-analysis (randomized controlled trials)

Funding

Industry + govt

Setting

Outpatient (any)

Synopsis

The investigators from 14 major trials of lipid lowering that used statins (eg, WOSCOPS, 4S, AFCAPS, GISSI, PROSPER, and so forth) pooled the data on 90,056 patients to provide more robust information on individual outcomes. Nine of the trials were secondary prevention studies. The median follow-up was 4.7 years (range = 2–6). Overall, the studies were composed mostly of men; approximately 21% had diabetes and 54% had cardiovascular disease. In other words, close to 1 in 5 adults in the United States would have been eligible to participate in these studies. Statins decreased all-cause mortality (8.5% vs 9.6%; number needed to treat (NNT; ie, the number of additional patients that need to be treated with a statin for 4.7 years to prevent 1 outcome) = 86; 95% CI, 65–126). The authors report that this translated to a 12% relative reduction for every mmol/L of low-density lipoprotein reduction. Similarly, statins reduced cardiovascular death (3.4% vs 4.4%; NNT = 109; 86–150). The rate of major coronary events was lower (NNT = 42; 36–49) with statins, as were the rates of revascularizations (NNT = 56; 47–68) and strokes (NNT = 162; 118–259). Additionally, statins were beneficial regardless of age or sex, although the magnitude of benefit was greater for those younger than 65 years (NNT = 68; 57–82; for older patients: NNT = 111, 86–155) and for men (NNT = 48; 42–57; for women: NNT = 326; 213–700). Although reductions in major coronary events are seen within the first year, they are greater with longer use and are proportional to the absolute risk at baseline. In other words, the highest risk patients derive the greatest benefit. These pooled data also did not find any association with developing incident cancers, in total or site specific. After 5 years, 0.01% more patients using statins will develop rhabdomyolysis ($P = .4$). The authors don't report on pooled drop-out rates or how many patients experience liver failure, hepatic enzyme elevation, myalgias, or arthralgias. A word of caution: Most, if not all, of these trials used targeted doses of statins and did not randomize patients to specific lipid levels. Since the effects of statins may be independent of their lipid-lowering effect, using the lipid levels inferred from these trials should be done with some trepidation.

Essential Evidence: Medicine that Matters, Edited by David Slawson, Allen Shaughnessy, Mark Ebell, and Henry Barry.

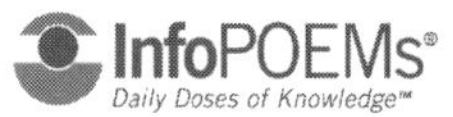

Cholesterol lowering cost-effective in high-risk elderly

Clinical question

What is the cost-effectiveness of pravastatin treatment of high-risk patients aged 65 years to 75 years?

Bottom line

From the viewpoint of a health system, it is cost-effective to treat high-risk patients older than 65 years with pravastatin (Pravachol) no matter what their level of initial cholesterol level. The increased cost of treatment is partially offset by savings in other areas. This analysis did not take into account any effect on the quality of the life extension by pravastatin. (LOE = 2c)

Reference

Tonkin AM, Eckermann S, White H, et al, for the LIPID Study Group. Cost-effectiveness of cholesterol-lowering therapy with pravastatin in patients with previous acute coronary syndromes aged 65–74 years compared with younger patients: Results from the LIPID study. Am Heart J 2006;151:1305–1312.

Study Design	Funding	Setting
Cost-effectiveness analysis	Unknown/not stated	Outpatient (any)

Synopsis

The Australian researchers conducting this study used data from the LIPID study conducted in the early 1990s to estimate the relative cost of treating high-risk patients with pravastatin to lower their risk of mortality and hospitalization. The perspective was from the viewpoint of the healthcare system. The 9014 patients had a history of either myocardial infarction or unstable angina, a cholesterol level ranging from 115 mg/dL to 271 mg/dL (4.0–7.0 mmol/L), and were randomly treated with placebo or pravastatin 40 mg daily for 6 years. This analysis evaluated the cost-effectiveness of the treatment in patients between the ages of 65 years and 75 years as compared with patients younger than 65 years. To determine cost the authors used actual data on hospitalizations, office visits, diagnostic tests, nursing home stays, and medications, expressed as Australian dollars and reflecting costs to the Australian healthcare system. No utilities were used to evaluate outcomes; that is, the researchers did not evaluate the effect of treatment on quality of life. The analysis was based on a decrease in all-cause mortality from 20.6% to 16.3% in older patients and from 9.8% to 7.5% in younger patients. This translates into an additional 4.7 months to 4.8 months of additional life in the average patient. The average cost-per-patient for treatment was A$4792 for older patients and A$4989 in younger patients. These costs were somewhat offset in both groups by decreases in the costs of other medications, hospitalizations, and other costs. The overall additional cost of treatment was lower for older patients (A$2140 for older patients, A$3539 for younger patients). For every 1000 patients aged 65 years to 74 years, pravastatin treatment for 6 years prevented 43 deaths at a cost of A$2.1 million, or A$55,474 per life saved. In the younger patient group, 31 deaths were prevented at a cost of A$3.5 million, or A$167,161 per life saved. These estimates were not adjusted for quality of life; thus, the quality of a life saved in the younger group could be better than that of a life saved in the older group. As a result, quality-adjusted life estimates, which takes more into account the viewpoint of the patient could be different from these estimates.

Essential Evidence: Medicine that Matters, Edited by David Slawson, Allen Shaughnessy, Mark Ebell, and Henry Barry.

Intensive lipid lowering of marginal benefit even if high-risk

Clinical question

What is the benefit of intensive lipid lowering in patients with stable coronary disease?

Bottom line

The benefit of intensive lipid therapy in patients with known heart disease is very modest: a number needed to treat (NNT) of 45 for 5 years to prevent any cardiovascular outcome. There was no difference in all-cause mortality between intensive and less intensive treatment groups (5.6% vs 5.7%), and the study was large enough and long enough to be able to detect such a benefit if one existed. Since the benefit of lipid lowering is greatest in patients with known disease, any benefit is certainly much less lower for patients without known disease who are at much lower risk. (LOE = 1b)

Reference

LaRosa JC, Grundy SM, Waters DD, et al, for the Treating to New Targets (TNT) Investigators. Intensive lipid lowering with atorvastatin in patients with stable coronary disease. N Engl J Med 2005;352:1425–1435.

Study Design	Funding	Allocation
Randomized controlled trial (double-blinded)	Industry	Uncertain

Setting

Outpatient (any)

Synopsis

How low should we go? Recent guidelines have been urging us to lower the low-density lipoprotein (LDL) of patients at very high risk of coronary artery disease to 70 mg/dL. In this study, 15,464 adults with a known coronary artery disease (angina with objective evidence of coronary artery disease, previous myocardial infarction [MI], or previous coronary revascularization) and an LDL between 130 mg/dL and 250 mg/dL were given 10 mg of atorvastatin daily for 8 weeks. Anyone with an LDL lower than 130 mg/dL (n = 10,003) at the end of this active run-in period entered the study and was randomized to atorvastatin at a dose of 10 mg or 80 mg per day. Patients were followed up for a median of 4.9 years. The higher dose of atorvastatin reduced the LDL cholesterol level more than the lower dose (to an average 77 mg/dL vs 101 mg/dL). The primary outcome was the usual cardiovascular combined outcome of death from coronary heart disease, nonfatal MI, resuscitation after cardiac arrest, or stroke. This outcome was slightly less common among patients receiving high-dose atorvastatin (8.7% vs 10.9%; $P < .001$; number needed to treat [NNT] = 45 for 5 years), largely because of fewer nonfatal MIs. However, there was no difference in the likelihood of death from any cause (5.6% vs 5.7%). Both doses of the drug were well tolerated, which isn't surprising given the active drug run-in period. Adverse events were more common in the high-dose atorvastatin group (8.1% vs 5.8%; $P < .001$; number needed to treat to harm [NNTH] = 43 for 5 years) as were discontinuation rates (7.2% vs 5.3%; $P < .001$; NNTH = 52 for 5 years). There were only 5 cases of rhabdomyolysis – 2 in one group and 3 in the other – among the 10,000 participants. These findings are consistent with those of another recent article (Arch Intern Med 2005;165:725–30; see POEM June 2005).

Essential Evidence: Medicine that Matters, Edited by David Slawson, Allen Shaughnessy, Mark Ebell, and Henry Barry.

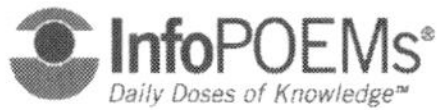

Varying effects of lipid drugs on overall mortality

Clinical question

What methods of lipid lowering decrease overall mortality in patients with hyperlipidemia?

Bottom line

Only statin lipid-lowering drugs have been shown to decrease overall mortality in patients with high cholesterol but without evidence of heart disease. However, most patients treated with one of these drugs will not benefit: 228 have to be treated for 3.3 years to prevent 1 additional death during this period. In patients with known heart disease, statins and fish oil both have been shown to decrease mortality. Niacin, resins, and diet have not been shown to decrease mortality. Fibrates (gemfibrozil and others) actually increase overall mortality and at the same time decrease cardiac mortality. (LOE = 1a)

Reference

Studer M, Briel M, Leimenstoll B, Glass TR, Bucher HC. Effect of different antilipidemic agents and diets on mortality. A systematic review. Arch Intern Med 2005;165:725–730.

Study Design

Meta-analysis (randomized controlled trials)

Funding

Self-funded or unfunded

Setting

Various (meta-analysis)

Synopsis

Do all lipid-lowering drugs make people live longer, on average? These researchers searched 4 databases to find randomized trials addressing this question. Two authors then independently determined whether each study was suitable for inclusion, only including studies that were randomized and were conducted over at least 3 months. They included studies that enrolled patients without evidence of heart disease – primary prevention as well as secondary prevention studies that enrolled patients with known heart disease. They included studies written in any language and ended up with 97 studies enrolling more than 275,000 patients. Only statins and n-3 fatty acids (fish oils or linolenic acid) decreased overall mortality and the effect of the n-3 fatty acids was only seen with patients with pre-existing heart disease. In primary prevention trials, fibrates (fenofibrate, clofibrate, gemfibrozil) increased mortality, with one additional death in every 132 patients treated for an average 4.4 years (number needed to treat to harm [NNTH] = 132; 95% CI, 69–662). Many patients have to be treated with a statin to prevent one additional death; the number needed to treat for 3.3 years was 228 (123–2958). In patients with known heart disease, 50 patients (38–78) would have to be treated with a statin to prevent one additional death and 44 patients (31–84) would need to be treated with fish oil to prevent one additional death, each over an average 4.4 years (excluding one low-quality study). Treatment with diet, resins (colestipol, cholestyramine), or niacin did not affect overall mortality.

Statins equivalent for CVD prevention

Clinical question

Are there any differences in outcomes among the major statins?

Bottom line

The overall effectiveness of statin therapy on the most important outcomes – decreasing mortality, heart attacks, and strokes – is not different among the 3 major statins. These are the results from a meta-analysis; no study has directly compared equivalent doses of 2 statins. (LOE = 1a)

Reference

Zhou Z, Rahme E, Pilote L. Are statins created equal? Evidence from randomized trials of pravastatin, simvastatin, and atorvastatin for cardiovascular disease prevention. Am Heart J 2006;151:273–281.

Study Design

Meta-analysis (randomized controlled trials)

Funding

Self-funded or unfunded

Setting

Outpatient (any)

Synopsis

The researchers conducted this analysis of the research on the benefit of statins in the prevention of cardiovascular disease (CVD). The statins under consideration were pravastatin (Pravachol), simvastatin (Zocor), and atorvastatin (Lipitor). They authors identified, through a search of MEDLINE and the Cochrane Controlled Trials Register databases, all randomized controlled trials of at least 1000 participants that evaluated CVD or mortality as an outcome over the course of at least 1 year. The used only English language studies. They took other short cuts in the systematic review process that likely had little effect on their conclusions; they did not perform duplicate searching or data abstraction. They identified 8 studies enrolling almost 64,000 people that compared 1 of the statins with either placebo or usual care. The authors did not include the single study that directly compared 2 statins since the marketing-friendly goal of that study was to compare the intensity of treatment rather than the relative effectiveness of the 2 drugs. All studies showed a similar degree of reduction in lipid levels. There was no difference among the statins in reducing fatal coronary heart disease, nonfatal myocardial infarctions, fatal and nonfatal strokes, all cardiovascular deaths, or mortality due to any cause.

Essential Evidence: Medicine that Matters, Edited by David Slawson, Allen Shaughnessy, Mark Ebell, and Henry Barry.

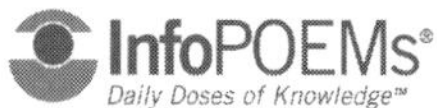

Intensive lipid lowering with statins unnecessary with stable CAD (IDEAL)

Clinical question

Is intensive lowering of serum lipids with statin drugs beneficial in patients with stable coronary artery disease?

Bottom line

The intensive reduction of low-density lipoprotein (LDL) levels to well below 100 mg/dL (2.5 mmol/L) did not result in a significant reduction in the recurrence of major coronary events or all-cause mortality among patients with stable coronary artery disease. Intensive lowering is associated with an increased risk of discontinuing medication because of adverse events and significant drug costs. Aiming for an LDL of approximately 100 mg/dL (2.5 mmol/L) seems optimal for the majority of patients with stable disease. (LOE = 1b–)

Reference

Pedersen TR, Faergeman O, Kastelein JJ, et al, for the Incremental Decrease in End Points Through Aggressive Lipid Lowering (IDEAL) Study Group. High-dose atorvastatin vs usual-dose simvastatin for secondary prevention after myocardial infarction. The IDEAL study: A randomized controlled trial. JAMA 2005;294:2437–2445.

Study Design	Funding	Allocation
Randomized controlled trial (single-blinded)	Industry	Uncertain

Setting

Outpatient (specialty)

Synopsis

Intensive lowering of LDL to well below 100 mg/dL (2.5 mmol/L) is beneficial for patients with acute coronary syndromes. It is uncertain, however, if similar treatment provides further benefit in stable coronary artery disease. These investigators enrolled 8888 adults from 190 ambulatory cardiology care and specialist practices in northern Europe. The patients were 80 years or younger, with a history of a definite myocardial infarction, and were randomly assigned (uncertain allocation concealment) to receive a high dose of atorvastatin (80 mg/d) or usual-dose simvastatin (20 mg/d). If, at 24 weeks of follow-up, plasma total cholesterol level was higher than 190 mg/dL (5.0 mmol/L), the dose of simvastatin could be increased to 40 mg/d. Follow-up occurred for nearly 100% of patients for 4.8 years. Individuals assessing outcomes were blinded to treatment group assignment. The primary outcome was recurrence of a major coronary event, defined as coronary death, hospitalization for nonfatal acute myocardial infarction, or cardiac arrest with resuscitation. During treatment, mean LDL levels were 104 mg/dL (2.7 mmol/L) in the simvastatin group and 81 mg/dL (2.1 mmol/L) in the atorvastatin group. Using intention-to-treat analysis, there was no statistical difference in the reoccurrence of a major coronary event between the 2 groups. The risk of death from any cause, including noncardiovascular causes, is also similar in both groups. The investigators report a number of different post hoc secondary outcomes showing benefit to intensive lipid lowering, but the important patient-oriented outcomes of living better and living longer are improved little, if at all, with intensive lowering. Discontinuation rates were higher in the atorvastatin group because of adverse events.

Essential Evidence: Medicine that Matters, Edited by David Slawson, Allen Shaughnessy, Mark Ebell, and Henry Barry.

JNC 7 report on prevention/evaluation/treatment of hypertension

Clinical question

What are the best methods to prevent, detect, evaluate, and treat hypertension?

Bottom line

(LOE = 2a)

Reference

Chobanian AV, Bakris GL, Black HR, et al. The seventh report of the Joint National Committee on prevention, detection, evaluation, and treatment of high blood pressure. JAMA 2003;289:2560–2572.

Study Design

Practice guideline

Setting

Various (guideline)

Synopsis

No surprises here. Key messages: 1. Systolic blood pressure (SBP) higher than 140 mm Hg is more important than diastolic blood pressure (DBP). 2. Anyone with an SBP of 120 to 139 mm Hg or a DBP of 80 to 89 mm Hg should be considered prehypertensive and encouraged to adopt a health-promoting lifestyle. There is no evidence, however, that this results in any long-term benefits. 3. Thiazide-type diuretics should be the initial drug used for almost everyone, except those patients with certain high-risk conditions: For those with stable coronary artery disease (CAD) – use a beta-blocker; unstable CAD – beta-blocker and angiotensin-converting enzyme (ACE) inhibitor; postmyocardial infarction – beta-blocker and ACE inhibitor; asymptomatic congestive heart failure (CHF) with proven ventricular dysfunction – beta-blocker and ACE inhibitor; symptomatic CHF – beta-blocker, ACE inhibitor, and aldosterone blocker; chronic renal disease – ACE inhibitor (it is okay to accept increase in creatinine up to 35% over baseline unless hyperkalemia develops). 4. Diuretics are preferred as a first-line treatment for patients with diabetes, unless they also have established renal disease (defined as glomerular filtration rate <60 mL/min; albuminuria >300 mg/d (positive on a urine dipstick; microalbuminuria alone does not warrant a change from diuretics); and patients with left ventricular hypertrophy alone with no evidence of ventricular dysfunction. Calcium channel blockers are NOT first-line agents for anyone. 5. Target goals are BP lower than 140/90 mm Hg for uncomplicated hypertension, and lower than 130/80 mm Hg for patients with diabetes or renal disease.

Essential Evidence: Medicine that Matters, Edited by David Slawson, Allen Shaughnessy, Mark Ebell, and Henry Barry.

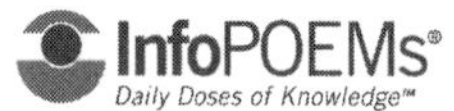

Work stress has no meaningful effect on blood pressure

Clinical question

Does work stress increase blood pressure?

Bottom line

Work stress has no meaningful effect on blood pressure. (LOE = 1b)

Reference

Guimont C, Brisson C, Dagenais GR, et al. Effects of job strain on blood pressure: a prospective study of male and female white-collar workers. Am J Public Health 2006;96:1436–1443.

Study Design

Cohort (prospective)

Funding

Foundation

Setting

Population-based

Synopsis

"I don't need medication; my blood pressure is only high because of my stressful job." How should you respond? This team of researchers observed more than 6000 white-collar workers (men and women) for 7.5 years (84% follow-up). They excluded anyone with known cardiovascular disease and hypertension at baseline. The participants completed a series of scales to assess job stress and other psychological demands of work. Additionally, the study team assessed each participant's vital signs, body mass index, tobacco use, exercise patterns, and so forth. Women had no difference in their blood pressure whether exposed to stress at baseline or at follow-up, or at both, or neither. Men who experienced no work stress at baseline or at follow-up also showed no change in blood pressure. The excited authors, however, point out a graded response: Stress levels present only at baseline were less important than stress levels only at follow-up, and when men's stress levels were present at both baseline and at follow-up, the systolic blood pressure increased a whopping 1.8 mm Hg. This is a perfect example of how researchers can confuse and mislead us with statistics. Yes, the difference was statistically significant, but the clinical difference was trivial.

Essential Evidence: Medicine that Matters, Edited by David Slawson, Allen Shaughnessy, Mark Ebell, and Henry Barry.

Pseudoephedrine has a minimal effect on blood pressure

Clinical question
Does pseudoephedrine (Sudafed) increase blood pressure in people or in patients with hypertension?

Bottom line
Overall, immediate-release pseudoephedrine produces a small increase in systolic blood pressure (1.5 mmHg) but has no effect on diastolic blood pressure. Sustained-release products do not affect blood pressure. Both types of products increase heart rate to a small degree. Unlike its cousin phenylpropanolamine, pseudoephedrine rarely causes large increases in blood pressure, although its effect on blood pressure is dose-related and a marked effect could occur with overdose. (LOE = 1a)

Reference
Salerno SM, Jackson JL, Berbano EP. Effect of oral pseudoephedrine on blood pressure and heart rate. Arch Intern Med 2005;165:1686–1694.

Study Design
Meta-analysis (randomized controlled trials)

Funding
Self-funded or unfunded

Setting
Outpatient (any)

Synopsis
The decongestant pseudoephedrine is pharmacologically related to phenylpropanolamine, the decongestant and anorectic banned from sale in the United States and other countries because of an increased risk of hemorrhagic stroke likely due to increased blood pressure. This meta-analysis evaluated the effect of pseudoephedrine on blood pressure as measured in 24 studies including 1285 patients. To identify studies for inclusion, the authors searched MEDLINE, EMBASE, the Cochrane Clinical Trials Registry, and references of reviewed articles for English-language research studies. They looked for extractable blood pressure in any study comparing pseudoephedrine with placebo, whether the studies addressed its safety or effectiveness for any number of conditions. Study quality was assessed independently by 2 reviewers. Immediate-release pseudoephedrine caused a slight, but statistically significant, increase in systolic blood pressure (1.53 mmHg; 95% CI, .49–2.56). Heart rate was also increased slightly, 2.3 beats per minute (1.42–3.19), but diastolic blood pressure was not affected, on average. Sustained-release pseudoephedrine had no effect on systolic or diastolic blood pressure but increased heart rate more so than the immediate-release version (4.48 beats/min; 3.31–5.64). In 7 trials of patients with known, stable hypertension, pseudoephedrine slightly increased systolic blood pressure by 1.2 mmHg but had no effect on diastolic blood pressure or heart rate. With regard to wide swings in blood pressure, of 1108 patients in 24 studies, only 2 patients experienced a large – 20 mmHg – increase in arterial pressure. One patient reported anxiety, a diastolic pressure of 100 mmHg, and a 25% increase in heart rate, and 1 patient reported anxiety and sinus tachycardia.

Essential Evidence: Medicine that Matters, Edited by David Slawson, Allen Shaughnessy, Mark Ebell, and Henry Barry.

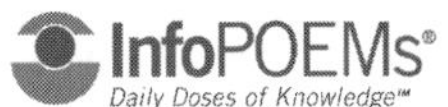

Habitual caffeine intake does not increase risk of hypertension in women

Clinical question

Does habitual caffeine intake increase the risk of hypertension in women?

Bottom line

Habitual caffeine consumption does not appear to increase the risk of hypertension in women. In particular, coffee and tea are not associated with increased risk. The development of hypertension is, however, significantly associated with the intake of cola drinks, including both sugared and diet versions. (LOE = 2b)

Reference

Winkelmayer WC, Stampfer MJ, Willett WC, Curhan GC. Habitual caffeine intake and the risk of hypertension in women. JAMA 2005;294:2330–2335.

Study Design

Cohort (prospective)

Funding

Government

Setting

Population-based

Synopsis

Caffeine intake acutely raises blood pressure, but the association between habitual intake and the risk of developing hypertension has been unclear. The investigators examined data obtained from 2 large-scale prospective cohort studies: – the Nurses' Health Studies (NHS) I and II. The NHS I cohort was assembled in 1976 with 121,700 female registered nurses, aged 30 to 55 years, reporting via self-completed questionnaire every 2 years. NHS II began in 1989 with 116,671 female registered nurses, aged 25 to 42 years, also reporting via self-completed questionnaire every 2 years. Follow-up for both cohorts occurred for more than 90% of participants. Questionnaires measured food and beverage intake and collected data on various health outcomes, including hypertension. Participants were not aware of the study hypothesis regarding a potential link between caffeine intake and hypertension. Health record reviews confirmed documented hypertension in a subset of women. In both cohorts, no significant linear association was detected between increasing caffeine consumption and risk of developing hypertension. In subgroup analysis with multivariate adjustments, habitual coffee and tea consumption did not increase the risk of hypertension, but a significant association between consumption of cola beverages (both sugared and diet) and the diagnosis of hypertension did exist.

Essential Evidence: Medicine that Matters, Edited by David Slawson, Allen Shaughnessy, Mark Ebell, and Henry Barry.

Home blood pressure monitoring valuable

Clinical question

What is the role of home blood pressure monitoring in patients with or without hypertension?

Bottom line

Blood pressure measurements taken at home with validated automatic monitors average lower than readings obtained in the office. They are also better prognostic indicators of the detrimental effects of hypertension. Before consigning patients to a diagnosis and treatment of hypertension, or before changing drug therapy, try a few days of at-home monitoring; it might avoid overdiagnosis and overtreatment. (LOE = 1a)

Reference

Verberk WJ, Kroon AA, Kessels AG, de Leeuw PW. Home blood pressure measurement. A systematic review. J Am Coll Cardiol 2005;46:743–751.

Study Design

Diagnostic test evaluation

Funding

Government

Setting

Outpatient (any)

Synopsis

Blood pressure can be measured in the office or at home using an automated self-measuring device or through the use of 24-hour ambulatory blood pressure monitoring. This systematic review evaluated the research on the use of home self-monitoring of blood pressure to determine its role in hypertension management. The reviewers searched 3 databases for research comparing self-measurement of blood pressure using validated self-measurement devices (see www.bhsoc.org for a list) with in-office monitoring. The report does not clearly outline how the articles were selected or abstracted, though they specifically excluded articles that evaluated patients with and without antihypertensive drug treatment without the possibility to distinguish both groups. Morning and evening readings over several days (the authors estimate 3 days, averaging the results from the second and third days) is necessary to accurately portray a patient's usual blood pressure. Blood pressures of untreated patients, taken at home, are lower than those measured in the office (on average 6.9 mm Hg systolic and 4.9 mm Hg diastolic), with the discrepancy in systolic blood pressure being more pronounced in older patients. Similarly, blood pressure readings at home were lower on average by 5.3 mm Hg systolic and 3.1 mm Hg diastolic, irrespective of age. Several studies, though their results are not clearly outlined in this paper, have shown that home blood pressure measurements correlate better with target organ damage and cardiovascular mortality and correlate well with 24-hour continuous blood pressure monitoring.

Essential Evidence: Medicine that Matters, Edited by David Slawson, Allen Shaughnessy, Mark Ebell, and Henry Barry.

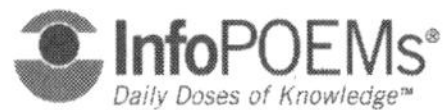

Office measurements usually overestimate blood pressure

Clinical question

How well do blood pressure measurements taken in the office correlate with a gold standard in-office measurement?

Bottom line

In this study, usual blood pressure readings in an office were frequently higher than standardized measurement, leading to incorrect labeling of blood pressure control in 1 of 5 patients. Several conclusions can be drawn from this study, which replicates the findings in other studies: First, retrain yourself to take an accurate blood pressure reading (see: http://www.theberries.ns.ca/SPRING2005a/taking_BP_technique.html). Second, train your office nurses how to do it correctly. Third, retrain them often, since other research has shown high recidivism. Fourth, check any patients with high blood pressure readings yourself, using good technique. (LOE = 1b)

Reference

Kim JW, Bosworth HB, Voils CI, et al. How well do clinic-based blood pressure measurements agree with the mercury standard? J Gen Intern Med 2005;20:647–649.

Study Design

Diagnostic test evaluation

Funding

Government

Setting

Outpatient (primary care)

Synopsis

The researchers conducting this study compared the blood pressure measurements recorded during a visit to an internal medicine clinic with those obtained from the same patients by a trained research assistant. Using a convenience sample of 100 patients, most of whom were taking antihypertensives, the researchers measured blood pressure either before the clinic visit or immediately afterward, on average approximately 24 minutes within the time of the clinic reading. The researchers were carefully trained and performed all the measurements according to the book; proper cuff size, arm at heart level, patients resting for 5 minutes, air pressure released slowly. They used a mercury sphygmomanometer with a random zero, meaning that the blood pressure numbers they obtained on the patients were not real but had to be converted to the real number by subtracting a number that was unique to each measurement. This research tool is designed to prevent blood pressure readings to be read where the researcher thinks the number should be. The clinic blood pressure measurements were performed by the office nurse. Overall, the agreement between the measurements on individual patients was good, with an intraclass correlation coefficient of .91 (95% CI, 0.62–0.86). However, using the degree of agreement statistic, clinic-based measurements were 8.3 mm Hg systolic and 7.1 mm Hg diastolic higher than the standard. A possible clinical impact, due to misclassification of blood pressure, could have occurred in 21% of patients who had controlled blood pressures as measured by the researcher but were uncontrolled according to the clinic measurement. The degree of overestimation more commonly occurred when blood pressures were in the normal range.

Essential Evidence: Medicine that Matters, Edited by David Slawson, Allen Shaughnessy, Mark Ebell, and Henry Barry.

Hypertension follow-up: 3 months = 6 months

Clinical question

Can patients with hypertension be seen every 6 months without loss of control, changes in patient satisfaction, or declines in adherence to treatment?

Bottom line

Seeing patients with controlled hypertension every 6 months, rather than every 3 months, resulted in similar blood pressure measurements both in the office and at home, with no changes in patients satisfaction or adherence to therapy. (LOE = 1b)

Reference

Birtwhistle RV, Godwin MS, Delva MD, et al. Randomised equivalence trial comparing three and six months of follow-up of patients with hypertension by family practitioners. BMJ 2004;328:204–206.

Study Design

Randomized controlled trial (nonblinded)

Setting

Outpatient (primary care)

Synopsis

Canadian, British, and American guidelines regarding the management of hypertension suggest an interval of 3 to 6 months for follow-up in patients with controlled hypertension. This study explored the difference between 3-month and 6-month follow-up in 609 patients with hypertension controlled for at least 3 months by at least 1 drug. Patients were randomized (allocation assignment concealed) to return every 3 or 6 months, with earlier follow-up if blood pressure was out of control or if drug therapy was changed. Analysis was by intention to treat. As one might expect, the 6-month group had significantly fewer office visits over the 3 years of the study (average = 16.2 vs 18.8), although they still were seen much more frequently than scheduled (they should have been seen an average of 6 and 12 times). Blood pressures measured at the end of each year in the office were not different among the 2 groups. Blood pressure measurements taken at home were similar to the doctors' measurements. At each period a similar percentage of patients (~20%) in each group were deemed by their doctor to have out-of-control blood pressure. Satisfaction with their care and self-reported adherence to therapy was similar in both groups. The study had the ability to find a true difference in blood pressure of $<10\%$ at a power of 0.8.

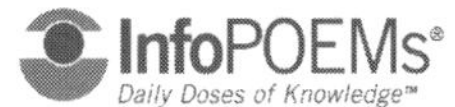

Patients with HTN + high lipids may benefit less from statins (ALLHAT)

Clinical question

Are statins beneficial for hypertensive patients with hypercholesterolemia?

Bottom line

Statin therapy did not reduce all-cause mortality or heart disease when compared to usual care in patients with treated hypertension and moderately elevated LDL cholesterol. We should strongly emphasize other alternatives, such as diet and exercise, before prescribing an expensive statin drug for our patients with well controlled hypertension and moderately elevated lipid levels. InfoRetriever has a helpful clinical decision tool that can calculate individual risk and benefit with additional treatment. (LOE = 2b−)

Reference

ALLHAT Officers and Coordinators. Major outcomes in moderately hypercholesterolemic, hypertensive patients randomized to pravastatin vs usual care. The Antihypertensive and Lipid-Lowering Treatment to prevent Heart Attack Trial (ALLHAT-LLT). JAMA 2002;288:2998–2907.

Study Design

Randomized controlled trial (nonblinded)

Setting

Outpatient (any)

Synopsis

Many studies have shown the benefit of lowering cholesterol with statins. As part of the ALLHAT trial, a sub-group of 10,355 patients, aged 55 years or older, with established hypertension and LDL cholesterol of 120 to 189 mg/dL (100 to 129 mg/dL if known heart disease) and triglycerides lower than 350 mg/dL were identified. These subjects were randomized to receive pravastatin, 20 to 40 mg/d, or usual care (concealed allocation assignment). In addition to hypertension, 14% of the patients had heart disease and 35% had type 2 diabetes. All subjects were advised to follow the Step I cholesterol diet. Practitioners treating patients in the pravastatin group had the option to prescribe other lipid-lowering interventions as deemed necessary. "Vigorous" cholesterol lowering therapy was discouraged in the usual care group unless deemed clinically necessary. Follow-up (98%) was for a mean of 4.9 years. Individuals assessing outcomes were not blind to treatment group assignment. Using intent-to-treat analysis, total cholesterol levels were reduced by 17% with pravastatin vs 8% with usual care. All-cause mortality rates were similar for the 2 groups, with 6-year mortality rates of 14.9% for pravastatin and 15.3% with usual care. Coronary heart disease event rates were also not significantly different between pravastatin and usual care (9.3% vs 10.4%). The study had an 84% power for detecting a 20% reduction in mortality. 70% of patients assigned to pravastatin reported taking 80% or more of their medication at year 6. By year 6, 26% of patients in the usual care group reported taking statin treatment. There were no significant differences in regards to age, sex, history of type 2 diabetes or heart disease status. Many critics believe the lack of benefit to statin therapy in this study was because only 70% of the patients on treatment vs 26% of patients not on treatment were taking statins after 6 years. This is in contrast to many other studies showing a clear benefit to statin therapy when almost none of the control patients received active treatment. However, epidemiologic studies have shown that few patients take cholesterol-lowering therapy long term.

Essential Evidence: Medicine that Matters, Edited by David Slawson, Allen Shaughnessy, Mark Ebell, and Henry Barry.

Excessive lowering of blood pressure causes more harm than good

Clinical question

Can aggressive lowering of blood pressure in patients with coronary artery disease be dangerous?

Bottom line

Lower is not always better. Despite a push toward lower blood pressure in many populations, bad outcomes (mortality, myocardial infarction, and stroke) are increased in patients with coronary artery disease (CAD) if their blood pressure consistently remains lower than 70 mmHg diastolic. (LOE = 1b)

Reference

Messerli FH, Mancia G, Conti CR, et al. Dogma disputed: can aggressively lowering blood pressure in hypertensive patients with coronary artery disease be dangerous? Ann Intern Med 2006;144:884–893.

Study Design

Cohort (prospective)

Funding

Industry

Setting

Outpatient (any)

Synopsis

Research has hinted at a J-shaped response to lowering blood pressure: As blood pressure is lowered, mortality and morbidity decrease, to a point, after which further lowering is associated with higher mortality and morbidity. Common guidelines and conventional wisdom do not take this risk into account and advocate various degrees of aggressive blood pressure control on the basis of other risk factors. This study is an analysis of the results of a study comparing the effectiveness of verapamil and trandolapril in hypertensive patients with CAD. In this analysis, the investigators evaluated the relationship between average diastolic blood pressure and the primary outcome of all-cause death, nonfatal stroke, and nonfatal myocardial infarction in the 22,576 patients enrolled in the study. The patients in this study were treated and monitored for a median 2.7 years and mortality and morbidity rates were not different between the 2 treatments. Blood pressure was divided into 10 mmHg increments and this outcome was evaluated at each level of control. As in other research, the J-curve is present in these data, associated with decreases in diastolic blood pressure. The best results were a diastolic blood pressure between 80 mmHg and 90 mmHg. A diastolic blood pressure between 70 mmHg and 80 mmHg was associated with slightly, but not significantly, increased bad outcomes, though patients with blood pressures of lower than 70 mmHg experienced bad outcomes at the same rate as those with readings higher than 100 mmHg.

Essential Evidence: Medicine that Matters, Edited by David Slawson, Allen Shaughnessy, Mark Ebell, and Henry Barry.

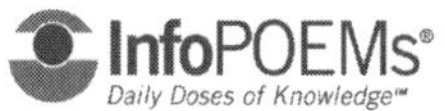

Diuretics clearly first line agent for HTN (ALLHAT)

Clinical question

Which agent is preferred as first-step therapy for hypertension?

Bottom line

Diuretics should be the preferred first line agent for almost all patients with hypertension, including those with diabetes, pre-existing heart disease. Many of the patients in this study requiring a step 2 agent were treated with an inexpensive, off-patent medication such as beta-blockers and reserpine. (LOE = 1b)

Reference

ALLHAT Officers and Coordinators. Major outcomes in high-risk hypertensive patients randomized to angiotensin-converting enzyme inhibitor or calcium channel blocker vs diuretic. The Antihypertensive and Lipid-Lowering Treatment to prevent Heart Attack Trial (ALLHAT). JAMA 2002;288:2981–2997.

Study Design

Randomized controlled trial (double-blinded)

Setting

Outpatient (any)

Synopsis

The ALLHAT trial included 33,357 patients, aged 55 years or older, with established hypertension (HTN) and at least 1 other heart disease risk factor. Patients were excluded with heart failure or an ejection fraction of less than 35%. An earlier arm of the study using doxazosin was discontinued after interim analysis showed that chlorthalidone was superior. Subjects were randomly assigned to receive chlorthalidone (Hygroton), 12.5 to 25 mg/d; amlodipine (Norvasc), 2.5 to 10 mg/d; or lisinopril (Prinivil) 10 to 40 mg/d. Follow-up (98%) ranged from 3.6 to 8 years (mean 4.9 years). The goal blood pressure in each group was <140/90 mmHg. The choice of a step 2 drug was either atenolol (Tenormin), clonidine (Catapres), or reserpine, or, when clinically indicated, low doses of open-label step 1 drugs. The step 3 drug was hydralazine. Control of hypertension was achieved in approximately two-thirds of participants (61% lisinopril; 66% amlodipine, and 68% chlorthalidone). The primary outcome of combined fatal heart disease or non-fatal MI occurred with equal frequency in all three groups. Likewise, there was no difference in all-cause mortality among the three treatment groups. However, compared with chlorthalidone, patients taking amlodipine were more likely to develop heart failure (10.2% vs 7.7%; NNTH = 40). Compared with chlorthalidone, patients taking lisinopril were more likely to develop cerebrovascular disease (33% vs 30.9%; NNTH = 50); stroke (6.3% vs 5.6%; NNTH = 143); or heart failure (8.7% vs 7.7%; NNTH = 100). The benefit of chlorthalidone was consistent across sub-groups including diabetes, heart disease and left ventricular hypertrophy. There were no differences noted in incidence of renal disease, glomerular filtration rates, or inverse creatinine slopes for lisinopril vs chlorthalidone. Interestingly, patients taking chlorthalidone were more likely to develop hypercholesterolemia and show evidence of insulin resistance with elevated levels of fasting blood glucose – all those supposedly bad things – and yet they lived longer and better! Pooled drop out rates at 5 years were similar among the three groups (chlorthalidone, 19.5%; amlodipine, 19.6%; and lisinopril, 27.4%), indicating that none of the agents offered a quality of life benefit.

Essential Evidence: Medicine that Matters, Edited by David Slawson, Allen Shaughnessy, Mark Ebell, and Henry Barry.

Meta-analysis supports diuretics as first line for HTN

Clinical question

What agent(s) is preferred as first-line treatment for hypertension?

Bottom line

It can't get clearer. Diuretics – the least expensive and most effective agents – should be the first-line treatment for almost everyone with hypertension, including patients with diabetes and asymptomatic left ventricular hypertrophy. Remember that the dose of the diuretic cannot be higher than an equivalent dose of 25 mg hydroclorothiazide. A higher dose creates an increased risk of mortality and morbidity without any additional benefit. (LOE = 1a)

Reference

Psaty BM, Lumley T, Furberg CD, et al. Health outcomes associated with various antihypertensive therapies used as first-line agents. A network meta-analysis. JAMA 2003;289:2534–2544.

Study Design

Meta-analysis (randomized controlled trials)

Setting

Various (meta-analysis)

Synopsis

Current evidence clearly supports using diuretics as the first-line treatment for hypertension in most patients, including those with diabetes, co-existing risk factors for cardiovascular disease (CVD), and asymptomatic left ventricular hypertrophy (see the Seventh Report of the Joint National Committee on Prevention, Detection, Evaluation, and Treatment of High Blood Pressure for exceptions). The authors combined 42 clinical trials including 192,478 patients randomized to 7 major treatment strategies, including placebo. Most recently included in the analysis were the Antihypertensive and Lipid-Lowering Treatment to Prevent Heart Attack Trial (ALLHAT) and the just-released Australian National Blood Pressure Study. None of the other first-line treatment strategies, including beta-blockers, angiotensin-converting enzyme (ACE) inhibitors, calcium channel blockers, alpha-blockers, and angiotensin receptor blockers were significantly better than low-dose diuretics for any outcome (despite the fact that most cost significantly more). Compared with calcium channel blockers, diuretics were associated with a reduced risk of CVD events and congestive heart failure (CHF). Compared with ACE inhibitors, diuretics were associated with reduced risks of CHF, CVD events, and stroke. Compared with beta-blockers, diuretics were associated with a reduced risk of CVD events. Blood pressure changes were similar with the different medications (so much for that as a surrogate marker). In the largest trial – the ALLHAT – low-dose diuretics were also shown to have the lowest rate of drop-outs due to intolerance and were also superior or equal to other agents including ACE inhibitors in patients with diabetes and asymptomatic left ventricular hypertrophy.

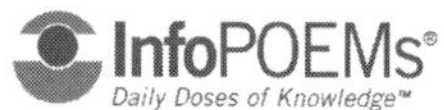

Outcomes for thiazides similar

Clinical question

Are health outcomes similar between chlorthalidone and other thiazide-type diuretics for treating hypertension?

Bottom line

The benefits are similar when treating hypertension with chlorthalidone or other thiazide-type diuretics. The dose should be in the low range (no more than 25 mg of hydrochlorothiazide). (LOE = 1a)

Reference

Psaty BM, Lumley T, Furberg CD. Meta-analysis of health outcomes of chlorthalidone-based vs nonchlorthalidone-based low-dose diuretic therapies. JAMA 2004;292:43–44.

Study Design

Meta-analysis (randomized controlled trials)

Setting

Various (meta-analysis)

Synopsis

In many of the large studies evaluating different therapies for hypertension, including the Antihypertensive and Lipid-Lowering Treatment to Prevent Heart Attack Trial (ALLHAT), chlorthalidone was used in the low-dose diuretic arm. Many clinicians are uncertain if the benefits of chlorthalidone are similar for other thiazide-type diuretics, including the more commonly prescribed hydrochlorothiazide. The authors previously published a meta-analysis (JAMA 2003: 289:2534–544) of various first-line agents for hypertension. In this review, however, they compare only placebo-controlled trials of low-dose diuretics that used chlorthalidone with those that used other low-dose diuretic therapies. A total of 5 trials enrolling 7146 participants were identified. Both treatments were equally superior to placebo in reducing both cardiovascular disease morbidity and mortality and all-cause mortality.

Essential Evidence: Medicine that Matters, Edited by David Slawson, Allen Shaughnessy, Mark Ebell, and Henry Barry.

ACEI better than diuretic in older men for hypertension

Clinical question
Are angiotensin-converting enzyme inhibitors or diuretics better in treating older hypertensive patients?

Bottom line
Enalapril is better than hydrochlorothiazide at preventing cardiovascular events in older men. These results contrast with results from ALLHAT, which found different outcomes between patients taking lisinopril and chlorthalidone in a group of patients 55 years and older with at least 1 cardiovascular risk factor. How to reconcile these findings? One possibility is that enalapril is more effective than lisinopril; another is that chlorthalidone is more effective than hydrochlorothiazide. Still another is that the design limitations of the current study (open label design, in particular) may have overestimated the effect of the "more modern" drug. We know that either is better than calcium channel blockers and alpha-blockers, both are cheaper than angiotensin receptor blockers, and that ACE inhibitors may be better in older, lower risk men. (LOE = 1b–)

Reference
Wing LM, Reid CM, Ryan P, et al. A comparison of outcomes with angiotensin-converting-enzyme inhibitors and diuretics for hypertension in the elderly. N Engl J Med 2003;348:583–592.

Study Design
Randomized controlled trial (single-blinded)

Setting
Outpatient (primary care)

Synopsis
The authors of this Australian study identified 6083 healthy older patients (aged 65 to 84 years) in 1594 family practices, and followed them up for a median of 4.1 years. Patients were assigned to either an angiotensin-converting enzyme (ACE) inhibitor group or a diuretic group. The recommended drugs were enalapril and hydrochlorothiazide, and physicians could add other drugs to achieve the blood pressure targets of 160/90 mm Hg, or 140/80 if tolerated. This was an open-label trial. Analysis was by intention to treat, and groups were similar at baseline. Loss to follow-up was minimal. Like life, this study was messy in terms of who got what. Of those in the ACE inhibitor group, 58% were still receiving an ACE inhibitor at the end of the study period, and 65% were on monotherapy. In the diuretic group, 62% were still receiving a diuretic and 67% were on monotherapy. Few patients required 3 or more drugs: 6% in the ACE inhibitor group and 5% in the diuretic group. The risk of death from any cause was similar between groups (15.7 vs 17.1 deaths per 1000 patient years). When they added cardiovascular events to deaths, there were slightly fewer in the ACE inhibitor group (56.1 vs 59.8 per 1000 patient years; number needed to treat = 270 to prevent 1 event over 1 year). Interestingly, there was no difference in the likelihood of cardiovascular events or all-cause mortality for women, but men had fewer cardiovascular events (but not all-cause deaths) when taking an ACE inhibitor.

Essential Evidence: Medicine that Matters, Edited by David Slawson, Allen Shaughnessy, Mark Ebell, and Henry Barry.

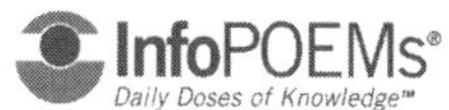

Atenolol of questionable efficacy for HTN

Clinical question

Does atenolol (Tenormin) reduce cardiovascular morbidity and mortality in patients with hypertension?

Bottom line

If these authors have identified all the relevant research, it appears that atenolol is more effective than placebo in lowering blood pressure. It is not more effective than other medications, however. Furthermore, it does not appear to reduce cardiovascular morbidity or mortality. (LOE = 1a–)

Reference

Carlberg B, Samuelsson O, Lindholm LH. Atenolol in hypertension: Is it a wise choice? Lancet 2004;364:1684–1689.

Study Design

Systematic review

Funding

Unknown/not stated

Setting

Various (meta-analysis)

Synopsis

The authors of this briefly described systematic review wanted to review the effect of atenolol on cardiovascular morbidity and mortality in patients with hypertension. A serious flaw in their study is that the search strategy may have prematurely restricted the field and therefore caused them to miss potentially relevant studies. Their search strategy only allowed them to include studies of atenolol versus placebo and 5 others that compared atenolol with other drugs. These studies included more than 23,000 patients who were evaluated for an average of 4.6 years. Compared with placebo, atenolol lowers blood pressure by approximately 10 mm Hg systolic and 6 mm Hg diastolic. Atenolol and the other drugs, however, had approximately the same effect on lowering blood pressure. In the placebo-controlled trials, atenolol had no effect on all-cause mortality, cardiovascular mortality, myocardial infarction, or stroke. In the studies against other drugs, one study (the Losartan Intervention for Endpoint reduction in hypertension study [LIFE]) included as many patients as the rest combined. The authors analyzed the studies with and without the LIFE data. When the LIFE study is included, there are no significant differences in all-cause mortality, cardiovascular mortality, myocardial infarction, or stroke. When the LIFE data is not included, atenolol increased all-cause mortality (number needed to treat to harm [NNTH] = 110 for 4.6 years; 95% CI, 59–798) and stroke (NNTH = 79 for 4.6 years; [CI, 51–176]). The authors included several studies with shaky study designs. One study was an unblinded trial, 2 recruited patients with transient ischemic stroke or minor stroke, and one only studied patients with left ventricular hypertrophy. Although most of the patients had hypertension, those studies are inappropriate to include as prevention trials. If we exclude these studies from the analysis, the authors' point that the data supporting atenolol's use are limited is well taken.

Essential Evidence: Medicine that Matters, Edited by David Slawson, Allen Shaughnessy, Mark Ebell, and Henry Barry.

Beta-blockers > placebo, not other drugs, in preventing HTN complications

Clinical question

Are beta-blockers more effective than other drugs in preventing stroke and myocardial infarction in patients with primary hypertension?

Bottom line

If these authors have identified all the relevant research, it appears that in comparison with placebo, beta-blockers do not reduce cardiovascular morbidity or mortality but decrease the risk of strokes. However, in comparison with other antihypertensive medications, beta-blockers are associated with a significantly higher risk of stroke. Most of the included studies used atenolol and the data on other beta-blockers are inconclusive. Before throwing the baby out with the bathwater, remember that some patients with hypertension will need beta-blockers to treat their comorbid coronary artery disease, congestive heart failure, and so forth. (LOE = 1a–)

Reference

Lindholm LH, Carlberg B, Samuelsson O. Should beta blockers remain first choice in the treatment of primary hypertension? A meta-analysis. Lancet 2005;366:1545–1553.

Study Design	Funding	Setting
Meta-analysis (randomized controlled trials)	Government	Various (meta-analysis)

Synopsis

The use of atenolol in treating hypertension has recently been questioned by the authors of this study. In this paper, they expanded their question to assess the effectiveness of all beta-blockers in the treatment of hypertension. To do this, they searched PubMed and the Cochrane Library using an explicit search strategy that may have limited their yield of important studies. Since none of the included studies were published before 1985, one might conclude that either no randomized controlled trials were done before 1985 or the authors' search strategy was inadequate. The authors also don't report looking for unpublished studies or whether they hand-searched the bibliographies of the studies they included. Finally, they don't discuss how the included studies were selected, if the quality of the studies were assessed, or how the data were extracted. Ultimately, they identified 13 randomized controlled trials (including nearly 106,000 patients) comparing beta-blockers with other antihypertensives. The duration of each study ranged from 2.6 to 10 years. They excluded 1 trial for not registering the number of patients treated with beta-blockers and 1 for "suboptimum registration of seven clinical events" and because there was a significant difference in blood pressure response between the treatment groups. All-cause mortality and the rate of myocardial infarction were similar regardless of treatment, however, the patients treated with beta-blockers had a higher risk of stroke (number needed to treat to harm [NNTH] = 461; 95% CI, 236–10,774). The data, however, were significantly heterogeneous across the studies. When looking at beta-blockers other than atenolol, the data are limited to 3 inconclusive studies. The authors also identified 7 trials (including more than 27,000 patients) of beta-blockers versus placebo or no therapy. The duration of each of these studies ranged from 2.1 to 5 years. Beta-blockers were more effective than placebo in preventing strokes, but not in preventing myocardial infarction or in improving all-cause mortality. There was no significant heterogeneity across these studies. Similarly, the data on beta-blockers other than atenolol are limited to 4 inconclusive studies.

Essential Evidence: Medicine that Matters, Edited by David Slawson, Allen Shaughnessy, Mark Ebell, and Henry Barry.

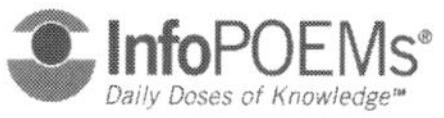

Renal function similarly affected by antihypertensives (ALLHAT)

Clinical question

Which drug class provides better renal protection in patients treated for hypertension?

Bottom line

It's blood pressure reduction, not the choice of drug, that prevents renal function decline in patients with hypertension, with or without diabetes. Neither the calcium channel blocker amlodipine (Norvasc) nor the angiotensin-converting enzyme inhibitor lisinopril (Prinivil) prevents the combined outcome of end-stage renal disease or a 50% decrease in renal function any better than the diuretic chlorthalidone (Hygroton). Results were the same in patients with already compromised renal function, as well as in patients with type 2 diabetes. (LOE = 1b)

Reference

Rahman M, Pressel S, Davis BR, et al. Renal outcomes in high-risk hypertensive patients treated with an angiotensin-converting enzyme inhibitor or a calcium channel blocker vs. a diuretic. A report from the antihypertensive and lipid-lowering treatment to prevent heart attack trial (ALLHAT). Arch Intern Med 2005;165:936–946.

Study Design	Funding	Setting
Randomized controlled trial (double-blinded)	Industry + govt	Outpatient (any)

Synopsis

This report is an analysis of the ALLHAT trial, which evaluated 33,357 patients, 55 years or older, with established hypertension and at least 1 other heart disease risk factor. An earlier arm of the study using doxazosin was discontinued after interim analysis showed that chlorthalidone was superior. Subjects were randomly assigned, in a double-blind fashion (concealed allocation assignment), to receive chlorthalidone (Hygroton) 12.5 to 25 mg per day; amlodipine (Norvasc) 2.5 to 10 mg per day; or lisinopril (Prinivil) 10 to 40 mg per day. Follow-up (98%) ranged from 3.6 years to 8 years (mean = 4.9). The goal blood pressure in each group was a reading lower than 140/90 mmHg. The choice of a step 2 drug was either atenolol (Tenormin), clonidine (Catapres), or reserpine, or, when clinically indicated, low doses of open-label step 1 drugs. The step 3 drug was hydralazine. Control of hypertension was achieved in approximately two thirds of participants (61% in the lisinopril group; 66% in the amlodipine group, and 68% in the chlorthalidone group). Study outcomes were assessed by individuals blinded to treatment group assignment. End-stage renal disease (ESRD) or a 50% or greater decline in renal function occurred in 1049 of the participants (3.1%). There was no significant differences in the overall rates of this outcome among the chlorthalidone, amlodipine, or lisinopril groups. There was also no difference when the researchers specifically evaluated only those patients with a mild decrease in renal function (a normalized glomerular filtration rate of 60–89 mL/min) or a moderate to severe decrease (<60 mL/min). At the end of the study, glomerular filtration rate was slightly higher, 3–6 mL/min, in the amlodipine-treated patients than in the chlorthalidone-treated patients; there was no difference between lisinopril and amlodipine.

Essential Evidence: Medicine that Matters, Edited by David Slawson, Allen Shaughnessy, Mark Ebell, and Henry Barry.

Screening program for abdominal aortic aneurysm ineffective

Clinical question

Does a screening program of older men decrease their risk of death from an abdominal aortic aneurysm?

Bottom line

A program of inviting older men for aortic abdominal aneurysm screening did not result in an overall reduction in deaths due to ruptured aneurysm. However, the ultrasound screening program reduced deaths in men aged 65 to 75 years. Aneurysm death rates were low in the population studied, and screening might be more effective in groups at higher risk of aneurysm. (LOE = 1b)

Reference

Norman PE, Jamrozik K, Lawrence-Brown MM, et al. Population based randomised controlled trial on impact of screening on mortality from abdominal aortic aneurysm. BMJ 2004;329:1259. Epub 2004 Nov 27.

Study Design	Funding	Allocation
Randomized controlled trial (nonblinded)	Government	Uncertain

Setting

Population-based

Synopsis

The overall case fatality rate of a ruptured abdominal aortic aneurysm (AAA) is approximately 80%. It would be great, then, if using ultrasound to screen older patients would identify patients at risk for rupture who could have repair successfully performed. This study began with a population of 41,000 men, aged 65 to 83 years, who registered to vote – which was compulsory – in Western Australia. The men were randomized by age and postal code to receive either a screening ultrasound or no screening. The men in the screened group were contacted up to 2 times by letter asking them to participate. The men were screened via ultrasound and given their results with a copy to give to their general practitioner, who then made all decisions regarding follow-up. Thus the study evaluated a common approach in the United States in which patients are solicited by newspaper advertisements to obtain screening from a traveling ultrasound provider making the rounds in the area. Analysis was by intention to treat: AAA rates were recorded for everyone in both groups, regardless of whether the men actually received screening ultrasound and independent of the follow-up prescribed by their general practitioner. Death rates were easy to determine in this study since Australia has a national electronic medical record that can track hospital deaths. Sixty-three percent of the men who were solicited for screening actually received the screening. The overall prevalence of any AAA was 7.2% in the 2 groups (aortic diameter at least 30 mm). Twice as many men in the screening group underwent elective surgery for AAA (P = .002). Overall death rates were not different between the screened and unscreened groups (mortality ratio = 0.61; 95% CI, 0.33–1.11). Death rates were lower in men between the ages of 65 and 75 years (mortality ratio = 0.19; 0.04–0.89). However, the expected death rate in the control group was approximately half what was expected, which leads to the following 2 speculations: First, it's possible that some men had previously been screened and treated for AAA before the study. Second, the low number of deaths in both groups makes it more difficult to find a difference that could conceivably be there.

Essential Evidence: Medicine that Matters, Edited by David Slawson, Allen Shaughnessy, Mark Ebell, and Henry Barry.

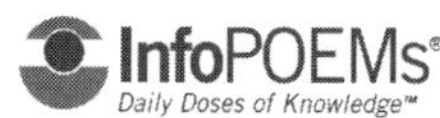

Fewer aneurysm deaths but not overall deaths with AAA screening

Clinical question

In older men, does screening for abdominal aortic aneurysm result in fewer overall deaths or deaths due to aneurysm over the next 5 years?

Bottom line

Offering screening to older men will decrease their risk of dying because of an abdominal aortic aneurysm but will not decrease their overall risk of dying over the next 4.3 years. This study evaluated screening in all men; other studies of screening have shown a benefit in men who smoke. (LOE = 1b)

Reference

Lindholt JS, Juul S, Fasting H, Henneberg EW. Screening for abdominal aortic aneurysms: single centre randomised controlled trial. BMJ 2005;330:750–752.

Study Design

Randomized controlled trial (single-blinded)

Funding

Foundation

Allocation

Uncertain

Setting

Population-based

Synopsis

The researchers conducting this Danish study enrolled all 12,639 men born in a single county. The men were between the ages of 64.3 years and 73.8 years (average = 67.7 years) at the time of the study. The men were randomly assigned to a control group or to be invited to undergo ultrasonography to screen for the presence of abdominal aortic aneurysm (AAA). Nonresponders to the invitation were reinvited once and 76.6% of all invited men underwent screening. Participants with an AAA of at least 5 cm diameter (0.5%) were referred to a vascular surgeon; men with small AAAs were screened yearly and referred if their aneurysm had increased to 5 cm diameter or more. There were 9 deaths due to AAA in the screened group and 27 deaths due to AAA in the control group over the 4.33 average years of follow-up. All-cause mortality in these older men was not affected by screening. These small numbers translate into a number needed to screen of 349 to prevent 1 AAA-related death over 4.3 years.

CABG not helpful before AAA or peripheral vascular surgery

Clinical question

In patients with significant, stable coronary disease, is coronary artery revascularization helpful before major vascular surgery?

Bottom line

Patients with significant, stable coronary artery disease do not benefit from revascularization before major peripheral vascular surgery. (LOE = 1b)

Reference

McFalls EO, Ward HB, Moritz TE, et al. Coronary-artery revascularization before elective major vascular surgery. N Engl J Med 2004;351:2795–2804.

Study Design

Randomized controlled trial (nonblinded)

Funding

Government

Allocation

Concealed

Setting

Inpatient (any location) with outpatient follow-up

Synopsis

Do you put patients through a risky procedure to make a second risky procedure safer? Tough question, when that first procedure may reduce long-term mortality. Patients undergoing either repair of an expanding abdominal aortic aneurysm or peripheral vascular surgery underwent angiography if they were felt to be at high risk for cardiovascular complications based standard guidelines. If one or more coronary arteries had a 70% stenosis they were randomized to either revascularization (59% got angioplasty, 41% coronary artery bypass graft) or no revascularization. Of 5859 patients initially enrolled, 1654 were not at high risk, 1025 required urgent surgery, 626 had prior revascularization, 731 had a severe coexisting illness, 633 were already in another study or declined to participate, and 680 were excluded for various other reasons. That left 510 for randomization; groups were balanced at the start of the study, and allocation to groups was concealed.Patients were followed for up to 6 years; the mean follow-up was 2.8 years. There were not surprisingly more deaths before surgery in the revascularization group (10 vs 1), no difference in the 30 days after the peripheral vascular surgery or AAA repair (7 vs 8), and no difference in long-term all-cause mortality (22% in the revascularization group vs 23% in the no revascularization group). The outcomes were the same for intention to treat and per protocol analyses.

Essential Evidence: Medicine that Matters, Edited by David Slawson, Allen Shaughnessy, Mark Ebell, and Henry Barry.

 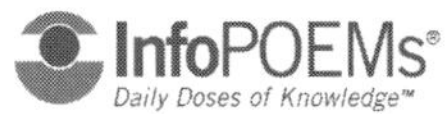

EVAR worse than open repair of AAA (EVAR Trial 1)

Clinical question

Is open repair better than endovascular repair for patients with abdominal aortic aneurysms?

Bottom line

Endovascular aneurysm repair (EVAR) offers no real advantage over traditional open repair in medically fit patients with abdominal aortic aneurysms. (LOE = 1b–)

Reference

EVAR trial participants. Endovascular aneurysm repair versus open repair in patients with abdominal aortic aneurysm (EVAR trial 1): randomised controlled trial. Lancet 2005;365:2179–2186.

Study Design

Randomized controlled trial (nonblinded)

Funding

Government

Allocation

Concealed

Setting

Inpatient (any location) with outpatient follow-up

Synopsis

In this multicenter study, patients 60 and older with abdominal aortic aneurysms at least 5.5 cm in diameter were randomly assigned (masked central allocation) to endovascular aneurysm repair (EVAR; n = 543) or traditional open repair (n = 539). The patients had to be "medically fit" for surgery. After repair of the aneurysm, the researchers evaluated the patients at 1, 3, and 12 months, and then yearly thereafter. While the study was unblinded, it is pretty hard to fudge the main outcome, all-cause mortality, assessed via intention to treat. The study was designed to be able to detect a 5% difference in all-cause mortality. The median duration of follow up was 2.9 years and only 5 patients were lost to follow up (2 in the EVAR group and 3 in the open repair group). The all-cause mortality rate was about 28% in each group. While there was a 3% absolute reduction in aneurysm-specific mortality in the first 30 days after EVAR (1.7% vs. 4.7%), EVAR cost more, didn't improve health-related quality of life, increased post-operative complications and increased the need for repeat procedures. So other than that, Mrs. Lincoln, how was the play?

Essential Evidence: Medicine that Matters, Edited by David Slawson, Allen Shaughnessy, Mark Ebell, and Henry Barry.

Bypass = angioplasty for severe leg ischemia, but costs more (BASIL)

Clinical question

Is bypass better than angioplasty in patients with severe ischemic disease of the legs?

Bottom line

Patients with advanced peripheral vascular disease who undergo either bypass surgery or balloon angioplasty have comparable amputation-free survival. Even though patients initially treated with angioplasty had a higher rate of re-intervention, the medical costs during the first year after treatment were one third higher in patients treated surgically. (LOE = 1b–)

Reference

Adam DJ, Beard JD, Cleveland T, et al, for the BASIL trial participants. Bypass versus angioplasty in severe ischaemia of the leg (BASIL): multicentre, randomised controlled trial. Lancet 2005;366:1925–1934.

Study Design

Randomized controlled trial (nonblinded)

Funding

Government

Allocation

Concealed

Setting

Inpatient (any location) with outpatient follow-up

Synopsis

Patients with severe peripheral vascular disease of a lower limb, defined as rest pain, ischemic ulcer, or gangrene, were randomly assigned (concealed allocation) to initial treatment with bypass surgery or balloon angioplasty (with no stents). To be eligible, the patients had to have confirmed infra-inguinal disease. Approximately one third of the patients presenting with severe disease were eligible to participate. The main outcomes were analyzed by intention to treat. Although this was an unblinded study, the outcomes, other than quality of life, are relatively free from measurement bias. However, decision-making about re-intervention and hospital resource use could have been influenced by any biases held by the performing surgeons. The researchers continued to follow each patient until the main end point (death or amputation) was reached. The study was designed to have 90% power to detect a 15% difference in 3-year amputation-free survival. Approximately two thirds of the patients were older than 70 years, nearly 80% were current or former smokers, and 40% had diabetes. Only 2% of the patients were lost to follow-up after randomization. Among the 228 patients initially managed surgically, 30 eventually died and 20 had an amputation; among the 224 initially treated with angioplasty, 28 died and 25 had an amputation. The patients treated with angioplasty had a significantly higher rate of re-intervention (26% vs 18%). The hospital costs during the first year after randomization for the patients treated surgically were approximately one third higher than the costs for the patients initially treated with angioplasty. In a post hoc analysis, patients treated with surgery seemed to do better after 2 years; the number of events after 2 years was small, though. Since post hoc analyses are fraught with problems, they should only be used to generate hypotheses.

Essential Evidence: Medicine that Matters, Edited by David Slawson, Allen Shaughnessy, Mark Ebell, and Henry Barry.

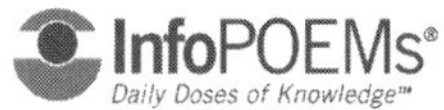

Sildenafil effective for primary pulmonary hypertension

Clinical question

Can sildenafil increase quality of life in patients with primary pulmonary hypertension?

Bottom line

Sildenafil in high doses produced significant improvements in fatigue and dyspnea scores and increased treadmill walking time by approximately 4 minutes in patients with primary pulmonary hypertension. It is an option – an expensive one – for the treatment of this disorder that has few good treatments. (LOE = 1b)

Reference

Sastry BK, Narasimhan C, Reddy NK, Raju BS. Clinical efficacy of sildenafil in primary pulmonary hypertension. A randomized, placebo-controlled, double-blind, crossover study. Am Coll Cardiol 2004;43:1149–1153.

Study Design

Cross-over trial (randomized)

Setting

Outpatient (specialty)

Synopsis

Just as it causes vasodilation to treat erectile dysfunction, sildenafil also inhibits the same enzyme in the lungs and can decrease pulmonary vascular resistance. This study evaluted the effect of sildenafil in 22 patients between the ages of 16 and 55 years with primary pulmonary hypertension and a New York Heart Association functional classification of II to III and pulmonary artery mean pressure of at least 30 mm Hg. Patients were randomly assigned to receive sildenafil 25 mg to 100 mg 3 times daily (depending on weight) or placebo for 6 weeks, followed by evaluation and then crossover to the other treatment for an additional 6 weeks. In this way each patient served as his or her own control, which allows conclusions to be drawn using a smaller number of patients. The use of nitrates or other vasodilators were not allowed during the study. Quality of life, measured by a chronic heart failure questionnaire, improved while taking sildenafil on the dyspnea score (22.0 vs 17.6 of a possible 35; $P < .05$) and fatigue score (22.2 vs 20.7 of a possible 28; $P < .05$), but the emotional function scale did not differ. Treadmill exercise time was unaffected by placebo when it was given first, but increased 3.8 minutes (from a baseline of 7.7 minutes) with sildenafil treatment. In patients who received sildenafil first, exercise time was increased 4.1 minutes but placebo treatment still resulted in a statistically significant 1.3 minutes. Cardiac index improved but pulmonary artery systolic pressure was not significantly affected. Note that this dosing regimen, at a cost of approximately $25 US per day, is very expensive (~$9000 US per year).

Sildenafil = bosentan in pulmonary hypertension (SERAPH)

Clinical question

Is sildenafil (Viagra) more effective than bosentan (Tracleer) in patients with class III pulmonary hypertension?

Bottom line

In this small study, sildenafil and bosentan had similar effects on patients with moderately severe pulmonary hypertension. (LOE = 1b)

Reference

Wilkins MR, Paul GA, Strange JW, et al. Sildenafil versus endothelin receptor antagonist for pulmonary hypertension (SERAPH) study. Am J Respir Crit Care Med 2005;171:1292–1297.

Study Design

Randomized controlled trial (double-blinded)

Funding

Foundation

Allocation

Concealed

Setting

Outpatient (specialty)

Synopsis

This team recruited consecutive patients with World Health Organization class III pulmonary hypertension. These patients could only walk 150 to 450 meters in 6 minutes. The researchers excluded patients with 3-fold elevations of liver enzymes, previous treatment with sildenafil (Viagra) or bosentan (Tracleer), and those in need of urgent therapy. The eligible patients were randomized (allocated via central computer) to receive sildenafil (n = 14) or bosentan (n = 12). The patients received bosentan 62.5 mg twice daily or sildenafil 50 mg twice daily for the first 4 weeks. Patients were then titrated up to sildenafil 50 mg 3 times daily or bosentan 125 mg twice daily (with a midday placebo tablet), for the next 12 weeks. The researchers evaluated a variety of intermediate outcomes (right ventricular mass, change in 6-minute walk distance, cardiac function, and so forth) and symptom scores via intention to treat. One patient treated with sildenafil died and another didn't finish the study. The researchers assigned worse case values for missing data. Although each treatment increased exercise capacity and quality of life, there were no differences between the treatments on any of the outcomes. The study was designed to detect tiny differences in right ventricle mass.

Essential Evidence: Medicine that Matters, Edited by David Slawson, Allen Shaughnessy, Mark Ebell, and Henry Barry.

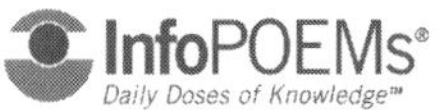

Testing for prothrombotic defects not necessary after first DVT

Clinical question

What risk factors predict recurrence after a first venous thrombotic event?

Bottom line

The risk of recurrence after a first venous thrombotic event (VTE) is increased in men, patients whose initial event is idiopathic, and women using oral contraceptives after the initial VTE. This study found no increased risk for recurrence in patients with prothrombotic abnormalities. Testing for prothrombotic abnormalities should be considered only in patients with a recurrent VTE. (LOE = 1b–)

Reference

Christiansen SC, Cannegieter SC, Koster T, Vandenbroucke JP, Rosendaal FR. Thrombophilia, clinical factors, and recurrent venous thrombotic events. JAMA 2005;293:2352–2361.

Study Design

Cohort (prospective)

Funding

Self-funded or unfunded

Setting

Inpatient (any location) with outpatient follow-up

Synopsis

The potential usefulness of screening for thrombophilia to prevent recurrence after a venous VTE is unknown. These investigators prospectively followed up 474 consecutive 18- to 70-year-old patients treated for a first confirmed VTE at participating hospitals and clinics in the Netherlands. Patients with a known malignancy were excluded. Complete follow-up occurred for 94% of the patients for an average of 7.3 years. Patients and clinicians were not blinded to outcome assessments. Recurrence of thrombotic events occurred in 90 patients, with the highest incidence during the first 2 years. Recurrence risk was statistically increased in men, patients whose initial event was idiopathic rather than provoked, and in women who used oral contraceptives after the initial VTE. There was no significant increased risk in patients with elevated levels of any prothrombotic abnormalities.

Management of antiphospholipid antibody syndrome

Clinical question

What is the optimal management of antiphospholipid antibody syndrome?

Bottom line

Patients who test positive for antiphospholipid antibodies are at an increased risk of thrombotic events. Similarly afflicted pregnant women are at an increased risk of fetal loss. Moderate-intensity anticoagulation with warfarin (target international normalized ratio (INR) = 2.0–3.0) prevents recurrent venous thrombosis. The optimal management of other thrombotic aspects of patients with antiphospholipid antibodies remains uncertain. (LOE = 1a–)

Reference

Lim W, Crowther MA, Eikelboom JW. Management of antiphospholipid antibody syndrome. A systematic review. JAMA 2006;295:1050–1057.

Study Design

Systematic review

Funding

Self-funded or unfunded

Setting

Various (meta-analysis)

Synopsis

Antiphospholipid antibodies are associated with an increased risk of thrombotic events and pregnancy morbidity. To fully evaluate this risk and potential treatments, the investigators systematically searched MEDLINE, the Cochrane Library, and reference lists from significant articles for randomized trials and cohort studies reporting on patients with antiphospholipid antibodies. The risk of developing a new thrombosis in otherwise healthy patients with antiphospholipid antibodies without prior thrombotic events is low (<1% per year). Among other patients with antiphospholipid antibodies, the risk of a new thrombotic event is moderately increased in women with recurrent fetal loss without prior thrombosis (up to 10% per year), and highest in patients with a history of venous thrombosis who have discontinued anticoagulant drugs within 6 months (>10% per year). Moderate-intensity anticoagulation (target INR = 2.0–3.0) significantly reduces the risk of recurrent thrombosis; no additional benefit is gained with high-intensity anticoagulation (target INR = >3.0). Evidence is lacking to make clear recommendations for patients with antiphospholipid antibodies without prior thrombosis, recurrent thrombosis despite anticoagulation, treatment of arterial thrombosis, and treatment of women with recurrent fetal loss.

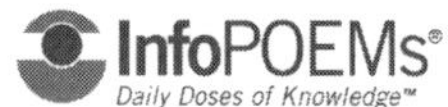

Fixed-dose, subcutaneous, unfractionated heparin effective for VTE

Clinical question

How safe and effective is fixed-dose subcutaneous unfractionated heparin in the treatment of venous thromboembolism?

Bottom line

In this study, fixed-dose weight-adjusted unfractionated heparin (UFH) administered subcutaneously was as safe and effective as low-molecular-weight heparin (LMWH) in the treatment of venous thromboembolism (VTE). Estimated drug costs for a 6-day course are $712 for LMWH and $37 for UFH. Most clinicians will want to see similar results from at least 1 additional well-done clinical trial, including more patients with symptomatic pulmonary embolism, before routinely treating VTE with subcutaneous UFH. (LOE = 1b)

Reference

Kearon C, Ginsberg JS, Julian JA, et al, for the Fixed-Dose Heparin (FIDO) Investigators. Comparison of fixed-dose weight-adjusted unfractionated heparin and low-molecular-weight heparin for acute treatment of venous thromboembolism. JAMA 2006;296:935–942.

Study Design	Funding	Allocation
Randomized controlled trial (single-blinded)	Foundation	Concealed

Setting

Outpatient (any)

Synopsis

These investigators randomly assigned (concealed allocation assignment) 708 patients, 18 years or older, with acute VTE to subcutaneous UFH (initial dose of 333 U/kg, followed by a fixed dose of 250 U/kg every 12 hours) or LMWH (dalteparin or enoxaparin, 100 IU/kg every 12 hours). The dose of subcutaneous UFH remained fixed for individual patients and was not changed during treatment as a result of anticoagulation profiles. The diagnosis of VTE included patients with acute deep vein thrombosis of the legs (81%) or symptomatic pulmonary embolism (19%). Oral warfarin was usually started on the same day as heparin in both groups and continued for a minimum of 3 months with doses adjusted to achieve an international normalized ratio (INR) of between 2.0 and 3.0. Heparin was continued for at least 5 days and until the INR was 2.0 or higher for 2 consecutive days. Individuals unaware of treatment group assignment assessed all outcomes, including study eligibility criteria. Follow-up occurred for more than 98% of subjects for 3 months. All eligible and consenting patients underwent final data analysis. The risk of recurrent VTE in the first 3 months after treatment was not significantly different between patients in the UFH group (3.8%) and those in the LMWH group (3.4%). The risk of major bleeding during the first 10 days of treatment was also similar between the UFH group (1.1%) and LMWH group (1.4%). Approximately 70% of patients in both groups received treatment entirely out of hospital. Overall, there were 18 deaths in the UFH group and 22 deaths in the LMWH group (difference not significant). Adverse events were unrelated to whether subjects were subtherapeutic or supratherapeutic.

Essential Evidence: Medicine that Matters, Edited by David Slawson, Allen Shaughnessy, Mark Ebell, and Henry Barry.

Compression stockings prevent post-thrombotic syndrome

Clinical question

Can off-the-shelf compression stockings prevent post-thrombotic syndrome in patients with a proximal deep vein thrombosis?

Bottom line

Post-thrombotic symptoms such as discomfort, swelling, and skin discoloration occur in up to one third of patients who have experienced a symptomatic proximal deep vein thrombosis. Use of below-the-knee graded compression stockings decreases the cumulative incidence of post-thrombotic symptoms by 50% over 2 years. Patients with a thrombosis should be advised to purchase these stockings following acute treatment. The stockings should be replaced every 6 months. (LOE = 2b)

Reference

Prandoni P, Lensing AW, Prins MH, et al. Below-knee elastic compression stockings to prevent the post-thrombotic syndrome. A randomized, controlled trial. Ann Intern Med 2005;141:249–256.

Study Design

Randomized controlled trial (nonblinded)

Allocation

Concealed

Setting

Outpatient (primary care)

Synopsis

Post-thrombotic syndrome occurs in 25% to 33% of patients following a symptomatic deep venous thrombosis (DVT). It occurs more commonly in elderly patients and in patients with recurrent DVT. The authors of this study enrolled 180 consecutive patients who presented with a first episode of symptomatic proximal DVT who received conventional anticoagulant treatment. Upon discharge, the patients were given nothing or below-the-knee elastic compression stockings to wear at least during the day for at least 2 years. The stockings, from an Italian company, provided 30 mm to 40 mm Hg of pressure at the ankle and were available in 5 sizes. In the United States, Jobst Support Hose with very firm support or other hose with surgical support provide a similar degree of compression. The investigators, who were unaware of treatment assignment, evaluated the patients every 3 months for at least 2 years, and up to 5 years. Using a self-developed and validated 33-point scale, investigators assigned a diagnosis of "mild" post-thrombotic syndrome to patients with scores of 5 to 14 on 2 consecutive visits, and "severe" post-thrombotic syndrome if they had a score greater than 15 on 2 consecutive examinations. Post-thrombotic syndrome occurred in 49.1% of unstockinged patients but only 24.5% of patients using the stockings (adjusted hazard ratio = 0.49; 95% CI, 0.29–0.84; P = .011). Over 2 years, one additional episode of the syndrome was avoided for every 4 patients who wore the stockings (number needed to treat = 4; 95% CI = 2.3–18.9).

Essential Evidence: Medicine that Matters, Edited by David Slawson, Allen Shaughnessy, Mark Ebell, and Henry Barry.

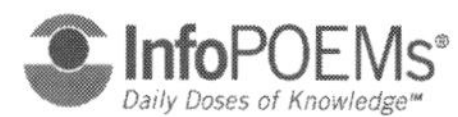

Routine use of vena cava filters doesn't reduce mortality

Clinical question

Does routine use of vena cava filters improve outcomes in patients with venous thromboembolism?

Bottom line

In a fairly high-risk group of patients with venous thromboembolism (VTE), vena cava filters reduce the risk of pulmonary embolism (PE), increase the risk of deep vein thrombosis (DVT), and do not alter the risk of death. However, this group was not typical of the group that is usually given these filters in clinical practice. (LOE = 1b)

Reference

PREPIC Study Group. Eight-year follow-up of patients with permanent vena cava filters in the prevention of pulmonary embolism. Circulation 2005;112:416–422.

Study Design

Randomized controlled trial (nonblinded)

Funding

Government

Setting

Inpatient (any location) with outpatient follow-up

Synopsis

Patients with acute proximal DVT with or without PE were randomized to permanent vena cava filter or usual treatment. All received warfarin for at least 3 months. Approximately one third were anticoagulated for only 3 months, one third for the entire 8-year follow-up period, and one third for an intermediate duration. The mean age of the 400 participants was 72 years, 95% were men, 36% had a PE, and 35% had a history of previous VTE. Although the study group is probably of higher-than-average risk among all patients with VTE, it is important to note that vena cava filters are generally only recommended for patients who have recurrent VTE despite adequate anticoagulation or those who cannot tolerate anticoagulation. Groups were balanced at the start of the study and analysis was by intention to treat. Patients and their physicians were aware of treatment assignment, but outcomes were adjudicated by a group blinded to treatment assignment. After 8 years, outcome data were available for all but 1 patient. Patients receiving a filter were less likely to have a PE (6.2% vs 15.1%; P = .008; number needed to treat = 11), but more likely to have a DVT (36% vs 27%; number needed to treat to harm = 11). There was no difference in the likelihood of post-thrombotic syndrome or death (50% in both groups).

Essential Evidence: Medicine that Matters, Edited by David Slawson, Allen Shaughnessy, Mark Ebell, and Henry Barry.

At least 6 months of anticoagulation optimal to prevent recurrent VTE

Clinical question

What is the optimal duration of anticoagulation following venous thromboembolism?

Bottom line

The optimal duration of anticoagulation following an initial venous thromboembolism (VTE) event is 6 months or more. The risk of a major bleeding event is most pronounced in the first month of treatment and the rate is similar to short-term (3 months or less) treatment. Since the magnitude of benefit appears to lessen beyond 6 months, physicians and patients should reassess individual risk/benefit profiles beyond this timeframe. (LOE = 1a)

Reference

Ost D, Tepper J, Mihara H, Lander O, Heinzer R, Fein A. Duration of anticoagulation following venous thromboembolism. A meta-analysis. JAMA 2005;294:706–715.

Study Design

Meta-analysis (randomized controlled trials)

Funding

Unknown/not stated

Setting

Various (meta-analysis)

Synopsis

Optimal duration of anticoagulation following venous thromboembolism (VTE) remains controversial. The investigators searched multiple databases, including the Cochrane database, clinical trial Web sites, and hand searches of reference lists. They included studies that were randomized controlled trials (in the English language) reporting the risk of recurrent VTE compared with the duration of anticoagulation in patients with an initial VTE event. Excluded studies were those reporting outcomes only on high-risk patients. Two reviewers independently assessed articles for both inclusion and exclusion criteria and study quality. A third reviewer adjudicated in cases of disagreement. Fifteen of 67 studies, enrolling a total of 5596 patients met inclusion criteria, and the overall quality of the individual studies was high. A formal evaluation for publication bias found minimal, if any, effect, and the overall findings of the multiple trials were consistent (homogenous). Long-term (median = 6 months) versus short-term (median = 1.75 months) therapy significantly reduced the risk of recurrent VTE events (number needed to treat = 50; 95% CI, 25–1000). Major bleeding events occurred most often in the first month of treatment and the overall risk was similar with long-term versus short-term therapy. Limited data suggests that extending anticoagulation beyond 6 months results in decreasing benefit.

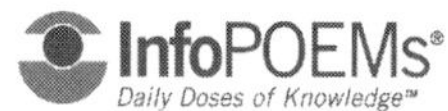

LMWH better than warfarin in preventing recurrent DVT in cancer patients

Clinical question

In patients with cancer and venous thromboembolism, is low-molecular-weight heparin more effective than warfarin in the prevention of recurrent emboli?

Bottom line

For every 13 cancer patients with an episode of venous thromboembolism (VTE) who receive 6 months of a low-molecular-weight heparin (dalteparin) instead of warfarin, there is 1 fewer recurrent episode of VTE. (LOE = 1b)

Reference

Lee AY, Levine MN, Baker RI, et al. Low-molecular-weight heparin versus a coumarin for the prevention of recurrent venous thromboembolism in patients with cancer. N Engl J Med 2003;349:146–153.

Study Design

Randomized controlled trial (single-blinded)

Setting

Outpatient (any)

Synopsis

Patients with cancer who have an episode of VTE, either deep vein thrombosis (DVT) or pulmonary embolism (PE), have an approximately 15% risk of recurrence during a 6-month follow-up period, even if treated appropriately with warfarin. All patients in this trial were given dalteparin in a dose of 200 IU/kg for 5 to 7 days. The 338 patients randomized to oral anticoagulation received a vitamin K antagonist (usually warfarin) for the remainder of the 6 months, adjusted to maintain the INR between 2.0 and 3.0. The 338 patients randomized (allocation concealed) to low-molecular-weight heparin received dalterparin in a dose of 200 IU/kg given once daily for the remainder of the first month, and then 150 IU/kg given once daily for the following 5 months. Groups were similar at baseline, with a mean age of 62 years, and 78% had metastatic disease. Approximately two thirds had a DVT alone, and one third had a PE with or without DVT. Patients were contacted at 2-week intervals during the 6-month follow-up period, and any suspected episodes of DVT or PE were investigated. At the end of the follow-up period, there were 14 DVTs, 8 nonfatal Pes, and 5 fatal PEs in the dalteparin group and 37 DVTs, 9 nonfatal PEs, and 7 fatal PEs in the oral anticoagulant group. The overall risk of VTE was significantly lower in the dalteparin group (8.0% vs 15.8%; P = .002, number needed to treat = 13). Major bleeding was more likely in the dalteparin group (19 vs 14 episodes), but this difference was not statistically significant. There was no difference in mortality between the groups (39% vs 41%; P = .53). The major limitation of the study was the failure to blind patients and physicians, although outcome adjudicators were masked to treatment assignment.

Best tests to rule in, rule out PE

Clinical question

In patients with suspected pulmonary embolism, which tests are effective in diagnosing or ruling out the condition?

Bottom line

Some tests are better at diagnosing pulmonary embolism (PE) and some are better at excluding it. To exclude PE in patients with a low likelihood of disease, use a lung scan, spiral computed tomography (CT) plus leg ultrasound, or D-dimer by ELISA. To diagnose PE in patients with a high likelihood of disease, use a ventilation perfusion scan, spiral CT, or leg ultrasound. (LOE = 1a)

Reference

Roy PM, Colombet I, Durieux P, Chatellier G, Sors H, Meyer G. Systematic review and meta-analysis of strategies for the diagnosis of suspected pulmonary embolism. BMJ 2005;331-259-68.

Study Design

Meta-analysis (other)

Funding

Self-funded or unfunded

Setting

Various (meta-analysis)

Synopsis

To evaluate the different diagnostic tests available to make the tricky identification of PE, the authors searched MEDLINE, Embase, and Pascal Biomed for English-language studies evaluating such tests. They also searched bibliographies and their personal libraries. Their search strategy did not include attempts to identify unpublished research and excluded articles not written in English, which are 2 minor limitations. Two reviewers independently selected studies for inclusion and extracted the data, and limited the studies they included to prospective studies that recruited consecutive patients, used pulmonary angiography as their reference standard, and for which the test being evaluated and the reference test were interpreted without knowledge of the results from the other study. The 48 studies selected for inclusion had an average prevalence of embolism of 30%. The results were reported in terms of likelihood ratio (LR): as a general rule, an test with an LR of less than 0.1 successfully excludes disease and a test with an LR of greater than 10 confidently identifies the disease. For exclusion of PE, negative LRs were: normal lung scan, 0.05 (95% CI, 0.03–0.1); negative spiral CT plus negative ultrasound, 0.04 (0.03–0.06); and a D-dimer concentration of less than 500 mcg/L by ELISA, 0.08 (0.04–0.18). At low probability, these tests lowered the likelihood of PE to less than 5%. D-dimer tests using other methods were not as effective, nor were leg ultrasound, magnetic resonance angiography, and echocardiography. For diagnosing PE, the LRs were: high probability ventilation perfusion scan, 18.3 (10.3–32.5); spiral CT, 24.1 (12.4–46.7); and leg ultrasound 16.2 (5.6–46.7). At high probability, these tests increased the likelihood of disease to 85%. Echocardiography is not useful and magnetic resonance angiography did not produce consistent results.

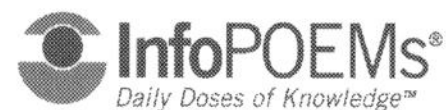

Clinical prediction rules accurate for PE diagnosis

Clinical question

Are clinical prediction rules accurate in the diagnosis of pulmonary embolism?

Bottom line

The clinical gestalt of experienced physicians and clinical prediction rules are similarly accurate in discriminating among patients with a low, medium, and high clinical/pre-test probability of pulmonary embolism (PE). The authors advocate the use of clinical prediction rules, particularly by less-experienced clinicians. (LOE = 1a)

Reference

Chunilal SD, Eikelboom JW, Attia J, et al. The rational clinical examination. Does this patient have pulmonary embolism? JAMA 2003;290:2849–2858.

Study Design

Systematic review

Setting

Other

Synopsis

Clinical prediction rules are commonly used to estimate the clinical probability of PE in selected patients. Experienced clinicians' gestalt is also similarly useful, but it is uncertain to what extent the 2 estimates are comparable. Three reviewers independently searched MEDLINE and bibliographies of pertinent articles to identify studies evaluating the accuracy of pretest probability assessment for PE using clinical gestalt versus clinical prediction rules. Included studies were those enrolling at least 50 or more consecutive, unselected patients; performance of clinical assessments blind to results of diagnostic testing; estimation of the pretest probability of PE using clinical gestalt or clinical prediction rule; and comparison of these 2 methods with acceptable gold standard methods for the diagnosis or exclusion of PE. From an initial identification of 1709 articles, 16 studies involving a total of 8306 patients met the inclusion criteria. Clinical gestalt strategy was used in 7 studies and, in the low-, moderate-, and high-risk categories, the rates of PE were 8% to 19%, 26% to 47%, and 46% to 91%, respectively. Clinical prediction rules were used in 10 studies and, in the low-, moderate-, and high-risk categories, the rates of PE were 3% to 28%, 16% to 46%, and 38% to 98%.

Essential Evidence: Medicine that Matters, Edited by David Slawson, Allen Shaughnessy, Mark Ebell, and Henry Barry.

Validated algorithm for evaluating suspected PE

Clinical question

What is the best work-up for suspected pulmonary embolism?

Bottom line

An algorithm that includes a careful, structured clinical assessment provides a safe, and presumably cost-effective, evaluation for patients with suspected pulmonary embolism (PE). The authors argue that omitting the lower extremity ultrasound is a reasonable option given its low yield in this study, although further evaluation of that step is needed in subsequent studies. (LOE = 1a)

Reference

Perrier A, Roy PM, Sanchez O, et al. Multidetector-row computed tomography in suspected pulmonary embolism. N Engl J Med 2005;352:1760–1768.

Study Design	**Funding**	**Setting**
Decision rule (validation)	Foundation	Emergency department

Synopsis

Helical CT initially used a single row of detectors; newer technology uses multiple rows. It is hoped that this will improve the sensitivity for detection of PE, since with single detector row CT approximately 30% of PEs are missed. With improved sensitivity it may be possible to forego the lower extremity ultrasound now recommended as an adjunct to single detector row helical CT. In this study, 1014 consecutive patients who presented with suspected PE were considered for inclusion; 756 met the inclusion criteria. The patients' clinical probability of PE was assessed using the Geneva score which includes signs, symptoms, chest radiograph findings, and blood gas results. Patients were classified as low, intermediate, or high probability, but the physicians could override the score if necessary. Patients with a low or intermediate probability had a D-dimer test; if negative, PE was ruled out. If the results were positive, these patients underwent multiple detector row helical CT and venous compression ultrasound of the lower extremities. Patients with a high clinical probability went directly to helical CT and venous ultrasound; if either result was positive, PE was diagnosed. If both results were negative in patients with high clinical probability they underwent pulmonary angiography. Patients with an inconclusive CT result were referred for either ventilation perfusion scanning or pulmonary angiography. Patients were followed up for 3 months, and only 4 were lost to follow-up. Of 82 patients with a high clinical probability of PE, 79 had a PE, and 78 of those were detected with the helical CT. Of 674 with a low or intermediate probability of PE, 115 (17%) had a PE. The algorithm performed well; of the 232 low/intermediate probability patients with a D-dimer < 500 mcg/L, none had a deep vein thrombosis, PE, or death during follow-up. Similarly, of 318 patients with a low/intermediate probability, D-dimer 500 mcg/L, and negative CT and venous ultrasound results, there were only 3 nonfatal thromboembolic events and 2 possible deaths from PE (1.7%; 95% CI, 0.7% to 3.9%). This is similar to the 3-month mortality of 1% to 2% seen in patients with suspected PE sent home after a normal pulmonary angiogram. It was rare that a clot was detected on lower extremity ultrasound in a patient with a normal CT result (3 of 324, 0.9%).

Essential Evidence: Medicine that Matters, Edited by David Slawson, Allen Shaughnessy, Mark Ebell, and Henry Barry.

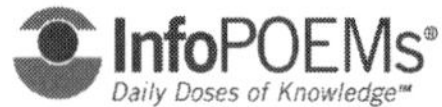

Optimal algorithm for evaluating suspected DVT

Clinical question

What is the best management strategy for patients with suspected deep vein thrombosis?

Bottom line

The most cost-effective algorithm for managing patients with suspected deep vein thrombosis (DVT) was identified, although several are nearly as good. The main message is that the best approach uses a combination of a validated clinical decision rule, D-dimer test, and venous ultrasound. (LOE = 1b)

Reference

Goodacre S, Stevenson M, Wailoo A, Sampson F, Sutton AJ, Thomas S. How should we diagnose suspected deep-vein thrombosis? QJM 2006;99:377–388.

Study Design

Cost-effectiveness analysis

Funding

Government

Setting

Various (meta-analysis)

Synopsis

These authors systematically reviewed the literature and identified 18 different strategies for managing patients with suspected DVT. They then evaluated a hypothetical group of 1000 patients using each algorithm, applying reasonable estimates of test accuracy, treatment effectiveness, and the cost of testing and treatment. This included the cost of applying a clinical decision rule, such as the Wells rule. They estimated a mean survival of 11.6 quality adjusted life years (QALYs) after diagnosis of DVT at age 60. The estimates were reasonable and most of the algorithms used some combination of the Wells rule, D-dimer, and venous ultrasound. The percentage of patients with proximal DVT who would be treated appropriately by the algorithms ranged from 90.1% to 99.5%, and the patients without DVT treated inappropriately ranged from 0.6% to 6.0%. The optimal algorithm used a latex D-dimer test as the initial screen. If patients were D-dimer negative and had a low or intermediate Wells score, DVT was considered ruled out. If they were D-dimer negative, but at high risk based on the Wells score, an above knee venous ultrasound was ordered. If the ultrasound was positive, they were treated; if negative, a repeat ultrasound was ordered. Patients who were D-dimer positive, underwent ultrasound: if positive, they were treated; if negative, they had repeat ultrasound. Several other algorithms were similarly cost-effective.

Essential Evidence: Medicine that Matters, Edited by David Slawson, Allen Shaughnessy, Mark Ebell, and Henry Barry.

Multidetector CT accurate for PE, but requires clinical context

Clinical question

How accurate is multidetector computed tomography for pulmonary embolism?

Bottom line

Patients with high or intermediate probability of pulmonary embolism (PE) and an abnormal result on computed tomographic angiography (CTA) or CTA combined with venous-phase imaging (CTA-CTV) are very likely to have PE. Those with low or intermediate probability and a negative CTA or CTA-CTV result are unlikely to have PE. All other patients – that is, those with discordant findings between the clinical examination and CTA or CTA-CTV – need either further testing or close clinical follow-up to confirm or exclude the diagnosis. Clinical evaluation using a validated decision rule remains an important part of the evaluation. (LOE = 2b)

Reference

Stein PD, Fowler SE, Goodman LR, et al, for the PIOPED II Investigators. Multidetector computed tomography for acute pulmonary embolism. N Engl J Med 2006;354:2317–2327.

Study Design

Diagnostic test evaluation

Funding

Government

Setting

Emergency department

Synopsis

CT technology continues to evolve, now moving from single slice CT to 4-slice or 16-slice multidetector scans. In this study, 824 patients with suspected PE underwent a standard clinical evaluation using the Wells clinical decision rule, CTA, CTA-CTV, ventilation perfusion (VQ) scanning, venous compression ultrasound of the legs, and pulmonary digital subtraction angiography (DSA), if necessary. Patients were drawn from a group of 7284 patients with suspected PE, but large numbers were excluded because they couldn't complete testing within 36 hours, had abnormal renal function, declined to participate, were using anticoagulants, or were otherwise unable to complete the protocol. The mean age of participants was 51 years, 65% were white, and 62% were women. Defined by the composite reference standard (high probability VQ scan, abnormal DSA result, or abnormal venous ultrasound and nondiagnostic VQ scan), 192 (23%) had a PE. Among those who'd had PE ruled out using this reference standard, only 2 had a likely PE during the 6-month follow-up. Also, 51 had CTA that was of insufficient quality and 87 had a CTA-CTV of poor quality, and they were excluded from the analysis. The CTA was 83% sensitive and 96% specific (positive likelihood ratio [LR+] = 19.6; negative likelihood ratio [LR–] = 0.18) and the CTA-CTV was 90% sensitive and 95% specific (LR+ = 16.5; LR– = 0.11). It's important to note that the predictive value of the tests depended on the clinical assessment. The Wells rule was used to stratify patients as high, intermediate, or low risk. The positive predictive value of CTA and CTA-CTV was 96%, but the negative predictive value was only 60% to 82% for those tests. However, for patients with a low clinical probability, the positive predictive value was only 57% to 58%, while the negative predictive value was a robust 96% to 97%. Values for positive and negative predictive value in intermedate probability patients were between 89% and 92%.

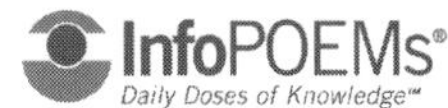

Negative CT scan to rule out PE equal to angiography

Clinical question

Can clinicians rely on a negative computed tomography scan to rule out suspected pulmonary embolism?

Bottom line

A negative computed tomography (CT) scan is as accurate as pulmonary angiography in ruling out suspected pulmonary embolism (PE). Clinicians should strongly consider using clinical decision rules to accurately assess the pretest probability of PE in a individual patient, and then interpret diagnostic tests in light of this probability. For example, a negative CT in a low-risk patient rules out PE, while a negative CT in a high-risk patient may require further confirmation. (LOE = 2a−)

Reference

Quiroz R, Kucher N, Zou KH, et al. Clinical validity of a negative computed tomography scan in patients with suspected pulmonary embolism. A systematic review. JAMA 2005;293:2012–2017.

Study Design	Funding	Setting
Systematic review	Government	Various (meta-analysis)

Synopsis

Previous studies question the value of using CT scanning alone to rule out suspected PE. These investigators thoroughly searched multiple databases – including MEDLINE, the Cochrane Registry of Controlled Trials, and Science Citation Index – and relevant journals for English language articles meeting selection criteria. Included studies used contrast-enhanced CT as the initial triage test to rule out the diagnosis of acute PE, had an appropriate clinical follow-up of at least 3 months, and a prospective design. The gold standard to establish the validity of testing to rule out PE was the rate of subsequent venous thromboembolic events (VTE) after anticoagulation therapy was withheld. Two reviewers independently abstracted data and a third party arbitrated discrepancies. From the initial search that found 22 studies, 15 studies evaluating a total of 3500 patients met the minimal inclusion criteria. Seven of these 15 met the criteria for level 1 diagnostic studies. Three different CT modalities were evaluated, including single-slice CT, multidetector-row (helical) CT, and electron-beam CT. Patient follow-up ranged from 3 months to 12 months. The overall negative likelihood ratio of a VTE after a negative CT scan for PE was 0.07 (95% CI, 0.05–0.11). There was no significant difference in the risk of a subsequent VTE based on the type of CT modality used. Compared with studies that used chest CT imaging only, the risk of subsequent VTEs in studies using additional imaging tests prior to chest CT was not significantly reduced. The reported negative likelihood ratio in this analysis compares favorably with that reported for pulmonary angiography (Henry JW, Relyea B, Stein PD. Chest 1995; 107:1375–78). A formal analysis found no evidence for significant publication bias, but there was some minimal heterogeneity among the results of the various trials.

Essential Evidence: Medicine that Matters, Edited by David Slawson, Allen Shaughnessy, Mark Ebell, and Henry Barry.

Determining major bleeding risk with warfarin for DVT

Clinical question

What is the risk of bleeding in patients receiving warfarin for thromboembolism?

Bottom line

In patients taking warfarin for the treatment of a deep vein thrombosis, approximately 1 in 45 (2.2%) will experience a major bleeding episode, and approximately 13% of these patients will die from the bleeding. The risk of bleeding decreases after the first 3 months to approximately 1 in 54 patients (1.9%). (LOE = 1a)

Reference

Linkins LA, Choi PT, Douketis JD. Clinical impact of bleeding in patients taking oral anticoagulant therapy for venous thromboembolism. Ann Intern Med 2003;139:893–900.

Study Design

Meta-analysis (randomized controlled trials)

Setting

Outpatient (any)

Synopsis

The authors of this meta-analysis combined the results of 29 randomized controlled trials and 4 prospective cohort studies. The studies were found through a search of 2 databases that was limited to those published in 1989 and later, since international normalized ratio (INR) was not used before 1989. Only articles in English were selected, and patients in the studies were treated with warfarin for at least 3 months. Two authors independently selected eligible studies; only one person extracted the data. Some of the data are a little tricky to understand; for example, to account for different lengths of treatment, the authors converted all outcomes into event rate per year. Major bleeding – bleeding that required hospitalization, transfusion, was intracranial or into a body cavity, or was fatal – occurred in approximately 1 in 14 patients per year (7.22 per 100 patient-years; 95% CI, 7.19–7.24). Intracranial bleeding occurred in approximately 1 in every 87 patients per year (1.15 per 100 patient-years; 95% CI, 1.14–1.16), or in approximately 9% of all major bleeding episodes. In the 2422 patients who received warfarin for more than 3 months, major bleeding occurred in 1 in every 45 patients during the first 3 months (2.23%), followed by 1 in 54 patients (1.9%) over the rest of the anticoagulation period (6–24 months). Approximately 1 in 8 patients will die following a major bleeding episode (fatality rate = 13.4%; 95% CI, 9.4%–17.4%).

Essential Evidence: Medicine that Matters, Edited by David Slawson, Allen Shaughnessy, Mark Ebell, and Henry Barry.

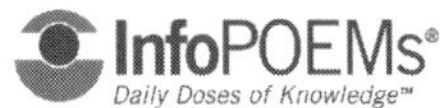

D-dimer useful for excluding DVT and PE

Clinical question

Can the d-dimer test be used to rule out suspected thromboembolism?

Bottom line

Although diagnostic tests often are good for both identifying and excluding disease, sometimes tests do one better than the other. A normal d-dimer test result can be relied upon to rule out suspected pulmonary embolism or deep vein thrombosis. It is not particularly helpful, by itself, to rule in the diagnosis. The results of this meta-analysis confirm an early meta-analysis (Ann Emerg Med 2002; 40:133–44). (LOE = 1a)

Reference

Stein PD, Hull RD, Patel KC, et al. D-dimer for the exclusion of acute venous thrombosis and pulmonary embolism. A systematic review. Ann Intern Med 2004;140:589–602.

Study Design

Meta-analysis (other)

Setting

Various (meta-analysis)

Synopsis

To answer the question concerning the role of d-dimer testing in patients with suspected deep vein thrombosis (DVT) or pulmonary embolism (PE), the authors of this meta-analysis identified 78 high-quality studies by searching MEDLINE and Embase for evaluative studies in all languages. They also performed a secondary analysis using an additional 30 studies with weaker study designs. As is now standard in meta-analyses, 2 authors determined what studies would be included and 2 authors independently extracted the data and then compared their results. Of the various methods of measuring d-dimer, enzyme-linked immunosorbent assay (ELISA) and quantitative rapid ELISA have the best test characteristics. For ruling out DVT, those tests have a sensitivity of 96% and a negative likelihood ratio of 0.09–0.12. Characteristics for ruling out PE are similar, with a sensitivity of 95% and a likelihood ratio of 0.12. In other words, this method of d-dimer testing accurately rules out DVT and PE. The test is not very useful, by itself, for identifying patients with DVT or PE, although it is helpful when combined with decision analysis or other testing (Arch Intern Med 2002;162;907–11).

Essential Evidence: Medicine that Matters, Edited by David Slawson, Allen Shaughnessy, Mark Ebell, and Henry Barry.

D-dimer < 250 ng/mL predicts low risk of VTE recurrence

Clinical question

Is a D-dimer level after a first spontaneous venous thromboembolism useful for predicting when it is safe to withdraw oral anticoagulation?

Bottom line

Patients with a first spontaneous venous thromboembolism (VTE) who terminate oral anticoagulation prophylaxis after at least 3 months have significantly less risk of VTE recurrence (3.7% vs 11.5%) if their D-dimer level is lower than 250 ng/mL. Now we need a well-constructed clinical decision rule that takes this information and integrates it with the risk of bleeding with continued prophylaxis for any specific individual, so each patients (and his or her clinician) can make an informed decision. (LOE = 2b)

Reference

Eichinger S, Minar E, Bialonczyk C, et al. D-dimer levels and risk of recurrent venous thromboembolism. JAMA 2003;290:1071–1074.

Study Design

Cohort (prospective)

Setting

Outpatient (specialty)

Synopsis

The optimal duration of oral anticoagulation after a first spontaneous VTE is unknown. The benefit of a reduced risk of VTE recurrence during anticoagulation must be balanced with the increased risk of bleeding. Since the D-dimer level is a marker for coagulation activation and an increased risk for VTE recurrence, the authors measured levels in 610 patients older than 18 years with a first spontaneous VTE. Patients were initially treated with oral anticoagulants for at least 3 months and D-dimer levels were obtained 3 weeks after discontinuation. Follow-up observations occurred at 3- to 6-month intervals for a mean duration of 38 months (up to 4 years). Thirty-seven (6%) of the patients were lost to follow up. A total of 79 (13%) patients had a recurrent VTE. The cumulative probability of recurrent VTE at 2 years was 3.7% (95% CI; 0.9%–6.5%) among patients with D-dimer levels lower than 250 ng/mL compared with 11.5% (95% CI; 8.0%–15%) among patients with higher levels (P = .001).

Essential Evidence: Medicine that Matters, Edited by David Slawson, Allen Shaughnessy, Mark Ebell, and Henry Barry.

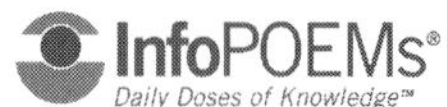

Restricted diet improves parental perception of hyperactive behavior

Clinical question

Does a diet that restricts food coloring and preservatives improve hyperactive behaviors in 3 year olds?

Bottom line

This study raises an interesting conundrum. Placing 3-year-old children on a diet that restricts food coloring and preservatives has no effect on hyperactive behaviors as observed by trained evaluators. However, the parents, who live with these kids for the remaining 23 hours of the day, report improvements in hyperactivity. There was no difference in results whether the child was hyperactive or atopic. (LOE = 2b)

Reference

Bateman B, Warner JO, Hutchinson E, et al. The effects of a double-blind, placebo-controlled, artificial food colourings and benzoate preservative challenge on hyperactivity in a general population sample of preschool children. Arch Dis Child 2004;89:506–511.

Study Design

Cross-over trial (randomized)

Setting

Outpatient (primary care)

Synopsis

These authors evaluated the effects of a restricted diet on 397 3-year-old children who were classified as hyperactive (HA) or not (HA-) and atopic (AT) or not (AT-), resulting in a 2 × 2 design. The study was split into 2 1-week treatment periods separated by 1-week washout periods. The children were to remain on a diet free of artificial coloring and benzoate preservatives for the entire 4 weeks. During the first week, the children were randomly assigned to receive a daily drink free of artificial coloring and sodium benzoate or an artificially colored and preserved drink identical in appearance. The children then were switched to the opposite drink during the second treatment period. Adults were unable to distinguish the taste of these beverages and the families and study personnel were all blinded to the specific treatment. Only 70% of the patients enrolled finished the study; 61 never started the study and 59 dropped out. Fifteen of the 59 parents who withdrew their child from the study did so because of behavioral changes. Nine of these withdrawals occurred during an active week and 6 during a placebo week. At the end of the study the parents were equally divided into those who did or did not correctly identify the drink order. Based on the parents ratings, their children were calmer during the week when no artificial coloring and preservatives were given. The trained observers, however, detected no significant differences during any of the treatment periods.

Essential Evidence: Medicine that Matters, Edited by David Slawson, Allen Shaughnessy, Mark Ebell, and Henry Barry.

Stimulants similarly effective for ADHD

Clinical question

Which drug therapy is more effective in children with attention-deficit hyperactivity disorder?

Bottom line

Stimulants have the best evidence of effectiveness in the treatment of children with attention-deficit hyperactivity disorder. The research does not give us a clear-cut choice among the stimulants or their formulations, so an empirical, trial-and-error approach is needed. Antidepressants may not be as effective. Behavioral therapy may add benefit to drug therapy, but is less effective than drug therapy when used alone. The role of atomoxetine (Strattera) is unclear because of few comparative studies or long-term studies. (LOE = 1a)

Reference

Brown RT, Amler RW, Freeman WS, et al. Treatment of attention-deficit/hyperactivity disorder: overview of the evidence. Pediatrics 2005;115:e749–e757.

Study Design	Funding	Setting
Systematic review	Other	Various (meta-analysis)

Synopsis

This report is from the American Academy of Pediatrics' Committee on Quality Improvement Subcommittee on Attention-Deficit/Hyperactivity Disorder. It is based on three evidence reviews performed by the McMaster Evidence-Based Practice Center, the Canadian Coordinating Office for Health Technology Assessment, the Multimodal Treatment Study for Children with ADHD, and the mysterious "supplemental reviews conducted by the subcommittee." The McMaster review seems to be the foundation for the report and is a well-described systematic review. Most of the results currently available are from short-term studies that compared the major stimulants used for attention-deficit hyperactivity disorder. Since the definition of what constitutes "improvement" varies among patients and research studies, study results could not be combined. Studies were not able to show, on average, a difference in treatment between methylphenidate (Ritalin), dextroamphetamine or its individual isomers, and pemoline (Cylert), or a difference in any formulations of the same drug. Similarly, there is no difference in the likelihood of adverse effects, though the studies are small. Studies of the antidepressants desipramine and imipramine compared with placebo show heterogeneous results. Nonpharmacologic intervention was not as effective as drug therapy, though behavioral therapy enhanced drug therapy in the Multimodal Treatment Study. Regarding the nonstimulant atomoxetine (Strattera), in a short-term study it is as effective as methylphenidate, with similar side effect profiles, causing similar appetite suppression and initial weight loss. It doesn't worsen insomnia but can cause daytime drowsiness and increase blood pressure in some adults and children. Atomexetine has a slow onset of action, taking up to 1 week to begin working, but seems to last longer throughout the day when it does work. Atomoxetine has been associated with an increased likelihood of suicidal ideation (0.4% vs 0.0% with placebo), according to the Food and Drug Administration (http://www.fda.gov/cder/drug/infopage/atomoxetine/default.htm).

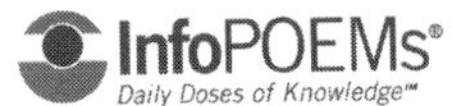

Responders to atomoxetine do well with lower doses

Clinical question

Can the dose of atomoxetine be lowered in children who respond to recommended doses?

Bottom line

In children who respond to the typical dose of atomoxetine (Strattera), a lowered dose of 0.5 mg per kg per day is similarly effective in maintaining scores on a validated measurement scale. (LOE = 1b)

Reference

Newcorn JH, Michelson D, Kratochvil C, Allen AJ, Ruff DD, Moore RJ, for the Atomoxetine Low-dose Study Group. Low-dose atomoxetine for maintenance treatment of attention-deficit/hyperactivity disorder. Pediatrics 2006;118:1701–1706.

Study Design

Randomized controlled trial (double-blinded)

Funding

Industry

Allocation

Uncertain

Setting

Outpatient (primary care)

Synopsis

The researchers conducting this study had previously conducted a study of the use of atomoxetine in children meeting the diagnostic criteria for attention-deficit/hyperactivity disorder (ADHD). The 229 children in this prior study who responded to full doses of atomoxetine, 1.2 mg per kg per day, were randomly assigned (concealed allocation uncertain) to continue their previously effective dose or to continue treatment at a dose of 0.5 mg/kg/day. The doses were only adjusted for weight changes over the 8 months of the study. The children had an average age of 10.5 years and had the combined subtype of ADHD; the majority were male. The primary measure was the Attention-Deficit/Hyperactivity Disorder Rating Scale-IV-Parent Version, an interviewer administered and scored list of 18 items. Relapse, defined as a return to 90% of baseline score, occurred over the course of the study in approximately 2.7% of children in each group. A similar percentage of children in each group also had scores that no longer met the criterion for response, but did not meet the relapse criterion (23% in the low-dose group vs 17% in the same-dose group; P = NS).

Anemia not prevented by iron in infants

Clinical question
Does prophylactic administration of iron prevent the development of anemia in infants?

Bottom line
Routine iron supplementation in infants, starting at 6 months of age, does not affect the prevalence of anemia when it is evaluated at the 9-month visit. Anemia in the infants in this study was related to maternal anemia during pregnancy, which was present in 43% of the mothers in this sample; the children were likely anemic since birth. (LOE = 1b)

Reference
Geltman PL, Meyers AF, Mehta SD, et al. Daily multivitamins with iron to prevent anemia in high-risk infants: a randomized clinical trial. Pediatrics 2004;114:86–93.

Study Design
Randomized controlled trial (double-blinded)

Setting
Outpatient (primary care)

Synopsis
The investigators of this study enrolled 376 healthy, full-term infants at their 6-month well visit. Approximately 90% of mothers received supplemental nutrition vouchers through the Special Supplemental Nutrition Program for Women, Infants, and Children, and 43% of the mothers were anemic during pregnancy. Iron status of the infants was not determined at this time. The children were randomized (allocation concealed) to receive a multivitamin with or without 10 mg of elemental iron for 3 months. Approximately 74% of the children were available 3 months to 6 months later for follow-up. At this visit, 84% of the children were either anemic (21% of total) or possibly iron deficient (defined by the number of indices, other than hemoglobin, that were abnormal). There was no statistical difference in the proportion of the children in either group who developed anemia, nor were there any differences in any specific anemia measure. The presence of anemia at ages 9 to 12 months was correlated with maternal anemia during pregnancy. The results were similar when including all patients, whether or not they were fully adherent to therapy (intention-to-treat analysis), or when analyzing only children who received iron daily. Since the children may have been anemic at the start of the study, another interpretation may be that 10 mg of iron is not sufficient to replete iron in anemic children.

Essential Evidence: Medicine that Matters, Edited by David Slawson, Allen Shaughnessy, Mark Ebell, and Henry Barry.

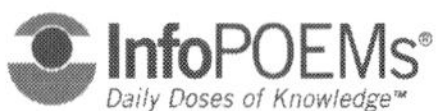

Anemia doesn't predict iron deficiency among toddlers

Clinical question

Does screening toddlers for anemia identify those with iron deficiency?

Bottom line

We cannot feel assured that a young child doesn't have iron deficiency if they show a normal hemoglobin level, and we can't be sure that he or she has iron deficiency anemia if the hemoglobin level is low. Screening for iron deficiency in toddlers by checking serum hemoglobin misses most children with a deficiency, and most of the children with anemia do not have an iron deficiency. (LOE = 1b)

Reference

White KC. Anemia is a poor predictor of iron deficiency among toddlers in the United States: For heme the bell tolls. Pediatrics 2005;115:315–320.

Study Design

Cohort (prospective)

Funding

Government

Setting

Population-based

Synopsis

An insuffcient level of iron (which is used in more than 200 enzymes in the body) is associated with developmental disabilities in young children. Measuring serum hemoglobin as an indicator of anemia is used to screen for iron deficiency in young children. The author of this study evaluated the correlation between anemia and iron deficiency by examining the findings of the National Health and Nutrition Survey (NHANES) conducted between 1988 and 1994. The NHANES is a stratified population sample performed across the United States. The survey included 1289 toddlers between the ages of 12 and 35 months, and all of these children underwent complete blood counts, as well as measures of iron stores: ferritin, transferrin saturation, and free erythrocyte protoporphyrin. Iron deficiency, identified in 10.9% of the children studied, was defined as at least 2 of the iron indices being below normal. Anemia was defined as a hemoglobin level of less than 11.0 g/dL.There was little relation in this sample between the presence of iron deficiency and anemia. Children with iron deficiency had an average hemoglobin level of 11.5 g/dL, which, although statistically lower than the average 12.1 g/dL in nondeficient toddlers, was still above the cutoff for anemia. Only 28% (95% CI, 20–38) of toddlers with low hemoglobin actually had iron deficiency. The ability of anemia to rule out iron deficiency was also low: the sensitivity of the test was only 30% (95% CI, 20–40). In other words, for every 100 toddlers studied, 9 will have anemia, and 9 will have iron deficiency, but only 3 of the children with iron deficiency will be anemic and only 3 of the children with anemia will be iron deficient; not a great overlap. Similar results have been shown in data from New Zealand, Britain, and Europe (see the Discussion section of this study).

Essential Evidence: Medicine that Matters, Edited by David Slawson, Allen Shaughnessy, Mark Ebell, and Henry Barry.

Long-term budesonide does not effect adrenal function in children

Clinical question
Does the use of chronic inhaled corticosteroids affect adrenal function in children?

Bottom line
A nagging worry about using inhaled corticosteroids in children has been relieved. In a study of more than 3 years, continuous use of budesonide (Pulmicort) had no effect on serum cortisol levels or cortisol response to adrenocorticotrophic hormone administration. (LOE = 1b)

Reference
Bacharier LB, Raissy HH, Wilson L, et al. Long-term effect of budesonide on hypothalamic-pituitary-adrenal axis function in children with mild to moderate asthma. Pediatrics 2004;113:1693–1699.

Study Design
Randomized controlled trial (nonblinded)

Setting
Outpatient (primary care)

Synopsis
Uncontrolled (eg, cross-sectional or retrospective) studies have suggested that chronic inhaled corticosteroid use in children may effect hypothalamic-pituitary-adrenal axis function. These authors evaluated this effect in 63 children with mild to moderate asthma who received standard doses of budesonide (400 mcg/day; n = 18) or either nedocromil (Tilade) or placebo (n = 45) for 36 months. At the time of enrollment children were approximately 9 years old. Serum cortisol levels and response to adrenocorticotrophic hormone (ACTH) stimulation were measured at baseline and at 12 and 36 months. At both measurements, response to ACTH stimulation was similar between the children receiving budesonide and those receiving nedocromil or placebo. Urinary excretion of cortisol over 24 hours was also not affected overall, although it was statistically lower (P = .05) if supplemental inhaled corticosteroid was used in the 4 months preceding the 36-month visit. Two caveats: (1) these 63 children may not be representative of all children with mild to moderate asthma, and (2) the analysis was by intention to treat,instead of by using only the children who had demonstrated continuous use of budesonide. Noncompliance with treatment might also be responsible for the lack of effect.

Essential Evidence: Medicine that Matters, Edited by David Slawson, Allen Shaughnessy, Mark Ebell, and Henry Barry.

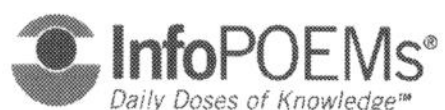

Amoxicillin for 3 days effective for pediatric pneumonia

Clinical question

Is 3 days of treatment with amoxicillin as effective as 5 days of the same therapy in children with non-severe pneumonia?

Bottom line

Outpatient treatment with 3 days of amoxicillin therapy produced similar results as 5 days of treatment in children with presumed pneumonia. In both groups, treatment failures occurred in 10% of children. (LOE = 1b)

Reference

ISCAP Study Group. Three day versus five day treatment with amoxicillin for non-severe pneumonia in young children: a multicentre randomised controlled trial. BMJ 2004;328:791–794.

Study Design

Randomized controlled trial (double-blinded)

Setting

Outpatient (primary care)

Synopsis

This study enrolled more than 2100 children between the ages of 2 months and 6 years with non-severe pneumonia. The diagnostic criteria were clinical: cough, rapid respiration, or difficulty breathing not deemed to be indicative of severe pneumonia. Fever was not a criterion. Patients were randomized (using concealed allocation) to receive either 3 days or 5 days of oral amoxicillin 30 mg to 50 mg per kg per day. Treatment failure was defined as retractions (chest indrawing), convulsions, drowsiness, the inability to drink, or a cutoff respiratory rate too high or an oxygen saturation too low on day 5. In the intention-to-treat analysis cure rates were similar between the 2 groups (90%), as were relapse rates within the next 7 to 9 days (5%). Cure rates were the same whether the children had wheezes and did not vary by age. Hospitalizations were infrequent but similar in the 2 groups (2%). The study had the power to find a 5% difference in treatment failures, assuming a 12% failure rate with the longer therapy.

Essential Evidence: Medicine that Matters, Edited by David Slawson, Allen Shaughnessy, Mark Ebell, and Henry Barry.

Educational programs effective for young asthmatics

Clinical question

Do educational programs for the self-management of asthma affect outcomes in children and adolescents?

Bottom line

Teaching children and adolescents how to manage their asthma improves their feeling of self-efficacy, improves lung function, decreases the number of days lost from school and the number of days with restricted activity, and decreases emergency visits. These were formal, multiple-session programs. Teaching methods focusing on individualized responses to changes in peak flow measurements had the strongest effects. (LOE = 1a)

Reference

Guevara JP, Wolf FM, Grum CM, Clark NM. Effects of educational interventions for self-management of asthma in children and adolescents: systematic review and meta-analysis. BMJ 2003;326:1308–1312.

Study Design

Meta-analysis (randomized controlled trials)

Setting

Outpatient (any)

Synopsis

An earlier meta-analysis (from 1992) of self-management education found no affect on children or adolescents; the analysis was based, however, on relatively few studies, and may not have had enough power to show a difference if one was truly there. The authors of the current meta-analysis searched several databases and identifed 32 randomized controlled trials enrolling a total of 3706 patients. They did a thorough job of searching the literature, including in their analysis articles published in any language. Their criterion for quality analysis was whether the investigators enrolling patients into the studies were unaware of the group to which the patients would be assigned (ie, concealed allocation); only 38% of the studies had a thorough description of this concealed allocation to treatment group and 10% clearly did not conceal allocation. However, results were similar when the high-quality studies were separately analyzed from lower-quality studies. The educational programs were diverse, and targeted children, adolescents, or both. These were not 2-minute this-what-you-do-with-your-peak-flow-meter lectures, but instead most of them used multiple sessions and focused on symptom-based strategies. In the 4 studies that evaluated it, the programs were associated with a moderate effect on lung function (standardized mean difference = 0.50; 95% CI, 0.25–0.75), translating into an approximately 10% increase in peak expiratory flow rate. Absences from school, night dusturbances, and the number of days with restricted activities were fewer in the children receiving the education, and children with moderate to severe asthma, as expected, experienced a greater effect. Children receiving the education reported a moderate improvement in their control of asthma. Visits to emergency departments were fewer in the educated patients, though hospitalization rate was not affected.

Essential Evidence: Medicine that Matters, Edited by David Slawson, Allen Shaughnessy, Mark Ebell, and Henry Barry.

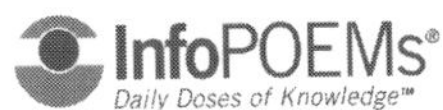

Nitazoxanide reduces rotavirus duration in hospitalized kids

Clinical question

Does nitazoxanide reduce the duration of rotavirus diarrhea in hospitalized children?

Bottom line

In this exploratory study, nitazoxanide (Alinia) reduced the duration of illness by nearly 2 days in children hospitalized with rotavirus diarrhea. It is unclear whether these findings would be similarly impressive in children who are less severely ill. (LOE = 2b–)

Reference

Rossignol JF, Abu-Zekry M, Hussein A, Santoro MG. Effect of nitazoxanide for treatment of severe rotavirus diarrhoea: randomised double-blind placebo-controlled trial. Lancet 2006;368:124–129.

Study Design

Randomized controlled trial (double-blinded)

Funding

Industry

Allocation

Concealed

Setting

Inpatient (ward only)

Synopsis

This is a preliminary study of 38 Egyptian patients younger than 12 years of age with watery diarrhea severe enough to require hospitalization. All of these children also had confirmed rotavirus infection. They were randomly assigned (concealed allocation) to receive 3 days of nitazoxanide or placebo. The majority of the children had 5 to 10 stools per day or more. Most of the hospitalized children were malnourished and had nearly 1 week of symptoms before admission. The dosing of nitazoxanide was 200 mg twice daily for children aged 4 years to 11 years, 100 mg twice daily for children aged 12 months to 47 months, and 0.375 mg per kg twice daily for those younger than 12 months. All patients remained in the hospital for 1 week after the start of treatment. The authors used an intention-to-treat analysis but removed children who also had other identified causes of diarrhea (like bacterial pathogens, Giardia lamblia, Entamoeba histolytica, and so forth). The children receiving nitazoxanide had a significant reduction in the duration of illness (31 hours compared with 75 hours in the control patients), though the authors don't define how this outcome was determined. The authors reported no significant adverse events in the treatment group and 2 minor adverse events in control children.

Essential Evidence: Medicine that Matters, Edited by David Slawson, Allen Shaughnessy, Mark Ebell, and Henry Barry.

Oral rotavirus vaccines safe and effective

Clinical question

Is an oral vaccine safe and effective for the prevention of a rotavirus infection in young children?

Bottom line

Oral vaccines have been developed that are safe and effective for the prevention of rotavirus in young children. This will be particularly useful in third world countries where this disease is a major cause of infant mortality. (LOE = 1b)

Reference

Ruiz-Palacios GM, Perez-Schael I, Velazquez FR, et al, for the Human Rotavirus Vaccine Study Group. Safety and efficacy of an attenuated vaccine against severe rotavirus gastroenteritis. N Engl J Med 2006;354:11–22.

Study Design

Randomized controlled trial (double-blinded)

Funding

Industry

Allocation

Uncertain

Setting

Population-based

Synopsis

The first vaccine for rotavirus (Rotashield) was withdrawn from the market because in rare cases it caused intussusception. This study evaluated a live attenuated vaccine (Rotarix) given in 2 oral doses 1 to 2 months apart, with the first dose given to patients between the ages of 6 weeks and 13 weeks. The study randomized more than 62,000 infants to the vaccine or placebo in Finland and in 11 South American and Central American countries. Allocation concealment and randomization procedures are not clearly described by the authors. The entire group was followed up for a median of 100 days to assess the safety of the vaccine, and a subgroup of 20,169 infants was followed up for 9 to 10 months to evaluate efficacy. There was no significant difference between groups in the likelihood of intussusception (9 in the vaccine group and 16 in the placebo group). Regarding efficacy, the risk of severe gastroenteritis of any cause (defined using a standard symptoms scale) was reduced from 52 to 31 episodes per 1000 infants per year (number needed to treat [NNT] = 48; 95% CI, 26–303) and the number of diarrhea-related hospitalizations was reduced from 42 to 25 episodes per 1000 infants per year (NNT = 56; 29–486). Both of these differences were statistically significant. A second study in the same issue of the journal reported similar findings for a second oral vaccine given in 3 doses called Rotateq (N Engl J Med 2006;354:23–33).

Essential Evidence: Medicine that Matters, Edited by David Slawson, Allen Shaughnessy, Mark Ebell, and Henry Barry.

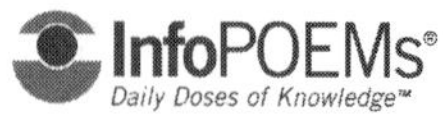

Intense diet-behavior-physical activity effective for obese children

Clinical question

Can a specific program of diet and exercise cause a sustained weight loss in children?

Bottom line

An intensive 3-month program of dietary counseling, a hypocaloric diet, and structured exercise can cause a weight loss in children that is sustained over 1 year. More important, the program seemed to increase the amount of exercise the children performed and this increase was sustained after the intervention was discontinued. (LOE = 2b)

Reference

Nemet D, Barkan S, Epstein Y, Friedland O, Kowen G, Eliakim A. Short- and long-term beneficial effects of a combined dietary-behavioral-physical activity intervention for the treatment of childhood obesity. Pediatrics 2005;115:443–449.

Study Design	Funding	Allocation
Randomized controlled trial (nonblinded)	Government	Uncertain

Setting

Outpatient (primary care)

Synopsis

The researchers conducting this study began with 54 obese children between the ages of 6 years and 16 years. The children were randomly assigned either to a control group that received a single nutrition counseling session or to an active treatment group. Active treatment consisted of heavy-duty dietary and exercise modification for 3 months. It is not clear that allocation to treatment groups was concealed and it is possible that children more likely to respond to treatment were preferentially enrolled. The dietary intervention consisted of 6 meetings over a 3-month period with parents and the child. These counseling sessions focused on food choices, nutritional information, and behavior change. The children were placed on a diet of approximately 30% less than the reported intake or 15% less than the estimated daily required intake. The exercise program was conducted 2 hours per week by physicians who were former members of the Israeli national track and field team and consisted of games focusing on endurance, with the children encouraged to add an extra 30 to 45 minutes of walking or other exercise per week. Analysis was per protocol and not by intention to treat, which is about the only way they could have done the analysis. Dropouts early during the intervention period and in the subsequent 1 year follow-up, dwindled the groups to 20 patients each. After 3 months of diet and exercise intervention, the children in the treatment group had lost an average 2.8 kg whereas the children in the control group gained an average 1.1 kg. Body mass index and body fat percentage also declined in the treated children. Over the 1 year of follow-up, children in the control group had gained an average 5.2 kg; the children in the treatment group gained an average 0.6 kg ($P < .05$). Body mass index increased in the control group but had decreased in the treated patients. Other significant differences at 1 year included lower body fat, amount of exercise activity, and endurance time on a treadmill. Both groups reported a decrease in screen time (that is, time spent watching television or playing video games) from an average 4.5 to 4.8 hours per day to 3.3 to 3.4 hours per day 1 year later.

Essential Evidence: Medicine that Matters, Edited by David Slawson, Allen Shaughnessy, Mark Ebell, and Henry Barry.

Evidence lacking for milk's benefit in children

Clinical question

Is abundant dietary calcium from dairy or other sources associated with better bone mineral density, bone mineral content, or lower fracture risk in children and young adults?

Bottom line

Although milk has a prominent place in the current recommendations for diet in children (see: www.mypyramid.com) there is a lack of convincing evidence that increased consumption of total dietary calcium generally, or dairy products specifically, provide even modest benefits for bone health in children and adolescents. (LOE = 1a)

Reference

Lanou AJ, Berkow SE, Barnard ND. Calcium, dairy products, and bone health in children and young adults: a reevaluation of the evidence. Pediatrics 2005;115:736–743.

Study Design

Systematic review

Funding

Other

Setting

Various (meta-analysis)

Synopsis

Current dietary guidelines in the U.S. recommend 2–3 cups (480 mL–720 mL) of milk daily for children. This review sought to determine whether there is sufficient evidence to support current recommendations of abundant intake of calcium in childhood to promote bone integrity, and whether milk or other dairy products are better than other calcium-containing foods or calcium supplements. Most studies were conducted with white preadolescent and adolescent girls. The review included 17 cross-sectional studies, 7 retrospective studies, 10 prospective studies, and 12 randomized controlled trials. Most studies assessed surrogate markers of bone health such as bone mineral density (BMD), bone mineral content (BMC), and calcium balance, although susceptibility to fractures was assessed in a few studies. There was no consistent evidence found for a relationship between dairy intake or total calcium intake and BMD, BMC, or fracture risk.

Essential Evidence: Medicine that Matters, Edited by David Slawson, Allen Shaughnessy, Mark Ebell, and Henry Barry.

Vaccine exposure does not increase risk of infectious disease hospitalization

Clinical question

Does exposure to multiple-antigen vaccine or aggregated vaccine increase the risk of infectious disease hospitalization?

Bottom line

There is no evidence for an increased risk of infectious-disease hospitalizations in children receiving multiple-antigen vaccines or aggregated vaccine exposure. (LOE = 1b)

Reference

Hviid A, Wohlfahrt J, Stellfeld M, Melbye M. Childhood vaccination and nontargeted infectious disease hospitalization. JAMA 2005;294:699–705.

Study Design

Cohort (prospective)

Funding

Government

Setting

Population-based

Synopsis

Many clinicians and laypersons are concerned that exposure to multiple-antigen vaccines and/or cumulative vaccine causes immune dysfunction secondary to an "overload" mechanism, resulting in an increased risk of subsequent infectious disease. The investigators monitored all children born in Denmark from January 1, 1990, through December 31, 2001. Individuals living in Denmark are given a unique identification number at birth allowing accurate linkage to information on childhood vaccinations, infectious disease hospitalizations, and potential confounding factors. Vaccines given during this time included the Haemophilus influenza type b (Hib), diphtheria-tetanus-inactivated pertussis, inactivated poliovirus, live attenuated oral polio virus, and mumps-measles-rubella. The effect of vaccination was evaluated in 3 different periods: within 14 days, 14 days through 3 months, and more than 3 months after vaccination. Appropriate statistical analyses accounted for potential confounders including sex, place of birth, birth weight, mother's age at birth, and month of birth. In the 805,206 children born during the study period, the investigators identified 84,317 cases of infectious disease hospitalization. Adequate follow-up occurred for more than 98% of the children. The only adverse association occurred between exposure to the Hib vaccine and subsequent hospitalization for acute upper respiratory tract infection (URI) more than 3 months after exposure (relative risk = 1.05; 95% CI, 1.01–1.08; number needed to treat to harm = 31,250; 19,531–156,250). Given that the authors tested 42 possible associations, it's likely they would find a significant difference in one of them by chance alone. In addition, there was no temporal or dose response relationship between Hib vaccination and hospitalization for URI, arguing against a causal relationship. No association was found between cumulative vaccine exposure and infectious diseases.

Dental restoration with amalgam (mercury) safe in children

Clinical question

Are amalgam dental restorations containing mercury safe for children?

Bottom line

Children who received dental restorative treatment with amalgam did not score significantly better or worse on neurobehavioral and neuropsychological assessments than children who received resin composite material. Children who receive restoration with resin may be more likely to need additional treatment. Studies evaluating outcomes for longer than 5 to 7 years are needed. (LOE = 1b–)

Reference

Bellinger DC, Trachtenberg F, Barregard L, et al. Neuropsychological and renal effects of dental amalgam in children. A randomized clinical trial. JAMA 2006;295:1775–1783.

Study Design

Randomized controlled trial (double-blinded)

Funding

Government

Allocation

Concealed

Setting

Population-based

Synopsis

Health risks associated with inhalation of mercury vapor released during amalgam dental restoration are unknown. The investigators identified 534 children, aged 6 to 10 years, with no known prior or existing amalgam restorations and at least 2 posterior teeth with dental caries requiring restoration. Eligible subjects randomly (concealed allocation assignment) underwent restoration with standard amalgam containing 50% elemental mercury or with a resin composite material (white filling) free of mercury. All individuals assessing outcomes remained blinded to treatment group assignment. Complete outcome data were available for at least 75% of enrolled children during the 5-year trial period, with an equal number of children unavailable in both treatment groups. Full assessment of intelligence, auditory memory, visual-motor integration, attention, and emotional state using previously validated scoring tools occurred at baseline prior to caries restoration, and at 3 years and 5 years. Children had a mean of 15 tooth surfaces restored during the 5-year period. Using intention-to-treat analysis, no statistically significant differences were found between children in the amalgam group and the composite group in any of the outcomes measured. Interestingly, there was a nonsignificant increase in IQ detected in children assigned to the amalgam group. The study was 80% powered to detect a 3-point difference in IQ scores between the treatment groups. A similar 7-year randomized trial enrolling 507 children from another setting published in the same journal issue (DeRouen TA, Martin MD, Leroux BG, et al. JAMA 2006;295:1784–1792) also reported no significant differences in neurobehavioral assessments between children receiving dental restorative treatment with amalgam and those receiving a resin composite. In the second study, children assigned to restoration with resin composite were more likely to require additional restorative treatment.

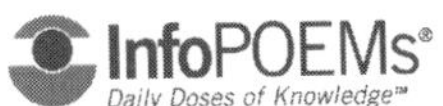

School-based violence prevention programs not proved

Clinical question

Are school-based violence prevention programs directed at high risk kids effective?

Bottom line

The studies included in this meta-analysis demonstrate modest reductions in aggressive behaviors, but that there is a need for larger, high quality studies. This is analogous to the studies of the DARE program: sounds good, doesn't work. (LOE = 1a–)

Reference

Mytton JA, DiGuiseppi, Gough DA, et al. School-based violence prevention programs: systematic review of secondary prevention programs. Arch Pediatr Adolesc Med 2002;156:752–762.

Study Design

Meta-analysis of randomized controlled trials

Setting

Other

Synopsis

The authors searched numerous databases and made a reasonable effort to locate unpublished randomized controlled studies of school-based violence prevention programs directed at children who had previously been identified as being at risk for aggressive behaviors. Two investigators independently extracted the data and when important elements were missing from the study, they contacted the authors. Unfortunately, they did not explicitly assess the quality of the studies. They ended up with 28 studies with 2096 children that met their criteria. None of them reported any data on violent injuries. While the studies demonstrated a 36% relative reduction in aggressive behaviors, there was significant and worrisome variation among the studies. They also found that larger studies found the least effect and that small studies showing harm or no benefit were lacking, suggesting that publication bias exists. That means that these small "negative" studies may have been rejected, creating a bias in the literature toward studies that show an effect.

Delayed prescription for AOM reduces unnecessary antibiotics

Clinical question

Will asking parents to delay filling a prescription for the treatment of acute otitis media reduce unnecessary antibiotic use?

Bottom line

A wait-and-see approach of asking parents of children given a diagnosis of acute otitis media (AOM) in the emergency department to delay filling a prescription significantly reduces unnecessary antibiotic use. Parents of children in the delayed group reported otalgia slightly, if any, more often than the parents of children in the standard group. All parents received explicit instructions to provide both ibuprofen and otic analgesic drops to their children. Children in the standard treatment group were more likely to have diarrhea. (LOE = 1b)

Reference

Spiro DM, Tay KY, Arnold DH, Dziura JD, Baker MD, Shapiro ED. Wait-and-see prescription for the treatment of acute otitis media: a randomized controlled trial. JAMA 2006;296:1235–1241.

Study Design	Funding	Allocation
Randomized controlled trial (single-blinded)	Foundation	Concealed

Setting

Emergency department

Synopsis

Previous studies evaluating the effects of asking parents to delay filling antibiotic prescriptions for children with AOM excluded children with high fever. These investigators enrolled 283 consecutive children, aged 6 months to 12 years, seen in an emergency department who were given a diagnosis of AOM. Exclusion criteria included: another bacterial infection, such as pneumonia; "toxic" appearance; immunocompromization; myringotomy tubes or perforated tympanic membrane; or antibiotic use within 7 days. Parents of children with AOM randomly received (concealed allocation assignment) verbal and written instructions "not to fill the antibiotic prescription unless your child either is not better or is worse 48 hours (2 days) after today's visit" (intervention group) or to "fill the antibiotic prescription and give the antibiotic to your child after today's visit" (standard group). Amoxicillin was prescribed for most patients. All subjects also received ibuprofen and otic analgesic drops (containing antipyrene and benzocaine) in standard doses. Individuals blinded to treatment group assignment assessed outcomes at 4 to 6 days, 11 to 14 days, and 30 to 40 days after enrollment. In addition, a research assistant called pharmacies 4 days after enrollment to confirm whether prescriptions were filled. Follow-up occurred for more than 94% of participants. Using intention-to-treat analysis, prescriptions were filled significantly less often for children in the wait-and-see group versus the standard group (62% vs 13%). The difference was also significant in the subgroup of children younger than 2 years of age (47% wait-and-see vs 5% standard). Verification of whether prescriptions were actually filled was assessed for 28% of the study population; the pharmacy confirmed parental report in almost all instances. Otalgia occurred for a slightly greater period (0.4 days) in the wait-and-see group, but the overall rate of otalgia after 4 days was similar in both groups. Unscheduled follow-up visits were similar in both groups. No serious adverse events occurred in either treatment group, but parents in the standard group reported significantly more diarrhea in their children (23% vs 8%; number needed to treat to harm = 7).

Essential Evidence: Medicine that Matters, Edited by David Slawson, Allen Shaughnessy, Mark Ebell, and Henry Barry.

Parent satisfaction okay with no treatment of AOM

Clinical question

Are parents whose children do not receive treatment for acute otitis media less satisfied with their child's care?

Bottom line

Parents don't seem to mind if their children are not treated with antibiotics. In this study comparing no treatment to immediate antibiotic treatment of acute otitis media, parent satisfaction scores were similar between the 2 groups, even though 21% of the no-treatment children eventually needed antibiotics. (LOE = 1b–)

Reference

McCormick DP, Chonmaitree T, Pittman C, et al. Nonsevere acute otitis media: a clinical trial comparing outcomes of watchful waiting versus immediate antibiotic treatment. Pediatrics 2005;115:1455–1465.

Study Design	Funding	Allocation
Randomized controlled trial (single-blinded)	Government	Uncertain

Setting

Outpatient (primary care)

Synopsis

Several studies have shown that not treating children initially with antibiotics for acute otitis media results in fewer eventual prescriptions and fewer adverse effects. This study again evaluated watchful waiting versus immediate antibiotic treatment, and also surveyed parents regarding their satisfaction with care. The researchers enrolled 223 infants and children with symptoms and otoscopic evidence of acute otitis media rated as not severe. Approximately 30% of the children were younger than 1 year, 25% were between the ages of 1 year and 2 years, and the rest were between the ages of 2 years and 13 years. The children were randomized (allocation concealment uncertain) to receive either high-dose amoxicillin, 90 mg per kg per day for 10 days, or no treatment. Children were concurrently treated with ibuprofen, a decongestant, and saline nose drops. They were also given an antihistamine, although this class of drugs was shown to be ineffective more than 20 years ago and were recently shown to extend the duration of middle ear effusion. Parents were instructed to return to the clinic if symptoms failed to improve or worsened, which occurred in 5% of antibiotic-treated children and 21% of no-antibiotic children (P = .001; number needed to treat with antibiotic to prevent one failure = 7). Treatment failure occurred significantly more often in children who had received antibiotics in the previous 30 days. On a questionnaire of satisfaction, which included questions regarding the parents' feelings toward medication side effects, extra time spent receiving care for the infection, difficulty giving the antibiotic, work absences, and overall satisfaction, the average score was not significantly different between the 2 groups of parents when measured on day 12 and day 30 of the study, with scores in both groups averaging about 44 of a possible 48. The study has many limitations: there is no mention whether the parent questionnaires were written in Spanish, which is important since the study was conducted in a predominantly Spanish-speaking area of the United States; the questionnaire was not validated; and there was unblinding of the investigators in a number of instances. Parents were also not given a delayed prescription to fill if symptoms didn't resolve, but were asked to return to the clinic for further evaluation.

Essential Evidence: Medicine that Matters, Edited by David Slawson, Allen Shaughnessy, Mark Ebell, and Henry Barry.

Parents prefer shared decision-making for AOM

Clinical question

Do parents with children with acute otitis media prefer to share in the decision to use antibiotics?

Bottom line

Presenting information about the pros and cons of antibiotic treatment for acute otitis media and letting parents decide whether and when to start treatment increases parents' satisfaction with their visit and could decrease antibiotic use. These results were found in wealthy, white, older parents and may not apply to other socioeconomic groups. (LOE = 2c)

Reference

Merenstein D, Diener-West M, Krist A, Pinneger M, Cooper LA. An assessment of the shared-decision model in parents of children with acute otitis media. Pediatrics 2005;116:1267–1275.

Study Design

Cross-sectional

Funding

Foundation

Setting

Outpatient (primary care)

Synopsis

The researchers conducting this study wished to determine to what extent parents would like to participate in the decision-making regarding the treatment of their child, given a scenario in which their child had acute otitis media. The parents in this study were not typical; they were older with an average age of 46 years), wealthy (76% had a family income >$75,000), well educated (87% attended college), mostly non-Hispanic white, and almost all had health insurance. During a visit to a family practice, 466 parents were asked to imagine their reaction to 1 of 3 clinical vignettes. All vignettes presented a mother taking her 2 1/2-year-old son to the doctor with a fever. The child is diagnosed with acute otitis media. In each vignette the doctor explains a desire to decrease antibiotic use and the lack of need for antibiotic use in most instances. In the "paternalistic" vignette the doctor clearly recommends antibiotics. In the "shared decision-making" vignettes the doctor makes no specific recommendation but gives a prescription for an antibiotic to be started in 2 days if the child is not better; in 1 of these vignettes acetaminophen is also recommended as treatment. Before reading the vignettes, 93% of parents reported that they felt that antibiotics were needed if an ear infection is present. After reading the vignettes, 82% reported being willing to wait 48 hours before starting treatment. However, 27% of the parents receiving the paternalistic vignette would start antibiotics immediately; only 7% receiving the shared decision-making vignettes would do so ($P < .001$). All reported similar degrees of satisfaction with the amount of information they received. Significantly more patients reported being satisfied with the shared decision-making approaches than with the paternalistic approach (76% satisfied in the paternalistic group vs 84% and 93% in the shared decision-making groups; $P < .001$).

Essential Evidence: Medicine that Matters, Edited by David Slawson, Allen Shaughnessy, Mark Ebell, and Henry Barry.

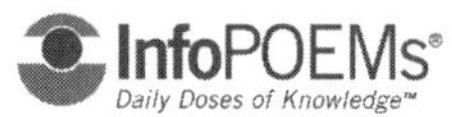

Tubes marginally effective in otitis media with effusion

Clinical question

Are ventilation tubes effective in managing children with otitis media with effusion?

Bottom line

Compared with watchful waiting, inserting pressure-equalizing tubes improves hearing in children with otitis media with effusion over the short term. Outcomes within 18 months, however, are the same. The tubes have no effect on language development. Watchful waiting is a reasonable option in most of these children. (LOE = 1a)

Reference

Rovers MM, Black N, Browning GG, Maw R, Zielhuis GA, Haggard MP. Grommets in otitis media with effusion: an individual patient data meta-analysis. Arch Dis Child 2005;90:480–485.

Study Design

Meta-analysis (randomized controlled trials)

Funding

Government

Setting

Various (meta-analysis)

Synopsis

This research team systematically reviewed several databases (including PubMed and Cochrane) looking for randomized controlled trials of ventilation tubes for children with otitis media with effusion. Ultimately, they included only the 7 studies (including a total of 1234 children) that were randomized to "a high standard" (ie, concealed allocation). They contacted the authors of the studies to get the individual patient data. After pooling all these data, the researchers looked at 3 outcomes: duration of the effusion, hearing, and language development. Since each of the studies had slightly different intermediate (6 and 9 months) and final (12 and 18 months) follow-up periods, the authors simply aggregated them. Children with tubes had a shorter duration of effusions (19.7 weeks vs 37 weeks; P = .001) than the control patients. At 6 months of follow-up, the mean hearing level was 26.6 dB in the children with tubes compared with 31.1 dB in the control group (P = .001). However, by the time of the final follow-up 12 months to 18 months later, there were no differences in hearing. Finally, the tubes had no effect on language development. The authors suggest that children attending daycare and/or those with worse hearing loss at baseline may benefit more from tubes, but this conclusion requires further study.

Essential Evidence: Medicine that Matters, Edited by David Slawson, Allen Shaughnessy, Mark Ebell, and Henry Barry.

Early tympanostomy tubes do not improve outcomes after 3 or more years

Clinical question

Does early insertion of tympanostomy tubes improve important clinical outcomes more than delayed insertion?

Bottom line

Early insertion of tympanostomy tubes does not improve long-term clinical outcomes of importance (speech acquisition and hearing) in children with persistent otitis media with effusion. Delaying 6 months for bilateral effusion and 9 months for unilateral effusion before revisiting the decision to insert tubes is the preferred approach to management, since it results in fewer procedures with equivalent outcomes. (LOE = 1b)

Reference

Paradise JL, Campbell TF, Dollaghan CA, et al. Developmental outcomes after early or delayed insertion of tympanostomy tubes. N Engl J Med 2005;353:576–586.

Study Design

Randomized controlled trial (single-blinded)

Funding

Industry + govt

Allocation

Concealed

Setting

Outpatient (any)

Synopsis

The initial report of this study's results found that early insertion of tympanostomy tubes in children with persistent otitis media with effusion did not improve outcomes at 3 years of age over delaying up to 9 months (see: Delaying tymp tubes doesn't worsen outcomes in effusion. N Engl J Med 2005;344:1179–87). In brief, children were enrolled before 2 months of age and underwent pneumatic otoscopy monthly until 3 years of age. If they had a persistent otitis media with effusion – defined as 90 days of bilateral effusion, 135 of unilateral effusion, or at least 67% of 180- and 270-day periods for bilateral and unilateral effusion in children with intermittent effusion – they were randomized to either immediate insertion of tympanostomy tubes or delaying 6 months to 9 months and only inserting tubes at that time if the effusion persisted. Outcome assessors were blinded to treatment assignment and allocation was concealed. At the end of the study, 85% in the early treatment group had received tubes, compared with only 41% in the delayed insertion group. Of course, the children who received immediate tubes could hear and speak better, right? Although that would make perfect sense, it is not what happened in this carefully done follow-up study that reports outcomes at 6 years of age. There was no difference between groups in tests of intelligence, speech complexity, hearing, auditory processing, behavior, or parental stress. With approximately 200 children in each group, the study had adequate statistical power to detect clinically meaningful differences if they existed.

Essential Evidence: Medicine that Matters, Edited by David Slawson, Allen Shaughnessy, Mark Ebell, and Henry Barry.

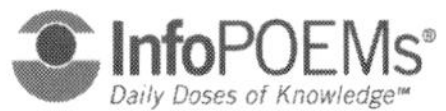

Prompt tympanostomy tube insertion doesn't improve 9 year outcomes

Clinical question

Does the delayed insertion of tympanostomy tubes impair the long-term outcomes in children with persistent middle-ear effusion?

Bottom line

Delayed tympanostomy tube insertion successfully helps many children avoid tubes and does not result in any developmental or other impairment. (LOE = 1b)

Reference

Paradise JL, Feldman HM, Campbell TF, et al. Tympanostomy tubes and developmental outcomes at 9 to 11 years of age. N Engl J Med 2007;356:248–261.

Study Design

Randomized controlled trial (single-blinded)

Funding

Government

Allocation

Concealed

Setting

Outpatient (any)

Synopsis

Many parents and clinicians still believe that there is a significant risk of permanent harm if tympanostomy tubes are not promptly inserted for children with persistent middle-ear effusion. In this study, which is a follow-up to a previously published POEM (N Engl J Med 2005;353:576), 429 children between the ages of 2 months and 3 years with middle-ear effusion for at least 90 days (bilateral) or 135 days (unilateral) were randomized to receive either prompt or delayed tympanostomy tube insertion. The delay was 6 months for bilateral effusion and 9 months for unilateral effusion. Allocation was concealed, groups were balanced at the start of the study, and analysis was by intention to treat. The researchers did an excellent job of following up: 195 of 216 in the early treatment group and 196 of 213 in the delayed treatment group underwent developmental testing between the ages of 9 years and 11 years. At the time of this final evaluation, 86% in the early treatment group had received tympanostomy tubes compared with only 49% in the delayed treatment group. There was no differences between groups in the results of a broad range of tests including evaluation of hearing, reading, oral fluency, auditory processing, phonological processing, behavior, or intelligence. There was also no difference between these groups and a group of children with ear problems that weren't bad enough to qualify them for the study.

Essential Evidence: Medicine that Matters, Edited by David Slawson, Allen Shaughnessy, Mark Ebell, and Henry Barry.

Bed and pillow covers ineffective for allergic rhinitis

Clinical question
Do impermeable bed and pillow covers improve symptoms of allergic rhinitis?

Bottom line
Impermeable bed and pillow covers do not improve symptoms more than conventional covers in patients with allergic rhinitis who are sensitive to dust mites. (LOE = 1b)

Reference
Terreehorst I, Hak E, Oosting AJ, et al. Evaluation of impermeable covers for bedding in patients with allergic rhinitis. N Engl J Med 2003;349:237–246.

Study Design
Randomized controlled trial (double-blinded)

Setting
Outpatient (specialty)

Synopsis
Impermeable bed and pillow covers reduce the exposure of allergic patients to dust mite allergens – but is that enough to improve symptoms? Previous studies have been small, poorly designed, and have provided conflicting results. In this trial, adults and children aged 8 to 50 years who were allergic to dust mites were randomized (allocation concealed) to receive either impermeable (n = 139) or permeable (n = 140) bed covers. They were recruited from specialty clinics, general practices, and by advertisements. Patients with pets in the home, using oral or high-dose inhaled steroids, and those taking cyclosporine or regular doses of antibiotics were excluded. Baseline and 12-month follow-up measurements were made between September and December, the peak months for Dutch dust mites. Nineteen patients in the control group and 24 in the impermeable cover group were lost to follow-up, most often because they moved or because of a protocol violation. The primary outcome was a 100-point allergy symptom severity score. The groups were similar at baseline, and analysis was by intention to treat for patients with a 12-month outcome measurement. Although allergen counts were significantly lower in the beds of patients with impermeable bed covers, and while both groups experienced an improvement in symptoms, there was no significant difference between groups in the degree of improvement (−9.8 points in the impermeable cover group vs −10.9 points in the control group; P = 0.8). There was also no signficant difference in daily symptom scores and in the results of the nasal allergen provocation test. The study was powered to detect at least a 25% reduction in the symptom score.

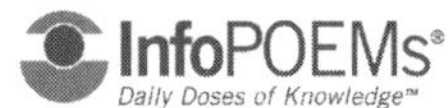

Risk scoring system predicts mortality in pediatric ICU

Clinical question

Can mortality in pediatric ICU patients be predicted using an easy scoring system?

Bottom line

Scoring systems can effectively predict mortality in children admitted to the ICU. The PIM, a point-of-care score, is easier to administer. (LOE = 1b)

Reference

Tibby SM, Taylor D, Festa M, et al. A comparison of three scoring systems for mortality risk among retrieved intensive care patients. Arch Dis Child 2002:87:421–425.

Study Design

Cohort (prospective)

Setting

Inpatient (ICU only)

Synopsis

These authors compared three different risk scoring systems in 928 critically ill children admitted to ICU. Two of the scoring systems, pre-ICU PRISM and PIM, use clinical data collected before admission to the ICU while the PRISM II also includes data from the first 24 hours after ICU admission. They were able to get complete scoring for only 24% using the pre-ICU PRISM, 88% for the PIM, and 60% using PRISM II. The authors calculated the area under the receiver operator characteristic curve (AUROCC) to determine which system was better at predicting mortality. All three systems performed reasonably well with AURROC between 0.83 and 0.87. They found, however, that all of the systems were not as good at predicting those at medium risk. The PIM was better in children with respiratory diseases.

Essential Evidence: Medicine that Matters, Edited by David Slawson, Allen Shaughnessy, Mark Ebell, and Henry Barry.

Petroleum jelly doesn't reduce recurrent pediatric epistaxis

Clinical question

Does petroleum jelly (Vaseline) reduce the likelihood that epistaxis will recur in children?

Bottom line

In this highly selected group of patients with recurrent epistaxis, petroleum jelly applied twice daily for 4 weeks did not reduce the number of bleeds in the subsequent 4 weeks. This should make you question this commonly recommended treatment. But don't abandon it just yet, since it may work in children with less severe disease in the primary care setting, and because there was potential for recall bias by parents in this study. (LOE = 2b)

Reference

Loughran S, Spinou E, Clement WA, et al. A prospective, single-blind, randomized controlled trial of petroleum jelly/Vaseline for recurrent paediatric epistaxis. Clin Otolaryngol 2004;29:266–269.

Study Design

Randomized controlled trial (single-blinded)

Setting

Outpatient (specialty)

Synopsis

Recurrent nosebleeds are a common problem in children. Many doctors advise the application of petroleum jelly (Vaseline) to the anterior nares, since bleeding is thought to result from drying, picking, rubbing, and all the other things children do to their noses. In this small but well-designed study, 105 children aged 1 to 14 years referred to otolaryngologists for recurrent epistaxis were identified. The median duration of symptoms was 12 months and the median duration of bleeds was 5 minutes. The children were randomized (allocation concealed) to receive 1 of 2 letters: instructions to apply Vaseline twice daily for 4 weeks and keep a nosebleed diary, or simply instructions to keep a nosebleed diary. Patients were assessed after 8 weeks, and the primary outcome was the percentage with recurrent bleeds in the previous 4 weeks. Analysis was by intention to treat and the physician assessing outcomes was blinded to treatment assignment and was careful not to ask about treatment adherence until the end of the visit. Groups were similar at baseline. They were also similar after the intervention: 27.5% in the treatment group and 33.9% in the control group ($P = 0.47$) had no bleeds during the 4 weeks prior to the visit and after the intervention. The study had limitations, though. Approximately 14% of patients never came in for evaluation (evenly split between groups) and most parents were noncompliant with the diaries. The researchers therefore used parental recall instead of the diaries to assess the primary outcome.

Essential Evidence: Medicine that Matters, Edited by David Slawson, Allen Shaughnessy, Mark Ebell, and Henry Barry.

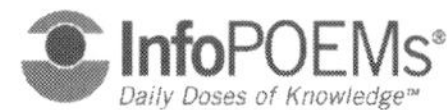

Effective and ineffective interventions for infant colic

Clinical question

What interventions are effective in the treatment of infantile colic?

Bottom line

Interventions with some evidence of effectiveness for infantile colic include hypoallergenic diets and formula, soy formula, decreased infant stimulation, herbal tea, and dicyclomine (Bentyl). Reports of severe adverse effects of dicyclomine in infants younger than 7 weeks caused a black box warning for use under the age of 6 months. The following interventions are essentially equal to or worse than placebo treatment: simethicone (Mylicon, Gas-X), scopolamine, lactase enzyme (Lactaid), fiber-enriched formula, increased carrying, car ride simulators, and sucrose. (LOE = 1a–)

Reference

Garrison MM, Christakis DA. Early childhood: colic, child development, and poisoning prevention. A systematic review of treatments for infant colic. Pediatrics 2000;106:184–190.

Study Design

Systematic review

Setting

Various (meta-analysis)

Synopsis

Numerous interventions are recommended for the treatment of colic, although few have been rigorously evaluated for their effectiveness. The authors performed a careful search of the literature. Of the RCTs evaluating pharmaceutical interventions, 3 studied simethicone, 3 dicyclomine, and 1 scopolamine. None of the three simethicone trials found any significant benefit over placebo. Dicyclomine performed significantly better than placebo in all 3 trials (number needed to treat [NNT] = 3). However, severe adverse effects have been attributed to dicyclomine use (apnea, seizures, and coma), especially in infants younger than 7 weeks. Thus, the manufacturer has contraindicated its use in infants younger than 6 months. The one trial of scopolamine found no benefit compared with placebo, but a higher incidence of adverse effects. Nine different trials evaluated various dietary interventions. In breastfeeding women, a maternal hypoallergenic diet free of milk, egg, wheat, and nut products reduced colic symptoms by 25% or more (NNT = 6) compared with a usual diet. In bottle-fed infants, both soy (NNT = 2) and hypoallergenic formula (NNT = 6) were more effective than regular formula. Treatment with lactase enzymes and fiber-enriched formula was no more effective than placebo. With regard to behavioral intervention, neither carrying the infant more often (ie, with a Snugli) nor the use of a car ride simulator (SleepTight) reduced symptoms significantly. Interestingly, advising parents to "reduce stimulation" reduceD symptoms (NNT = 2). Two naturopathic interventions were evaluated. One RCT comparing herbal tea (containing chamomile, vervain, licorice, fennel, and balm-mint) with placebo tea given at the onset of colic episodes, with a maximum dose of 150 mL up to 3 times per day, found a significant reduction in the number of infants meeting the criteria for colic (NNT = 3). One RCT evaluating sucrose found a significant benefit compared with placebo that lasted less than 30 minutes.

Essential Evidence: Medicine that Matters, Edited by David Slawson, Allen Shaughnessy, Mark Ebell, and Henry Barry.

Ear thermometry is unreliable in detecting fever

Clinical question
How reliable is ear thermometry in detecting fever in children?

Bottom line
Ear thermometry will only detect approximately two thirds of febrile children. Although it is fast and easy, the use of ear thermometry should be limited to those situations in which it doesn't matter if fever is present. (LOE = 1a–)

Reference
Dodd SR, Lancaster GA, Craig JV, Smyth RL, Williamson PR. In a systematic review, infrared ear thermometry for fever diagnosis in children finds poor sensitivity. J Clin Epidemiol 2006;59:354–357.

Study Design
Systematic review

Funding
Unknown/not stated

Setting
Outpatient (any)

Synopsis
In 2002, these authors published a systematic review (Lancet 2002;360:603–609) that demonstrated wide variability in the agreement between ear thermometry and rectal thermometry in children. In this study, they used the same review to determine the reliability of ear thermometry in detecting fever in children. To do this, they systematically searched numerous databases and tried to find unpublished studies. Two authors independently assessed the quality of the 23 included studies (of nearly 4100 children) and 2 authors independently extracted the data. The sensitivity of ear thermometry ranged from 0 to 100%. The specificity ranged from 58% to 100%. The most conservative pooled estimates, however, were 64% and 95%, respectively. In other words, ear thermometry is not very reliable in detecting fever.

Essential Evidence: Medicine that Matters, Edited by David Slawson, Allen Shaughnessy, Mark Ebell, and Henry Barry.

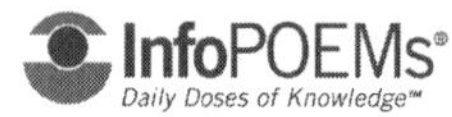

Acetaminophen, ibuprofen comparable for pain, fever in children

Clinical question

Do acetaminophen and ibuprofen have equivalent efficacy in treating fever and pain in children?

Bottom line

In this meta-analysis, single doses of acetaminophen (paracetamol) and ibuprofen are comparable for the relief of pain in children. Single doses of ibuprofen are minimally better than acetaminophen in relief of fever. These data also find no difference in safety between the drugs. These data are specious, however, since most febrile or painful conditions require multiple doses and any toxicity from the medication is more likely to appear after multiple doses rather than a single dose. Some argue that ibuprofen is preferable over acetaminophen because of its longer duration of action; this study didn't address this theory. (LOE = 1a)

Reference

Perrott DA, Piira T, Goodenough B, Champion GD. Efficacy and safety of acetaminophen vs ibuprofen for treating children's pain or fever: a meta-analysis. Arch Pediatr Adolesc Med 2004;158:521–526.

Study Design

Meta-analysis (randomized controlled trials)

Setting

Various (meta-analysis)

Synopsis

These authors systematically searched MEDLINE, EMBASE, the Cochrane Library, and numerous other databases for randomized clinical trials of acetaminophen and ibuprofen for treating pain or fever in children younger than 18 years. They also hand-searched the bibliographies, textbooks, and other sources to identify potential studies. Two authors, blinded to all but the data, independently coded all data with near-perfect agreement (median kappa = 0.75; minimum = 0.75). Any disagreements were resolved by consensus. They didn't assess the quality of the studies. The main outcomes were achieving 50% reduction in pain, reduction in temperature, and safety of the drugs. They classified side effects as minor if they didn't result in withdrawal from the study. Seventeen studies were included in this analysis.Virtually all of the studies were small (fewer than 40 patients) and only assessed response after a single dose. Only 3 pain studies were included (92 patients taking 7 to 15 mg/kg acetaminophen; 94 patients taking 4 to 10 mg/kg ibuprofen) and they found no significant differences between the 2 drugs. Ten studies addressed fever (539 children taking 10 to 15 mg/kg acetaminophen; 539 taking 5 to 10 mg/kg ibuprofen), and found that ibuprofen was slightly more effective than acetaminophen. The safety data were variable, in part due to differences in reporting. There was no significant difference in minor or major side effects, although the confidence intervals were fairly wide. There was no heterogeneity among the studies.

Essential Evidence: Medicine that Matters, Edited by David Slawson, Allen Shaughnessy, Mark Ebell, and Henry Barry.

Cough suppressants ineffective in children

Clinical question

Do cough suppressants improve the sleep of children with respiratory infections, or the sleep of their parents?

Bottom line

In this single dose study, placebo worked just as well as either dextromethorphan or diphenhydramine to decrease cough frequency or severity in children. Also, the active drugs provided no additional benefit on parents' report of their own or their child's sleep. This is both bad news and good news. The bad news is that these drugs don't work any better than placebo (which, actually, was reported to work pretty well). The good news is that when parents feel the need to do something when their child has a cold all products work equally well. (LOE = 1b–)

Reference

Paul IM, Yoder KE, Crowell KR, et al. Effect of dextromethorphan, diphenhydramine, and placebo on nocturnal cough and sleep quality for coughing children and their parents. Pediatrics 2004;114:e85–e90.

Study Design

Randomized controlled trial (double-blinded)

Setting

Outpatient (primary care)

Synopsis

When a young child coughs at night, parents don't get much sleep. Although the American Academy of Pediatrics recommends against antitussives because of their lack of demonstrated benefit, these products fly off pharmacy shelves in the winter months. This study identified 100 children experiencing rhinitis and cough symptoms for 1 week or less, who didn't have asthma or allergies; in other words, children with a cold. The average age was slightly older than 4 years (range = 2–16 years). The children were randomized (allocation concealment uncertain) to receive a single dose of placebo, diphenhydramine (Diphen), or dextromethorphan (Benylin), for the single night of the study. Using a 7-point Likert scale, parents were asked to rate the effect of treatment on the child's cough frequency, as well as the effect on their own sleep and that of the child. As compared with ratings obtained for the night before the study night, parents overall reported a significant decrease in cough frequency and severity (from "somewhat" to "occasional" on the descriptive scale). The combined symptom score decreased from 19.8 to 8.9 (of a possible 30) with any treatment ($P < .01$). Parents also reported a significant improvement in both their sleep and their childrens' sleep. However, the results were not different whether the child was treated with either drug or placebo. Adverse effects were reported equally in all 3 study groups. The study had the power to find a 1-point change in scores of the 3 arms, if one truly existed.

Essential Evidence: Medicine that Matters, Edited by David Slawson, Allen Shaughnessy, Mark Ebell, and Henry Barry.

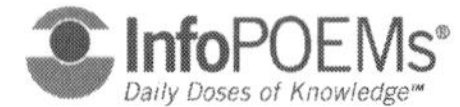

Delayed prescriptions for URIs reduce antibiotic use

Clinical question

Do delayed prescriptions reduce antibiotic use in upper respiratory tract infections?

Bottom line

Delayed prescriptions for upper respiratory tract infections reduces the use of antibiotics; patient satisfaction, however, may be worse. (LOE = 1a−)

Reference

Arroll B, Kenealy T, Kerse N. Do delayed prescriptions reduce antibiotic use in respiratory tract infections? A systematic review. Br J Gen Pract 2003;53:871–877.

Study Design

Systematic review

Setting

Outpatient (primary care)

Synopsis

For this systematic review, the authors included controlled trials of studies in which the intervention was a delayed prescription compared with an immediate prescription for patients with upper respiratory tract infections. They searched several databases (MEDLINE, Embase, Cochrane) and searched for unpublished studies. Two of the authors independently assessed the quality of the trials (randomization, concealment of allocation, co-interventions, losses to follow-up, and so forth). Disagreements among the reviewers were resolved by discussion and consensus. The authors were only able to find 5 controlled trials, 4 of which were randomized. All the randomized controlled trials had Jadad scores above 3, indicating reasonable to good quality. Since the authors found significant heterogeneity among the studies, they refrained from pooling the data. However, each study demonstrated significant reduction in the rate of antibiotic use. In 2 of the studies, however, patient satisfaction was significantly worse, and in 3 studies the symptoms were worse among those receiving a delayed prescription.

Essential Evidence: Medicine that Matters, Edited by David Slawson, Allen Shaughnessy, Mark Ebell, and Henry Barry.

Amoxicillin for 3 days effective for pediatric pneumonia

Clinical question

Is 3 days of treatment with amoxicillin as effective as 5 days of the same therapy in children with non-severe pneumonia?

Bottom line

Outpatient treatment with 3 days of amoxicillin therapy produced similar results as 5 days of treatment in children with presumed pneumonia. In both groups, treatment failures occurred in 10% of children. (LOE = 1b)

Reference

ISCAP Study Group. Three day versus five day treatment with amoxicillin for non-severe pneumonia in young children: a multicentre randomised controlled trial. BMJ 2004;328:791–794.

Study Design

Randomized controlled trial (double-blinded)

Setting

Outpatient (primary care)

Synopsis

This study enrolled more than 2100 children between the ages of 2 months and 6 years with non-severe pneumonia. The diagnostic criteria were clinical: cough, rapid respiration, or difficulty breathing not deemed to be indicative of severe pneumonia. Fever was not a criterion. Patients were randomized (using concealed allocation) to receive either 3 days or 5 days of oral amoxicillin 30 mg to 50 mg per kg per day. Treatment failure was defined as retractions (chest indrawing), convulsions, drowsiness, the inability to drink, or a cutoff respiratory rate too high or an oxygen saturation too low on day 5. In the intention-to-treat analysis cure rates were similar between the 2 groups (90%), as were relapse rates within the next 7 to 9 days (5%). Cure rates were the same whether the children had wheezes and did not vary by age. Hospitalizations were infrequent but similar in the 2 groups (2%). The study had the power to find a 5% difference in treatment failures, assuming a 12% failure rate with the longer therapy.

Essential Evidence: Medicine that Matters, Edited by David Slawson, Allen Shaughnessy, Mark Ebell, and Henry Barry.

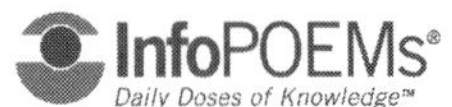

Herbal tea effective for symptoms of acute pharyngitis

Clinical question

Can herbal tea help reduce the symptoms of pain associated with acute pharyngitis?

Bottom line

An herbal tea containing a mixture of traditional demulcents (soothing agents) was more effective than a placebo tea in the short-term relief of pain in patients with acute pharyngitis. The effect does not last long – less than 30 minutes – so requires frequent tea drinking throughout the day. On the occasion of my next sore throat, I'm going to reach for an analgesic and a topical anesthetic, but herbal tea may be useful for patients who prefer a more active approach and who wish to avoid the partially anesthetized mouth feel. (LOE = 1b)

Reference

Brinckmann J, Sigwart H, van Houten Taylor L. Safety and efficacy of a traditional herbal medicine (Throat Coat) in symptomatic temporary relief of pain in patients with acute pharyngitis: a multicenter, prospective, randomized, double-blinded, placebo-controlled study. J Altern Complement Med 2003;9:285–298.

Study Design

Randomized controlled trial (double-blinded)

Setting

Outpatient (any)

Synopsis

Demulcents is a general category of products that are soothing and relieve irritation. They are not topical anesthetics, but have been used for many years to treat sore throat. This study evaluated the effectiveness of a demulcent mixture containining licorice root, elm inner bark, marshmallow root, and licorice root aqueous dry extract (an herbal tea called Throat Coat). Sixty patients with acute pharyngitis by any cause were randomly assigned to use the herbal tea or a similar-tasting and -smelling placebo tea 4 to 6 times daily for as long as symptoms remained. No other treatment was allowed. Treatment allocation was concealed from the enrolling physician. Patients rated pain relief after 1 minute then every 5 minutes for 30 minutes, then at 3 and 24 hours after the first dose, and then daily using a scale from 0 to 10. Analysis was by intention to treat and compared the degree of change in pain scores at each period, as well as the total amount of pain relief using the total area under the curve of pain changes. Details on exactly what statistics were used are sketchy, which is odd considering the great detail in which other aspects of the study were reported. Changes from baseline pain after the first dose were significantly different than placebo at 5 and 10 minutes. The sum of pain intensity differences occurring in the first 30 minutes of treatment was approximately twice as good in the treatment group ($P = .041$). Pain relief was also greater in treated patients at 10 minutes after the first dose. By intention-to-treat analysis, however, total pain relief over the first 30 minutes was not different between the 2 groups.

Steroids provide brief relief of pain in mononucleosis

Clinical question

Does dexamethasone reduce throat pain in acute mononucleosis?

Bottom line

Dexamethasone provides improvement in throat pain in children with acute mononucleosis but the effect lasts less than 24 hours. (LOE = 1b–)

Reference

Roy M, Bailey B, Amre DK, et al. Dexamethasone for the treatment of sore throat in children with suspected infectious mononucleosis: a randomized, double-blind, placebo-controlled, clinical trial. Arch Pediatr Adolesc Med 2004;158:250–254.

Study Design

Randomized controlled trial (double-blinded)

Setting

Emergency department

Synopsis

The investigators enrolled children between the ages of 8 and 18 years with suspected mononucleosis in this small study. The 40 children were randomly assigned (masked allocation) to receive a single oral dose of dexamethasone (0.3 mg/kg, maximum 15 mg) or a matched placebo. Pain was measured using a 100-mm visual analog scale, with a 20 mm or greater difference chosen as the main outcome. Pain was assessed 12, 24, 48, and 72 hours after treatment, and then one final time on day 7. Analysis was by intention to treat.To assess the quality of blinding, the investigators tried to guess whether participants received dexamethasone or placebo after patients completed the pain scale (they couldn't). At the 12-hour assessment, 12 of 20 in the dexamethasone group improved (at least 20 mm on the scale) compared with 5 of 19 taking placebo (number needed to treat = 4; P = .03). At 24 hours, half the patients treated with dexamethasone (11/20) had pain relief compared with one third (6/20) taking placebo. The study did not have sufficient power to detect whether this difference was real or not. Assessments after the first 24 hours were virtually identical.

Essential Evidence: Medicine that Matters, Edited by David Slawson, Allen Shaughnessy, Mark Ebell, and Henry Barry.

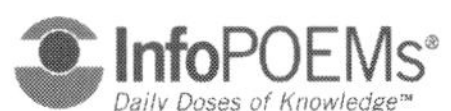

Echinacea purpurea ineffective for treating URI in kids

Clinical question

How effective and safe is echinacea in the treatment of upper respiratory tract infections in children?

Bottom line

Echinacea purpurea extract (above ground plant only), prepared and used at the doses in this study was ineffective in treating upper respiratory tract infections (URIs) in children. Although it was generally safe to use, more parents reported a rash on their child and 2 children had a serious allergic-type reaction. Interestingly, children using echinacea were less likely to have recurrent URI (number needed to treat = 9). (LOE = 1b)

Reference

Taylor JA, Weber W, Standish L, et al. Efficacy and safety of echinacea in treating upper respiratory tract infections in children. A randomized controlled trial. JAMA 2003;290:2824–2830.

Study Design

Randomized controlled trial (double-blinded)

Setting

Outpatient (primary care)

Synopsis

Although the average child has 6 to 8 colds per year, each lasting 7 to 10 days, commonly used medications such as decongestants, antihistamines, and cough suppressants lack efficacy in those younger than 12 years. Echinacea is widely used for the prevention and treatment of URIs in adults, but there is limited data on efficacy and safety of use in children. Data were obtained and analyzed on a total of 707 URIs that occurred in 407 children. At the onset of each URI, subjects were randomly given (concealed allocation assignment) either dried pressed Echinacea purpurea juice (obtained from the above-ground herb, harvested at flowering, extracted in an alcohol-free preparation combined with syrup), or identical placebo. Dosing was age-based on the recommendations of the manufacturer and was continued until all symptoms had resolved, up to a maximum of 10 days. Parents recorded the severity of symptoms and adverse events in a daily logbook. The patients, parents, practitioners and research staff were all unaware of treatment group assignment. Ninety-four percent of the subjects were followed up for a total of 4 months. Using intention-to-treat analysis, there were no differences in duration of URIs or in the overall estimate of severity of URI symptoms between the 2 treatment groups. Other over-the-counter cold remedies were administered by parents at the same rate in both groups, but antipruitics and analgesics other than acetaminophen were administered more often to children treated with echinacea (9.8% vs 5.1%; P = .03). After limiting the analysis to the URIs in which patients received at least 80% of the study medication (per protocol analysis), there were still no differences found between the 2 groups. Children assigned to echinacea were less likely to have a second URI than those in the placebo group (52.3% vs 64.4%; P = .015; number needed to treat = 9). Adverse events were reported similarly in each group, although rash was reported more often in children receiving echinacea (7.1% vs 2.7%). Two children receiving echinacea had the sudden onset of stridor requiring emergency treatment with steroids.

Yogurt prevents antibiotic-associated diarrhea

Clinical question

Is yogurt effective in the prevention of antibiotic-associated diarrhea?

Bottom line

Vanilla-flavored yogurt containing active bacterial cultures is effective in decreasing the incidence and duration of antibiotic-associated diarrhea. Tell your patients to look for yogurt that contains active cultures. If they can't find it, consider probiotic agents. (LOE = 2b)

Reference

Beniwal RS, Arena VC, Thomas L, et al. A randomized trial of yogurt for prevention of antibiotic-associated diarrhea. Dig Dis Science 2003;48:2077–2082.

Study Design

Randomized controlled trial (nonblinded)

Setting

Inpatient (any location) with outpatient follow-up

Synopsis

Probiotic agents are effective in preventing antibiotic-associated diarrhea. Controversy exists about whether commercially available yogurt products are similarly effective. A total of 202 hospitalized patients receiving oral or intravenous antibiotics were randomized (concealed allocation assignment) to either vanilla-flavored yogurt (8 ounces twice daily for 8 days) or usual care without yogurt supplementation. The authors do not specify the brand or type of yogurt but note that manufacturer-supplied nutritional data indicated that the product contained active cultures of Lactobacillus acidophilus, L. bulgaricus, and Streptococcus thermophilus. The mean age of the study group was 70 years. All patients were followed up for a total of 8 days. Individuals assessing outcomes were not blinded to treatment group assignment. Antibiotic-associated diarrhea was defined as the new onset of more than 2, less-than-formed bowel movements per day representing a change in prior bowel patterns. Using intention-to-treat analysis, patients receiving yogurt reported less frequent diarrhea (12% vs 24%; P = .04; number needed to treat = 12). In addition, subjects ingesting yogurt daily reported significantly less total diarrheal days (23 vs 60). No side effects were reported other than boredom: Yogurt-fed subjects yearned for fruit-flavored yogurt to break the monotony ("I'm sick and tired of vanilla yogurt! Don't you have any other flavors?!").

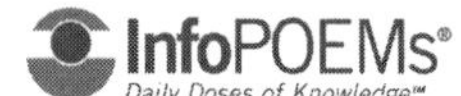

Probiotics helpful for antibiotic-associated diarrhea

Clinical question

Can probiotics prevent antibiotic-associated diarrhea and assist in the treatment of Clostridium difficile disease?

Bottom line

The probiotics Saccharomyces boulardii and Lactobacillus rhamnosus GG both prevent antibiotic-associated diarrhea (AAD), as does a combination of 2 or more probiotics. S. boulardii, given in addition to vancomycin or metronidazole, is also an effective treatment for Clostridium difficile disease (CDD). (LOE = 1a–)

Reference

McFarland LV. Meta-analysis of probiotics for the prevention of antibiotic associated diarrhea and the treatment of Clostridium difficile disease. Am J Gastroenterol 2006;101:812–822.

Study Design

Meta-analysis (randomized controlled trials)

Funding

Unknown/not stated

Setting

Various (meta-analysis)

Synopsis

A variety of probiotics have been proposed to help reestablish the gut flora, prevent AAD, and treat CDD. This meta-analysis identified any blinded randomized controlled trials (RCTs) on MEDLINE and Google Scholar and evaluated their quality. There were 25 RCTs of AAD prevention including 2810 patients and 6 RCTs of CDD treatment including 354 patients. Studies were generally of good quality. There was considerable heterogeneity regarding population and results for studies of prevention of AAD. Although there was no difference in outcomes for studies in adults or children or by duration of therapy, a greater benefit was seen for studies using a higher dose. S. boulardii and L. rhamnosus GG, both studied in 6 RCTs, were most effective (combined relative risk = 0.37 and 0.31, respectively) as were studies using a mixture of 2 probiotics. In most studies of the treatment of CDD, patients were also given vancomycin or metronidazole and the outcome was the likelihood of recurrence of CDD. Results of the 6 studies were homogeneous and a combined estimate of effect showed a relative risk of recurrent CDD of 0.59 (95% CI, 0.41–0.81). S. boulardii seemed to be the most effective probiotic. Adverse effects in both sets of studies were minimal. These studies took place largely in immunocompetent patients and should not be generalized to immunocompromised patients.

Essential Evidence: Medicine that Matters, Edited by David Slawson, Allen Shaughnessy, Mark Ebell, and Henry Barry.

Probiotics effective in preventing acute diarrhea, but not traveler's diarrhea

Clinical question

Are probiotics effective in the prevention of acute diarrhea?

Bottom line

Probiotics reduce the risk of antibiotic-associated diarrhea and other types of acute diarrhea, but not the risk of traveler's diarrhea, in both children and adults. The protective effect does not vary among different probiotic strains nor by mode of delivery. (LOE = 1a)

Reference

Sazawal S, Hiremath G, Dhingra U, Malik P, Deb S, Black RE. Efficacy of probiotics in prevention of acute diarrhea: A meta-analysis of masked, randomized, placebo-controlled trials. Lancet Infect Dis 2006;6:374–382.

Study Design

Meta-analysis (randomized controlled trials)

Funding

Government

Setting

Various (meta-analysis)

Synopsis

Probiotics are effective in the treatment of acute infectious diarrhea in adults and children. However, evidence for the role of probiotics in preventing acute diarrhea is less certain. These investigators thoroughly searched multiple databases – including MEDLINE, the Cochrane Registry, and references of published review articles – and personally contacted researchers known to be working in the field. Only randomized double-blind placebo-controlled trials in either English or French were included in the analysis. Three individuals separately evaluated articles for eligibility and quality; disagreements were resolved by consensus discussion. A total of 34 trials including 4844 patients, aged 6 months to 71 years, met the inclusion criteria. Overall, probiotics reduced the risk of acquiring diarrhea by 33% (95% CI, 22%–44%; number needed to treat = 15, 11–22). In subgroup analyses, probiotics significantly reduced the risk of antibiotic-associated diarrhea and acute diarrhea of other types, but did not reduce the risk of traveler's diarrhea. Probiotics were more effective in children than in adults, and the protective effect did not vary significantly among different probiotic strains or by mode of delivery (ie, capsules, tablets, granules, or powder). A formal analysis found no evidence of significant publication bias.

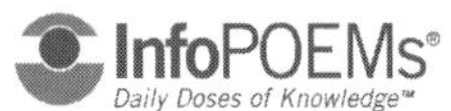

Popular diets equally effective for losing weight

Clinical question

Which of 4 popular diets (Atkins, Zone, Weight Watchers, and Ornish) is most effective for losing weight and reducing cardiac risk factors?

Bottom line

All 4 popular diets (Atkins, Zone, Weight Watchers, and Ornish) are equally effective for helping adults lose weight and reduce cardiac risk factors. Since success in this study directly correlated with self-adherence to the diet, it makes sense to help patients choose the diet that is "easiest" for them to follow, and not preferentially encourage one over another. (LOE = 1b–)

Reference

Dansinger ML. Gleason JA, Griffith JL, Selker HP, Schaefer EJ. Comparison of the Atkins, Ornish, Weight Watchers, and Zone die for weight loss and heart disease risk reduction. A randomized trial. JAMA 2005;293:43–53.

Study Design	Funding	Allocation
Randomized controlled trial (single-blinded)	Government	Concealed

Setting

Outpatient (specialty)

Synopsis

Every week it seems that somebody else writes another diet book and claims that they have "the best" method for losing weight and keeping it off. In fact, there is very little data addressing the health effects of popular diets and even less comparing different diets directly to each other. The investigators enrolled 160 overweight or obese (mean BMI 35; range 27–42) adults, aged 22 to 72 years, with known hypertension, dyslipidemia, or fasting hyperglycemia. Subjects were randomized (concealed allocation assignment) to either Atkins (carbohydrate restriction), Zone (macronutrient balance), Weight Watchers (calorie restriction), or Ornish (fat restriction) diet groups. Individuals assessing outcomes were blind to treatment group assignment. The study attrition rate as a result of patient drop outs was high: the number of participants who did not complete the study at months 2, 6, and 12 were 34 (21%), 61 (38%), and 67 (42%), respectively. The most common reason cited by subjects for withdrawing was that the assigned diet was too hard to follow or was not resulting in enough weight loss. Although the results were not statistically significant (P = 0.08), more subjects discontinued the Atkins (48%) and Ornish diets (50%) than the less extreme Zone (35%) and Weight Watchers (35%) diets. Using intention-to-treat analysis, all 4 diets resulted in similar weight loss at 1 year with no statistically significant difference between the diets. In each of the diet groups, approximately 25% and 10% of subjects sustained a weight loss of more than 5% and 10% of initial body weight, respectively, at one year. Cardiac risk factor improvement was directly proportional to the amount of weight loss and was similar among the diet groups. Self-reported dietary adherence directly correlated with the amount of weight loss and reduction in cardiac risk factors. The study was powered to have an 80% chance of detecting a weight change of 2% from baseline or a 3% difference between diets.

Essential Evidence: Medicine that Matters, Edited by David Slawson, Allen Shaughnessy, Mark Ebell, and Henry Barry.

Mediterranean diet associated with lower all cause mortality

Clinical question

Does a Mediterranean diet reduce mortality?

Bottom line

This excellent study lends further strength to the association between a Mediterranean diet (rich in vegetables, legumes, fruits, nuts, cereals, olive oil, fish, and alcohol and low in meat) and a reduction in all-cause mortality. Salut! (LOE = 2b)

Reference

Trichopoulou A, Costacou T, Bamia C, Trichopoulos D. Adherence to a Mediterranean diet and survival in a Greek population. N Engl J Med 2003;348:2599–2608.

Study Design

Cohort (prospective)

Setting

Population-based

Synopsis

It's hard to go wrong with a diet containing pasta, olive oil, and red wine, and it may even make you live longer! There have been numerous ecologic studies suggesting that a Mediterranean diet high in vegetables, legumes, fruits, nuts, cereals, olive oil, fish, and alcohol; moderate in cheese and yogurt; and low in saturated lipids, meat, and poultry is associated with greater longevity. This is the largest prospective study to date of this hypothesis. The researchers identified 25,917 community-dwelling Greeks, and excluded 3874 with coronary heart disease, diabetes mellitus, or cancer at enrollment. They did a detailed assessment of diet and lifestyle, and rated the participants adherence to the Mediterranean diet on a scale from 0 (not at all) to 9 (perfect adherence – lots of veggies, seafood, wine, and pasta!) The median follow-up was 3.7 years. This was not a randomized trial, so the outcomes were adjusted for age, sex, smoking status, body mass index, and energy expenditure. The mean body mass index was 28.1 for men and 28.8 for women, making them a slightly pudgy group; 60% were women and more than half of all participants had never smoked. Other than the ratio of monounsaturated lipids to saturated lipids, individual dietary factors were not associated with mortality. However, every 2-point increase in the Mediterranean diet score was associated with a 25% reduction in the risk of death from any cause, a 33% reduction in the risk of death from coronary heart disease, and a 24% reduction in the risk of death from cancer. The benefit was greater in women, in persons older than 55 years, in never-smokers, in heavier folks, and in sedentary persons.

Essential Evidence: Medicine that Matters, Edited by David Slawson, Allen Shaughnessy, Mark Ebell, and Henry Barry.

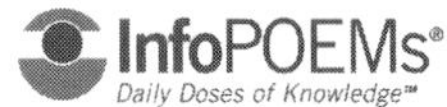

Omega 3 fatty acids do not affect mortality

Clinical question

Does supplementation with omega 3 fatty acids decrease mortality, cardiovascular disease, or cancer in adults?

Bottom line

Overall, omega 3 fatty acid supplementation does not decrease mortality or cardiovascular disease as compared with placebo. This study combined both primary and secondary prevention; that is, it included people with and without coronary heart disease. (LOE = 1a)

Reference

Hooper L, Thompson RL, Harrison RA, et al. Risks and benefits of omega 3 fats for mortality, cardiovascular disease, and cancer: systematic review. BMJ 2006;332:752–760.

Study Design

Systematic review

Funding

Government

Setting

Various (meta-analysis)

Synopsis

The authors of this review, which is an update of a previous Cochrane review, identified 48 randomized controlled trials and 41 cohort studies evaluating the effect of fish oil supplementation on overall mortality, cardiovascular disease, and cancer in adults. They identified these studies using the usual rigorous Cochrane methodology and analyzed the results from randomized trials separately from cohort data. The studies included patients with and without pre-existing coronary heart disease. As a result, the authors of this study combined both primary and secondary prevention research. Omega 3 fatty acids were given either as supplements or as a recommendation to eat more oily fish. In randomized trials enrolling more than 30,000 patients, omega 3 supplementation did not significantly reduce mortality (relative risk [RR] = 0.87; 95% CI, 0.73–1.03) or the likelihood of a cardiovascular event (RR = 1.09; 0.87–1.37). Long-chain omega 3 fatty acids did not produce different results than short-chain fats. Cancer was neither increased nor decreased in either clinical trials or cohort studies. The lack of benefit demonstrated in this study conflicts with the results of an earlier meta-analysis of the effect in patients with coronary heart disease (Am J Med 2002;112:298–304). However, this is the second study published after that meta-analysis that did not find a benefit overall.

Essential Evidence: Medicine that Matters, Edited by David Slawson, Allen Shaughnessy, Mark Ebell, and Henry Barry.

Diet and exercise prevent diabetes in high-risk patients

Clinical question

Do diet and exercise delay the development of diabetes in high-risk patients?

Bottom line

Diet and exercise are effective in delaying the diagnosis of diabetes in patients at increased risk. (LOE = 2b)

Reference

Lindstrom J, Ilanne-Parikka P, Peltonen M, et al, for the Finnish Diabetes Prevention Study Group. Sustained reduction in the incidence of type 2 diabetes by lifestyle intervention: follow-up of the Finnish Diabetes Prevention Study. Lancet 2006;368:1673–1679.

Study Design

Randomized controlled trial (nonblinded)

Funding

Industry + foundation

Allocation

Unconcealed

Setting

Outpatient (any)

Synopsis

In the Finnish Diabetes Prevention Study, 522 men and women, aged between 40 years and 65 years and at high risk for developing diabetes, were randomly assigned either to a tailored diet-and-exercise regimen or to usual care. To be eligible, the patients had to have a body mass index greater than 25 and have impaired glucose tolerance. The original study lasted a median of 4 years. The cumulative incidence of diabetes in the intervention group was 11% compared with 23% in the control group (number needed to treat = 8; 95% CI 6–16). In this report, the researchers provide 3 additional years of observations on the patients who had not developed diabetes by the end of the original study. No specific diet or exercise information was provided to the patients during this follow-up period. After a total of 7 years of follow-up, 75 patients in the intervention group and 110 patients in the control group developed diabetes. The cumulative incidence rate was 4.3 per 100 person-years in the intervention group, and 7.4 in the control group. The authors estimate that one would need to treat 22 patients with diet and exercise to prevent 1 patient per year from developing diabetes.

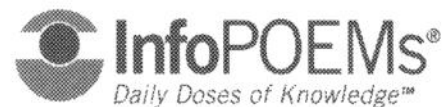

Restricted diet improves parental perception of hyperactive behavior

Clinical question

Does a diet that restricts food coloring and preservatives improve hyperactive behaviors in 3 year olds?

Bottom line

This study raises an interesting conundrum. Placing 3-year-old children on a diet that restricts food coloring and preservatives has no effect on hyperactive behaviors as observed by trained evaluators. However, the parents, who live with these kids for the remaining 23 hours of the day, report improvements in hyperactivity. There was no difference in results whether the child was hyperactive or atopic. (LOE = 2b)

Reference

Bateman B, Warner JO, Hutchinson E, et al. The effects of a double-blind, placebo-controlled, artificial food colourings and benzoate preservative challenge on hyperactivity in a general population sample of preschool children. Arch Dis Child 2004; 89:506–511.

Study Design

Cross-over trial (randomized)

Setting

Outpatient (primary care)

Synopsis

These authors evaluated the effects of a restricted diet on 397 3-year-old children who were classified as hyperactive (HA) or not (HA-) and atopic (AT) or not (AT-), resulting in a 2 × 2 design. The study was split into 2 1-week treatment periods separated by 1-week washout periods. The children were to remain on a diet free of artificial coloring and benzoate preservatives for the entire 4 weeks. During the first week, the children were randomly assigned to receive a daily drink free of artificial coloring and sodium benzoate or an artificially colored and preserved drink identical in appearance. The children then were switched to the opposite drink during the second treatment period. Adults were unable to distinguish the taste of these beverages and the families and study personnel were all blinded to the specific treatment. Only 70% of the patients enrolled finished the study; 61 never started the study and 59 dropped out. Fifteen of the 59 parents who withdrew their child from the study did so because of behavioral changes. Nine of these withdrawals occurred during an active week and 6 during a placebo week. At the end of the study the parents were equally divided into those who did or did not correctly identify the drink order. Based on the parents ratings, their children were calmer during the week when no artificial coloring and preservatives were given. The trained observers, however, detected no significant differences during any of the treatment periods.

Essential Evidence: Medicine that Matters, Edited by David Slawson, Allen Shaughnessy, Mark Ebell, and Henry Barry.

Variable support for CAM therapies for anxiety

Clinical question

Which complementary and alternative medicines are effective in the treatment of anxiety disorders?

Bottom line

The majority of complementary and alternative medicines lack valid evidence of effectiveness in the treatment of anxiety disorders. Some supporting evidence was found for inositol, acupuncture, massage (only in children), autogenic therapy, bibliotherapy, dance/movement therapy, exercise, meditation, music, and relaxation therapy. Many common herbal and homoeopathy treatments lack any evidence of effectiveness. (LOE = 2a)

Reference

Jorm AF, Christensen H, Griffiths KM, Parslow RA, Rodgers B, Blewitt KA. Effectiveness of complementary and self-help treatments for anxiety disorders. Med J Aust 2004;181:S29–S46.

Study Design

Systematic review

Funding

Government

Setting

Various (meta-analysis)

Synopsis

Anxiety disorders are estimated to affect 5% to 15% of patients each year. Less than one fifth of these people consult a health professional and many report using various self-help methods. The investigators searched PubMed, PsychLit and the Cochrane Registry of Controlled Trials (CRCT) to review the effectiveness of complementary and alternative treatments on anxiety. Articles were included if they reported treatment of individuals selected as having an anxiety disorder. Independent studies were assessed for validity using standard criteria. No mention is made whether the search for, and evaluation of, the articles was done independently by more than one person, and there is no discussion of possible publication bias. Very limited, if any, evidence of effectiveness was found for the following treatments: Bach flower essences, berocca, ginger, gotu kola, homeopathy, lemongrass leaves, licorice, magnesium, passion flower, St. John's wort, valerian, vitamin C, aromatherapy, hydrotherapy, humor, prayer, yoga, caffeine reduction, nicotine avoidance, and a carbohydrate-rich/protein-poor diet. Limited evidence was found for effectiveness for inositol, acupuncture, massage (only in children), autogenic therapy, bibliotherapy, dance/movement therapy, exercise, meditation, music, and relaxation therapy. Kava and 5-hydroxyl-L-tryptophan were effective but not recommended because of the risk of severe side effects (liver toxicity and eosinophilia-myalgia syndrome, respectively).

Essential Evidence: Medicine that Matters, Edited by David Slawson, Allen Shaughnessy, Mark Ebell, and Henry Barry.

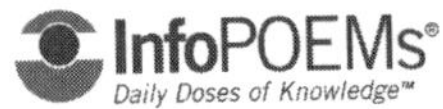

Antioxidants do not prevent dementia

Clinical question

Are antioxidants associated with a decreased risk of Alzheimer's disease?

Bottom line

In this study and in at least one other cohort study (Engelhart MJ. JAMA 2002;287:3223–29), antioxidant consumption in the elderly was not associated with protection against developing dementia. At least one randomized controlled trial (Sano M. NEJM 1997;336:1216–22) demonstrated that vitamin E may slow the progression of moderately severe Alzheimer's disease. (LOE = 2b)

Reference

Luchingser JA, Tang MX, Shea S, Mayeaux R. Antioxidant vitamin intake and risk of Alzheimer disease. Arch Neurol 2003;60:203–208.

Study Design

Cohort (prospective)

Setting

Outpatient (any)

Synopsis

In this cohort study, patients completed diaries of diet and vitamin supplementation (vitamin C, vitamin E, carotene). The researchers evaluated the patients at baseline and only included those who were free of dementia. After an average of 4 years of follow-up of 980 patients, they compared antioxidant consumption with subsequent development of dementia using standardized criteria. A total of 242 of these patients developed Alzheimer's disease. After adjusting for educational level and other covariates that might affect cognition, they found no association between antioxidant use and the development of dementia. Some limitations of this study include the role of recall bias since patients had to report on their dietary intake from the previous year. For those of us who can't recall what we had for breakfast (or even if we ate breakfast), this would be a major challenge.

Essential Evidence: Medicine that Matters, Edited by David Slawson, Allen Shaughnessy, Mark Ebell, and Henry Barry.

Lowering homocysteine with B vitamins doesn't improve cognition

Clinical question

Does supplementation to reduce homocysteine levels with folate, vitamin B12, and vitamin B6 have a beneficial effect on cognition in older adults?

Bottom line

There is no evidence from this well-designed study that vitamin supplementation to lower homocysteine levels has any beneficial effect on cognition. Although cognition actually appeared to worsen with the use of vitamins in one of the tests, this may be a spurious finding given the large number of comparisons made by the researchers. (LOE = 1b)

Reference

McMahon JA, Green TJ, Skeaff CM, Knight RG, Mann JI, Williams SM. A controlled trial of homocysteine lowering and cognitive performance. N Engl J Med 2006;354:2764–2772.

Study Design

Randomized controlled trial (double-blinded)

Funding

Government

Allocation

Concealed

Setting

Population-based

Synopsis

Observational studies have found an association between higher levels of serum homocysteine and Alzheimer's disease and cognitive impairment. However, it is not clear whether this association is causal, or whether lowering homocysteine levels improves cognition. In this trial, community-dwelling healthy adults older than 65 years with a plasma homocysteine level of at least 13 micromoles per liter were recruited. The authors excluded those with impaired renal function, with known cognitive impairment, who were taking folate or B vitamins, or who were taking medications that might interfere with folate metabolism. After an extensive battery of baseline cognitive tests, patients were randomly assigned to receive either 1000 mcg folate, 500 mcg vitamin B12 (cobalamin), and 10 mg vitamin B6 (pyridoxine) daily or matching placebo. The 276 patients underwent cognitive testing after 1 and 2 years; of 138 who began the study in each group, 126 in the placebo group and 127 in the treatment group had data available for analysis. The mean age of participants was 73 years and 44% were female (37% in the vitamin group, 52% in the placebo group; P = .02). The vitamins had the expected effect on homocysteine levels, reducing them approximately 16 to 12 micromoles per liter in the treatment group during the 2-year study. The homocysteine levels did not change in the placebo group. There was no improvement on cognition. In fact, the average score on the Wechsler Paragraph Recall test was worse in the vitamin group, although this difference disappeared after adjustment for sex and education. The vitamin group also did worse on the Reitan Trail Making Test, a difference that persisted after adjustment for sex and education.

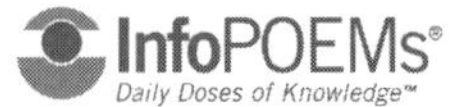

Vitamin E, donepezil ineffective for mild cognitive impairment

Clinical question

Does Vitamin E or donepezil (Aricept) prevent progression from mild cognitive impairment to Alzheimer's disease?

Bottom line

Vitamin E does not slow progression of mild cognitive impairment to full-fledged Alzheimer's disease. Donepezil provides an early benefit that is gone by 3 years. A secondary analysis found that donepezil appeared more beneficial for patients with the apolipoprotein E4 (APOE) gene. This finding requires prospective confirmation before we begin to test all patients with mild cognitive impairment for APOE and use it to guide therapy. (LOE = 1b)

Reference

Petersen RC, Thomas RG, Grundman M, et al. Vitamin E and donepezil for the treatment of mild cognitive impairment. N Engl J Med 2005;352:2379–2388.

Study Design

Randomized controlled trial (double-blinded)

Funding

Industry + govt

Allocation

Concealed

Setting

Outpatient (any)

Synopsis

Mild cognitive impairment (MCI) is an intermediate stage between normal cognition and Alzheimer's disease often characterized by deficits of memory. In this study, researchers identified 769 patients with MCI, defined as impaired memory on standardized tests, a Mini Mental State (MMS) test score between 24 and 30, and age 55 years to 90 years. These patients were randomly assigned to receiver either 2000 IU vitamin E, 10 mg donepezil (Aricept), or placebo daily; all patients received a multivitamin containing 15 IU vitamin E. MMS scores, age, and APOE gene status was considered when patients were allocated to treatment groups, but appears to have been concealed from the investigators. Analysis was by intention to treat and outcomes were blindly assessed. At the end of the 3-year study, 212 of the 769 patients who began the study had progressed to Alzheimer's disease (a rate of 16% per year). Taking vitamin E or donepezil did not have any effect on the likelihood of progression to Alzheimer's at 3 years. There was a decreased risk of progression to Alzheimer's in the donepezil group at 12 months compared with placebo (14.7% vs 6.3%; P = .04; number needed to treat [NNT] = 12), but this did not persist at 36 months. There was also no significant difference in MMS scores or other measures of cognition at 3 years. Patients with the APOE gene were much more likely to progress to Alzheimer's disease, and if you only consider that group, then the benefit of donepezil persists for the full 3 years of the study.

Essential Evidence: Medicine that Matters, Edited by David Slawson, Allen Shaughnessy, Mark Ebell, and Henry Barry.

Light therapy as effective as fluoxetine for seasonal affective disorder

Clinical question

Is light therapy an acceptable alternative to antidepressants for patients with seasonal affective disorder?

Bottom line

Light therapy and fluoxetine (Prozac) are equally effective treatment options for patients with seasonal affective disorder (SAD). Patient preference and an individual assessment of risks and benefits should guide treatment selection. (LOE = 1b)

Reference

Lam RW, Levitt AJ, Levitan RD, et al. The CAN-SAD Study: A randomized controlled trial of the effectiveness of light therapy and fluoxetine in patients with winter seasonal affective disorder. Am J Psychiatry 2006;163:805–812.

Study Design

Randomized controlled trial (double-blinded)

Funding

Industry + govt

Allocation

Concealed

Setting

Outpatient (specialty)

Synopsis

Both light therapy and antidepressants are effective in the treatment of SAD, but few studies have directly compared the 2 treatments. These investigators identified 96 adults (mean age = 42 years) meeting DSM-IV criteria for major depressive disorder with a seasonal (winter) pattern with scores greater than 23 on the 24-item Hamilton Depression Rating Scale (HAM-D). Subjects were randomized in double-blind fashion (concealed allocation assignment) to 8 weeks of treatment with either 10,000-lux light treatment plus placebo or 100-lux light treatment (placebo light) plus fluoxetine 20mg per day. Light treatment occurred for 30 minutes as soon as possible after awakening, between 7:00 AM and 8:00 AM. Individuals blinded to treatment group assignment assessed outcomes using the HAM-D. A significant clinical response included a 50% or greater reduction from baseline in HAM-D scores. Follow-up occurred for 96% of subjects for 8 weeks. Using intention-to-treat analysis, there were no significant differences between the light and fluoxetine treatment groups in clinical response rates (67% for both conditions) or remission rates (50% vs 54%, respectively). There were also no significant differences in either outcome noted between the 2 treatment groups for a subset of severely depressed patients. The placebo light, although dim, may have some clinical effect, possibly by accentuating the benefit of fluoxetine. More fluoxetine-treated patients complained of agitation, sleep disturbance, and palpitations. However, treatment emergent adverse event rates and drop-out rates were similar in both groups.

Essential Evidence: Medicine that Matters, Edited by David Slawson, Allen Shaughnessy, Mark Ebell, and Henry Barry.

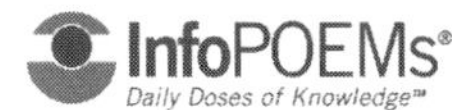

Acupuncture effective for chronic back pain

Clinical question

Is acupuncture effective in treating acute or chronic low back pain?

Bottom line

Acupuncture is an effective treatment for decreasing pain in patients with chronic low back pain. It doesn't seem to be a placebo effect; acupuncture produces a significantly greater effect on pain than sham acupuncture. There is not enough research to allow a conclusion for the treatment of acute low back pain. (LOE = 1a)

Reference

Manheimer E, White A, Berman B, Forys K, Ernst E. Meta-analysis: Acupuncture for low back pain. Ann Intern Med 2005;142:651–663.

Study Design

Meta-analysis (randomized controlled trials)

Funding

Industry + govt

Setting

Various (meta-analysis)

Synopsis

Acupuncture is becoming more common in Western medicine, with many traditionally trained physicians crosstrained in its use. This meta-analysis assembled 22 randomized controlled trials comparing acupuncture with no treatment, sham acupuncture, or another active treatment such as massage or analgesics in the treatment of chronic low back pain. Sham acupuncture is used to convince patients they are receiving acupuncture and consists of inserting acupuncture needles either superficially or at inappropriate sites, or by using the acupuncture needle tube or other blunt device to provide pressure without actual penetration. The studies (in any language) were identified by searching 7 databases, contacting experts, handsearching a Japanese acupuncture journal, and using previous review articles. Two authors independently selected the studies and abstracted the data. Results of sham-controlled studies were homogeneous. One study of the 5 studies that compared acupuncture with no additional therapy produced heterogeneous results favoring no treatment as compared with acupuncture. Publication bias could not be assessed. For patients with chronic low back pain, lasting at least 3 months, acupuncture was more effective than sham acupuncture, sham transcutaneous nerve stimulation (TENS), and no treatment for short-term pain relief. It was not significantly better or worse than massage, medication therapy, or actual TENS treatment, and was significantly less effective than spinal manipulation. It provided long-term pain relief as compared with sham TENS or no treatment but was not different from sham acupuncture or active TENS. There is not enough data on the effectiveness of acupuncture for acute back pain to provide a conclusion. Three studies evaluated the use of acupuncture in the treatment of antenatal low back pain; all 3 studies found a benefit, though their results could not be combined.

Essential Evidence: Medicine that Matters, Edited by David Slawson, Allen Shaughnessy, Mark Ebell, and Henry Barry.

Tai chi improves symptoms of osteoarthritis

Clinical question
Can a specifically designed tai chi exercise program improve symptoms and physical functioning in women with osteoarthritis?

Bottom line
A specifically designed tai chi program for older women with osteoarthritis decreased pain and joint stiffness and improved physical functioning, balance, and abdominal muscle strength in the women who continued the exercises. The results may be a bit inflated because the researchers evaluating the outcomes may have known which patients had received treatment. (LOE = 1b−)

Reference
Song R, Lee EO, Lam P, Bae SC. Effects of tai chi exercise on pain, balance, muscle strength, and perceived difficulties in physical functioning in older women with osteoarthritis: a randomized clinical trial. J Rheumatol 2003;30:2039–2044.

Study Design
Randomized controlled trial (nonblinded)

Setting
Outpatient (specialty)

Synopsis
Tai chi is a martial art that involves slow, continuous, and gentle motions including isometric exercise, relaxation, stretching, and correct body posturing. A series of 12 Sun-style tai chi exercises have been developed to meet the specific needs of patients with arthritis. Patients in this study were older women in South Korea with radiologic and clinical evidence of osteoarthritis (OA) who were not in an exercise program. The investigators started with 72 women, but only 43 women completed the 12 weeks of the study. Approximately half the patients completing the study considered themselves to be in poor or very poor health. The average body mass index iof the women was 25. They were randomly assigned (using concealed allocation) to regular care without exercise or tai chi training. The tai chi group members participated in classes 3 times a week for the first 2 weeks, followed by weekly classes supplemented with twice weekly home exercise for 20 minutes for the next 10 weeks. The analysis only included the 43 women who completed all 12 weeks of the study. Using the Korean version of the Western Ontario and McMaster Universities Osteoarthritis Index, joint pain, stiffness, and physical functioning all were significantly different in the exercise group. Balance on one foot was significantly increased (by 7 seconds vs −1 seconds; $P < .05$) as was abdominal muscle strength (an increase of 2 sit-ups vs 0; $P < .05$). Muscle strength and endurance, flexibility, and weight were not affected. A concern: The investigators evaluating the outcomes may not have been blinded to the treatment the patients received.

Essential Evidence: Medicine that Matters, Edited by David Slawson, Allen Shaughnessy, Mark Ebell, and Henry Barry.

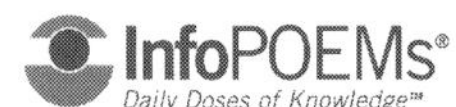

Acupuncture effective for OA of the knee

Clinical question

Is acupuncture effective in decreasing pain and improving function in patients with osteoarthritis of the knee?

Bottom line

Acupuncture, as compared with sham acupuncture treatment or no treatment, decreases pain scores by an average of 40% and improves function similarly in patients who stick with it. The acupuncture used in this study was based on the Traditional Chinese Medicine meridian theory and was used for the entire 6 months of the study. (LOE = 1b)

Reference

Berman BM, Lao L, Langenberg P, Lee WL, Gilpin AM, Hochberg MC. Effectiveness of acupuncture as adjunctive therapy in osteoarthritis of the knee: a randomized, controlled trial. Ann Intern Med 2004;141:901–910.

Study Design	Funding	Allocation
Randomized controlled trial (double-blinded)	Government	Concealed

Setting

Outpatient (any)

Synopsis

This is the largest and most rigorous study to date of the effect of acupuncture in the treatment of osteoarthritis. The authors enrolled 570 patients who had radiologic and clinical evidence of osteoarthritis of the knee and who had not had any intra-articular injections. The patients were assigned to 1 of 3 treatment groups: (1) "true acupuncture" based on Traditional Chinese Medicine meridian theory to treat knee joint pain; (2) a sham treatment that mimicked true acupuncture, except that the needles weren't actually inserted (the acupuncture guiding tubes were tapped at sham points, followed by affixing needles, without insertion, at these sites with adhesive tape); and (3) a control group that received 6 2-hour group education sessions lead by a patient education specialist, with follow-up mailed educational materials. Treatment was rendered twice a week for 8 weeks, tapering over the next month to 1 treatment per month, which was continued through the end of the study. This design addresses 2 issues that have plagued previous acupuncture research by providing a sham treatment, as well as a no-treatment group. At week 14, pain scores using the Western Ontario and McMaster University Osteoarthritis Index (WOMAC) decreased from an initial average score of 8.9 (of a possible 20) by 3.6 units (40% improvement) in the true acupuncture group compared with a 2.7 unit increase in the sham group and a 1.5 unit decrease in the education group. This change with true acupuncture was statistically significant compared with the other 2 groups. Pain scores continued to improve in all 3 groups over the course of the study, though true acupuncture scores continued to improve statistically more than the other 2 groups. Functional deficit diminished from an average 32 units (of a possible 68 at baseline) to 19 units at the end of the study, an almost 40% improvement that was statistically better than the other 2 groups. Patient global assessment scores also improved in the acupuncture group to a statistically greater extent than in either other group. Distance during the 6-minute walk and 36-Item Short-Form Health Survey scores improved more with true and sham acupuncture treatment than with education, but the results were similar between those 2 groups.

Essential Evidence: Medicine that Matters, Edited by David Slawson, Allen Shaughnessy, Mark Ebell, and Henry Barry.

Acupuncture ineffective for fibromyalgia

Clinical question

Is standardized acupuncture effective in decreasing symptoms in patients with fibromyalgia?

Bottom line

A standardized acupuncture protocol was no better than sham acupuncture in relieving pain or improving other symptoms in patients with significant fibromyalgia symptoms. Patients in all groups reported slightly better scores. Acupuncture is just one aspect of traditional Chinese medicine, however, and this fairly artificial study does not help us understand if this approach is effective. (LOE = 1b)

Reference

Assefi NP, Sherman KJ, Jacobsen C, Goldberg J, Smith WR, Buchwald D. A randomized clinical trial of acupuncture compared with sham acupuncture in fibromyalgia. Ann Intern Med 2005;143:10–19.

Study Design

Randomized controlled trial (double-blinded)

Funding

Government

Allocation

Concealed

Setting

Outpatient (any)

Synopsis

The researchers recruited by advertisement 100 people with a diagnosis of fibromyalgia, who had a global pain score of 4 or more (average = 7) on a visual analog scale of 0 (no pain) to 10 (worst pain ever), and who agreed to maintain current treatment during the study. Using concealed allocation, the patients were randomized to receive either traditional Chinese Medicine acupuncture according to a standardized (ie, not individualized) protocol (n = 25) or 1 of 3 sham acupuncture treatments (n = 25 patients each) administered by 8 practitioners. The participants were treated twice weekly for 12 weeks with acupuncture only. The study, in its attempt to maintain consistency of the acupuncture treatment, resulted in artificial treatment, since acupuncture is just one aspect of traditional Chinese medicine and the clinician usually adjusts treatment to the specific patients. Using intention-to-treat analysis, no differences were found in any outcome; pain intensity and fatigue intensity improved similarly in all 4 groups, as did sleep quality and overall well-being. Scores of general health status, as measured by the Short Form 36-item Health Survey, did not change in any of the 4 groups.

Essential Evidence: Medicine that Matters, Edited by David Slawson, Allen Shaughnessy, Mark Ebell, and Henry Barry.

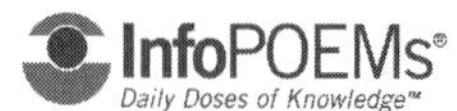

Acupuncture better than sham treatment for neck pain

Clinical question

Is acupuncture more effective than sham treatments for patients with neck pain?

Bottom line

If this systematic review identified all the relevant literature, there is moderate evidence that acupuncture is more effective than some sham treatments or inactive therapies in relieving neck pain at the end of treatment and at 3 months of follow up. The overall quality of the research, however, is poor. (LOE = 1a–)

Reference

Trinh K, Graham N, Gross A, et al. Acupuncture for neck disorders. Spine 2007;32:236–243.

Study Design

Meta-analysis (other)

Funding

Self-funded or unfunded

Setting

Outpatient (any)

Synopsis

The authors of this Cochrane review searched multiple databases looking for trials (randomized and quasi-randomized) of acupuncture compared with sham acupuncture or other inactive treatment in the treatment of adults with neck pain. The authors do not describe looking for unpublished studies. At least 2 authors independently assessed articles for inclusion and extracted the data. Additionally, at least 2 authors independently assessed the methodologic quality of the included studies. In each of these quality steps, they used a consensus process to reconcile discrepancies. Finally, they also rated the overall strength of evidence. Overall, most of the studies were of poor quality and did not have enough power to detect modest differences in treatment effect. In general, the authors found modest evidence that acupuncture was effective in reducing pain. Of the 10 small trials (with a total 661 patients) included, only 4 were of high quality. One underpowered study found no difference between acupuncture and sham electro-acupuncture. The remaining trials were fairly consistent in finding some benefit with acupuncture (range of numbers needed to treat from the studies = 2–17). The authors don't address this, but it is possible that publication bias in favor of studies with positive results will not reflect what we are likely to see in the real world.

Vitamin E not helpful, perhaps harmful

Clinical question

In patients with or without heart disease, does vitamin E supplementation decrease mortality?

Bottom line

Vitamin E supplementation does not decrease all-cause mortality in patients with or without pre-existing heart disease. At higher doses it can actually be harmful, although the deleterious effect is small (number needed to treat to harm = 250). (LOE = 1b)

Reference

Miller ER 3rd, Pastor-Barriuso R, Dalal D, Riemersma RA, Appel LJ, Guallar E. Meta-analysis: high-dosage vitamin E supplementation may increase all-cause mortality. Ann Intern Med 2005;142:37–46.

Study Design

Meta-analysis (randomized controlled trials)

Funding

Government

Setting

Outpatient (any)

Synopsis

The antioxidant property of vitamin E has led many to use it to prevent cardiovascular or cancer-related mortality. However, several studies and several previous meta-analyses have shown either no benefit or a slight increase in mortality with its use. The authors of this study performed a literature search in the usual way, searching MEDLINE, the Cochrane Clinical Trials Database, and reference lists and files. They included 19 randomized studies of almost 136,000 patients comparing vitamin E with a control or placebo group for at least 1 year and with at least 10 deaths in the trial. Study subjects varied and included elderly patients, healthy adults, and patient with cardiovascular disease. Study results were analyzed by intention to treat. The method of data extraction was not explained and studies were not graded or selected on the basis of quality. In the studies the baseline death rate was approximately 10%. Overall, there was no difference in all-cause mortality between the control group and placebo group. However, when comparing low-dose versus high-dose vitamin E (less than 400 IU/day vs 400 IU/day or more), differences were found. In the studies of lower doses, there was no benefit or detriment to vitamin E supplementation (relative risk = 0.98; 95% CI, 0.96–1.01). When high dose supplementation was studied separately, the risk was slightly but significantly higher in the supplemented group, with a number needed to treat to harm of 250 (143–998). The effect of vitamin E supplementation was not different when the results were evaluated by patient's sex or average age, or by the length of follow-up.

Essential Evidence: Medicine that Matters, Edited by David Slawson, Allen Shaughnessy, Mark Ebell, and Henry Barry.

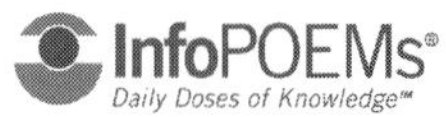

Vitamin E doesn't lower women's risk of cardiovascular disease or cancer

Clinical question

Is vitamin E effective in reducing the risk of cardiovascular disease and cancer among healthy women?

Bottom line

Vitamin E does not reduce the risk of cardiovascular disease, cancer, or total mortality among healthy women 45 years or older. (LOE = 1b)

Reference

Lee IM, Cook NR, Gaziano JM, et al. Vitamin E in the primary prevention of cardiovascular disease and cancer. The Women's Health Study: A randomized controlled trial. JAMA 2005;294:56–65.

Study Design

Randomized controlled trial (double-blinded)

Funding

Industry + govt

Allocation

Concealed

Setting

Population-based

Synopsis

Evidence from observational trials suggests that vitamin E may be effective in preventing cardiovascular disease and cancer in women. In the Women's Health Study, the investigators randomized (concealed allocation assignment) 39,876 healthy women, 45 years or older, to receive either (1) 600 IU natural-source vitamin E every other day, (2) placebo and 100 mg aspirin every other day, or (3) placebo only in a 2 × 2 factorial design. Individuals blinded to treatment group assignment assessed outcomes. Follow-up occurred for an average of 10.1 years for more than 97% of the subjects. Using intention-to-treat analysis, vitamin E did not significantly reduce the risk of major cardiovascular events, including myocardial infarction, ischemic stroke, or hemorrhagic stroke. Although vitamin E slightly reduced the risk of cardiovascular death (number needed to treat for 10.1 years = 586; 95% CI, 306–6058), all-cause mortality was not significantly reduced. Vitamin E did not significantly reduce the risk of any cancer, including breast, lung, and colorectal cancers. Cancer mortality was not significantly lower in any group.

Essential Evidence: Medicine that Matters, Edited by David Slawson, Allen Shaughnessy, Mark Ebell, and Henry Barry.

Vitamin E has no effect on cardiovascular disease

Clinical question
Does vitamin E have a role in the treatment or prevention of heart disease?

Bottom line
Vitamin E has no effect on the cardiovascular system. It is not useful for the prevention or treatment of heart disease. (LOE = 1a)

Reference
Shekelle PG, Morton SC, Jungvig LK, et al. Effect of supplemental vitamin E for the prevention and treatment of cardiovascular disease. J Gen Intern Med 2004;19:380–389.

Study Design
Meta-analysis (randomized controlled trials)

Setting
Various (meta-analysis)

Synopsis
This systematic review started with a search of 11 databases to find research on vitamin E or its relatives. The authors did a nice job of locating the 8173 studies in any language, and of narrowing this number to 84 controlled trials of vitamin E that evaluated clinical outcomes. In 6 studies ranging from 2 years to 7 years of follow-up, vitamin E supplementation did not affect mortality when used as either secondary or primary prevention. Cardiovascular death rates were not different when the 5 large studies were combined. Vitamin E therapy also had no effect on rates of fatal or nonfatal myocardial infarction. Vitamin E also did not increase the risk of any outcomes, which is reassuring. These studies evaluated thousands of patients. However, most of the studies were of low quality (Jadad score = < 3 of a possible 5).

Essential Evidence: Medicine that Matters, Edited by David Slawson, Allen Shaughnessy, Mark Ebell, and Henry Barry.

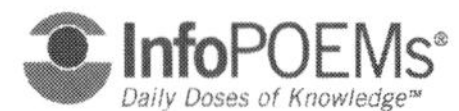

Antioxidants don't prevent GI cancers, and may increase overall mortality

Clinical question

Do antioxidants prevent gastrointestinal cancers?

Bottom line

Antioxidants do not prevent gastrointestinal cancers. In fact, in pooled results of high-quality studies, antioxidants increased overall mortality. (LOE = 1a)

Reference

Bjelakovic G, Nikolova D, Simonetti RG, Gluud C. Antioxidant supplements for prevention of gastrointestinal cancers: a systematic review and meta-analysis. Lancet 2004;364:1219–1228.

Study Design

Meta-analysis (randomized controlled trials)

Funding

Foundation

Setting

Various (meta-analysis)

Synopsis

This is a Cochrane Review that follows their usual rigorous methods of searching, identification of unpublished data, and data extraction. The authors included all trials that randomized participants to supplementation with antioxidants (beta-carotene, vitamins A, C, and E, and selenium, as different combinations or separately) versus placebo, and that reported the incidence of gastrointestinal cancers. The authors assessed the methodological quality of trials and calculated whether the findings were consistent across trials. A total of 14 randomized controlled trials with 170,525 patients were evaluated. The number of patients in each trial ranged from 226 to nearly 40,000. Half the studies of cancer incidence were of good quality; 7 of the 9 that also reported mortality were of good quality. None of the supplements protected against esophageal cancer, gastric cancer, colorectal cancer, or pancreatic cancer. In the high-quality studies, antioxidants increased overall mortality (8.0% vs 6.6%). This translates to a number needed to treat to harm of 69 for 1 additional death (95% CI, 58–85). It is interesting to note that 4 trials of selenium (3 with unclear or poor methodology) reduced the incidence of gastrointestinal cancer (odds ratio = 0.49; 95% CI, 0.36–0.67). Selenium should be evaluated in randomized trials with sound methods.

Essential Evidence: Medicine that Matters, Edited by David Slawson, Allen Shaughnessy, Mark Ebell, and Henry Barry.

Antioxidants don't prevent colorectal cancer

Clinical question

Can colorectal cancer risk be decreased with antioxidant supplements?

Bottom line

Antioxidant supplementation for up to 6 years does not decrease the risk of colorectal adenomatous polyps and thus, by extension, does not reduce the risk of colorectal cancer. Vitamin E may increase the risk of colorectal adenoma. (LOE = 1a–)

Reference

Bjelakovic G, Nagorni A, Nikolova D, Simonetti RG, Bjelakovic M, Gluud C. Meta-analysis: antioxidant supplements for primary and secondary prevention of colorectal adenoma. Aliment Pharmacol Ther 2006;24:281–291.

Study Design

Meta-analysis (randomized controlled trials)

Funding

Self-funded or unfunded

Setting

Outpatient (any)

Synopsis

The researchers conducted this analysis using standard methodology and searched 5 databases for all randomized trials comparing beta-carotene, vitamin A, vitamin C, vitamin E, or selenium with no treatment or placebo on the development of colorectal adenoma, a cancer precursor. They also searched for unpublished studies. They report that they used The Cochrane Collaboration methodology for conducting the meta-analysis but they don't give details of how they chose studies for inclusion or how they abstracted the data. They assessed the research for quality, identifying the studies as high quality or low quality according to study design. There was no publication bias.The 8 trials used in this analysis included a total of 17,260 participants, though most of the patients (88%) were in a single high-quality study. This study enrolled patients without previous adenoma; the rest of the studies enrolled participants with previously removed colorectal adenomas (6 studies) or previous colorectal cancer (1 study). Overall, there was no benefit of antioxidant supplementation on the development of colorectal adenoma. High-quality studies showed no effect or a slight increase of risk of adenoma with antioxidants; the small, low-quality studies found a benefit with antioxidants. When analyzed separately, none of the individual antioxidants had a beneficial effect on adenoma rates. Vitamin E, used in the largest study, produced a statistically significant increase in the risk of colorectal adenoma (relative risk = 1.7; 95% CI, 1.1–2.8).

Essential Evidence: Medicine that Matters, Edited by David Slawson, Allen Shaughnessy, Mark Ebell, and Henry Barry.

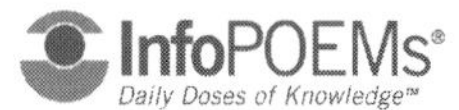

Green tea consumption is associated with reduced mortality

Clinical question

Can green tea consumption reduce the risk of premature mortality?

Bottom line

Green tea consumption is associated with reduced cardiovascular and all-cause mortality, but not cancer mortality. Women appear to benefit more than men: Men's mortality was significantly reduced only in those consuming more than 5 cups per day. Furthermore, there appears to be no benefit of green tea consumption in smokers. (LOE = 2b–)

Reference

Kuriyama S, Shimazu T, Ohmori K, et al. Green tea consumption and mortality due to cardiovascular disease, cancer, and all causes in Japan: the Ohsaki study. JAMA 2006;296:1255–1265.

Study Design

Cohort (prospective)

Funding

Government

Setting

Population-based

Synopsis

These investigators analyzed data from a large population-based cohort of 40,530 persons living in northeastern Japan where green tea is widely consumed. Beginning in 1994, healthy adults aged 40 years to 79 years, received a questionnaire inquiring about the frequency of intake of 4 beverages (green tea, oolong tea, black tea, and coffee) and 36 food items. Individuals reported green tea consumption in 5 categories: never, occasionally, 1 to 2 cups per day, 3 to 4 cups per day, and 5 or more cups per day. Validation with daily food diaries occurred randomly for 113 participants. Researchers investigated causes of death by reviewing public records, but the authors do no state whether blinding to green tea consumption occurred. Follow-up occurred for up to 11 years for all-cause mortality for 86% of participants and for up to 7 years for cause-specific mortality for 90% of participants. Statistical analysis controlled for potential confounding variables, including: age; job status; body mass index; exercise; history of hypertension, diabetes, or gastric ulcer; smoking; alcohol consumption; and other food consumption. Green tea consumption was significantly associated with reduced cardiovascular and all-cause mortality. Drinking more than 1 cup per day was associated with reduced mortality in women; however, drinking less than 5 cups per day of green tea was not associated with reduced mortality in men. Consuming green tea was not associated with a significant reduction in cancer mortality. Interestingly, the inverse relationship between green tea consumption and cardiovascular mortality was significant only in participants who never smoked. The authors report that the consumption of black tea or oolong tea was not associated with reduced mortality, but don't make any mention of coffee's association with mortality.

DHEA, testosterone not effective in aging patients

Clinical question

Do DHEA and testosterone have anti-aging properties?

Bottom line

There is no evidence that supplementation with dehydroepiandrosterone (DHEA) or testosterone has any meaningful clinical benefit for older patients with low serum levels of those hormones. (LOE = 1b)

Reference

Nair KS, Rizza RA, O'Brien P, et al. DHEA in elderly women and DHEA or testosterone in elderly men. N Engl J Med 2006;355:1647–1659.

Study Design

Randomized controlled trial (double-blinded)

Funding

Government

Allocation

Concealed

Setting

Outpatient (any)

Synopsis

Because their level often declines as we age, supplementation with DHEA and testosterone are widely promoted by some of our more entrepreneurial colleagues as anti-aging drugs. In this study, men older than 60 years with a DHEA level of less than 1.57 mcg/mL (4.3 umol/L) and a testosterone level of less than 103 ng/dL (3.6 nmol/L) and women older than 60 years with a DHEA level of less than 0.95 mcg/mL (2.6 umol/L) were included. All participants were generally healthy; men with elevated prostate-specific antigen or prostate nodules were excluded. Patients were randomly assigned by concealed allocation to receive active drug or placebo; analysis included all patients who had data collected for at least 12 months, with the last value carried forward. Ninety-two men (mean age = 67 years) were randomized to receive either DHEA 75 mg per day or matching placebo tablet, or to transdermal testosterone 5 mg per day or matching placebo patch. Sixty women (mean age = 69 years) were randomized to receive DHEA 50 mg per day or matching placebo tablet. Loss to follow-up was minimal and the drugs were well tolerated. As expected, supplementation increased the mean serum levels of DHEA in men and women and of testosterone in men. At 24 months, there was no change from baseline regarding quality of life, measures of physical performance, or muscle strength. Men had a small decrease in fat-free mass (slightly more than 1%) and both groups had small increases in bone mineral density at the femoral neck. Given the large number of comparisons, these "benefits" are likely to be simply due to chance. Overall, there was no consistent or clinically meaningful benefit to supplementation. The authors state that the study had a 90% power to detect clinically meaningful differences between groups, but they do not tell us what they considered to be clinically meaningful.

Essential Evidence: Medicine that Matters, Edited by David Slawson, Allen Shaughnessy, Mark Ebell, and Henry Barry.

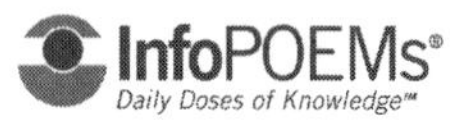

Lowering homocysteine does not reduce cardiovascular disease (HOPE 2)

Clinical question

Is supplementation to lower homocysteine levels an effective treatment for cardiovascular disease or disease prevention?

Bottom line

Supplementation with folic acid and B vitamins is ineffective for adults 55 years and older with known cardiovascular disease (CVD) or diabetes. A second report in the same issue found that similar supplementation in patients with a recent acute myocardial infarction was not helpful and may actually increase the risk of a bad cardiovascular outcome (relative risk = 1.22; 95% CI, 1.0–1.5). (LOE = 1b)

Reference

Lonn E, Yusuf S, Arnold MJ, et al, for the Heart Outcomes Prevention Evaluation (HOPE) 2 Investigators. Homocysteine lowering with folic acid and B vitamins in vascular disease. N Engl J Med 2006;354:1567–1577.

Study Design	Funding	Allocation
Randomized controlled trial (double-blinded)	Government	Concealed

Setting

Outpatient (any)

Synopsis

An elevated level of homocysteine is an independent predictor of the risk of developing CVD. The leap that many physicians and patients have made (unsubstantiated by any evidence) is that lowering homocysteine levels through the use of B vitamins and folic acid supplements will therefore prevent or treat CVD. The current study is the first to evaluate this hypothesis in a prospective, randomized trial. The authors enrolled 5522 patients older than 54 years with known coronary, cerebrovascular, or peripheral vascular disease, or diabetes plus one additional risk factor for CVD. They then randomized the patients (allocation concealed) to receive either 2.5 mg folic acid, 50 mg vitamin B6, and 1 mg vitamin B12 or matching placebo daily. Patients came from countries in which folate fortification of food is mandatory (United States and Canada) and not mandatory (Brazil, Western Europe, and Slovakia). Compliance with treatment was good: More than 90% and patients were followed up for a mean of 5 years. Groups were balanced at the start of the study and analysis was by intention to treat. As expected, homocysteine levels dropped and vitamin levels increased in the active treatment group. However, there was no difference between groups in the combined risk of cardiovascular death, myocardial infarction, or stroke (18.8% vs 19.8%; relative risk = 0.95; 95% CI, 0.84–1.07). There was also no difference regarding this combination of outcomes in patients in the top tertile of homocysteine levels (23.9% vs 24%). There was no difference in outcomes between countries that did or did not fortify foods with folate. Regarding individual outcomes, there were slightly fewer strokes (4.0% vs 5.3%), but more hospitalizations for unstable angina (9.7% vs 7.9%) with supplementation. The study was powered to detect a 17% to 20% relative reduction in the risk of the primary outcome. A second report in the same issue of the journal also failed to find any benefit for secondary prevention of cardiovascular events in patients with a recent acute myocardial infarction (N Engl J Med 2006;345:1578–1588). In fact, they found evidence of possible harm from B vitamin supplementation in this group of high-risk patients.

Essential Evidence: Medicine that Matters, Edited by David Slawson, Allen Shaughnessy, Mark Ebell, and Henry Barry.

Folic acid supplementation does not reduce cardiovascular disease risk nor mortality

Clinical question
Does folic acid supplementation decrease morbidity or mortality from cardiovascular diseases?

Bottom line
The available evidence does not support the use of folic acid supplementation as secondary prevention of cardiovascular disease events, stroke, or all-cause mortality among patients with preexisting vascular diseases. (LOE = 1a)

Reference
Bazzano LA, Reynolds K, Holder KN, He J. Effect of folic acid supplementation on risk of cardiovascular diseases. A meta-analysis of randomized controlled trials. JAMA 2006;296:2720–2726.

Study Design
Meta-analysis (randomized controlled trials)

Funding
Government

Setting
Various (meta-analysis)

Synopsis
These investigators searched MEDLINE, reference lists from relevant studies, and contacted experts in the field to identify trials investigating the effect of folic acid supplementation on cardiovascular disease risk. No language restrictions were applied. Inclusion criteria included randomized controlled trials of folic acid supplementation with a duration of at least 6 months. Two investigators independently performed the search and identified reports meeting inclusion criteria. Discrepancies were resolved by consensus discussion with a third investigator. From an initial pool of 165 potentially relevant studies, the authors included a total of 12 trials representing data from 16,958 patients with preexisting cardiovascular or renal disease. The dosage of folic acid in the intervention groups ranged from 0.5 mg per day to 15 mg per day. All trials reported a reduction in homocysteine levels. However, compared with control patients, there was no significant reduction in the risk of total cardiovascular disease events, stroke, or all-cause mortality among patients using folic acid supplementation. A formal analysis found no evidence for publication bias or significant heterogeneity among the various trials (no significant differences in reported outcomes among the various individual trials). The longest follow-up period for any of the individual trials was 5 years, so it is possible that a benefit could occur with more prolonged use. Multiple large trials are currently underway addressing this issue.

Essential Evidence: Medicine that Matters, Edited by David Slawson, Allen Shaughnessy, Mark Ebell, and Henry Barry.

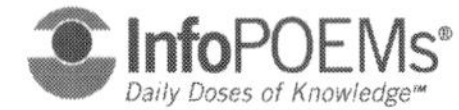

Herbs may reduce cholesterol, no data on clinical outcomes

Clinical question

Can herbal supplements reduce cholesterol?

Bottom line

The herbal supplements fenugreek, red yeast rice, artichoke, and guggul may reduce cholesterol, although the quality and consistency of studies is poor. There is no evidence that using these herbs improves clinical outcomes, although they do appear to be safe. (LOE = 1b–)

Reference

Coon JST, Ernst E. Herbs for serum cholesterol reduction: a systematic review. J Fam Pract 2003;52:468–478.

Study Design

Systematic review

Setting

Various (meta-analysis)

Synopsis

There is reasonably good evidence that garlic modestly lowers cholesterol, but we have no reason to believe it improves patient-oriented outcomes. This thorough review of the literature looked at other herbs, such as fenugreek, red yeast rice, artichoke, and guggul (whatever that is; it sounds like a character from the Lord of the Rings to me). They found 25 studies, but 13 had a Jadad score of 2 or lower on a scale from 0 to 5, and all but a few were quite small. Results were mixed, and in many cases the herb lowered cholesterol levels, but no more than placebo. None of the studies measured patient-oriented outcomes.

Essential Evidence: Medicine that Matters, Edited by David Slawson, Allen Shaughnessy, Mark Ebell, and Henry Barry.

Herbal tea effective for symptoms of acute pharyngitis

Clinical question

Can herbal tea help reduce the symptoms of pain associated with acute pharyngitis?

Bottom line

An herbal tea containing a mixture of traditional demulcents (soothing agents) was more effective than a placebo tea in the short-term relief of pain in patients with acute pharyngitis. The effect does not last long – less than 30 minutes – so requires frequent tea drinking throughout the day. On the occasion of my next sore throat, I'm going to reach for an analgesic and a topical anesthetic, but herbal tea may be useful for patients who prefer a more active approach and who wish to avoid the partially anesthetized mouth feel. (LOE = 1b)

Reference

Brinckmann J, Sigwart H, van Houten Taylor L. Safety and efficacy of a traditional herbal medicine (Throat Coat) in symptomatic temporary relief of pain in patients with acute pharyngitis: a multicenter, prospective, randomized, double-blinded, placebo-controlled study. J Altern Complement Med 2003;9:285–298.

Study Design

Randomized controlled trial (double-blinded)

Setting

Outpatient (any)

Synopsis

Demulcents is a general category of products that are soothing and relieve irritation. They are not topical anesthetics, but have been used for many years to treat sore throat. This study evaluated the effectiveness of a demulcent mixture containining licorice root, elm inner bark, marshmallow root, and licorice root aqueous dry extract (an herbal tea called Throat Coat). Sixty patients with acute pharyngitis by any cause were randomly assigned to use the herbal tea or a similar-tasting and -smelling placebo tea 4 to 6 times daily for as long as symptoms remained. No other treatment was allowed. Treatment allocation was concealed from the enrolling physician. Patients rated pain relief after 1 minute then every 5 minutes for 30 minutes, then at 3 and 24 hours after the first dose, and then daily using a scale from 0 to 10. Analysis was by intention to treat and compared the degree of change in pain scores at each period, as well as the total amount of pain relief using the total area under the curve of pain changes. Details on exactly what statistics were used are sketchy, which is odd considering the great detail in which other aspects of the study were reported. Changes from baseline pain after the first dose were significantly different than placebo at 5 and 10 minutes. The sum of pain intensity differences occurring in the first 30 minutes of treatment was approximately twice as good in the treatment group ($P = .041$). Pain relief was also greater in treated patients at 10 minutes after the first dose. By intention-to-treat analysis, however, total pain relief over the first 30 minutes was not different between the 2 groups.

Essential Evidence: Medicine that Matters, Edited by David Slawson, Allen Shaughnessy, Mark Ebell, and Henry Barry.

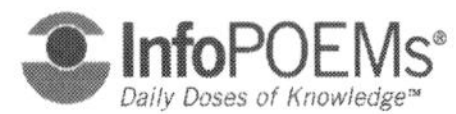

Petroleum jelly doesn't reduce recurrent pediatric epistaxis

Clinical question

Does petroleum jelly (Vaseline) reduce the likelihood that epistaxis will recur in children?

Bottom line

In this highly selected group of patients with recurrent epistaxis, petroleum jelly applied twice daily for 4 weeks did not reduce the number of bleeds in the subsequent 4 weeks. This should make you question this commonly recommended treatment. But don't abandon it just yet, since it may work in children with less severe disease in the primary care setting, and because there was potential for recall bias by parents in this study. (LOE = 2b)

Reference

Loughran S, Spinou E, Clement WA, et al. A prospective, single-blind, randomized controlled trial of petroleum jelly/Vaseline for recurrent paediatric epistaxis. Clin Otolaryngol 2004;29:266–269.

Study Design

Randomized controlled trial (single-blinded)

Setting

Outpatient (specialty)

Synopsis

Recurrent nosebleeds are a common problem in children. Many doctors advise the application of petroleum jelly (Vaseline) to the anterior nares, since bleeding is thought to result from drying, picking, rubbing, and all the other things children do to their noses. In this small but well-designed study, 105 children aged 1 to 14 years referred to otolaryngologists for recurrent epistaxis were identified. The median duration of symptoms was 12 months and the median duration of bleeds was 5 minutes. The children were randomized (allocation concealed) to receive 1 of 2 letters: instructions to apply Vaseline twice daily for 4 weeks and keep a nosebleed diary, or simply instructions to keep a nosebleed diary. Patients were assessed after 8 weeks, and the primary outcome was the percentage with recurrent bleeds in the previous 4 weeks. Analysis was by intention to treat and the physician assessing outcomes was blinded to treatment assignment and was careful not to ask about treatment adherence until the end of the visit. Groups were similar at baseline. They were also similar after the intervention: 27.5% in the treatment group and 33.9% in the control group (P = 0.47) had no bleeds during the 4 weeks prior to the visit and after the intervention. The study had limitations, though. Approximately 14% of patients never came in for evaluation (evenly split between groups) and most parents were noncompliant with the diaries. The researchers therefore used parental recall instead of the diaries to assess the primary outcome.

Saline nasal irrigation effective for frequent sinusitis

Clinical question

Does daily nasal irrigation with hypertonic saline improve symptoms in patients with frequent sinus infections?

Bottom line

This is an inexpensive, easy, and effective treatment for a condition considered intractable by many. Daily nasal irrigation using 2% saline was a highly effective treatment for patients with frequent sinusitis. (LOE = 1b–)

Reference

Rabago D, Zgierska A, Mundt M, et al. Efficacy of daily hypertonic saline nasal irrigation among patients with sinusitis: a randomized controlled trial. J Fam Pract 2002;51:1049–1055.

Study Design

Randomized controlled trial (nonblinded)

Setting

Outpatient (primary care)

Synopsis

Sinus infections are often recurrent and can be difficult to treat. The Yogic tradition advocates daily rinsing of the nasal passage with a hypertonic saline solution as a way to clean things out. Previous studies, although promising, have been small and poorly designed. In this primary care clinical trial, the authors identified patients with either 2 episodes of acute sinusitis or 1 episode of chronic sinusitis per year for 2 consecutive years. Their mean age was 42 years, 74% were women, only 5% were smokers, and most had recurrent episodes of acute sinusitis rather than chronic sinusitis. They randomized these patients to either usual care (n = 24) or to an experimental group (n = 52) that received instruction in using the SinuCleanse nasal cup with 2% saline buffered with baking soda. Subjects completed a daily diary to record adherence to the nasal irrigation protocol, filled out a symptom survey every 2 weeks, and a more extensive set of outcome measures at 1.5, 3, and 6 months. Groups were similar at baseline. Although not blinded, allocation to groups was appropriately concealed, randomization was valid, and analysis was by intention-to-treat. At 6 months, there was a clinically and statistically greater improvement in the Rhinosinusitis Disability Index and the Single Item Symptom Severity Assessment for patients using nasal irrigation. There were also significant improvements in sinus headache, frontal pain, frontal pressure, and nasal congestion, and a reduction in antibiotic and nasal spray use. Although 10 subjects reported side effects (eg, nasal irritation, nasal burning, and nosebleeds) all 44 experimental subjects who completed the final questions about satisfaction said they would continue to use nasal irrigation.

Essential Evidence: Medicine that Matters, Edited by David Slawson, Allen Shaughnessy, Mark Ebell, and Henry Barry.

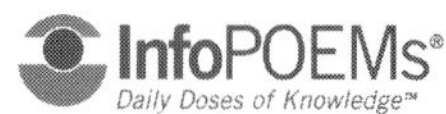

Forcing fluids during a respiratory infection unsupported by studies

Clinical question

What is the evidence that drinking plenty of fluids is effective and not harmful?

Bottom line

There is no research evaluating whether drinking plenty of fluids is beneficial to patients with respiratory infections. Although the benefit seems to be self-evident, there is a theoretical risk of harm. Antidiuretic hormone secretion increases in both adults and children with lower respiratory tract infections who drink large amounts of fluids, and hyponatremia has been documented in these situations in cohort and case studies. There is weak evidence to support either continuing the practice or stopping the practice. (LOE = 1a–)

Reference

Guppy MPB, Mickan SM, Del Mar CB. "Drink plenty of fluids": a systematic review of evidence for this recommendation in acute respiratory infections. BMJ 2004;328:499–500.

Study Design

Systematic review

Setting

Various (meta-analysis)

Synopsis

The unpleasant symptoms of respiratory tract infections are often accompanied by the frustration that there is little one can do to hasten recovery. In other words, it's difficult to do nothing. Now we have a study suggesting that even the most benign do-nothing-by-doing-something-innocuous is not so harmless after all. The authors of this study attempted to determine whether drinking extra fluids while experiencing a respiratory tract infection is evidence-based or a medical myth. With appropriate rigor they searched several databases, examined references of relevant papers and contacted experts in an attempt to cough up studies on the subject. As might be expected, there has been no fevered rush to research this topic and they came up dry when looking for randomized controlled trials. They found 2 studies reporting hyponatremia at rates of 31% and 45% for children with moderate to severe pneumonia but without signs of dehydration, and several case series in which children developed hyponatremia during a respiratory infection that responded to fluid restriction.

Essential Evidence: Medicine that Matters, Edited by David Slawson, Allen Shaughnessy, Mark Ebell, and Henry Barry.

Zinc nasal gel reduces duration of common cold

Clinical question

Does zinc nasal gel reduce the duration of the common cold?

Bottom line

Zinc nasal gel was effective in this small study, reducing the duration of cold symptoms by 1.7 days. It was well tolerated, although minor adverse effects were more common in the treatment group. (LOE = 1b)

Reference

Mossad SB. Effect of zincum gluconicum nasal gel on the duration and symptom severity of the common cold in otherwise healthy adults. QJM 2003;96:35–43.

Study Design

Randomized controlled trial (double-blinded)

Setting

Outpatient (any)

Synopsis

Zinc lozenges have been shown effective in 6 randomized trials and ineffective in 8 others. Meta-analyses are equivocal. Advocates for zinc suggest that the delivery vehicle may be part of the problem, and this trial evaluates a zinc nasal gel. Eighty patients were recruited from advertisements, and were included if they were aged 18 to 55 years, had symptoms of a cold for 24 to 48 hours, and had 2 major and at least 1 minor symptom or 1 major and at least 3 minor symptoms. Major symptoms included nasal drainage and sore throat; minor symptoms included nasal congestion, sneezing, scratchy throat, hoarseness, cough, headache, muscle aches, and oral temperature above 98.6 F. These seem reasonable, although the definition of fever is too low. Patients with diabetes, with a noncorrected deviated nasal septum or recurrent sinusitis, and smokers were excluded. Patients were randomized with concealed allocation to either zincum gluconicum (Zenullose or Zicam) 120 microliters via metered dose applicator or matching placebo. Patients and investigators were masked, and after 1 day patients could not guess whether they were in the active treatment or control groups. The primary outcome was the time to resolution of all cold symptoms. Patients completed a diary of symptoms and adverse effects twice a day, rating each on a scale from 0 (none) to 3 (severe). They measured a lot of secondary outcomes, but we'll focus on the primary outcome. The groups were similar at the start of the study, with 40 patients in each group. Two patients in the control group were lost to follow-up, and because there were no follow-up data, were excluded from the analysis. Three in the treatment group and 1 in the control group were diagnosed with an illness other than the common cold and discontinued treatment, but were still included in the analysis (appropriately). The time to resolution of all symptoms was shorter in the treatment group (4.3 vs 6 days; P = .002), and the time to resolution was also shorter for all individual symptoms, except headache, muscle aches, and fever. There was no statistically significant difference between groups for each adverse effect. More patients in the treatment group had any adverse effect (31% vs 14%), although no test of statistical significance is reported for this comparison, which is a bit suspicious.

Essential Evidence: Medicine that Matters, Edited by David Slawson, Allen Shaughnessy, Mark Ebell, and Henry Barry.

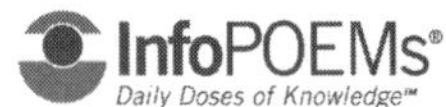

Echinacea purpurea ineffective for treating URI in kids

Clinical question

How effective and safe is echinacea in the treatment of upper respiratory tract infections in children?

Bottom line

Echinacea purpurea extract (above ground plant only), prepared and used at the doses in this study was ineffective in treating upper respiratory tract infections (URIs) in children. Although it was generally safe to use, more parents reported a rash on their child and 2 children had a serious allergic-type reaction. Interestingly, children using echinacea were less likely to have recurrent URI (number needed to treat = 9). (LOE = 1b)

Reference

Taylor JA, Weber W, Standish L, et al. Efficacy and safety of echinacea in treating upper respiratory tract infections in children. A randomized controlled trial. JAMA 2003;290:2824–2830.

Study Design

Randomized controlled trial (double-blinded)

Setting

Outpatient (primary care)

Synopsis

Although the average child has 6 to 8 colds per year, each lasting 7 to 10 days, commonly used medications such as decongestants, antihistamines, and cough suppressants lack efficacy in those younger than 12 years. Echinacea is widely used for the prevention and treatment of URIs in adults, but there is limited data on efficacy and safety of use in children. Data were obtained and analyzed on a total of 707 URIs that occurred in 407 children. At the onset of each URI, subjects were randomly given (concealed allocation assignment) either dried pressed Echinacea purpurea juice (obtained from the above-ground herb, harvested at flowering, extracted in an alcohol-free preparation combined with syrup), or identical placebo. Dosing was age-based on the recommendations of the manufacturer and was continued until all symptoms had resolved, up to a maximum of 10 days. Parents recorded the severity of symptoms and adverse events in a daily logbook. The patients, parents, practitioners and research staff were all unaware of treatment group assignment. Ninety-four percent of the subjects were followed up for a total of 4 months. Using intention-to-treat analysis, there were no differences in duration of URIs or in the overall estimate of severity of URI symptoms between the 2 treatment groups. Other over-the-counter cold remedies were administered by parents at the same rate in both groups, but antipruitics and analgesics other than acetaminophen were administered more often to children treated with echinacea (9.8% vs 5.1%; P = .03). After limiting the analysis to the URIs in which patients received at least 80% of the study medication (per protocol analysis), there were still no differences found between the 2 groups. Children assigned to echinacea were less likely to have a second URI than those in the placebo group (52.3% vs 64.4%; P = .015; number needed to treat = 9). Adverse events were reported similarly in each group, although rash was reported more often in children receiving echinacea (7.1% vs 2.7%). Two children receiving echinacea had the sudden onset of stridor requiring emergency treatment with steroids.

Essential Evidence: Medicine that Matters, Edited by David Slawson, Allen Shaughnessy, Mark Ebell, and Henry Barry.

Echinacea doesn't shorten or lessen cold symptoms

Clinical question

Is Echinacea purpurea effective in the treatment of cold symptoms?

Bottom line

A product containing the freeze-dried extract of the above-ground part of Echinacea purpurea was ineffective in decreasing the duration or severity of the common cold. These results contradict findings of 2 meta-analyses which documented some benefit with other extracts. (LOE = 1b–)

Reference

Yale SH, Liu K. Echinacea purpurea therapy for the treatment of the common cold. Arch Intern Med 2004;164:1237–1241.

Study Design

Randomized controlled trial (double-blinded)

Setting

Outpatient (any)

Synopsis

This study evaluated the effectiveness of a freeze-dried extract prepared from the above-ground parts of the Echinacea purpurea plant (EchinaFresh). All formulations of echinacea are not the same: 2 different species are in common use – E purpurea and E augustifolia – and different parts of the plant, such as the whole plant, root, or upper parts are used to make extracts. The participants in this study were solicited by advertisements. The investigators enrolled 128 adults, primarily women, with an average age of 38 years, within 24 hours of the onset of cold symptoms. Only 10% were smokers. The average duration of symptoms was 15 hours. The patients were randomized to receive either placebo or echinacea 100 mg 3 times daily as long as they had symptoms, for up to 14 days. The patients were asked not to take other symptom-relief products, except acetaminophen. Daily symptoms scores, which consisted of 4 points on each of 8 symptom scales (nasal discharge, cough, and so forth), were not different at any time between the 2 groups. The time to complete resolution of symptoms also was not shortened by echinacea. The study was large enough to find a 25% difference in symptoms or a 3-day difference in duration.

Essential Evidence: Medicine that Matters, Edited by David Slawson, Allen Shaughnessy, Mark Ebell, and Henry Barry.

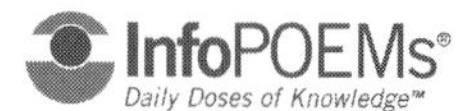

Black cohosh ineffective for vasomotor symptoms

Clinical question

Do soy, black cohosh, or a naturopathic multibotanical provide greater relief from vasomotor symptoms than placebo in menopausal or perimenopausal women?

Bottom line

Neither soy, black cohosh, or a naturopathic multibotanical was effective in decreasing the duration or severity of vasomotor symptoms. These results are similar to other research findings. (LOE = 1b)

Reference

Newton KM, Reed SD, LaCroix AZ, Grothaus LC, Ehrlich K, Guiltinan J. Treatment of vasomotor symptoms of menopause with black cohosh, multibotanicals, soy, hormone therapy, or placebo. Ann Intern Med 2006;145:869–879.

Study Design

Randomized controlled trial (double-blinded)

Funding

Government

Allocation

Concealed

Setting

Outpatient (any)

Synopsis

Women in this US study were members of a managed care organization and were recruited by mail. The 351 women were perimenopausal or menopausal and had at least 2 menopausal symptoms daily, with at least 6 moderate to severe symptoms over a 2-week period. The women were randomly assigned, using concealed allocation, to receive 1 of the following treatments daily for 1 year: black cohosh 160 mg (Cimipure); a multibotanical frequently used by naturopaths (Progyne) containing black cohosh and 9 other products; the same multibotanical with dietary soy counseling; conjugated estrogens 0.625 mg; or placebo. Analysis was by intention to treat. Vasomotor symptoms per day, symptom intensity, or scores on the Wiklund Vasomotor Symptom Subscale did not differ between herbal interventions and placebo at 3, 6, or 12 months or on average over all follow-up points. However, symptom intensity was significantly worse for patients treated with the multibotanical plus soy diet at 1 year ($P = .016$). This small study was designed to find a effect of herbs halfway between the expected effects of hormone and placebo therapy, and small changes in symptoms conceivably could have been missed. However, none of the treatments approached the effectiveness of estrogen therapy.

Essential Evidence: Medicine that Matters, Edited by David Slawson, Allen Shaughnessy, Mark Ebell, and Henry Barry.

Acupuncture ineffective for hot flashes

Clinical question
Is acupuncture an effective treatment for perimenopausal and postmenopausal hot flashes?

Bottom line
Acupuncture is not an effective treatment for menopausal hot flashes. (LOE = 1b)

Reference
Vincent A, Barton DL, Mandrekar JN, et al. Acupuncture for hot flashes: randomized, sham-controlled clinical study. Menopause 2007;14:45–52.

Study Design
Randomized controlled trial (single-blinded)

Funding
Foundation

Allocation
Uncertain

Setting
Outpatient (specialty)

Synopsis
In this single-blinded study, 103 perimenopausal and postmenopausal women aged 45 years to 59 years were randomized to acupuncture or sham procedure twice weekly for 5 weeks. Perimenopausal status was defined as menstrual irregularity or amenorrhea for at least 3 months, and postmenopausal status as amenorrhea for at least 12 months. Women were eligible if they reported at least 5 hot flashes daily and were not taking estrogen, soy, progesterone, vitamin E, black cohosh, gabapentin, or antidepressants used for treating hot flashes. Other exclusion criteria were the use of coumadin, certain skin disorders, the presence of a pacemaker or prosthetic joint, diabetic neuropathy, and active chemotherapy. A single acupuncturist with more than 5000 hours experience provided the treatments. Women used a daily diary to note the number of hot flashes and the severity of each (from 1 [mild] to 3 [severe]). The sum of the severity scores for each hot flash provided a daily hot flash score. The authors used survival curve statistics with an intention-to-treat analysis, and performed an appropriate power analysis. There were no differences between groups at baseline, 6 weeks, or 12 weeks.

Essential Evidence: Medicine that Matters, Edited by David Slawson, Allen Shaughnessy, Mark Ebell, and Henry Barry.

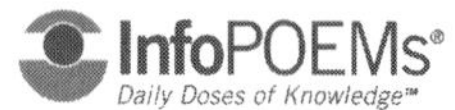

Lactobacillus doesn't prevent post-antibiotic vaginitis

Clinical question

Can lactobacillus preparations, whether given orally, vaginally, or both, prevent post-antibiotic vaginal candidiasis?

Bottom line

Lactobacillus, whether given orally, vaginally, or both, had no effect on the development of culture-proven vaginal candidiasis. Lactobacillus probiotics have been shown effective, however, in decreasing antibiotic-associated diarrhea (Aliment Pharmacol Ther 2002;16:1461-67). (LOE = 1b)

Reference

Pirotta M, Gunn J, Chondros P, et al. Effect of lactobacillus in preventing post-antibiotic vulvovaginal candidiasis: a randomised controlled trial. BMJ 2004;329:548–551.

Study Design

Randomized controlled trial (double-blinded)

Allocation

Concealed

Setting

Outpatient (primary care)

Synopsis

Probiotics, commensal microorganisms given to antagonize the activity of pathogenic microorganisms, have been used to replace bacterial flora wiped out by antibiotics with the aim of preventing antibiotic-associated diarrhea or vaginal candidiasis. The investigators of this study evaluated the role of products containing Lactobacillus spp. to prevent vaginal candidiasis in 278 nonpregnant women who required a short course of antibiotics for a nongynecological infection. The actual antibiotics were not specified. The women were randomly assigned, using concealed allocation, to receive an oral powder containing Lactobacillus spp (Lactobac), a vaginal pessary containing Lactobacillus (Femilac), both treatments, or placebo. The women took the powder twice daily 20 minutes before meals and used one pessary at night for 10 nights during the 6-day course of antibiotics and for 4 days after. Viability of the lactobacilli was confirmed. Candida was cultured in 23% of women, a rate consistent with other research. There was no difference in the rate of vaginal candidiasis in women receiving one or both forms of probiotic or placebo. The study was stopped early because of lack of benefit.

Essential Evidence: Medicine that Matters, Edited by David Slawson, Allen Shaughnessy, Mark Ebell, and Henry Barry.

Immersion exercise reduces leg edema in pregnancy

Clinical question

Does immersion exercise reduce dependent edema in pregnant women?

Bottom line

Water immersion exercise is an option for managing leg edema in otherwise uncomplicated pregnancies. (LOE = 2b)

Reference

Hartmann S, Huch R. Response of pregnancy leg edema to a single immersion exercise session. Acta Obstet Gynecol Scand 2005;84:1150–1153.

Study Design

Cohort (prospective)

Funding

Unknown/not stated

Setting

Outpatient (specialty)

Synopsis

Dependent edema is common in pregnancy. In this study 9 women with marked edema and otherwise uncomplicated pregnancies participated in a 45-minute immersion exercise session in water. Lower leg volumes were measured before and after the session, including the foot and 10 cm of the lower leg. Mean volume decreased by 112 mL on the left leg and 84 mL on the right leg ($P = .007$). The women also had a subjective impression of reduction in edema. The authors did not report the duration of the effect or other patient-oriented outcomes.

Essential Evidence: Medicine that Matters, Edited by David Slawson, Allen Shaughnessy, Mark Ebell, and Henry Barry.

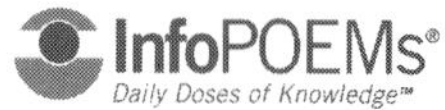

Diet and exercise prevent diabetes in high-risk patients

Clinical question

Do diet and exercise delay the development of diabetes in high-risk patients?

Bottom line

Diet and exercise are effective in delaying the diagnosis of diabetes in patients at increased risk. (LOE = 2b)

Reference

Lindstrom J, Ilanne-Parikka P, Peltonen M, et al, for the Finnish Diabetes Prevention Study Group. Sustained reduction in the incidence of type 2 diabetes by lifestyle intervention: follow-up of the Finnish Diabetes Prevention Study. Lancet 2006;368:1673–1679.

Study Design

Randomized controlled trial (nonblinded)

Funding

Industry + foundation

Allocation

Unconcealed

Setting

Outpatient (any)

Synopsis

In the Finnish Diabetes Prevention Study, 522 men and women, aged between 40 years and 65 years and at high risk for developing diabetes, were randomly assigned either to a tailored diet-and-exercise regimen or to usual care. To be eligible, the patients had to have a body mass index greater than 25 and have impaired glucose tolerance. The original study lasted a median of 4 years. The cumulative incidence of diabetes in the intervention group was 11% compared with 23% in the control group (number needed to treat = 8; 95% CI 6–16). In this report, the researchers provide 3 additional years of observations on the patients who had not developed diabetes by the end of the original study. No specific diet or exercise information was provided to the patients during this follow-up period. After a total of 7 years of follow-up, 75 patients in the intervention group and 110 patients in the control group developed diabetes. The cumulative incidence rate was 4.3 per 100 person-years in the intervention group, and 7.4 in the control group. The authors estimate that one would need to treat 22 patients with diet and exercise to prevent 1 patient per year from developing diabetes.

Essential Evidence: Medicine that Matters, Edited by David Slawson, Allen Shaughnessy, Mark Ebell, and Henry Barry.

Treating prediabetes does not affect progression

Clinical question

Does treatment of postprandial hyperglycemia in patients with early, asymptomatic diabetes delay progression to frank fasting hyperglycemia?

Bottom line

The jury is still out regarding the identification and treatment of patients with prediabetes. According to this study, a similar percentage of patients with early diabetes will develop frank diabetes whether or not they receive therapy to lower postprandial glucose levels. A larger, though shorter, study has shown a difference, but it looks like early benefit is lost over time. (LOE = 1b–)

Reference

Kirkman MS, Shankar RR, Shankar S. Treating postprandial hyperglycemia does not appear to delay progression of early type 2 diabetes. Diabetes Care 2006;29:2095–2101.

Study Design

Randomized controlled trial (nonblinded)

Funding

Industry + govt

Allocation

Uncertain

Setting

Outpatient (specialty)

Synopsis

Researchers conducting this US-based study enrolled 219 adults with obesity, a history of gestational diabetes, or a family history of diabetes. The patients did not have a diagnosis of diabetes but had a fasting plasma glucose level between 105 mg/dL and 140 mg/dL (5.5 mmol/L–7.8 mmol/L) and a 2-hour postload of plasma glucose of at least 200 mg/dL (11.1 mmol/L). After a 2-day admission for extensive testing, patients were randomly assigned, concealed allocation uncertain, to receive either placebo or acarbose (Precose) titrated to a maximum dose of 100 mg 3 times daily. The maximum dose was achieved by 91% of patients. The patients had their fasting glucose level measured every 3 months for up to 5 years. Approximately 43% of the patients did not complete the study. Since the dropout rates were similar in both groups, it is likely that the patients represent a highly motivated group of people. Additionally, given the frequent side effects of acarbose, patients receiving placebo were probably aware of that fact and may have been more rigorous with nondrug efforts to reduce the risk of diabetes. This increased effort might be responsible for the lower than expected development of diabetes in the placebo-treated patients. Though postprandial glucose levels were decreased by acarbose, over the 5 years of the study a similar proportion of patients in both groups developed frank fasting hyperglycemia, approximately 30% in both groups (29% vs 34%). The study was small and the results would only be significant if the treatment decreased the development of diabetes by half as compared with typical rates of development. The results conflict with the shorter-duration STOP-NIDDM study which found, after an average 3 years, that 32% of treated patients had diabetes as compared with 42% of placebo-treated patients (Lancet 2002;359:2072–2077). A nonsignificant difference in diabetes also occurred at 3 years in the current study, though the difference was lost by the end of the study.

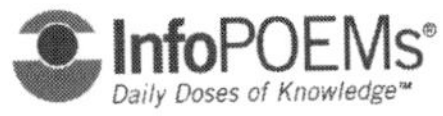

Rosiglitazone delays developing diabetes mellitus (DREAM)

Clinical question

Does rosiglitazone delay the development of diabetes in patients with impaired glucose tolerance or impaired fasting glucose levels?

Bottom line

Patients at increased risk of developing diabetes were less likely to develop diabetes if taking rosiglitazone (Avandia) than if given a placebo. We don't know how well rosiglitazone compares with other interventions also known to delay diabetes: diet and exercise, metformin, or acarbose. We also don't know if clinically relevant outcomes are improved. (LOE = 1b)

Reference

DREAM (Diabetes REduction Assessment with ramipril and rosiglitazone Medication) Trial Investigators; Gerstein HC, Yusuf S, Bosch J, et al. Effect of rosiglitazone on the frequency of diabetes in patients with impaired glucose tolerance or impaired fasting glucose: a randomised controlled trial. Lancet 2006;368:1096–1105.

Study Design

Randomized controlled trial (double-blinded)

Funding

Industry + govt

Allocation

Concealed

Setting

Outpatient (any)

Synopsis

To be eligible for this study, patients had to have a fasting blood glucose level between 6.1 mmol/L and 7 mmol/L (110 mg/dL to 126 mg/dL); impaired glucose tolerance, defined as a glucose level between 7.8 mmol/L and 11.1 mmol/L (140 mg/dL to 200 mg/dL) measured 2 hours after a 75-g glucose load; or both. Additionally, they had to demonstrate at least 80% compliance with taking rosiglitazone during a 17-day run-in period. The authors excluded patients with diabetes and cardiovascular disease. All patients received diet and exercise advice, which is very different than a formal diet and exercise intervention. More than 5200 patients received rosiglitazone 4 mg daily for the first 2 months, then 8 mg daily for the remainder of the study, or placebo. The researchers evaluated the patients sequentially for a median of 3 years. The main outcome – diabetes or death – was evaluated by intention-to-treat analysis. At the end of the study, 11.6% of patients taking rosiglitazone developed this composite end point compared with 26% of the control patients (number needed to treat [NNT] = 7; 95% CI, 6–8). Since there was no difference in deaths, this NNT was entirely due to delayed development of diabetes. Only 10.6% of the patients taking rosiglitazone developed diabetes compared with 25% of the control patients (NNT = 7; 6–8). Approximately 25% of the patients taking rosiglitazone stopped taking the medication, compared with 21.5% of those taking placebo (number needed to treat to harm [NNTH] = 30; 18–95). Additionally, 0.5% of the patients taking rosiglitazone developed congestive heart failure compared with 0.1% of the control patients (NNTH = 220; 123–619). A word of precaution: Knowler and colleagues (NEJM 2002;346:393–403) compared lifestyle changes with metformin and placebo, and found that lifestyle changes were more effective than metformin. Since the DREAM study omitted the most effective intervention, we really don't know how rosiglitazone stacks up.

Hypertension control most important aspect of diabetes care

Clinical question

What is the role of blood pressure control in patients with type 2 diabetes?

Bottom line

(LOE = 1a)

Reference

Vijan S, Hayward RA. Treatment of hypertension in type 2 diabetes mellitus: blood pressure goals, choice of agents, and setting priorities in diabetes care. Ann Intern Med 2003;138:593–602. Snow V, Weiss KB, Mottur-Pilson C, et al. The evidence base for tight blood pressure control in the management of type 2 diabetes mellitus. Ann Intern Med 2003;138:587–592.

Study Design

Practice guideline

Setting

Various (guideline)

Synopsis

Aggressive control of blood pressure, with a goal of achieving <135/<80 mmHg, is the single most important management aspect for patients with type 2 diabetes. Unlike aggressive blood glucose control, blood pressure control has been shown to decrease clinically relevant macrovascular and microvascular events that occur with diabetes, as well as prolong life. From the report: "We do not intend to suggest that glycemic control is an ineffective intervention, but rather that treatment of hypertension should be prioritized and stressed as the most important intervention for the average population of persons with type 2 diabetes." Angiotensin-converting enzyme inhibitors offer no advantage over thiazide diuretics, and second-choice agents should be beta-blockers or calcium-channel blockers.

Essential Evidence: Medicine that Matters, Edited by David Slawson, Allen Shaughnessy, Mark Ebell, and Henry Barry.

Fenofibrate doesn't prevent coronary events in diabetes mellitus (FIELD)

Clinical question

In patients with type 2 diabetes, does fenofibrate prevent coronary events?

Bottom line

In this study, patients with type 2 diabetes treated with fenofibrate (Antara, Lofibra, Tricor) had no significant reduction in coronary events compared with patients treated with placebo. There was a small reduction, however, in nonfatal myocardial infarctions, total cardiovascular disease, and revascularization. (LOE = 1b)

Reference

Keech A, Simes RJ, Barter P, et al, for the FIELD study investigators. Effects of long-term fenofibrate therapy on cardiovascular events in 9795 people with type 2 diabetes mellitus (the FIELD study): randomised controlled trial. Lancet 2005;366:1849–1861.

Study Design	Funding	Allocation
Randomized controlled trial (double-blinded)	Industry + govt	Concealed

Setting

Outpatient (any)

Synopsis

In this study, nearly 10,000 patients between the ages of 50 and 75 years with type 2 diabetes mellitus were randomly assigned to receive 200 mg micronized fenofibrate every day or a matching placebo. The patients all had a total cholesterol level between 3.0 mmol/L and 6.5 mmol/L (115 and 250 mg/dL), plus either a total cholesterol/HDL cholesterol ratio of 4.0 or higher, or a triglyceride level between 1.0 mmol/L and 5.0 mmol/L (88 and 440 mg/dL), with no clear indication for, or treatment with, lipid-modifying therapy at the start of the study. After randomization, the patients were seen every 4 to 6 months for up to 5 years. Subsequent decisions about adding other medications were left to the discretion of the treating physician. The study was designed to have enough power to detect modest differences in the rate of events.The outcomes for this study were analyzed by intention to treat and were assessed by evaluators unaware of the treatment group. The median follow up was 5 years and the researchers were able to account for more than 99% of the patients. The patients treated with placebo were more likely to receive subsequent nonstudy lipid-lowering medications (17% vs 8%). There was no significant difference in coronary events (6% vs 5%) between groups, although patients treated with placebo had more nonfatal myocardial infarctions (8.4% vs 6.4%; number needed to treat [NNT] = 100; 95% CI, 58–406). Patients taking fenofibrate also were less likely to have a cardiovascular event (NNT = 69; 95% CI, 36–1060) or revascularization (NNT = 67; 95% CI, 40–194). A systematic review* of fibrates has shown a significant increase in all-cause mortality (number needed to treat to harm = 132 for 4.4 years). In this study, there was also a nonsignificant increase in all-cause mortality (14.2/1000 vs 12.9/1000; P = .18). *Studer M, Briel M, Leimenstoll B, Glass TR, Bucher HC. Effect of different antilipidemic agents and diets on mortality. A systematic review. Arch Intern Med 2005;165:725–30

Essential Evidence: Medicine that Matters, Edited by David Slawson, Allen Shaughnessy, Mark Ebell, and Henry Barry.

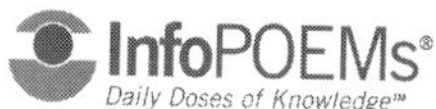

Home glucose monitoring makes little difference in type 2 diabetes

Clinical question

In patients with type 2 diabetes who are not using insulin, does home monitoring of blood glucose improve care?

Bottom line

Intensive monitoring of blood glucose in patients with type 2 diabetes not using insulin results in a small decrease in hemoglobin A1c (HbA1c) levels but does not change fasting blood glucose levels. Urine glucose monitoring works just as well. More casual monitoring of blood glucose, such as once a day, has not been studied. There is a strong possibility that the weak study design was largely responsible for the difference seen in the study. Blood glucose monitoring is expensive: At the intense level of monitoring used in some of these studies (6 times a day), the cost of the monitoring strips alone can be $2000 US per year. (LOE = 1a)

Reference

Welschen LM, Bloemendal E, Nijpels G, Dekker JM, Heine RJ, Stalman WA, Bouter LM. Self-monitoring of blood glucose in patients with type 2 diabetes who are not using insulin. Diabetes Care 2005;28:1510–1517.

Study Design

Meta-analysis (randomized controlled trials)

Funding

Self-funded or unfunded

Setting

Outpatient (any)

Synopsis

The researchers conducting this meta-analysis started by searching 3 databases for randomized controlled studies evaluating blood glucose self-monitoring with typical care in patients with type 2 diabetes who were not using insulin. They also searched the reference lists of identified studies for other studies. They did not attempt to find unpublished studies, research that's usually rejected because it doesn't find a difference. Two authors independently reviewed the studies for inclusion and evaluated the methodologic quality, and 2 authors independently extracted the data. The study quality was moderate for 4 of the studies and high for 2 of the studies. However, patients in the 6 studies included in this analysis were not blinded. Concealed allocation was either not done or not described in any of the studies, allowing the very real possibility that the patients in the blood glucose monitoring groups were different from those in the control groups. They were also highly motivated patients; patients doing the self-monitoring checked blood glucose levels from twice every other day to 6 times per day, 6 days per week. The comparison groups in the study either did no self-monitoring or monitored urine glucose. In the 5 studies that compared blood glucose monitoring with no monitoring, HbA1c levels were nominally but significantly lower in the blood glucose monitoring group (−.39%; 95% CI, −0.56 to −0.21) after approximately 6 months of follow-up. Blood glucose monitoring did not produce better HbA1c levels than urine glucose monitoring. Fasting blood glucose levels were not different in the 2 studies that evaluated it, and quality of life was not different with blood glucose monitoring in the 2 studies that evaluated it. In one study of more than 700 patients in which it was monitored, no serious hypoglycemic episodes occurred in any patient.

Essential Evidence: Medicine that Matters, Edited by David Slawson, Allen Shaughnessy, Mark Ebell, and Henry Barry.

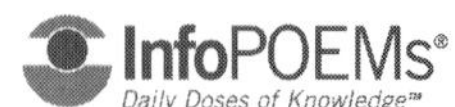

Rosiglitazone more likely to succeed as monotherapy clinical outcomes no better

Clinical question

Which oral diabetes drug is most likely to help patients avoid the need for a second drug?

Bottom line

Patients taking rosiglitazone (Avandia) are a bit less likely than those taking metformin to require a second drug after 5 years. However, there is much better evidence to support the benefit of metformin with regard to cardiovascular events. The results of this study should not change the current practice of beginning treatment with metformin whenever possible in patients with type 2 diabetes. (LOE = 1b)

Reference

Kahn SE, Haffner SM, Heise MA, et al, for the ADOPT Study Group. Glycemic durability of rosiglitazone, metformin or glyburide monotherapy. N Engl J Med 2006;355:2427–2443.

Study Design	Funding	Allocation
Randomized controlled trial (double-blinded)	Industry	Uncertain

Setting

Outpatient (any)

Synopsis

Because thiazolidinediones are thought to preserve beta-cell function to some extent, some diabetologists argue that they should be the initial treatment choice in patients with type 2 diabetes. In this study, 4351 patients (most of whom were white) between the ages of 30 and 75 years with newly diagnosed type 2 diabetes were randomly assigned to receive either 4 mg rosiglitazone, 500 mg metformin, or 2.5 mg glyburide once a day. Analysis was by intention to treat and allocation to groups appears to have been properly concealed. The dose was increased as needed to achieve a fasting blood glucose level of less than 140 mg/dL (7.8 mmol/L); the maximum doses were 4 mg rosiglitazone twice daily, 1 g metformin twice daily, or 7.5 mg glyburide twice daily. Patients with significant cardiovascular disease or contraindications to the study medications were excluded. The number of withdrawals during the study was higher in the glyburide group, due in part to an increased number of adverse events in that group. The primary outcome of this study was a disease-oriented end point: whether the patient required a second drug to control their blood sugar, with failure defined as a fasting blood sugar reading higher than 180 mg/dL (10 mmol/L). At the end of the study, 15% of patients taking rosiglitazone, 21% taking metformin, and 34% taking glyburide had failed monotherapy. Interestingly, the number of patients studied and the length of the study were both increased beyond 4 years because the authors were having difficulty proving that the sponsor's drug (rosiglitazone) was better than metformin on the primary outcome. Regarding patient-oriented outcomes, there was no difference in all-cause mortality, but there were somewhat fewer cardiovascular events (largely heart failure) with glyburide and metformin than with rosiglitazone. Weight gain was more common with rosiglitazone, it increased LDL cholesterol, and it was associated with more edema and use of loop diuretics than metformin or glyburide.

Essential Evidence: Medicine that Matters, Edited by David Slawson, Allen Shaughnessy, Mark Ebell, and Henry Barry.

ACE inhibitors beneficial in diabetics

Clinical question

Are ACE inhibitors or angiotensin receptor blockers beneficial in patients with diabetes who have microalbuminuria or macroalbuminuria?

Bottom line

Treatment with an angiotensin converting enzyme inhibitor, but not angiotensin receptor blockers, delay mortality in patients with diabetes who also have microalbuminuria (and pre-existing heart disease) or frank albuminuria. This benefit occurs regardless of whether patients were also hypertensive. Angiotensin receptor blockers have been demonstrated to prevent a decline in renal function and decrease the likelihood of end-stage renal disease in high-risk patients. This analysis does not provide good evidence that screening for and treating microalbuminuria in patients with diabetes but without heart disease is effective. (LOE = 1a)

Reference

Strippoli GF, Craig M, Deeks JJ, Schena FP, Craig JC. Effects of angiotensin converting enzyme inhibitors and angiotensin II receptor antagonists on mortality and renal outcomes in diabetic nephropathy: systematic review. BMJ 2004;329:828. Epub 2004 Sep 30.

Study Design

Meta-analysis (randomized controlled trials)

Funding

Government

Setting

Outpatient (any)

Synopsis

Angiotensin converting enzyme inhibitors (ACE inhibitors) and angiotensin II receptor blockers (ARBs) are recommended for use in patients with diabetes with either microalbuminuria or frank albuminuria, regardless of blood pressure status. This meta-analysis summarized the current data on the effectiveness of these drugs in preventing overall mortality and end-stage renal disease, reducing the likelihood of a decline in renal function, and, less important, the progression from microalbuminuria to frank albuminuria. The investigators searched several databases using Cochrane Collaboration search strategies. Study selection, data extraction, and quality assessment were performed in the usual manner. They ended up with 43 randomized studies enrolling 7545 patients. Most of the research compares an ACE inhibitor with placebo in patients with microalbuminuria and pre-existing heart disease (the Micro-HOPE study). Treatment with an ACE inhibitor decreases overall mortality (8.50% vs 12.12%). The number needed to treat is 44 for approximately 4.5 years, though the range is very large (95% CI, 24.2–938). ARBs, studied on similar numbers of patients but for shorter time periods, have not shown any effect on mortality. ACE inhibitors do not decrease the development of end-stage renal disease, although the rate was low to begin with (4.3%) in the studied patients. ARBs have been demonstrated to have an effect in patients at high risk (19.3%) of developing end-stage renal disease. Similarly, ARBs but not ACE inhibitors have been demonstrated to have an effect on progression of renal disease as measured by the doubling of serum creatinine. Both types of drugs decrease the number of patients with microalbuminuria who progress to macroalbuminuria, although the significance of this outcome is not known. There is not enough research that directly compares the 2 types of drugs to provide guidance regarding which is better.

Essential Evidence: Medicine that Matters, Edited by David Slawson, Allen Shaughnessy, Mark Ebell, and Henry Barry.

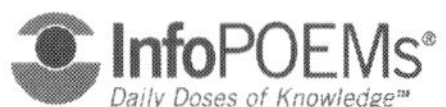

ARB no better than ACEI for prevention of nephropathy progression

Clinical question

Are angiotensin receptor blockers as good as angiotensin-converting enzyme inhibitors at preventing the progression of nephropathy?

Bottom line

Enalapril (Vasotec) was at least as effective as telmisartan (Micardis) and showed a trend toward greater benefit in preventing decline in glomerular filtration rate. Although this study measured a disease-oriented end point, its results are consistent with the body of literature that supports the less expensive angiotensin-converting enzyme (ACE) inhibitors as the drug of choice over angiotensin receptor blockers (ARBs). (LOE = 1b)

Reference

Barnett AH, Bain SC, Bouter P, et al. Angiotensin-receptor blockade versus converting-enzyme inhibition in Type 2 diabetes and nephropathy. N Engl J Med 2004;351:1952–1961.

Study Design

Randomized controlled trial (double-blinded)

Funding

Industry

Allocation

Uncertain

Setting

Outpatient (any)

Synopsis

This study is what we call a DOE (disease-oriented evidence) since it measured progression of nephropathy instead of the patient-oriented outcome of renal failure or need for dialysis. However, the results are worth knowing about because we so often hear of the potential DOE-related advantages of ARBs over the older, less expensive, and less often promoted ACE inhibitors. In this study 250 diabetic subjects with mild to moderate hypertension and evidence of early nephropathy (urinary albumin excretion rate between 11 and 999 mcg/minute and a serum creatinine less than 1.6 mg/dL) were randomized to receive either telmisartan 40 mg per day or enalapril 10 mg per day. If tolerated, the dose was increased to 80 mg and 20 mg respectively after one month. Blood pressure medicines other than an ACE inhibitor or ARB could be added at the discretion of the treating physician to control blood pressure. The primary outcome was the glomerular filtration rate. There was a high dropout rate, and the last observation was appropriately carried forward for the analysis. The results for only those patients with complete data were also reported. In both cases, there was almost no difference in glomerular filtration rate for the first 2 years, with a trend toward greater benefit for enalapril that almost became significant at 4 years and declined slightly at 5 years.

Essential Evidence: Medicine that Matters, Edited by David Slawson, Allen Shaughnessy, Mark Ebell, and Henry Barry.

Pioglitazone ineffective in secondary prevention of macrovascular complications (PROactive)

Clinical question

Is pioglitazone (Actos) effective in the secondary prevention of macrovascular complications in adults with type 2 diabetes?

Bottom line

In patients with type 2 diabetes and comorbid macrovascular disease, 3 years of intensive diabetes care using pioglitazone did not significantly prevent further complications or mortality compared with placebo. (LOE = 1b)

Reference

Dormandy JA, Charbonnel B, Eckland DJ, et al, for the PROactive investigators. Secondary prevention of macrovascular events in patients with type 2 diabetes in the PROactive Study (PROspective pioglitAzone Clinical Trial In macroVascular Events): a randomised controlled trial. Lancet 2005;366:1279–1289.

Study Design	Funding	Allocation	Setting
Randomized controlled trial (double-blinded)	Industry	Concealed	Outpatient (any)

Synopsis

In the United Kingdom Prospective Diabetes Study, tight glycemic control with sulfonylureas, metformin, or insulin didn't prevent macrovascular complications in adult patients with type 2 diabetes. However, obese patients taking metformin did better independent of glycemic control. In the PROactive study, adult patients with type 2 diabetes were eligible if they had a baseline glycohemoglobin level higher than 6.5% and if they had evidence of extensive cardiovascular disease. The research team randomly assigned more than 5200 patients (concealed allocation) to receive pioglitazone 15 mg daily or placebo in addition to their usual regimen. They increased the pioglitazone by 15 mg each month to reach a target dose of 45 mg daily. The trial required that therapy be maximized in each group to bring the glycohemoglobin level to 6.5% or lower and to optimize antiplatelet therapy, lipid levels, and blood pressure. The primary outcome, assessed via intention to treat and adjudicated by assessors masked to treatment group, was the composite of all-cause mortality, nonfatal myocardial infarction, stroke, acute coronary syndrome, endovascular or surgical intervention in the coronary or leg arteries, and amputation above the ankle.After a median follow-up of almost 3 years, the composite of the outcomes occurred in 20% of patients taking pioglitazone and 22% of patients taking placebo ($P = .095$). Overall mortality rates were similar between the groups (6.8% vs 7.1%). Approximately 16% of the patients in each group discontinued the medication. Patients taking pioglitazone were more likely to be admitted to the hospital for congestive heart failure (number needed to treat to harm = 62; 95% CI, 36–224). Fewer patients taking pioglitazone experienced the main secondary end point, the composite of all-cause mortality, nonfatal myocardial infarction, and stroke (11.6% vs 13.6%; number needed to treat = 49; 95% CI, 27–408). For the primary purpose of the study, pioglitazone was no better than placebo. For the secondary outcomes, for every patient who benefits, one will need to be admitted for congestive heart failure.

Cancer linked to some diabetes treatments

Clinical question

Is there a relationship between cancer-related mortality and treatments for type 2 diabetes mellitus?

Bottom line

Death due to cancer seems to be more prevalent in patients with type 2 diabetes treated with either insulin or a sulfonylurea than in patients treated with metformin (Glucophage). It may be that hyperinsulinemia increases cancer risk, or that metformin is protective. Another explanation could be that, although cancer is related to certain medication use, it is not caused by their use. We need a controlled study to answer these questions. (LOE = 2b)

Reference

Bowker SL, Majumdar SR, Veugelers P, Johnson JA. Increased cancer-related mortality for patients with type 2 diabetes who use sulfonylureas or insulin. Diabetes Care 2006;29:254–258.

Study Design	Funding	Setting
Cohort (retrospective)	Foundation	Population-based

Synopsis

Insulin resistance and the resulting hyperinsulinemia has been linked to a number of disorders, especially, of course, to type 2 diabetes mellitus. The sequela of the metabolic syndrome are also a consequence, and there is some evidence that cancer is related. Insulin and insulin-like growth factor are required at all stages of cell growth, cancerous or not. Data from the United Kingdom Prospective Diabetes Study (UKPDS) suggest the possibility of an increase in all-cause mortality for patients with type 2 diabetes treated with insulin. The researchers conducting this provocative study identified 10,309 new users of metformin or sulfonylureas in Canada using a drug plan database. They monitored the patients for an average 5.4 years using a computerized vital statistics file. All patients were followed up. The patients were an average 63.4 years old, and 55% were men. In this type of study, no intervention particular to the study was performed; the patients were treated by their individual physicians as they saw fit and the outcomes of the patients were determined over time. Since the patients were not specifically assigned to therapy, imbalances could have (and did) occur. The average age of the patients who were started on a sulfonylurea was 5 years older than the metformin-treated patients (66.9 years vs 61.8 years; $P < .0001$). A greater proportion of men were in the sulfonylurea group (58.6% vs 53.5%; $P < .0001$) and more patients initially started on metformin eventually were given insulin (16.3% vs 9.2%; $P < .0001$). All of these imbalances can be adjusted statistically, though an ideal study would randomly assign patients to prevent such imbalances. A total of 407 cancer-related deaths (3.9%) occurred in the whole group. Before statistical adjustment, 3.5% of patients receiving metformin died of a cancer-related illness compared with 4.9% patients in the sulfonylurea-treated group ($P = .001$). After statistical adjustment, deaths were still 30% higher in the group treated with a sulfonylurea than in the group taking metformin (hazard ratio [HR] = 1.3; 95% CI, 1.1–1.6; $P = .012$). In addition, cancer-related mortality was almost twice as high in patients treated with insulin, regardless of other treatment (HR = 1.9; 1.5–2.4).

Essential Evidence: Medicine that Matters, Edited by David Slawson, Allen Shaughnessy, Mark Ebell, and Henry Barry.

Duloxetine decreases pain of diabetic neuropathy

Clinical question
Does duloxetine reduce pain in patients with diabetic peripheral neuropathy?

Bottom line
In this study, duloxetine (Cymbalta) 60 mg daily was more effective than placebo in reducing pain from neuropathy in patients with diabetes. Higher doses of duloxetine didn't provide much additional benefit. The biases in this study favor treatment, so it is likely that the real benefit is less than what these investigators observed. Finally, we don't know if duloxetine is any more effective than other treatments used for painful diabetic neuropathy. (LOE = 2b–)

Reference
Wernicke JF, Pritchett YL, D'Souza DN, et al. A randomized controlled trial of duloxetine in diabetic peripheral neuropathic pain. Neurology 2006;67:1411–1420.

Study Design
Randomized controlled trial (double-blinded)

Funding
Industry

Allocation
Concealed

Setting
Outpatient (any)

Synopsis
Patients with diabetic peripheral neuropathy and glycosylated hemoglobin levels no higher than 12% were randomly assigned to receive placebo (n = 108), duloxetine 60 mg daily (n = 114), or duloxetine 60 mg twice daily (n = 112). The patients recorded their assessment of pain severity (on a scale from 0 to 10) in a daily diary. The main outcome – the weekly average pain score from the diary – was evaluated by a modified intention-to-treat analysis. In other words, they only included patients who completed the study. In general, this tends to bias the results in favor of the interventions. The patients had comparable pain levels at the beginning of the study. Patients in each group improved by the end of the study: those taking placebo improved by 1.4 points, those taking duloxetine 60 mg daily improved by 2.7 points, and those taking duloxetine 60 mg twice daily improved by 2.8 points. The largest reduction in pain was seen by the second week of treatment. In general, a reduction of 2 points is considered clinically important. This degree of reduction was observed in 42% of patients taking placebo, 63% of patients taking duloxetine 60 mg daily, and 69% of patients taking twice-daily duloxetine. Compared with placebo, one would need to treat 5 patients with once-daily duloxetine (95% CI, 3–17) for 1 patient to benefit. The number needed to treat for twice-daily duloxetine is 4 (3–8). A large proportion of patients dropped out of the study (21% in the placebo group and 25% and 30% in the 2 duloxetine groups), which reinforces my concerns about bias.

Essential Evidence: Medicine that Matters, Edited by David Slawson, Allen Shaughnessy, Mark Ebell, and Henry Barry.

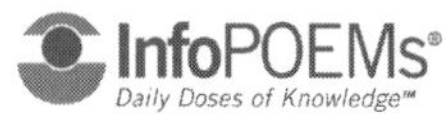

Weight loss interventions have little effect on quality of life

Clinical question

Do weight loss interventions improve health-related quality of life?

Bottom line

Based on the existing research, weight loss interventions have little effect on health-related quality of life. The overall quality of the existing research, however, is poor. (LOE = 1a)

Reference

Maciejewski ML, Patrick DL, Williamson DF. A structured review of randomized controlled trials of weight loss showed little improvement in health-related quality of life. J Clin Epidemiol 2005;58:568–578.

Study Design

Systematic review

Funding

Unknown/not stated

Setting

Outpatient (any)

Synopsis

The authors systematically searched several databases using a sensible search strategy. However, they excluded research not published in English and didn't describe any attempts at finding unpublished studies. After obtaining the initial bazillion articles, the authors applied exclusion criteria (studies of children or pregnant women) and whittled the batch down to a few hundred studies. The authors then read the abstracts to exclude nonrandomized studies and those not addressing quality of life. This left them with 34 eligible trials. The authors independently extracted the data and assessed the quality of the studies. In general, the studies suffered from several methodologic shortcomings that typically bias the findings in favor of the intervention. The included trials ranged in duration from 6 weeks to 2 years and evaluated a variety of interventions: medications, surgeries, behavior modifications. Only 9 of the 34 studies showed improvement in general health-related quality of life. There was no overall effect at all on depression, either.

Essential Evidence: Medicine that Matters, Edited by David Slawson, Allen Shaughnessy, Mark Ebell, and Henry Barry.

Popular diets equally effective for losing weight

Clinical question

Which of 4 popular diets (Atkins, Zone, Weight Watchers, and Ornish) is most effective for losing weight and reducing cardiac risk factors?

Bottom line

All 4 popular diets (Atkins, Zone, Weight Watchers, and Ornish) are equally effective for helping adults lose weight and reduce cardiac risk factors. Since success in this study directly correlated with self-adherence to the diet, it makes sense to help patients choose the diet that is "easiest" for them to follow, and not preferentially encourage one over another. (LOE = 1b–)

Reference

Dansinger ML, Gleason JA, Griffith JL, Selker HP, Schaefer EJ. Comparison of the Atkins, Ornish, Weight Watchers, and Zone die for weight loss and heart disease risk reduction. A randomized trial. JAMA 2005;293:43–53.

Study Design	Funding	Allocation
Randomized controlled trial (single-blinded)	Government	Concealed

Setting

Outpatient (specialty)

Synopsis

Every week it seems that somebody else writes another diet book and claims that they have "the best" method for losing weight and keeping it off. In fact, there is very little data addressing the health effects of popular diets and even less comparing different diets directly to each other. The investigators enrolled 160 overweight or obese (mean BMI 35; range 27–42) adults, aged 22 to 72 years, with known hypertension, dyslipidemia, or fasting hyperglycemia. Subjects were randomized (concealed allocation assignment) to either Atkins (carbohydrate restriction), Zone (macronutrient balance), Weight Watchers (calorie restriction), or Ornish (fat restriction) diet groups. Individuals assessing outcomes were blind to treatment group assignment. The study attrition rate as a result of patient drop outs was high: the number of participants who did not complete the study at months 2, 6, and 12 were 34 (21%), 61 (38%), and 67 (42%), respectively. The most common reason cited by subjects for withdrawing was that the assigned diet was too hard to follow or was not resulting in enough weight loss. Although the results were not statistically significant ($P = 0.08$), more subjects discontinued the Atkins (48%) and Ornish diets (50%) than the less extreme Zone (35%) and Weight Watchers (35%) diets. Using intention-to-treat analysis, all 4 diets resulted in similar weight loss at 1 year with no statistically significant difference between the diets. In each of the diet groups, approximately 25% and 10% of subjects sustained a weight loss of more than 5% and 10% of initial body weight, respectively, at one year. Cardiac risk factor improvement was directly proportional to the amount of weight loss and was similar among the diet groups. Self-reported dietary adherence directly correlated with the amount of weight loss and reduction in cardiac risk factors. The study was powered to have an 80% chance of detecting a weight change of 2% from baseline or a 3% difference between diets.

Essential Evidence: Medicine that Matters, Edited by David Slawson, Allen Shaughnessy, Mark Ebell, and Henry Barry.

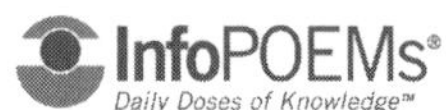

Intense diet-behavior-physical activity effective for obese children

Clinical question

Can a specific program of diet and exercise cause a sustained weight loss in children?

Bottom line

An intensive 3-month program of dietary counseling, a hypocaloric diet, and structured exercise can cause a weight loss in children that is sustained over 1 year. More important, the program seemed to increase the amount of exercise the children performed and this increase was sustained after the intervention was discontinued. (LOE = 2b)

Reference

Nemet D, Barkan S, Epstein Y, Friedland O, Kowen G, Eliakim A. Short- and long-term beneficial effects of a combined dietary-behavioral-physical activity intervention for the treatment of childhood obesity. Pediatrics 2005;115:443–449.

Study Design

Randomized controlled trial (nonblinded)

Funding

Government

Allocation

Uncertain

Setting

Outpatient (primary care)

Synopsis

The researchers conducting this study began with 54 obese children between the ages of 6 years and 16 years. The children were randomly assigned either to a control group that received a single nutrition counseling session or to an active treatment group. Active treatment consisted of heavy-duty dietary and exercise modification for 3 months. It is not clear that allocation to treatment groups was concealed and it is possible that children more likely to respond to treatment were preferentially enrolled. The dietary intervention consisted of 6 meetings over a 3-month period with parents and the child. These counseling sessions focused on food choices, nutritional information, and behavior change. The children were placed on a diet of approximately 30% less than the reported intake or 15% less than the estimated daily required intake. The exercise program was conducted 2 hours per week by physicians who were former members of the Israeli national track and field team and consisted of games focusing on endurance, with the children encouraged to add an extra 30 to 45 minutes of walking or other exercise per week. Analysis was per protocol and not by intention to treat, which is about the only way they could have done the analysis. Dropouts early during the intervention period and in the subsequent 1 year follow-up, dwindled the groups to 20 patients each.After 3 months of diet and exercise intervention, the children in the treatment group had lost an average 2.8 kg whereas the children in the control group gained an average 1.1 kg. Body mass index and body fat percentage also declined in the treated children. Over the 1 year of follow-up, children in the control group had gained an average 5.2 kg; the children in the treatment group gained an average 0.6 kg ($P < .05$). Body mass index increased in the control group but had decreased in the treated patients. Other significant differences at 1 year included lower body fat, amount of exercise activity, and endurance time on a treadmill. Both groups reported a decrease in screen time (that is, time spent watching television or playing video games) from an average 4.5 to 4.8 hours per day to 3.3 to 3.4 hours per day 1 year later.

Essential Evidence: Medicine that Matters, Edited by David Slawson, Allen Shaughnessy, Mark Ebell, and Henry Barry.

Rimonabant minimally effective for weight loss

Clinical question

Is rimonabant effective for reducing weight in obese or overweight patients?

Bottom line

Rimonabant (Acomplia) is minimally effective for obese or overweight patients for achieving sustained weight loss. Less than half the subjects initially enrolled in this study completed the protocol at 1 year. Of those remaining in the study, only one fourth lost a clinically significant amount of weight (10% or more) and, as with other weight-loss drugs, the patients who stopped taking the medicine after 1 year regained the weight. (LOE = 1b–)

Reference

Pi-Sunyer FX, Aronne LJ, Heshmati HM, Devin J, Rosenstock J, for the RIO-North America Study Group. Effect of rimonabant, a cannabinoid-1 receptor blocker, on weight and cardiometabolic risk factors in overweight or obese patients. RIO-North America: A randomized controlled trial. JAMA 2006;295:761–775.

Study Design

Randomized controlled trial (double-blinded)

Funding

Industry

Allocation

Uncertain

Setting

Outpatient (specialty)

Synopsis

Rimonabant (Acomplia) is a selective cannabinoid-1 receptor blocker that reduces appetite and may promote weight loss in patients who are obese or overweight. The investigators enrolled 3500 obese (body mass index [BMI] >= 30) or overweight (BMI > 27) adults from 64 US and Canadian clinical research centers. After a 4-week period during which all patients received placebo plus diet, compliant patients (87%) randomly received (uncertain allocation concealment) 20 mg rimonabant per day, 5 mg rimonabant per day, or placebo. During the second year of the study rimonabant-treated patients were re-randomized to receive placebo or continue to take the same rimonabant dose. All patients were also placed on a 600 kcal per day deficit diet. The authors do not specify whether outcomes were measured by individuals blinded to treatment group assignment. At 1 year, slightly more than half the initial patients completed the study protocol; the rest withdrew because of lack of efficacy, adverse events, poor compliance, or patient request. Using modified intention-to-treat analysis (including only patients who took at least one dose of the medicine), patients in the 20 mg rimonabant group lost significantly more weight than those receiving placebo (−6.3 kg vs −1.6 kg; overall difference = 4.7 kg/10.3 pounds). The percentage of patients achieving a clinically relevant (10% or greater) weight loss was 25.2% for patients receiving 20 mg rimonabant and 8.5% for patients in the placebo group (number needed to treat for 1 year = 17); the difference between 5 mg rimonabant and placebo was not significant. Patients switching from the 20 mg rimonabant group to the placebo group during year 2 experienced weight gain while those who continued to take 20 mg rimonabant did not.

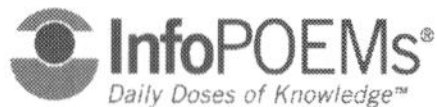

Topiramate beneficial for binge eating disorder with obesity

Clinical question

Is topiramate effective in the treatment of binge eating disorder associated with obesity?

Bottom line

Topiramate appears effective in the treatment of binge eating disorder associated with obesity. Nearly half of the total patients in this study, however, dropped out for various reasons including adverse events, lack of treatment efficacy, or treatment nonadherence for unclear reasons. (LOE = 2b–)

Reference

McElroy SL, Arnold LM, Shapira NA, et al. Topiramate in the treatment of binge eating disorder associated with obesity: a randomized, placebo-controlled trial. Am J Psychiatry 2003;160:255–261.

Study Design

Randomized controlled trial (double-blinded)

Setting

Outpatient (specialty)

Synopsis

Binge eating disorder is characterized by recurrent episodes of binge eating without the weight loss associated with bulimia nervosa or anorexia nervosa. Topiramate is approved for the treatment of epilepsy but is also associated with stabilization of mood disorders and anorexia and weight loss. Sixty-one patients (53 women and 8 men) meeting DSM-IV-TR criteria for binge eating disorder and obesity (body mass index > 30 kg/m^2) were enrolled in a 14-week trial. Patients were randomized (concealed allocation assignment) to either topiramate (initial dose 25 mg each evening titrated to a maximum of 600 mg/day) or matching placebo. Outcomes were assessed by patient self report. Using intention-to-treat analysis, patients receiving topiramate reported a significantly greater rate of reduction in binge frequency, binge day frequency, and improved scores on global impression severity and obsessive compulsive scales. Patients taking topiramate also lost an average of 5.9 kg of weight; those taking placebo lost an average of 1.2 kg. Only 58% of patients completed all 14 weeks of treatment. Nine patients (3 taking placebo, 6 taking topiramate) discontinued treatment because of adverse events. The most common reasons for discontinuing topiramate were headache and paresthesia.

Essential Evidence: Medicine that Matters, Edited by David Slawson, Allen Shaughnessy, Mark Ebell, and Henry Barry.

Bariatric surgery effective for morbid obesity

Clinical question

How effective is bariatric surgery in the treatment of morbid obesity in association with diabetes, hyperlipidemia, hypertension, and obstructive sleep apnea?

Bottom line

Bariatric surgery is highly effective in treating common comorbidities of morbid obesity including diabetes, hyperlipidemia, hypertension, and obstructive sleep apnea. Operative mortality rates for various procedures, though very low, vary by as much as tenfold. Additional studies are needed on long-term morbidity, mortality, and quality of life. Most of the current studies measure outcomes at 2 years or less. (LOE = 2a)

Reference

Buchwald H, Avidor Y, Braunwald E, et al. Bariatric surgery. A systematic review and meta-analysis. JAMA 2004;292:1724–1737.

Study Design	Funding	Setting
Meta-analysis (other)	Industry	Various (meta-analysis)

Synopsis

Nearly 5% of the US population is morbidly obese and many of these individuals are afflicted with other comorbidities (eg, type 2 diabetes, hyperlipidemia, hypertension, sleep apnea, degenerative arthritis, depression, and so forth). The investigators conducted a systematic review of published observational and interventional trials focusing on the impact of bariatric surgery specifically on diabetes, hyperlipidemia, hypertension, and obstructive sleep apnea. The search strategy for relevant articles was thorough and included MEDLINE, the Cochrane Library Registry of Clinical Trials, Current Contents, and reference lists of recent reviews. Extracted studies could be of any design and had to have enrolled at least 10 patients undergoing bariatric surgery. Surgical procedures were grouped into the following categories: gastric banding, gastric bypass, gastroplasty, biliopancreatic diversion or duodenal switch, and mixed/other. A total of 136 studies enrolling 22,094 patients were included. Of these, only 5 were randomized controlled trials. The majority of the subjects were women (72.6%) with a mean age of 39 years and a baseline mean body mass index of 46.9. The mean percentage of excess weight loss was 61.2% for all patients, including 47.5% undergoing gastric banding; 61.6%, gastric bypass; 68.2%, gastroplasty; and 70.1%, biliopancreatic diversion or duodenal switch. Mortality in the first 30 days was 0.1% for gastric banding and gastroplasty, 0.5% for gastric bypass, and 1.1% for biliopancreatic diversion or duodenal switch operations. Resolution or significant improvement of disease was as follows: diabetes, 86%; hyperlipidemia, 70%; hypertension, 78.5%; and obstructive sleep apnea, 83.6%. Data from the 5 randomized controlled trials, which only enrolled 621 patients (2.8% of the total), were consistent with the overall analysis. The majority of the studies reported outcomes measured at 2 years or less, but outcomes were similar in those studies reporting outcomes after more than 2 years.

Essential Evidence: Medicine that Matters, Edited by David Slawson, Allen Shaughnessy, Mark Ebell, and Henry Barry.

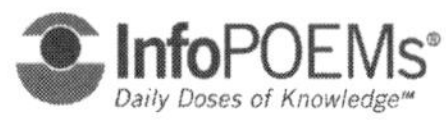

Bed and pillow covers ineffective for allergic rhinitis

Clinical question

Do impermeable bed and pillow covers improve symptoms of allergic rhinitis?

Bottom line

Impermeable bed and pillow covers do not improve symptoms more than conventional covers in patients with allergic rhinitis who are sensitive to dust mites. (LOE = 1b)

Reference

Terreehorst I, Hak E, Oosting AJ, et al. Evaluation of impermeable covers for bedding in patients with allergic rhinitis. N Engl J Med 2003;349:237–246.

Study Design

Randomized controlled trial (double-blinded)

Setting

Outpatient (specialty)

Synopsis

Impermeable bed and pillow covers reduce the exposure of allergic patients to dust mite allergens – but is that enough to improve symptoms? Previous studies have been small, poorly designed, and have provided conflicting results. In this trial, adults and children aged 8 to 50 years who were allergic to dust mites were randomized (allocation concealed) to receive either impermeable (n = 139) or permeable (n = 140) bed covers. They were recruited from specialty clinics, general practices, and by advertisements. Patients with pets in the home, using oral or high-dose inhaled steroids, and those taking cyclosporine or regular doses of antibiotics were excluded. Baseline and 12-month follow-up measurements were made between September and December, the peak months for Dutch dust mites. Nineteen patients in the control group and 24 in the impermeable cover group were lost to follow-up, most often because they moved or because of a protocol violation. The primary outcome was a 100-point allergy symptom severity score. The groups were similar at baseline, and analysis was by intention to treat for patients with a 12-month outcome measurement. Although allergen counts were significantly lower in the beds of patients with impermeable bed covers, and while both groups experienced an improvement in symptoms, there was no significant difference between groups in the degree of improvement (−9.8 points in the impermeable cover group vs −10.9 points in the control group; P = 0.8). There was also no signficant difference in daily symptom scores and in the results of the nasal allergen provocation test. The study was powered to detect at least a 25% reduction in the symptom score.

Essential Evidence: Medicine that Matters, Edited by David Slawson, Allen Shaughnessy, Mark Ebell, and Henry Barry.

Pollen blocker cream effective for allergic rhinitis

Clinical question

Is a pollen blocker cream effective in preventing allergic rhinitis?

Bottom line

Alergol, a European petrolatum product that sounds suspiciously like Vaseline, when applied 4 times a day to the nares, results in a significant improvement in provoked nasal allergic symptoms. The study was done in a carefully controlled manner and results may not be the same in practice. Other than an exceedingly small risk of lipid pneumonia, however, coating the inside of the nose with petrolatum is a nontoxic, nonsystemic approach to try in patients with allergic rhinitis. (LOE = 2b)

Reference

Schwetz S, Olze H, Melchisedech S, Grigorov A, Latza R. Efficacy of pollen blocker cream in the treatment of allergic rhinitis. Arch Otolaryngol Head Neck Surg 2004; 130:979–984.

Study Design

Cross-over trial (randomized)

Funding

Industry

Setting

Outpatient (specialty)

Synopsis

Alergol is a petrolatum-based ointment containing highly refined long-chain hydrocarbons. Since petrolatum is simply long-chain hydrocarbons, how this product differs from Vaseline and other petroleum jellies is not clear to me. In this study, the authors enrolled 91 white patients in Russia and Germany who were allergic to house dust mites, animal dander, or pollen for at least 2 years. The study compared Alergol with a placebo of a carboxymethylcellulose gel, which is aqueous and doesn't last long. This was a crossover study, so patients received, in a random fashion, treatment with both products. The patients applied one product 4 times a day for 3 days, and then, after 1 day of no therapy, they used the other product for 3 days. Efficacy was assessed using a nasal provocation test using the allergen at a concentration previously demonstrated to elicit symptoms in each patient. Sneezing, nasal discharge, and "other related symptoms" (tearing, ear itch, and so forth) were each assigned a value from 0 to 2 (maximum score = 6). This scoring method has not been validated, but it seems straightforward. Scores fell from a median of 4 to a median of 1 following the use of Alergol; symptoms after using placebo fell from 4 to 3 (both statistically significant). Nasal airflow rates were not different between the 2 treatments. Symptoms were slightly lower with either treatment given in the second 3-day phase, perhaps reflecting that patients became better at applying the products with time.

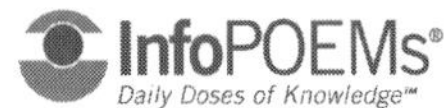

Montelukast alone ineffective for allergic rhinitis

Clinical question

Is montelukast an effective treatment for allergic rhinitis?

Bottom line

Montelukast (Singulair) alone is not an effective treatment for allergic rhinitis, although when combined with a nonsedating antihistamine the efficacy is probably similar to that of a topical nasal corticosteroid alone. (LOE = 1a)

Reference

Grainger J, Drake-Lee A. Montelukast in allergic rhinitis: a systematic review and meta-analysis. Clin Otolaryngol 2006;31:360–367.

Study Design

Meta-analysis (randomized controlled trials)

Funding

Unknown/not stated

Setting

Outpatient (any)

Synopsis

Montelukast is a leukotriene inhibitor that has become a standard treatment for allergic rhinitis. In this systematic review, the authors did a comprehensive search of the literature and identified 20 randomized controlled trials with blinded outcome assessment of montelukast for the treatment of allergic rhinitis in adults. Twelve studies compared montelukast with placebo, 6 with an antihistamine, and 4 with a topical nasal corticosteroid. Fifteen were parallel group studies with between 38 and 1992 patients; 5 were cross-over studies with between 12 and 37 patients. Montelukast produced a consistent, statistically significant 3.4% decrease in nasal symptom scores. However, a 10% to 15% decrease is considered the minimum clinically significant improvement. The improvement was slightly greater (4.4%) for the subgroup of patients with asthma. Results were similar for those studies that used the same outcome measure (the Rhinosinusitis Quality of Life Questionnaire). Comparisons with fexofenadine 180 mg (Allegra, 1 study) or loratadine 10 mg (Claritin, 5 studies) found a 3% greater improvement in nasal symptom scores for the antihistamine groups compared with montelukast. Topical nasal corticosteroids were also significantly more effective than montelukast (8.4% greater improvement; 95% CI, 6% to 11%). Montelukast plus antihistamine was similarly effective to nasal corticosteroid in 2 studies.

Petroleum jelly doesn't reduce recurrent pediatric epistaxis

Clinical question

Does petroleum jelly (Vaseline) reduce the likelihood that epistaxis will recur in children?

Bottom line

In this highly selected group of patients with recurrent epistaxis, petroleum jelly applied twice daily for 4 weeks did not reduce the number of bleeds in the subsequent 4 weeks. This should make you question this commonly recommended treatment. But don't abandon it just yet, since it may work in children with less severe disease in the primary care setting, and because there was potential for recall bias by parents in this study. (LOE = 2b)

Reference

Loughran S, Spinou E, Clement WA, et al. A prospective, single-blind, randomized controlled trial of petroleum jelly/Vaseline for recurrent paediatric epistaxis. Clin Otolaryngol 2004;29:266–269.

Study Design

Randomized controlled trial (single-blinded)

Setting

Outpatient (specialty)

Synopsis

Recurrent nosebleeds are a common problem in children. Many doctors advise the application of petroleum jelly (Vaseline) to the anterior nares, since bleeding is thought to result from drying, picking, rubbing, and all the other things children do to their noses. In this small but well-designed study, 105 children aged 1 to 14 years referred to otolaryngologists for recurrent epistaxis were identified. The median duration of symptoms was 12 months and the median duration of bleeds was 5 minutes. The children were randomized (allocation concealed) to receive 1 of 2 letters: instructions to apply Vaseline twice daily for 4 weeks and keep a nosebleed diary, or simply instructions to keep a nosebleed diary. Patients were assessed after 8 weeks, and the primary outcome was the percentage with recurrent bleeds in the previous 4 weeks. Analysis was by intention to treat and the physician assessing outcomes was blinded to treatment assignment and was careful not to ask about treatment adherence until the end of the visit. Groups were similar at baseline. They were also similar after the intervention: 27.5% in the treatment group and 33.9% in the control group ($P = 0.47$) had no bleeds during the 4 weeks prior to the visit and after the intervention. The study had limitations, though. Approximately 14% of patients never came in for evaluation (evenly split between groups) and most parents were noncompliant with the diaries. The researchers therefore used parental recall instead of the diaries to assess the primary outcome.

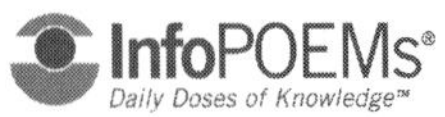

Lutein improves vision with macular degeneration in men

Clinical question

Does lutein supplementation improve vision in men with age-related macular degeneration?

Bottom line

Supplementation with lutein 10 mg daily in men with age-related macular degeneration resulted in improved visual acuity. Antioxidant therapy did not offer an additional benefit. Other studies of antioxidant therapy generally have yielded no benefit, though a combination of antioxidants and zinc did show benefit (Arch Ophthalmol 2001;119:1417–436). (LOE = 1b)

Reference

Richer S, Stiles W, Statkute L, et al. Can lutein supplementation improve vision in men with atrophic age-related macular degeneration? Double-masked, placebo-controlled, randomized trial of lutein and antioxidant supplementation in the intervention of age-related macular degeneration: the Veterans LAST (lutein antioxidant supplementation trial). Optometry 2004;75:216–230.

Study Design

Randomized controlled trial (double-blinded)

Allocation

Concealed

Setting

Outpatient (specialty)

Synopsis

Atrophic age-related macular degeneration (ARMD) accounts for 90% of all ARMD. Aging and smoking are the most significant risk factors for ARMD. Lutein, an essential catotenoid pigment and also an antioxidant, is found in fruits and vegetables and low intake of these foods is related to low levels of macular pigment and a higher risk of ARMD. The authors of this study enrolled 90 patients, 96% male, with an average age of 75 years, and ARMD diagnosed for an average 4.5 years. The patients were randomized (allocation concealed) to receive lutein (FloraGlo) 10 mg daily, lutein plus antioxidants, minerals, and other nutrients (OcuPower), or placebo for 12 months. Measured at 4, 8, and 12 months, visual acuity improved by approximately 1 line on the eye chart (average 5.4 Snellen equivalent letters) in the lutein-treated patients; somewhat less in the combination-treated group (3.5 Snellen equivalent letters) and decreased slightly in the placebo-treated patients. Glare recovery time, a measure of macular function, decreased significantly over the 12 months in the lutein-treated group, decreasing from 100 seconds to 65 seconds in right eyes and from 80 to 60 seconds in left eyes (a glare recovery of less than 60 seconds is normal). Glare recovery times decreased similarly in the combination-treated group, but decreased less with placebo (15–20 second decrease). Night driving was not affected in any of the 3 groups.

Essential Evidence: Medicine that Matters, Edited by David Slawson, Allen Shaughnessy, Mark Ebell, and Henry Barry.

Three indicators herald bacterial conjunctivitis in adults

Clinical question

What signs and symptoms predict the presence of bacterial infection in adults with conjunctivitis?

Bottom line

Eyes glued shut upon waking predicts the presence of bacterial infection, whereas a complaint of itching or a history of conjunctivitis indicates a nonbacterial cause. These results do not apply to children with conjunctivitis or to patients who wear contacts. (LOE = 1b)

Reference

Rietveld RP, ter Riet G, Bindels PJ, Sloos JH, van Weert HC. Predicting bacterial cause in infectious conjunctivitis: cohort study on informativeness of combinations of signs and symptoms. BMJ 2004;329:206–208.

Study Design

Cohort (prospective)

Setting

Outpatient (primary care)

Synopsis

Clinicians typically have the same chance of correctly diagnosing bacterial conjunctivitis as does a flipped coin. To determine what signs and symptoms are associated with either the presence or absence bacterial infection, the researchers enrolled 184 consecutive adult patients of general practitioners in the Netherlands who presented with a red eye and either purulent discharge or sticking of the eyelids. They did not study children or contact lens wearers. Clinicians documented the presence of a number of different signs and symptoms, and then obtained a conjunctival sample for culture. The prevalence of bacterial culture was 32%. After analysis of the individual signs and symptoms, the authors determined that eyes glued shut in the morning was predictive of bacterial cause, whereas a history of previous episodes of conjunctivitis or a history of itching predicted a nonbacterial cause. Bilateral glued eyes was the highest predictor (odds ratio = 14.99; 95% CI, 4.36–51.53), and 77% of patients with this indicator and without the other 2 indicators had bacterial conjunctivitis. At the other extreme, only 4% of subjects complaining of itching and a history of conjunctivitis without glued eyes had a bacterial cause.

Essential Evidence: Medicine that Matters, Edited by David Slawson, Allen Shaughnessy, Mark Ebell, and Henry Barry.

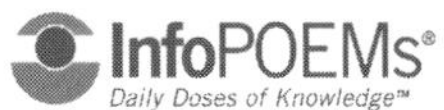

Antibiotics for conjunctivitis decreases symptom duration

Clinical question

In adults or children with acute infective conjunctivitis, are antibiotics effective in decreasing the length and severity of symptoms?

Bottom line

Treatment with an antibiotic, either immediately or after 3 days without symptom improvement, shortened the duration of acute conjunctivitis but did not decrease the severity of symptoms. Delaying the antibiotic reduced the need for antibiotics by almost 50% with similar symptom control and no more repeat visits than immediate antibiotic use. These results were the same for conjunctivitis with and without an identified bacterial cause. (LOE = 1b)

Reference

Everitt HA, Little PS, Smith PW. A randomised controlled trial of management strategies for acute conjunctivitis in general practice. BMJ 2006;333:321–326

Study Design

Randomized controlled trial (nonblinded)

Funding

Government

Allocation

Concealed

Setting

Outpatient (primary care)

Synopsis

The investigators enrolled 307 adults and children seen in 30 general practices in England who presented with uncomplicated acute infective conjunctivitis. The patients were randomly assigned, using concealed allocation, to receive immediate antibiotic treatment with chloramphenicol eye drops, delayed antibiotic treatment, or no treatment. The delayed antibiotic treatment was a prescription for chloramphenicol that could be picked up if symptoms were not better after 3 days, which occurred 53% of the time. The main outcomes of this study were the duration of moderately bad symptoms, average severity score for the 3 days following diagnosis, and belief in the effectiveness of antibiotics. The duration of moderate symptoms was shorter for both the immediate antibiotic group and the delayed antibiotic group: 3.3 days and 3.9 days, respectively, versus 4.8 days. The average severity of symptoms on days 1 to 3 did not differ among the groups. Approximately half the patients were cultured for the presence of bacteria, and significant bacterial growth was found in 50%. However, the duration and severity of symptoms was not different in patients with bacterial infection and those without. Nine percent of patients returned within 2 weeks; significantly fewer patients in the delayed antibiotic group returned within 2 weeks. Patients receiving immediate antibiotic treatment were more likely than patients not receiving treatment to believe antibiotics were effective (number needed to treat = 5). This belief could have lead these patients to underestimate their symptoms, which might have been responsible for the shorter duration. A better way to control for this belief would be to use placebo eye drops instead of no eye drops.

Essential Evidence: Medicine that Matters, Edited by David Slawson, Allen Shaughnessy, Mark Ebell, and Henry Barry.

Diet high in beta carotene, vitamins C and E, and zinc may reduce risk of macular degeneration

Clinical question

Is a high dietary intake of beta carotene, vitamins C and E, and zinc associated with a reduced risk of age-related macular degeneration?

Bottom line

A high dietary intake of beta carotene, vitamins C and E, and zinc reduces the risk of age-related macular degeneration (AMD). (LOE = 2b–)

Reference

van Leeuwen R, Boekhoorn S, Vingerling JR, et al. Dietary intake of antioxidants and risk of age-related macular degeneration. JAMA 2005;294:3101–3107.

Study Design

Cohort (prospective)

Funding

Government

Setting

Population-based

Synopsis

High-dose supplementation with beta carotene, vitamins C and E, and zinc slows the progression of AMD. It remains uncertain, however, whether regular dietary intake from normal daily foods is similarly effective. The investigators assessed dietary intake of all 10,275 residents, aged 55 years or older, of Rotterdam, the Netherlands. Of these, 6780 (66%) took part in the ophthalmologic evaluation. Dietary intake was assessed by a questionnaire that was further validated with 2-week food diaries. From a baseline cohort of 5836 patients with no AMD in either eye, 4170 (71%) were available for full follow-up at 8 years. Of these, 560 persons (13.4%) were found to have incident AMD. Individuals blinded to dietary intake status performed all outcome assessments. An above-median intake of all 4 nutrients – beta carotene, vitamins C and E, and zinc – was associated with a 35% reduced risk (hazard ratio = 0.65; 95% CI, 0.46–0.92) of AMD. Statistical adjustments for potential confounders (eg, smoking, serum lipid levels, blood pressure) did not change the results.

Essential Evidence: Medicine that Matters, Edited by David Slawson, Allen Shaughnessy, Mark Ebell, and Henry Barry.

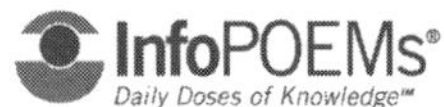

Parent satisfaction okay with no treatment of AOM

Clinical question
Are parents whose children do not receive treatment for acute otitis media less satisfied with their child's care?

Bottom line
Parents don't seem to mind if their children are not treated with antibiotics. In this study comparing no treatment to immediate antibiotic treatment of acute otitis media, parent satisfaction scores were similar between the 2 groups, even though 21% of the no-treatment children eventually needed antibiotics. (LOE = 1b–)

Reference
McCormick DP, Chonmaitree T, Pittman C, et al. Nonsevere acute otitis media: a clinical trial comparing outcomes of watchful waiting versus immediate antibiotic treatment. Pediatrics 2005;115:1455–1465.

Study Design	Funding	Allocation
Randomized controlled trial (single-blinded)	Government	Uncertain

Setting
Outpatient (primary care)

Synopsis
Several studies have shown that not treating children initially with antibiotics for acute otitis media results in fewer eventual prescriptions and fewer adverse effects. This study again evaluated watchful waiting versus immediate antibiotic treatment, and also surveyed parents regarding their satisfaction with care. The researchers enrolled 223 infants and children with symptoms and otoscopic evidence of acute otitis media rated as not severe. Approximately 30% of the children were younger than 1 year, 25% were between the ages of 1 year and 2 years, and the rest were between the ages of 2 years and 13 years. The children were randomized (allocation concealment uncertain) to receive either high-dose amoxicillin, 90 mg per kg per day for 10 days, or no treatment. Children were concurrently treated with ibuprofen, a decongestant, and saline nose drops. They were also given an antihistamine, although this class of drugs was shown to be ineffective more than 20 years ago and were recently shown to extend the duration of middle ear effusion. Parents were instructed to return to the clinic if symptoms failed to improve or worsened, which occurred in 5% of antibiotic-treated children and 21% of no-antibiotic children (P = .001; number needed to treat with antibiotic to prevent one failure = 7). Treatment failure occurred significantly more often in children who had received antibiotics in the previous 30 days. On a questionnaire of satisfaction, which included questions regarding the parents' feelings toward medication side effects, extra time spent receiving care for the infection, difficulty giving the antibiotic, work absences, and overall satisfaction, the average score was not significantly different between the 2 groups of parents when measured on day 12 and day 30 of the study, with scores in both groups averaging about 44 of a possible 48. The study has many limitations: there is no mention whether the parent questionnaires were written in Spanish, which is important since the study was conducted in a predominantly Spanish-speaking area of the United States; the questionnaire was not validated; and there was unblinding of the investigators in a number of instances. Parents were also not given a delayed prescription to fill if symptoms didn't resolve, but were asked to return to the clinic for further evaluation.

Essential Evidence: Medicine that Matters, Edited by David Slawson, Allen Shaughnessy, Mark Ebell, and Henry Barry.

Parents prefer shared decision-making for AOM

Clinical question

Do parents with children with acute otitis media prefer to share in the decision to use antibiotics?

Bottom line

Presenting information about the pros and cons of antibiotic treatment for acute otitis media and letting parents decide whether and when to start treatment increases parents' satisfaction with their visit and could decrease antibiotic use. These results were found in wealthy, white, older parents and may not apply to other socioeconomic groups. (LOE = 2c)

Reference

Merenstein D, Diener-West M, Krist A, Pinneger M, Cooper LA. An assessment of the shared-decision model in parents of children with acute otitis media. Pediatrics 2005;116:1267–1275.

Study Design

Cross-sectional

Funding

Foundation

Setting

Outpatient (primary care)

Synopsis

The researchers conducting this study wished to determine to what extent parents would like to participate in the decision-making regarding the treatment of their child, given a scenario in which their child had acute otitis media. The parents in this study were not typical; they were older with an average age of 46 years), wealthy (76% had a family income >$75,000), well educated (87% attended college), mostly non-Hispanic white, and almost all had health insurance. During a visit to a family practice, 466 parents were asked to imagine their reaction to 1 of 3 clinical vignettes. All vignettes presented a mother taking her 2 1/2-year-old son to the doctor with a fever. The child is diagnosed with acute otitis media. In each vignette the doctor explains a desire to decrease antibiotic use and the lack of need for antibiotic use in most instances. In the "paternalistic" vignette the doctor clearly recommends antibiotics. In the "shared decision-making" vignettes the doctor makes no specific recommendation but gives a prescription for an antibiotic to be started in 2 days if the child is not better; in 1 of these vignettes acetaminophen is also recommended as treatment. Before reading the vignettes, 93% of parents reported that they felt that antibiotics were needed if an ear infection is present. After reading the vignettes, 82% reported being willing to wait 48 hours before starting treatment. However, 27% of the parents receiving the paternalistic vignette would start antibiotics immediately; only 7% receiving the shared decision-making vignettes would do so ($P < .001$). All reported similar degrees of satisfaction with the amount of information they received. Significantly more patients reported being satisfied with the shared decision-making approaches than with the paternalistic approach (76% satisfied in the paternalistic group vs 84% and 93% in the shared decision-making groups; $P < .001$).

Essential Evidence: Medicine that Matters, Edited by David Slawson, Allen Shaughnessy, Mark Ebell, and Henry Barry.

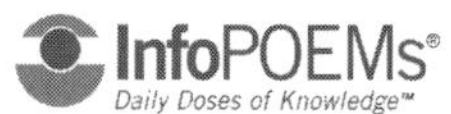

Delayed prescription for AOM reduces unnecessary antibiotics

Clinical question

Will asking parents to delay filling a prescription for the treatment of acute otitis media reduce unnecessary antibiotic use?

Bottom line

A wait-and-see approach of asking parents of children given a diagnosis of acute otitis media (AOM) in the emergency department to delay filling a prescription significantly reduces unnecessary antibiotic use. Parents of children in the delayed group reported otalgia slightly, if any, more often than the parents of children in the standard group. All parents received explicit instructions to provide both ibuprofen and otic analgesic drops to their children. Children in the standard treatment group were more likely to have diarrhea. (LOE = 1b)

Reference

Spiro DM, Tay KY, Arnold DH, Dziura JD, Baker MD, Shapiro ED. Wait-and-see prescription for the treatment of acute otitis media: a randomized controlled trial. JAMA 2006;296:1235–1241.

Study Design	Funding	Allocation
Randomized controlled trial (single-blinded)	Foundation	Concealed

Setting

Emergency department

Synopsis

Previous studies evaluating the effects of asking parents to delay filling antibiotic prescriptions for children with AOM excluded children with high fever. These investigators enrolled 283 consecutive children, aged 6 months to 12 years, seen in an emergency department who were given a diagnosis of AOM. Exclusion criteria included: another bacterial infection, such as pneumonia; "toxic" appearance; immunocompromization; myringotomy tubes or perforated tympanic membrane; or antibiotic use within 7 days. Parents of children with AOM randomly received (concealed allocation assignment) verbal and written instructions "not to fill the antibiotic prescription unless your child either is not better or is worse 48 hours (2 days) after today's visit" (intervention group) or to "fill the antibiotic prescription and give the antibiotic to your child after today's visit" (standard group). Amoxicillin was prescribed for most patients. All subjects also received ibuprofen and otic analgesic drops (containing antipyrene and benzocaine) in standard doses. Individuals blinded to treatment group assignment assessed outcomes at 4 to 6 days, 11 to 14 days, and 30 to 40 days after enrollment. In addition, a research assistant called pharmacies 4 days after enrollment to confirm whether prescriptions were filled. Follow-up occurred for more than 94% of participants. Using intention-to-treat analysis, prescriptions were filled significantly less often for children in the wait-and-see group versus the standard group (62% vs 13%). The difference was also significant in the subgroup of children younger than 2 years of age (47% wait-and-see vs 5% standard). Verification of whether prescriptions were actually filled was assessed for 28% of the study population; the pharmacy confirmed parental report in almost all instances. Otalgia occurred for a slightly greater period (0.4 days) in the wait-and-see group, but the overall rate of otalgia after 4 days was similar in both groups. Unscheduled follow-up visits were similar in both groups. No serious adverse events occurred in either treatment group, but parents in the standard group reported significantly more diarrhea in their children (23% vs 8%; number needed to treat to harm = 7).

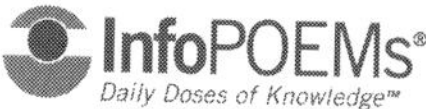

Tubes marginally effective in otitis media with effusion

Clinical question

Are ventilation tubes effective in managing children with otitis media with effusion?

Bottom line

Compared with watchful waiting, inserting pressure-equalizing tubes improves hearing in children with otitis media with effusion over the short term. Outcomes within 18 months, however, are the same. The tubes have no effect on language development. Watchful waiting is a reasonable option in most of these children. (LOE = 1a)

Reference

Rovers MM, Black N, Browning GG, Maw R, Zielhuis GA, Haggard MP. Grommets in otitis media with effusion: an individual patient data meta-analysis. Arch Dis Child 2005;90:480–485.

Study Design

Meta-analysis (randomized controlled trials)

Funding

Government

Setting

Various (meta-analysis)

Synopsis

This research team systematically reviewed several databases (including PubMed and Cochrane) looking for randomized controlled trials of ventilation tubes for children with otitis media with effusion. Ultimately, they included only the 7 studies (including a total of 1234 children) that were randomized to "a high standard" (ie, concealed allocation). They contacted the authors of the studies to get the individual patient data. After pooling all these data, the researchers looked at 3 outcomes: duration of the effusion, hearing, and language development. Since each of the studies had slightly different intermediate (6 and 9 months) and final (12 and 18 months) follow-up periods, the authors simply aggregated them. Children with tubes had a shorter duration of effusions (19.7 weeks vs 37 weeks; P = .001) than the control patients. At 6 months of follow-up, the mean hearing level was 26.6 dB in the children with tubes compared with 31.1 dB in the control group (P = .001). However, by the time of the final follow-up 12 months to 18 months later, there were no differences in hearing. Finally, the tubes had no effect on language development. The authors suggest that children attending daycare and/or those with worse hearing loss at baseline may benefit more from tubes, but this conclusion requires further study.

Essential Evidence: Medicine that Matters, Edited by David Slawson, Allen Shaughnessy, Mark Ebell, and Henry Barry.

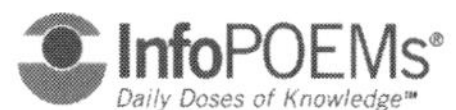

Early tympanostomy tubes do not improve outcomes after 3 or more years

Clinical question

Does early insertion of tympanostomy tubes improve important clinical outcomes more than delayed insertion?

Bottom line

Early insertion of tympanostomy tubes does not improve long-term clinical outcomes of importance (speech acquisition and hearing) in children with persistent otitis media with effusion. Delaying 6 months for bilateral effusion and 9 months for unilateral effusion before revisiting the decision to insert tubes is the preferred approach to management, since it results in fewer procedures with equivalent outcomes. (LOE = 1b)

Reference

Paradise JL, Campbell TF, Dollaghan CA, et al. Developmental outcomes after early or delayed insertion of tympanostomy tubes. N Engl J Med 2005;353:576–586.

Study Design

Randomized controlled trial (single-blinded)

Funding

Industry + govt

Allocation

Concealed

Setting

Outpatient (any)

Synopsis

The initial report of this study's results found that early insertion of tympanostomy tubes in children with persistent otitis media with effusion did not improve outcomes at 3 years of age over delaying up to 9 months (see: Delaying tymp tubes doesn't worsen outcomes in effusion. N Engl J Med 2005;344:1179–87). In brief, children were enrolled before 2 months of age and underwent pneumatic otoscopy monthly until 3 years of age. If they had a persistent otitis media with effusion – defined as 90 days of bilateral effusion, 135 of unilateral effusion, or at least 67% of 180- and 270-day periods for bilateral and unilateral effusion in children with intermittent effusion – they were randomized to either immediate insertion of tympanostomy tubes or delaying 6 months to 9 months and only inserting tubes at that time if the effusion persisted. Outcome assessors were blinded to treatment assignment and allocation was concealed. At the end of the study, 85% in the early treatment group had received tubes, compared with only 41% in the delayed insertion group. Of course, the children who received immediate tubes could hear and speak better, right? Although that would make perfect sense, it is not what happened in this carefully done follow-up study that reports outcomes at 6 years of age. There was no difference between groups in tests of intelligence, speech complexity, hearing, auditory processing, behavior, or parental stress. With approximately 200 children in each group, the study had adequate statistical power to detect clinically meaningful differences if they existed.

Prompt tympanostomy tube insertion doesn't improve 9 year outcomes

Clinical question

Does the delayed insertion of tympanostomy tubes impair the long-term outcomes in children with persistent middle-ear effusion?

Bottom line

Delayed tympanostomy tube insertion successfully helps many children avoid tubes and does not result in any developmental or other impairment. (LOE = 1b)

Reference

Paradise JL, Feldman HM, Campbell TF, et al. Tympanostomy tubes and developmental outcomes at 9 to 11 years of age. N Engl J Med 2007;356:248–261.

Study Design

Randomized controlled trial (single-blinded)

Funding

Government

Allocation

Concealed

Setting

Outpatient (any)

Synopsis

Many parents and clinicians still believe that there is a significant risk of permanent harm if tympanostomy tubes are not promptly inserted for children with persistent middle-ear effusion. In this study, which is a follow-up to a previously published POEM (N Engl J Med 2005;353:576), 429 children between the ages of 2 months and 3 years with middle-ear effusion for at least 90 days (bilateral) or 135 days (unilateral) were randomized to receive either prompt or delayed tympanostomy tube insertion. The delay was 6 months for bilateral effusion and 9 months for unilateral effusion. Allocation was concealed, groups were balanced at the start of the study, and analysis was by intention to treat. The researchers did an excellent job of following up: 195 of 216 in the early treatment group and 196 of 213 in the delayed treatment group underwent developmental testing between the ages of 9 years and 11 years. At the time of this final evaluation, 86% in the early treatment group had received tympanostomy tubes compared with only 49% in the delayed treatment group. There was no differences between groups in the results of a broad range of tests including evaluation of hearing, reading, oral fluency, auditory processing, phonological processing, behavior, or intelligence. There was also no difference between these groups and a group of children with ear problems that weren't bad enough to qualify them for the study.

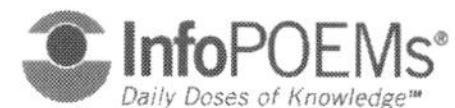

Saline nasal irrigation effective for frequent sinusitis

Clinical question
Does daily nasal irrigation with hypertonic saline improve symptoms in patients with frequent sinus infections?

Bottom line
This is an inexpensive, easy, and effective treatment for a condition considered intractable by many. Daily nasal irrigation using 2% saline was a highly effective treatment for patients with frequent sinusitis. (LOE = 1b–)

Reference
Rabago D, Zgierska A, Mundt M, et al. Efficacy of daily hypertonic saline nasal irrigation among patients with sinusitis: a randomized controlled trial. J Fam Pract 2002;51:1049–1055.

Study Design
Randomized controlled trial (nonblinded)

Setting
Outpatient (primary care)

Synopsis
Sinus infections are often recurrent and can be difficult to treat. The Yogic tradition advocates daily rinsing of the nasal passage with a hypertonic saline solution as a way to clean things out. Previous studies, although promising, have been small and poorly designed. In this primary care clinical trial, the authors identified patients with either 2 episodes of acute sinusitis or 1 episode of chronic sinusitis per year for 2 consecutive years. Their mean age was 42 years, 74% were women, only 5% were smokers, and most had recurrent episodes of acute sinusitis rather than chronic sinusitis. They randomized these patients to either usual care (n = 24) or to an experimental group (n = 52) that received instruction in using the SinuCleanse nasal cup with 2% saline buffered with baking soda. Subjects completed a daily diary to record adherence to the nasal irrigation protocol, filled out a symptom survey every 2 weeks, and a more extensive set of outcome measures at 1.5, 3, and 6 months. Groups were similar at baseline. Although not blinded, allocation to groups was appropriately concealed, randomization was valid, and analysis was by intention-to-treat. At 6 months, there was a clinically and statistically greater improvement in the Rhinosinusitis Disability Index and the Single Item Symptom Severity Assessment for patients using nasal irrigation. There were also significant improvements in sinus headache, frontal pain, frontal pressure, and nasal congestion, and a reduction in antibiotic and nasal spray use. Although 10 subjects reported side effects (eg, nasal irritation, nasal burning, and nosebleeds) all 44 experimental subjects who completed the final questions about satisfaction said they would continue to use nasal irrigation.

Essential Evidence: Medicine that Matters, Edited by David Slawson, Allen Shaughnessy, Mark Ebell, and Henry Barry.

Intranasal steroids alone effective for acute uncomplicated sinusitis

Clinical question

Are intranasal steroids alone effective in the treatment of acute uncomplicated rhinosinusitis?

Bottom line

The vast majority of patients with acute uncomplicated rhinosinusitis improve in 2 to 4 weeks without any specific treatment. Treatment with mometasone furoate nasal spray (Nasonex) 200 ug twice daily significantly reduces the time to resolution compared with amoxicillin alone or placebo. Patients who "must do something" may still find it easier and cheaper to try other modalities such as nasal saline. (LOE = 1b)

Reference

Meltzer EO, Bachert C, Staudinger H. Treating acute rhinosinusitis: Comparing efficacy and safety of mometasone furoate nasal spray, amoxicillin, and placebo. J Allergy Clin Immunol 2005;116:1289–1295.

Study Design

Randomized controlled trial (double-blinded)

Funding

Industry

Allocation

Concealed

Setting

Outpatient (specialty)

Synopsis

Intranasal steroids used with antibiotics are more effective in the treatment of recurrent sinus infections than antibiotics alone. The benefit of intranasal steroids alone for uncomplicated sinusitis is uncertain. The investigators randomized (concealed allocation assignment) 981 subjects with acute uncomplicated sinusitis to 1 of 4 treatment groups: (1) mometasone furoate nasal spray (MFN) 200 ug once daily; (2) MFN 200 ug twice daily; (3) amoxicillin 500 mg 3 times daily; or (4) placebo. Exclusion criteria included fever greater than 101 F/ 38.3 C, severe unilateral facial or tooth pain, facial swelling, dental involvement, or a worsening of symptoms after initial improvement. These criteria likely excluded subjects with a significant bacterial infection. Fourteen-day follow-up occurred for 90% of subjects. Patients blinded to treatment group assignment self-reported outcomes. Using intention-to-treat analysis, the major symptom score (sum of scores for rhinorrhea, postnasal drip, nasal congestion, headache, and facial pain/pressure) was significantly reduced for those patients receiving MFN twice daily compared with those receiving amoxicillin and placebo. Both amoxicillin and MFN once daily were similarly more effective than placebo. At 2 weeks of follow-up, however, patients in all 4 treatment groups reported more than a 50% reduction in their major symptom score. Patients receiving MFN twice daily were less likely to met criteria for treatment failure or to discontinue treatment early because of failure to improve.

Essential Evidence: Medicine that Matters, Edited by David Slawson, Allen Shaughnessy, Mark Ebell, and Henry Barry.

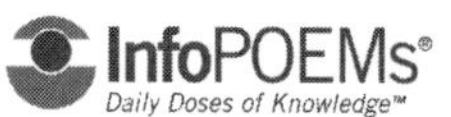

Herbal tea effective for symptoms of acute pharyngitis

Clinical question

Can herbal tea help reduce the symptoms of pain associated with acute pharyngitis?

Bottom line

An herbal tea containing a mixture of traditional demulcents (soothing agents) was more effective than a placebo tea in the short-term relief of pain in patients with acute pharyngitis. The effect does not last long – less than 30 minutes – so requires frequent tea drinking throughout the day. On the occasion of my next sore throat, I'm going to reach for an analgesic and a topical anesthetic, but herbal tea may be useful for patients who prefer a more active approach and who wish to avoid the partially anesthetized mouth feel. (LOE = 1b)

Reference

Brinckmann J, Sigwart H, van Houten Taylor L. Safety and efficacy of a traditional herbal medicine (Throat Coat) in symptomatic temporary relief of pain in patients with acute pharyngitis: a multicenter, prospective, randomized, double-blinded, placebo-controlled study. J Altern Complement Med 2003;9:285–298.

Study Design

Randomized controlled trial (double-blinded)

Setting

Outpatient (any)

Synopsis

Demulcents is a general category of products that are soothing and relieve irritation. They are not topical anesthetics, but have been used for many years to treat sore throat. This study evaluated the effectiveness of a demulcent mixture containining licorice root, elm inner bark, marshmallow root, and licorice root aqueous dry extract (an herbal tea called Throat Coat). Sixty patients with acute pharyngitis by any cause were randomly assigned to use the herbal tea or a similar-tasting and -smelling placebo tea 4 to 6 times daily for as long as symptoms remained. No other treatment was allowed. Treatment allocation was concealed from the enrolling physician. Patients rated pain relief after 1 minute then every 5 minutes for 30 minutes, then at 3 and 24 hours after the first dose, and then daily using a scale from 0 to 10. Analysis was by intention to treat and compared the degree of change in pain scores at each period, as well as the total amount of pain relief using the total area under the curve of pain changes. Details on exactly what statistics were used are sketchy, which is odd considering the great detail in which other aspects of the study were reported. Changes from baseline pain after the first dose were significantly different than placebo at 5 and 10 minutes. The sum of pain intensity differences occurring in the first 30 minutes of treatment was approximately twice as good in the treatment group ($P = .041$). Pain relief was also greater in treated patients at 10 minutes after the first dose. By intention-to-treat analysis, however, total pain relief over the first 30 minutes was not different between the 2 groups.

Essential Evidence: Medicine that Matters, Edited by David Slawson, Allen Shaughnessy, Mark Ebell, and Henry Barry.

Steroids provide brief relief of pain in mononucleosis

Clinical question
Does dexamethasone reduce throat pain in acute mononucleosis?

Bottom line
Dexamethasone provides improvement in throat pain in children with acute mononucleosis but the effect lasts less than 24 hours. (LOE = 1b–)

Reference
Roy M, Bailey B, Amre DK, et al. Dexamethasone for the treatment of sore throat in children with suspected infectious mononucleosis: a randomized, double-blind, placebo-controlled, clinical trial. Arch Pediatr Adolesc Med 2004;158:250–254.

Study Design
Randomized controlled trial (double-blinded)

Setting
Emergency department

Synopsis
The investigators enrolled children between the ages of 8 and 18 years with suspected mononucleosis in this small study. The 40 children were randomly assigned (masked allocation) to receive a single oral dose of dexamethasone (0.3 mg/kg, maximum 15 mg) or a matched placebo. Pain was measured using a 100-mm visual analog scale, with a 20 mm or greater difference chosen as the main outcome. Pain was assessed 12, 24, 48, and 72 hours after treatment, and then one final time on day 7. Analysis was by intention to treat.To assess the quality of blinding, the investigators tried to guess whether participants received dexamethasone or placebo after patients completed the pain scale (they couldn't). At the 12-hour assessment, 12 of 20 in the dexamethasone group improved (at least 20 mm on the scale) compared with 5 of 19 taking placebo (number needed to treat = 4; P = .03). At 24 hours, half the patients treated with dexamethasone (11/20) had pain relief compared with one third (6/20) taking placebo. The study did not have sufficient power to detect whether this difference was real or not. Assessments after the first 24 hours were virtually identical.

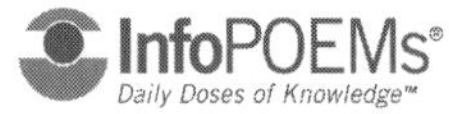

Gargling with water prevents colds

Clinical question

Is gargling with water or povidone-iodine effective in preventing upper respiratory tract infections?

Bottom line

Gargling with water effectively reduces the risk of developing an upper respiratory tract infection (URTI). Nine individuals will need to gargle with water for 1 minute 3 times daily for 60 days to prevent 1 additional person from developing a URTI. Gargling with povidone-iodine was no more effective than usual care. (LOE = 1b–)

Reference

Satomura K, Kitamura T, Kawamura T, et al, for the Great Cold Investigators-I. Prevention of upper respiratory tract infections by gargling. A randomized trial. Am J Prev Med 2005;29:302–307.

Study Design

Randomized controlled trial (single-blinded)

Funding

Foundation

Allocation

Concealed

Setting

Outpatient (primary care)

Synopsis

Regular gargling with water or povidone-iodine solution may remove nasal-pharyngeal acquired viruses before they result in a URTI. These investigators randomized (allocation assignment concealed) 387 adults, aged 18 to 65 years, to gargling with water, gargling with povidone-iodine, or usual care. Subjects in the first 2 groups gargled with approximately 20 mL of water or povidone-iodine for approximately 15 seconds 3 times consecutively, at least 3 times daily. Follow-up occurred for 60 days from December 2002 to March 2003 for 99% of subjects. Outcomes were reported by individuals (the study subjects) not blinded to treatment group assignment. Using intention-to-treat analysis, 130 subjects (34%) acquired a URTI, including 50 in the control group, 34 in the water group, and 46 in the povidone-iodine group. Only the difference between the water group and usual care group was significant (number needed to treat = 9 for 60 days).

Essential Evidence: Medicine that Matters, Edited by David Slawson, Allen Shaughnessy, Mark Ebell, and Henry Barry.

Delayed prescriptions for URIs reduce antibiotic use

Clinical question
Do delayed prescriptions reduce antibiotic use in upper respiratory tract infections?

Bottom line
Delayed prescriptions for upper respiratory tract infections reduces the use of antibiotics; patient satisfaction, however, may be worse. (LOE = 1a–)

Reference
Arroll B, Kenealy T, Kerse N. Do delayed prescriptions reduce antibiotic use in respiratory tract infections? A systematic review. Br J Gen Pract 2003;53:871–877.

Study Design
Systematic review

Setting
Outpatient (primary care)

Synopsis
For this systematic review, the authors included controlled trials of studies in which the intervention was a delayed prescription compared with an immediate prescription for patients with upper respiratory tract infections. They searched several databases (MEDLINE, Embase, Cochrane) and searched for unpublished studies. Two of the authors independently assessed the quality of the trials (randomization, concealment of allocation, co-interventions, losses to follow-up, and so forth). Disagreements among the reviewers were resolved by discussion and consensus. The authors were only able to find 5 controlled trials, 4 of which were randomized. All the randomized controlled trials had Jadad scores above 3, indicating reasonable to good quality. Since the authors found significant heterogeneity among the studies, they refrained from pooling the data. However, each study demonstrated significant reduction in the rate of antibiotic use. In 2 of the studies, however, patient satisfaction was significantly worse, and in 3 studies the symptoms were worse among those receiving a delayed prescription.

Essential Evidence: Medicine that Matters, Edited by David Slawson, Allen Shaughnessy, Mark Ebell, and Henry Barry.

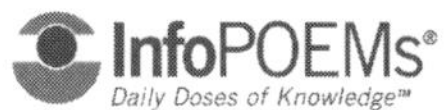

Forcing fluids during a respiratory infection unsupported by studies

Clinical question

What is the evidence that drinking plenty of fluids is effective and not harmful?

Bottom line

There is no research evaluating whether drinking plenty of fluids is beneficial to patients with respiratory infections. Although the benefit seems to be self-evident, there is a theoretical risk of harm. Antidiuretic hormone secretion increases in both adults and children with lower respiratory tract infections who drink large amounts of fluids, and hyponatremia has been documented in these situations in cohort and case studies. There is weak evidence to support either continuing the practice or stopping the practice. (LOE = 1a−)

Reference

Guppy MPB, Mickan SM, Del Mar CB. "Drink plenty of fluids": a systematic review of evidence for this recommendation in acute respiratory infections. BMJ 2004;328:499–500.

Study Design

Systematic review

Setting

Various (meta-analysis)

Synopsis

The unpleasant symptoms of respiratory tract infections are often accompanied by the frustration that there is little one can do to hasten recovery. In other words, it's difficult to do nothing. Now we have a study suggesting that even the most benign do-nothing-by-doing-something-innocuous is not so harmless after all. The authors of this study attempted to determine whether drinking extra fluids while experiencing a respiratory tract infection is evidence-based or a medical myth. With appropriate rigor they searched several databases, examined references of relevant papers and contacted experts in an attempt to cough up studies on the subject. As might be expected, there has been no fevered rush to research this topic and they came up dry when looking for randomized controlled trials. They found 2 studies reporting hyponatremia at rates of 31% and 45% for children with moderate to severe pneumonia but without signs of dehydration, and several case series in which children developed hyponatremia during a respiratory infection that responded to fluid restriction.

Essential Evidence: Medicine that Matters, Edited by David Slawson, Allen Shaughnessy, Mark Ebell, and Henry Barry.

Zinc nasal gel reduces duration of common cold

Clinical question

Does zinc nasal gel reduce the duration of the common cold?

Bottom line

Zinc nasal gel was effective in this small study, reducing the duration of cold symptoms by 1.7 days. It was well tolerated, although minor adverse effects were more common in the treatment group. (LOE = 1b)

Reference

Mossad SB. Effect of zincum gluconicum nasal gel on the duration and symptom severity of the common cold in otherwise healthy adults. QJM 2003;96:35–43.

Study Design

Randomized controlled trial (double-blinded)

Setting

Outpatient (any)

Synopsis

Zinc lozenges have been shown effective in 6 randomized trials and ineffective in 8 others. Meta-analyses are equivocal. Advocates for zinc suggest that the delivery vehicle may be part of the problem, and this trial evaluates a zinc nasal gel. Eighty patients were recruited from advertisements, and were included if they were aged 18 to 55 years, had symptoms of a cold for 24 to 48 hours, and had 2 major and at least 1 minor symptom or 1 major and at least 3 minor symptoms. Major symptoms included nasal drainage and sore throat; minor symptoms included nasal congestion, sneezing, scratchy throat, hoarseness, cough, headache, muscle aches, and oral temperature above 98.6 F. These seem reasonable, although the definition of fever is too low. Patients with diabetes, with a noncorrected deviated nasal septum or recurrent sinusitis, and smokers were excluded. Patients were randomized with concealed allocation to either zincum gluconicum (Zenullose or Zicam) 120 microliters via metered dose applicator or matching placebo. Patients and investigators were masked, and after 1 day patients could not guess whether they were in the active treatment or control groups. The primary outcome was the time to resolution of all cold symptoms. Patients completed a diary of symptoms and adverse effects twice a day, rating each on a scale from 0 (none) to 3 (severe). They measured a lot of secondary outcomes, but we'll focus on the primary outcome. The groups were similar at the start of the study, with 40 patients in each group. Two patients in the control group were lost to follow-up, and because there were no follow-up data, were excluded from the analysis. Three in the treatment group and 1 in the control group were diagnosed with an illness other than the common cold and discontinued treatment, but were still included in the analysis (appropriately). The time to resolution of all symptoms was shorter in the treatment group (4.3 vs 6 days; P = .002), and the time to resolution was also shorter for all individual symptoms, except headache, muscle aches, and fever. There was no statistically significant difference between groups for each adverse effect. More patients in the treatment group had any adverse effect (31% vs 14%), although no test of statistical significance is reported for this comparison, which is a bit suspicious.

Essential Evidence: Medicine that Matters, Edited by David Slawson, Allen Shaughnessy, Mark Ebell, and Henry Barry.

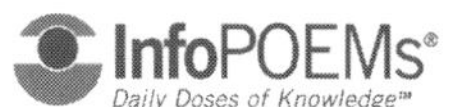

Echinacea purpurea ineffective for treating URI in kids

Clinical question

How effective and safe is echinacea in the treatment of upper respiratory tract infections in children?

Bottom line

Echinacea purpurea extract (above ground plant only), prepared and used at the doses in this study was ineffective in treating upper respiratory tract infections (URIs) in children. Although it was generally safe to use, more parents reported a rash on their child and 2 children had a serious allergic-type reaction. Interestingly, children using echinacea were less likely to have recurrent URI (number needed to treat = 9). (LOE = 1b)

Reference

Taylor JA, Weber W, Standish L, et al. Efficacy and safety of echinacea in treating upper respiratory tract infections in children. A randomized controlled trial. JAMA 2003;290:2824–2830.

Study Design

Randomized controlled trial (double-blinded)

Setting

Outpatient (primary care)

Synopsis

Although the average child has 6 to 8 colds per year, each lasting 7 to 10 days, commonly used medications such as decongestants, antihistamines, and cough suppressants lack efficacy in those younger than 12 years. Echinacea is widely used for the prevention and treatment of URIs in adults, but there is limited data on efficacy and safety of use in children. Data were obtained and analyzed on a total of 707 URIs that occurred in 407 children. At the onset of each URI, subjects were randomly given (concealed allocation assignment) either dried pressed Echinacea purpurea juice (obtained from the above-ground herb, harvested at flowering, extracted in an alcohol-free preparation combined with syrup), or identical placebo. Dosing was age-based on the recommendations of the manufacturer and was continued until all symptoms had resolved, up to a maximum of 10 days. Parents recorded the severity of symptoms and adverse events in a daily logbook. The patients, parents, practitioners and research staff were all unaware of treatment group assignment. Ninety-four percent of the subjects were followed up for a total of 4 months. Using intention-to-treat analysis, there were no differences in duration of URIs or in the overall estimate of severity of URI symptoms between the 2 treatment groups. Other over-the-counter cold remedies were administered by parents at the same rate in both groups, but antipruitics and analgesics other than acetaminophen were administered more often to children treated with echinacea (9.8% vs 5.1%; P = .03). After limiting the analysis to the URIs in which patients received at least 80% of the study medication (per protocol analysis), there were still no differences found between the 2 groups. Children assigned to echinacea were less likely to have a second URI than those in the placebo group (52.3% vs 64.4%; P = .015; number needed to treat = 9). Adverse events were reported similarly in each group, although rash was reported more often in children receiving echinacea (7.1% vs 2.7%). Two children receiving echinacea had the sudden onset of stridor requiring emergency treatment with steroids.

Essential Evidence: Medicine that Matters, Edited by David Slawson, Allen Shaughnessy, Mark Ebell, and Henry Barry.

Antibiotics slightly effective for purulent rhinitis

Clinical question

In patients with short-term colored rhinitis, is antibiotic treatment more effective than placebo treatment?

Bottom line

Antibiotic treatment of patients with purulent rhinitis of less than 10 days duration increased the number of patients who had resolution of the rhinitis 5 days to 7 days later. On average, almost 60% of patients improved without treatment; antibiotics produced 1 more patient who benefited for every 6 patients who were treated. (LOE = 1a)

Reference

Arroll B, Kenealy T. Are antibiotics effective for acute purulent rhinitis? Systematic review and meta-analysis of placebo controlled randomised trials. BMJ 2006;333:279. Epub 2006 Jul 21.

Study Design

Meta-analysis (randomized controlled trials)

Funding

Self-funded or unfunded

Setting

Outpatient (any)

Synopsis

When does a cold turn into a bonafide bacterial infection? Traditional wisdom suggests the presence of colored nasal discharge heralds the onset of bacterial invasion, although this notion has been disputed for years. To address this issue, the researchers conducting this study combined the results of 6 studies that evaluated the use of antibiotics in patients with purulent rhinitis. To find the research, the authors searched 3 databases and contacted authors of identified studies to obtain additional studies. Two researchers independently evaluated the articles for inclusion. Four studies contributed data on the benefits of antibiotics. Combining those data for 598 adults and children, patients receiving antibiotics were slightly more likely (20%) to be improved at days 5 to 8 than those receiving placebo (number needed to treat = 5.8; 95% CI, 4.1–10.3). Amoxicillin, co-trimoxazole, and cephalexin were used in the studies. Adverse effects were more common in the treated patients, with numbers needed to treat to harm of 12 to 78 in the significant studies.

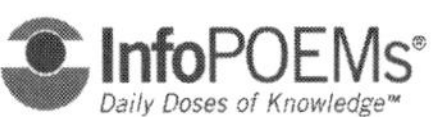

Echinacea doesn't shorten or lessen cold symptoms

Clinical question

Is Echinacea purpurea effective in the treatment of cold symptoms?

Bottom line

A product containing the freeze-dried extract of the above-ground part of Echinacea purpurea was ineffective in decreasing the duration or severity of the common cold. These results contradict findings of 2 meta-analyses which documented some benefit with other extracts. (LOE = 1b–)

Reference

Yale SH, Liu K. Echinacea purpurea therapy for the treatment of the common cold. Arch Intern Med 2004;164:1237–1241.

Study Design

Randomized controlled trial (double-blinded)

Setting

Outpatient (any)

Synopsis

This study evaluated the effectiveness of a freeze-dried extract prepared from the above-ground parts of the Echinacea purpurea plant (EchinaFresh). All formulations of echinacea are not the same: 2 different species are in common use – E purpurea and E augustifolia– and different parts of the plant, such as the whole plant, root, or upper parts are used to make extracts. The participants in this study were solicited by advertisements. The investigators enrolled 128 adults, primarily women, with an average age of 38 years, within 24 hours of the onset of cold symptoms. Only 10% were smokers. The average duration of symptoms was 15 hours. The patients were randomized to receive either placebo or echinacea 100 mg 3 times daily as long as they had symptoms, for up to 14 days. The patients were asked not to take other symptom-relief products, except acetaminophen. Daily symptoms scores, which consisted of 4 points on each of 8 symptom scales (nasal discharge, cough, and so forth), were not different at any time between the 2 groups. The time to complete resolution of symptoms also was not shortened by echinacea. The study was large enough to find a 25% difference in symptoms or a 3-day difference in duration.

Essential Evidence: Medicine that Matters, Edited by David Slawson, Allen Shaughnessy, Mark Ebell, and Henry Barry.

Yogurt prevents antibiotic-associated diarrhea

Clinical question

Is yogurt effective in the prevention of antibiotic-associated diarrhea?

Bottom line

Vanilla-flavored yogurt containing active bacterial cultures is effective in decreasing the incidence and duration of antibiotic-associated diarrhea. Tell your patients to look for yogurt that contains active cultures. If they can't find it, consider probiotic agents. (LOE = 2b)

Reference

Beniwal RS, Arena VC, Thomas L, et al. A randomized trial of yogurt for prevention of antibiotic-associated diarrhea. Dig Dis Science 2003;48:2077–2082.

Study Design

Randomized controlled trial (nonblinded)

Setting

Inpatient (any location) with outpatient follow-up

Synopsis

Probiotic agents are effective in preventing antibiotic-associated diarrhea. Controversy exists about whether commercially available yogurt products are similarly effective. A total of 202 hospitalized patients receiving oral or intravenous antibiotics were randomized (concealed allocation assignment) to either vanilla-flavored yogurt (8 ounces twice daily for 8 days) or usual care without yogurt supplementation. The authors do not specify the brand or type of yogurt but note that manufacturer-supplied nutritional data indicated that the product contained active cultures of Lactobacillus acidophilus, L. bulgaricus, and Streptococcus thermophilus. The mean age of the study group was 70 years. All patients were followed up for a total of 8 days. Individuals assessing outcomes were not blinded to treatment group assignment. Antibiotic-associated diarrhea was defined as the new onset of more than 2, less-than-formed bowel movements per day representing a change in prior bowel patterns. Using intention-to-treat analysis, patients receiving yogurt reported less frequent diarrhea (12% vs 24%; P = .04; number needed to treat = 12). In addition, subjects ingesting yogurt daily reported significantly less total diarrheal days (23 vs 60). No side effects were reported other than boredom: Yogurt-fed subjects yearned for fruit-flavored yogurt to break the monotony ("I'm sick and tired of vanilla yogurt! Don't you have any other flavors?!").

Essential Evidence: Medicine that Matters, Edited by David Slawson, Allen Shaughnessy, Mark Ebell, and Henry Barry.

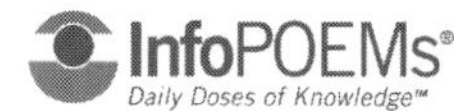

Probiotics helpful for antibiotic-associated diarrhea

Clinical question

Can probiotics prevent antibiotic-associated diarrhea and assist in the treatment of Clostridium difficile disease?

Bottom line

The probiotics Saccharomyces boulardii and Lactobacillus rhamnosus GG both prevent antibiotic-associated diarrhea (AAD), as does a combination of 2 or more probiotics. S. boulardii, given in addition to vancomycin or metronidazole, is also an effective treatment for Clostridium difficile disease (CDD). (LOE = 1a–)

Reference

McFarland LV. Meta-analysis of probiotics for the prevention of antibiotic associated diarrhea and the treatment of Clostridium difficile disease. Am J Gastroenterol 2006;101:812–822.

Study Design

Meta-analysis (randomized controlled trials)

Funding

Unknown/not stated

Setting

Various (meta-analysis)

Synopsis

A variety of probiotics have been proposed to help reestablish the gut flora, prevent AAD, and treat CDD. This meta-analysis identified any blinded randomized controlled trials (RCTs) on MEDLINE and Google Scholar and evaluated their quality. There were 25 RCTs of AAD prevention including 2810 patients and 6 RCTs of CDD treatment including 354 patients. Studies were generally of good quality. There was considerable heterogeneity regarding population and results for studies of prevention of AAD. Although there was no difference in outcomes for studies in adults or children or by duration of therapy, a greater benefit was seen for studies using a higher dose. S. boulardii and L. rhamnosus GG, both studied in 6 RCTs, were most effective (combined relative risk = 0.37 and 0.31, respectively) as were studies using a mixture of 2 probiotics. In most studies of the treatment of CDD, patients were also given vancomycin or metronidazole and the outcome was the likelihood of recurrence of CDD. Results of the 6 studies were homogeneous and a combined estimate of effect showed a relative risk of recurrent CDD of 0.59 (95% CI, 0.41–0.81). S. boulardii seemed to be the most effective probiotic. Adverse effects in both sets of studies were minimal. These studies took place largely in immunocompetent patients and should not be generalized to immunocompromised patients.

Essential Evidence: Medicine that Matters, Edited by David Slawson, Allen Shaughnessy, Mark Ebell, and Henry Barry.

Probiotics effective in preventing acute diarrhea, but not traveler's diarrhea

Clinical question

Are probiotics effective in the prevention of acute diarrhea?

Bottom line

Probiotics reduce the risk of antibiotic-associated diarrhea and other types of acute diarrhea, but not the risk of traveler's diarrhea, in both children and adults. The protective effect does not vary among different probiotic strains nor by mode of delivery. (LOE = 1a)

Reference

Sazawal S, Hiremath G, Dhingra U, Malik P, Deb S, Black RE. Efficacy of probiotics in prevention of acute diarrhea: A meta-analysis of masked, randomized, placebo-controlled trials. Lancet Infect Dis 2006;6:374–382.

Study Design

Meta-analysis (randomized controlled trials)

Funding

Government

Setting

Various (meta-analysis)

Synopsis

Probiotics are effective in the treatment of acute infectious diarrhea in adults and children. However, evidence for the role of probiotics in preventing acute diarrhea is less certain. These investigators thoroughly searched multiple databases – including MEDLINE, the Cochrane Registry, and references of published review articles – and personally contacted researchers known to be working in the field. Only randomized double-blind placebo-controlled trials in either English or French were included in the analysis. Three individuals separately evaluated articles for eligibility and quality; disagreements were resolved by consensus discussion. A total of 34 trials including 4844 patients, aged 6 months to 71 years, met the inclusion criteria. Overall, probiotics reduced the risk of acquiring diarrhea by 33% (95% CI, 22%–44%; number needed to treat = 15, 11–22). In subgroup analyses, probiotics significantly reduced the risk of antibiotic-associated diarrhea and acute diarrhea of other types, but did not reduce the risk of traveler's diarrhea. Probiotics were more effective in children than in adults, and the protective effect did not vary significantly among different probiotic strains or by mode of delivery (ie, capsules, tablets, granules, or powder). A formal analysis found no evidence of significant publication bias.

Essential Evidence: Medicine that Matters, Edited by David Slawson, Allen Shaughnessy, Mark Ebell, and Henry Barry.

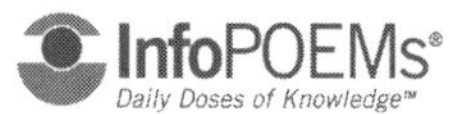

Nitazoxanide reduces rotavirus duration in hospitalized kids

Clinical question

Does nitazoxanide reduce the duration of rotavirus diarrhea in hospitalized children?

Bottom line

In this exploratory study, nitazoxanide (Alinia) reduced the duration of illness by nearly 2 days in children hospitalized with rotavirus diarrhea. It is unclear whether these findings would be similarly impressive in children who are less severely ill. (LOE = 2b−)

Reference

Rossignol JF, Abu-Zekry M, Hussein A, Santoro MG. Effect of nitazoxanide for treatment of severe rotavirus diarrhoea: randomised double-blind placebo-controlled trial. Lancet 2006;368:124–129.

Study Design

Randomized controlled trial (double-blinded)

Funding

Industry

Allocation

Concealed

Setting

Inpatient (ward only)

Synopsis

This is a preliminary study of 38 Egyptian patients younger than 12 years of age with watery diarrhea severe enough to require hospitalization. All of these children also had confirmed rotavirus infection. They were randomly assigned (concealed allocation) to receive 3 days of nitazoxanide or placebo. The majority of the children had 5 to 10 stools per day or more. Most of the hospitalized children were malnourished and had nearly 1 week of symptoms before admission. The dosing of nitazoxanide was 200 mg twice daily for children aged 4 years to 11 years, 100 mg twice daily for children aged 12 months to 47 months, and 0.375 mg per kg twice daily for those younger than 12 months. All patients remained in the hospital for 1 week after the start of treatment. The authors used an intention-to-treat analysis but removed children who also had other identified causes of diarrhea (like bacterial pathogens, Giardia lamblia, Entamoeba histolytica, and so forth). The children receiving nitazoxanide had a significant reduction in the duration of illness (31 hours compared with 75 hours in the control patients), though the authors don't define how this outcome was determined. The authors reported no significant adverse events in the treatment group and 2 minor adverse events in control children.

Essential Evidence: Medicine that Matters, Edited by David Slawson, Allen Shaughnessy, Mark Ebell, and Henry Barry.

Oral rotavirus vaccines safe and effective

Clinical question

Is an oral vaccine safe and effective for the prevention of a rotavirus infection in young children?

Bottom line

Oral vaccines have been developed that are safe and effective for the prevention of rotavirus in young children. This will be particularly useful in third world countries where this disease is a major cause of infant mortality. (LOE = 1b)

Reference

Ruiz-Palacios GM, Perez-Schael I, Velazquez FR, et al, for the Human Rotavirus Vaccine Study Group. Safety and efficacy of an attenuated vaccine against severe rotavirus gastroenteritis. N Engl J Med 2006;354:11–22.

Study Design

Randomized controlled trial (double-blinded)

Funding

Industry

Allocation

Uncertain

Setting

Population-based

Synopsis

The first vaccine for rotavirus (Rotashield) was withdrawn from the market because in rare cases it caused intussusception. This study evaluated a live attenuated vaccine (Rotarix) given in 2 oral doses 1 to 2 months apart, with the first dose given to patients between the ages of 6 weeks and 13 weeks. The study randomized more than 62,000 infants to the vaccine or placebo in Finland and in 11 South American and Central American countries. Allocation concealment and randomization procedures are not clearly described by the authors. The entire group was followed up for a median of 100 days to assess the safety of the vaccine, and a subgroup of 20,169 infants was followed up for 9 to 10 months to evaluate efficacy. There was no significant difference between groups in the likelihood of intussusception (9 in the vaccine group and 16 in the placebo group). Regarding efficacy, the risk of severe gastroenteritis of any cause (defined using a standard symptoms scale) was reduced from 52 to 31 episodes per 1000 infants per year (number needed to treat [NNT] = 48; 95% CI, 26–303) and the number of diarrhea-related hospitalizations was reduced from 42 to 25 episodes per 1000 infants per year (NNT = 56; 29–486). Both of these differences were statistically significant. A second study in the same issue of the journal reported similar findings for a second oral vaccine given in 3 doses called Rotateq (N Engl J Med 2006;354:23–33).

Essential Evidence: Medicine that Matters, Edited by David Slawson, Allen Shaughnessy, Mark Ebell, and Henry Barry.

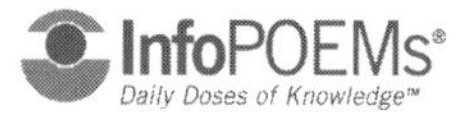

Ondansetron effective for gastroenteritis with vomiting

Clinical question

Is ondansetron safe and effective for dehydrated children with gastroenteritis?

Bottom line

Ondansetron (Zofran) given to children who are mildly to moderately dehydrated because of diarrhea and vomiting improves their ability to comply with oral rehydration and reduces the need for intravenous hydration. (LOE = 1b)

Reference

Freedman SB, Adler M, Seshadri R, Powell EC. Oral ondansetron for gastroenteritis in a pediatric emergency department. N Engl J Med 2006;354:1698–1705.

Study Design

Randomized controlled trial (double-blinded)

Funding

Government

Allocation

Concealed

Setting

Emergency department

Synopsis

Although oral rehydration is the treatment of choice for children with gastroenteritis, it can be a challenge when the child can't keep anything down. This leads to overuse of intravenous hydration, particularly given the time pressures in the emergency department. These authors considered for inclusion any mildly to moderately dehydrated child who'd had at least 1 episode of diarrhea and 1 episode of vomiting in the previous 4 hours. Those with a body weight of less than 8 kg (17 pounds), who were severely dehydrated using standardized symptoms (eg, clammy or cool skin, very dry mucosa, no tears, moderate tachycardia, no urine for at least 6 hours, limp, and lethargic), and those with significant comorbodities were excluded. Of the 243 children asked to enroll, 215 underwent randomization (allocation concealed) to ondansetron or placebo. The dose of ondansetron was 2 mg for children who weighed between 8 kg and 15 kg, 4 mg for those who weighed 15 kg to 30 kg, and 8 mg for those who weighed more than 30 kg. The dose was repeated if children vomited within 15 minutes of taking the medicine. The mean age of children was 28 months, 57% were male, and they had a mean of 9 episodes of vomiting and 6 episodes of diarrhea in the previous 24 hours. Groups were similar at baseline, and analysis was by intention to treat. Children receiving ondansetron were less likely to vomit while being given liquids (14% vs 35%; $P = .001$; number needed to treat [NNT] = 5), had fewer vomiting episodes (0.18 vs 0.65; $P < .001$), and were less likely to require intravenous rehydration (14% vs 31%; $P = .003$; NNT = 5). There was no difference in the number of children requiring hospitalization or the percentage returning to the emergency department. The drug was well tolerated, although there was a mean of 0.9 additional episodes of diarrhea for children randomized to ondansetron.

Essential Evidence: Medicine that Matters, Edited by David Slawson, Allen Shaughnessy, Mark Ebell, and Henry Barry.

Omeprazole 20 mg = 40 mg for primary care acid-related dyspepsia

Clinical question
Is 40 mg omeprazole more effective than 20 mg for primary care patients with dyspepsia?

Bottom line
Omeprazole (Prilosec) 20 mg is highly effective for the treatment of acid-related dyspepsia. There was no advantage to higher doses, and relapse following the initial 2-week treatment period was common. (LOE = 1b)

Reference
Meineche-Schmidt V. Empiric treatment with high and standard dose of omeprazole in general practice: 2-week randomized placebo-controlled trial and 12-month follow-up of healthcare consumption. Am J Gastroenterol 2004;99:1050–1058.

Study Design
Randomized controlled trial (double-blinded)

Funding
Industry

Allocation
Concealed

Setting
Outpatient (primary care)

Synopsis
A common primary care strategy for patients with dyspepsia and no alarm symptoms is to prescribe a proton-pump inhibitor. This pragmatic study took place in a Danish primary care research network with 103 participating physicians and 829 patients. Adults presenting with dyspepsia (that their physician thought was acid-related) and no alarm symptoms were randomized to omeprazole 40 mg per day, omeprazole 20 mg per day, or placebo. Alarm symptoms were defined as rectal bleeding or hematemesis, unintended weight loss, vomiting, dysphagia, jaundice, or other signs of serious disease. Groups were similar at baseline, with a mean age of 50 years; 58% were women. Allocation was concealed and outcomes were blindly assessed, with analysis by intention to treat. Patients were treated for 2 weeks, and then medications were discontinued. During the remaining year of observation, in which 92% of the patients participated, the author tracked the time until symptom relapse and the consumption of healthcare resources. The most common symptoms in both groups were epigastric pain, regurgitation, heartburn, bloating, and pain at night. Symptoms were rated as moderate by 63% of patients and severe by 15%. At 2 weeks, sufficient relief was reported more often in the 40 mg and 20 mg groups than in the placebo group (71%, 69.6%, and 43%, respectively), as was complete relief (66.4%, 63%, and 34.9%). The number needed to treat was between 3 and 4 for both outcomes. Results were similar for Helicobacter pylori-positive and H pylori-negative patients. Most patients in all 3 groups had a relapse of symptoms during the year following their initial treatment.

Essential Evidence: Medicine that Matters, Edited by David Slawson, Allen Shaughnessy, Mark Ebell, and Henry Barry.

 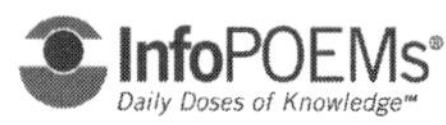

Omeprazole, ranitidine effective for HP negative dyspepsia (CADET-HN)

Clinical question

What is the most effective treatment for patients with Helicobacter pylori negative dyspepsia?

Bottom line

Omeprazole (and to a lesser extent, ranitidine) are somewhat effective for patients with Helicobacter pylori (HP) negative dyspepsia, even if patients with a primary complaint of heartburn or reflux are excluded. The benefit did not persist through the next 5 months when patients could use medications as needed rather than in a scheduled manner. Ranitidine was more cost-effective than omeprazole. It still makes sense to try ranitidine first for these patients, then stepping up to omeprazole if their symptoms are not improved adequately, particularly since this is a benign, self-limited condition. (LOE = 1b)

Reference

Veldhuyzen van Zanten SJ, Chiba N, Armstrong D, et al. A randomized trial comparing omeprazole, ranitidine, cisapride, or placebo in Helicobacter pylori negative, primary care patients with dyspepsia: The CADET-HN study. Am J Gastroenterol 2005;100:1477–1488.

Study Design	Funding	Allocation	Setting
Randomized controlled trial (double-blinded)	Industry	Concealed	Outpatient (primary care)

Synopsis

Previous studies have shown that patients with HP positive dyspepsia benefit from eradication of the infection. This study included patients with epigastric pain and a variety of other symptoms (bloating, nausea, early satiety, heartburn, and acid regurgitation) who were HP negative. Patients were excluded with heartburn as a primary symptom, who had symptoms consistent with irritable bowel syndrome, or with red flags for complicated ulcer disease. For the first 2 weeks of the study, the 512 participants recorded their symptoms without treatment. They were then randomized (allocation concealed) to receive either omeprazole (Prilosec) 20 mg once daily, ranitidine (Zantac) 150 mg twice daily, cisapride (Propulsid) 20 mg twice daily, or placebo. Patients and outcome assessors were properly blinded and analysis was by intention to treat. Patients took the study medications as directed for the first 4 weeks of the study, and after that were able to take them on an as-needed basis for the final 5 months of the study with an antacid as a rescue medication. The primary outcome was the Global Overall Severity score, a validated 7-point scale, at 4 weeks. Treatment success at 4 weeks was seen in 51% of those taking omeprazole, 36% taking ranitidine, 31% taking cisapride, and 23% taking placebo. Omeprazole was significantly more effective than all the other treatments and placebo (number needed to treat [NNT] compared with placebo = 3; compared with ranitidine = 7). However, there was no significant difference in the percentage of responders between groups at 6 months: 44% for omeprazole, 41% for ranitidine, 40% for cisapride, and 35% for placebo. A subgroup analysis of responders at 4 weeks who remained responders at 6 months remained higher for omeprazole than for ranitidine or placebo (31% vs 21% vs 13.5%; P = .001).

Essential Evidence: Medicine that Matters, Edited by David Slawson, Allen Shaughnessy, Mark Ebell, and Henry Barry.

4 drugs for 1 day eliminates H. pylori

Clinical question

Is a 1-day treatment of Helicobacter pylori as effective as a 7-day regimen in patients with dyspepsia?

Bottom line

A 4-drug, single day treatment was as effective as 7 days of treatment with 3 drugs in eradicating Helicobacter pylori and symptoms in patients with H. pylori-positive dyspepsia. (LOE = 1b)

Reference

Lara LF, Cisneros G, Gurney M, et al. One-day quadruple therapy compared with 7-day triple therapy for Helicobacter pylori infection. Arch Intern Med 2003;163:2079–2084.

Study Design

Randomized controlled trial (nonblinded)

Setting

Outpatient (any)

Synopsis

The researchers recruited 160 adult patients with dyspepsia scoring 3 or higher (of a possible 20) on the Glasgow Dyspepsia Severity Score (GDSS) and had a postive urea breath test, signifying the presence of H. pylori. Patients were randomized to receive either a 4-drug cocktail for 1 day or treatment with 3 drugs for 7 days. Allocation may not have been concealed from the enrolling researcher (patients randomized to receive the 7-day treatment were an average 7 years older than the other patients and less likely to smoke). The 1-day regimen consisted of 2 tablets of 262 mg bismuth subsalicylate (Pepto-Bismol), 500 mg metronidazole (Flagyl), and 2 g amoxicillin (suspension), all taken 4 times over the course of the day, along with 60 mg lansoprazole (Prevacid) taken once. The control group took 500 mg clarithromycin (Biaxin), 1 g amoxicillin, and 30 mg lansoprazole twice daily for 7 days. The urea breath test was readministered 5 weeks after the start of treatment to the 150 patients who returned. Eradication rates were similar in the 2 groups: 95% in the 1-day group and 90% in the 7-day group. Treatment success rates were also similar between the 2 groups: The GDSS scores dropped an average of 7.5 points in both groups (from a baseline of 7 to 11). Side effects were tallied at the 5-week follow-up rather than during or immediately after treatment and may not be particularly accurate.

Essential Evidence: Medicine that Matters, Edited by David Slawson, Allen Shaughnessy, Mark Ebell, and Henry Barry.

 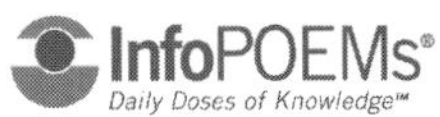

Aspirin + PPI safer than clopidogrel if history of GI bleed

Clinical question

What is the best antithrombotic for patients with a history of upper gastrointestinal bleeding?

Bottom line

For patients with a history of bleeding peptic ulcer, the combination of aspirin and a proton pump inhibitor twice a day was safer in terms of bleeding side effects than clopidogrel. While esomeprazole was used in this study, generic omeprazole 20 mg give twice a day provides nearly the same degree of acid suppression at a much lower cost. This study calls into question the overall safety of clopidogrel, which has been promoted as not increasing the risk of bleeding significantly. (LOE = 1b)

Reference

Chan FK, Ching JY, Hung LC, et al. Clopidogrel versus aspirin and esomeprazole to prevent recurrent ulcer bleeding. N Engl J Med 2005;352:238–244.

Study Design

Randomized controlled trial (double-blinded)

Funding

Government

Allocation

Concealed

Setting

Inpatient (any location) with outpatient follow-up

Synopsis

Clopidogrel (Plavix) has been recommended by the American College of Cardiology as the preferred drug for patients who require an antithrombotic agent to prevent heart disease but who also have a history of bleeding peptic ulcer. This study compared clopidogrel with the combination of aspirin and esomeprazole in this setting. Patients with a source of upper gastrointestinal bleeding (52% gastric ulcer, 34% duodenal ulcer, 8% both, 6% other erosions) who had healing confirmed endoscopically were randomized to clopidogrel 75 mg daily plus esomepraozle placebo twice daily or aspirin 80 mg daily plus esomeprazole 20 mg twice daily. Groups were fairly well balanced at the outset, allocation was concealed, and analysis was by intention-to-treat. Patients were treated for 12 months. The primary outcome (hematemesis, melena, or a decrease in hemoglobin of at least 2 gm/dl accompanied by endoscopic evidence of ulcer or erosion) was seen in 8.6% of the clopidogrel group and 0.7% of the aspirin plus esomeprazole group (p = 0.001, number needed to treat [NNT] = 13). Three patients in the clopidogrel group had severe bleeding complications not related to the gastrointestinal tract compared with none in the aspirin group, including two intraventricular hemorrhages, one of which was fatal. There were more deaths in the clopidogrel group (8 vs 4) but this difference was not statistically significant. There was no difference between groups in the likelihood of adverse cardiovascular events (9 vs 11).

A PPI test does not improve diagnosis of GERD

Clinical question

Is a response to a proton pump inhibitor a useful diagnostic strategy to determine gastroesophageal reflux?

Bottom line

Of patients who present with typical reflux symptoms, 70% will actually have gastroesophageal reflux disease (GERD). A 2-week trial to determine the response to a proton pump inhibitor (PPI) will not identify a significant proportion of patients who have true GERD. If a patient has typical reflux symptoms, begin treatment, since an early lack of response does not rule out true GERD. (LOE = 1c)

Reference

Aanen MC, Weusten BL, Numans ME, De Wit NJ, Baron A, Smout AJ. Diagnostic value of the proton pump inhibitor test for gastro-oesophageal reflux disease in primary care. Aliment Pharmacol Ther 2006;24:1377–1384.

Study Design

Diagnostic test evaluation

Funding

Industry

Setting

Outpatient (primary care)

Synopsis

A short course of a PPI is often used to determine whether a patient with typical reflux symptoms truly has GERD. To evaluate the diagnostic accuracy of the PPI test, the researchers enrolled 74 patients (average age = 51 years) with typical reflux symptoms. Approximately 1 in 5 patients smoked and 74% drank alcohol. Following 24-hour esophageal pH monitoring, all 74 patients then took esomeprazole 40 mg (Nexium) for 2 weeks, recording daily whether symptoms were suppressed. A positive response to the PPI test was considered to be a symptom association probability less than 95%, a symptom index of less than 50%, and a symptom severity index of less than 10%. These various outcomes are commonly used to evaluate GERD. The prevalence of GERD was 70% using the symptom association probability score, meaning that 70% of patients with refluxlike symptoms had GERD. The sensitivity of the PPI test was 91% (95% CI, 78%–96%) and the specificity was 26% (10%–49%). In this high prevalence population, the positive predictive value was 75% (62%–85%) and the negative predictive value was 54% (22%–81%). Using these results, the likelihood ratio for the PPI test was 1.2, similar to the likelihood ratio for the presence of typical symptoms.

Essential Evidence: Medicine that Matters, Edited by David Slawson, Allen Shaughnessy, Mark Ebell, and Henry Barry.

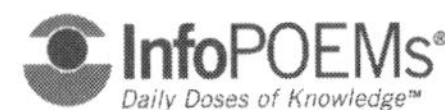

Lifestyle changes of little benefit in GERD

Clinical question

What lifestyle changes are effective in patients with gastroesophageal reflux disease?

Bottom line

Decreasing gastroesophageal reflux disease (GERD) symptoms with lifestyle changes requires an empirical approach; the research literature gives very little guidance regarding nondrug approaches. Neither smoking cessation, alcohol avoidance, nor any food avoidances have been shown to make, on average, a difference in symptoms, although existing studies are small and of poor quality. Elevating the head of the bed may be effective. Weight loss may also be effective. Of course, if patients find something that works, encourage them to continue doing it. (LOE = 3a–)

Reference

Kaltenbach T, Crockett S, Gerson LB. Are lifestyle measures effective in patients with gastroesophageal reflux disease? Arch Intern Med 2006;166:965–971.

Study Design

Systematic review

Funding

Foundation

Setting

Outpatient (any)

Synopsis

This systematic review assembled all English-language research on the value of lifestyle changes on the symptoms of GERD. Their search was severely flawed by limiting to only English-language articles and only searching one database back to the year 1975. Once the studies were identified, 2 authors independently reviewed every study; that is, they did not limit their review by quality of the study. Although smoking was associated with an increase in GERD symptoms, short-term (1–2 days) smoking cessation was not shown to decreased GERD symptoms in 3 low-quality studies. Alcohol use may or may not be associated with reflux symptoms. There is insufficient research supporting recommendations to abstain from citrus juices, carbonated beverages, coffee and caffeine, chocolate, spicy foods, fatty foods, or late evening meals. One study supports the effectiveness of raising the head of the bed, though other studies have not found a difference. Another study supported a wedge to elevate the head. Several studies have shown some association between weight loss or left lateral decubitus sleeping position and improved symptoms.

Essential Evidence: Medicine that Matters, Edited by David Slawson, Allen Shaughnessy, Mark Ebell, and Henry Barry.

All PPIs equivalent for treatment of GERD

Clinical question

Is there any difference between proton pump inhibitors for the treatment of gastroesophageal reflux disease?

Bottom line

There is no significant difference between equivalent doses of proton pump inhibitors, including equivalent doses of esomeprazole (Nexium) and omeprazole (Prilosec OTC). The decision to choose one over another should be based first on cost and second on individual patient response. (LOE = 1a)

Reference

Klok RM, Postma MJ, Van Hout BA, Brouwers JR. Meta-analysis: comparing the efficacy of proton pump inhibitors in short-term use. Aliment Pharmacol Ther 2003;17:1237–1245.

Study Design

Meta-analysis (randomized controlled trials)

Funding

Unknown/not stated

Setting

Various (meta-analysis)

Synopsis

This meta-analysis identified all double-blinded randomized controlled trials comparing one proton pump inhibitor with another for the treatment of gastroesphageal reflux disease (GERD), using endoscopic healing as the referece standard for treatment success. A total of 19 studies with more than 9000 patients were identified, most lasting 4 weeks. No difference in effectiveness was seen for the following comparisons: pantoprazole 40 mg vs omeprazole 20 mg; pantoprazole 20 mg vs omeprazole 20 mg; lansoprazole 30 mg vs omeprazole 20 mg; lansoprazole 15 mg vs omeprazole 20 mg; lansoprazole 30 mg vs omeprazole 40 mg; lansoprazole 30 mg vs pantoprazole 40 mg; rabeprazole 20 mg vs omeprazole 20 mg; rabeprazole 10 mg vs omeprazole 20 mg; and omeprazole 20 mg vs esomeprazole 20 mg. Only one comparison found a statistically significant difference between groups in the treatment of GERD: esomeprazole 40 mg vs omeprazole 20 mg (80% vs 67% response rate; P = .04; number needed to treat = 7). However, as noted above, a comparison in 1306 patients of equivalent doses of 20 mg esomeprazole vs 20 mg omeprazole found no difference in endoscopic healing. Furthermore, the response rates for omeprazole 20 mg in the 2 studies comparing it with esomeprazole 40 mg were 65% and 67% – considerably lower than in other comparisons looking at this dose, in which the success rate was between 70% and 91%. This would make esomeprazole look more effective in comparison. Thus, although this comparison has never been made directly, it seems very likely that 40 mg omeprazole ($38 per month over the counter) would be similar in effectiveness to 40 mg of esomeprazole ($124 per month).

Essential Evidence: Medicine that Matters, Edited by David Slawson, Allen Shaughnessy, Mark Ebell, and Henry Barry.

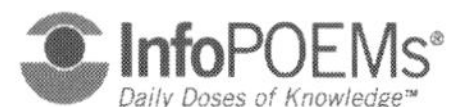

Acetaminophen does not affect liver function in alcoholics

Clinical question

Does acetaminophen affect liver function in alcoholic patients?

Bottom line

In this randomized, two-day study, 4 grams of acetaminophen per day did not affect liver function. These results do not rule out the possibility of acetaminophen-induced liver failure in alcoholic patients, especially those patients with pre-existing liver disease, but they cast doubt on the case reports that serve as the basis for this medical myth. (LOE = 1b)

Reference

Kuffer EK, Dart RC, Bogdan GM, Hill RE, Caper E, Darton L. Effect of maximal daily doses of acetaminophen on the liver of alcoholic patients. Arch Intern Med 2001;161:2247–2252.

Study Design

Randomized controlled trial (double-blinded)

Setting

Rehab unit

Synopsis

Medical myths, especially if they seem to make sense, seem to come alive and sometimes even achieve immortality. Acetaminophen toxicity in alcoholics is a newly hatched medical myth, nurtured by sketchy evidence, whose growth has been hard to arrest. The question is important, since, if we warn alcohol-using patients away from acetaminophen, chances are great that they will reach for a nonsteroidal antiinflammatory drug, which may have much more common adverse effects in this group. There are several ways to investigate this connection. One research method would be to try to determine chronic acetaminophen use in alcoholics and figure out which ones subsequently developed hepatic failure. Another method, which was used in this study, is to evaluate disease-oriented outcomes (change in liver function) in a group of patients and compare the results with patients receiving placebo. The invesigators of this study studied 201 people entering an alcohol detoxification facility. The enrolling investigator was not aware of the treatment to which the patient would be assigned (allocation was concealed). Alcoholics without evidence of liver dysfunction were given either placebo or acetaminophen 1 g four times a day for two days. Liver function testing was performed on the second day and again after another two days to determine whether acetaminophen at this dose would have an effect. Liver enzyme concentrations changed over baseline in both groups but were not different between the patients receiving placebo or actaminophen. A similar number of patients in both groups developed a short-lived increase in liver enzymes.

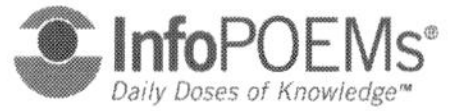

Evaluation of abnormal liver chemistries

Clinical question

What is the best approach to evaluation of the patient with abnormal liver chemistries?

Bottom line

Algorithms based on expert opinion are presented for the evaluation of abnormal liver chemistry tests. (LOE = 5)

Reference

AGA Clinical Practice Committee. AGA medical position statement: evaluation of liver chemistry tests. Gastroenterology 2002;123:1364–1366.

Study Design

Practice guideline

Setting

Other

Synopsis

This is not an evidence-based guideline. Since there are no clinical trials comparing different management strategies, we don't have much high-quality evidence on which to base such a guideline. They recommend that patients with a mild elevation in the alanine aminotransferase or aspartate aminotransferase (less than 5 times the upper limit of normal) have a careful history and physical examination and discontinue any hepatotoxic medications or alcohol consumption. Consider repeating the liver chemistries if laboratory error is suspected. If the diagnosis remains unclear, the following set of tests is recommended: liver chemistries, prothrombin time, albumin, complete blood count with platelets, hepatitis A, B and C serologies (HAV-IgM, HBsAg, HBcIgM, HCV antibody or HCV-RNA), serum iron, total iron binding capacity, and ferritin. Positive serologies require further laboratory evaluation. Asymptomatic patients with negative serology and without hepatic decompensation should discontinue alcohol, hepatotoxic drugs, lose weight, and improve diabetic control, then repeat chemistries in 6 months. Patients with negative serology and a higher index of suspicion should be considered for ultrasound, antinuclear antibody, anti-smooth muscle antibody, ceruloplasmin, and alpha-1-antitrypsin. Patients with an abnormal alkaline phosphatase should undergo an ultrasound if they have abnormal liver chemistries, or a gamma glutamyl transferase (GGT) if the results are normal. If the GGT result is abnormal, they should have an ultrasound, review of medications, and antimicrosomal antibody. Patients with an abnormal serum bilirubin should have a history and physical examination and liver chemistries first. Patients with unconjugated bilirubin and normal alkaline phosphatase and chemistries should have hemolysis studies and a review of medications; many will have Gilbert's syndrome. Patients with a conjugated hyperbilirubinemia or abnormal alkaline phosphatase and liver chemistries should have an ultrasound. If ductal dilitation is seen, they should have endoscopic retrograde cholangio-pancreatography or magnetic resonance cholangio-pancreatography.

Essential Evidence: Medicine that Matters, Edited by David Slawson, Allen Shaughnessy, Mark Ebell, and Henry Barry.

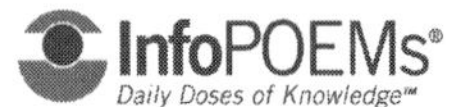

Enteral nutrition preferred in pancreatitis

Clinical question

Should parenteral nutrition be used preferentially over enteral nutrition in patients with acute pancreatitis?

Bottom line

Nasojejunal enteral nutrition in patients with acute pancreatitis results in fewer infections, surgical interventions, and possibly shorter hospital stays than parenteral nutrition. (LOE = 1b−)

Reference

Marik PE, Zaloga GP. Meta-analysis of parenteral nutrition versus enteral nutrition in patients with acute pancreatitis. BMJ 2004;328:1407–1410.

Study Design

Meta-analysis (randomized controlled trials)

Setting

Various (meta-analysis)

Synopsis

Total gut rest has been the standard for patients with acute pancreatitis, with parenteral nutrition used when needed. This meta-analysis combined the results of 6 studies, enrolling a total of 263 patients, that compared enteral and parenteral nutrition with regard to effectiveness and safety. The authors conducted an appropriate search for research trials, with 2 authors independently searching 4 databases. They examined bibliographies of identified articles were examined and queried experts. Results from the studies were independently extracted by 2 authors from the trials. Four of the 6 studies were of low quality (Jadad score = <3). Enteral nutrition via nasojejunal tube produced superior results, with significantly fewer infections (relative risk [RR] = 0.45; number needed to treat = 7; 95% CI, 5–16). Complications other than infections were not different between the 2 modes of nutrition. The need for surgical interventions, evaluated in 4 studies, were significantly less in patients fed enterally (RR = 0.48; 95% CI, .23–.99). Length of hospital stay, overall, was shorter in the enteral nutrition group, though there was significant heterogeneity among the studies. Mortality was similar in the 2 groups. Why is nasojejunal enteral nutrition better? Enteral nutrition prevents atrophy of gut lymphoid tissue, bacterial overgrowth in the intestine, and increased intestinal permeability, while the jejunal delivery results in little increase in enzyme output from the pancreas.

Essential Evidence: Medicine that Matters, Edited by David Slawson, Allen Shaughnessy, Mark Ebell, and Henry Barry.

Antibiotic prophylaxis reduces mortality in hospitalized cirrhotics

Clinical question

Does antibiotic prophylaxis improve outcomes in hospitalized cirrhotic patients?

Bottom line

Antibiotic prophylaxis reduces the risk of death in hospitalized cirrhotic patients. (LOE = 1a)

Reference

Soares-Weiser K, Brezis M, Tur-Kaspa R, et al. Antibiotic prophylaxis of bacterial infections in cirrhotic inpatients: a meta-analysis of randomized controlled trials. Scand J Gastroenterol 2003;38:193–200.

Study Design

Meta-analysis (randomized controlled trials)

Setting

Inpatient (any location)

Synopsis

Cirrhotic patients often develop nosocomial bacterial infections, most often urinary tract infections, peritonitis, pneumonia, and primary bacteremia. In this excellent systematic review, the authors carefully searched the literature for relevant placebo-controlled randomized trials, and identified 13 of them. Trials varied in duration of follow-up from hospitalization only to 12 months; antibiotics used included cefotaxime, ciprofloxacin, norfloxacin, imipenem, and several combinations; and only 5 of 13 reported adequate concealment of allocation. The latter is a very important characteristic of good clinical trials; not concealing allocation tends to signficantly overestimate treatment effects. Inclusion criteria varied: some studies included cirrhotic patients with low-protein ascitic fluid, and others included cirrhotic patients with gastrointestinal bleeding. When combining data for all studies, the authors found a significant benefit of antibiotic prophylaxis on all-cause mortality (relative risk = 0.70; 95% CI, 0.56–0.89). In terms of absolute risk, the pooled mortality rate was 15.9% in the antibiotic group and 21.6% in the placebo or no treatment group (absolute risk reduction = 5.7%; P = .003, number needed to treat = 17.5). The benefit was consistent across groups with differing inclusion criteria, with or without adequate allocation concealment, with or without exclusions after randomization, and with different durations of follow-up and disease severity. Although quinolones were the most widely used drugs, the authors were unable to draw conclusions regarding dose or duration of treatment. Doses studied included ciprofloxacin 500 mg per day, norfloxacin 800 mg per day, and norfloxacin 400 mg per day.

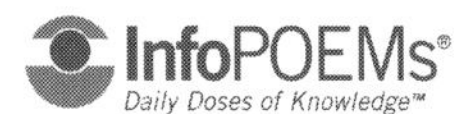

Many unnecessary Pap smears are performed after hysterectomy

Clinical question

How often are women undergoing Pap smear screening even though they are not at risk of cervical cancer?

Bottom line

Many American women who have had a hysterectomy with removal of the cervix for benign disease continue to undergo routine Papanicolaou (Pap) test despite a lack of supporting evidence and a clear recommendation from the United States Preventive Services Task Force against routine screening. Conversely, the vast majority of American women who die from cervical cancer were either underscreened or never screened for cervical disease, most likely as a result of real or perceived cost barriers. The money saved by not inappropriately performing Pap tests on low-risk women would pay for the cost of screening the 17 million women in the United States who are currently underscreened for cervical cancer (J Womens Health and Gender Based Med 2002;11:103–9.). (LOE = 2b)

Reference

Sirovich BE, Welch HG. Cervical cancer screening among women without a cervix. JAMA 2004;291:2990–2993.

Study Design

Cross-sectional

Setting

Population-based

Synopsis

Since 1996, the United States Preventive Services Task Force has suggested that routine Pap tests are unnecessary for women who have undergone hysterectomy with removal of the cervix for benign disease, placing them no longer at risk of cervical cancer. Many clinicians still perform Pap tests on these women, purportedly to screen for vaginal cancer. Since the risk of vaginal cancer is so low, however, women currently screened for cervical cancer with an intact cervix are not routinely screened for vaginal cancer. To determine the frequency of inappropriate screening, the authors used data from a survey conducted by the Centers for Disease Control and Prevention from 1992 to 2002 reporting the proportion of women with a hysterectomy who had a subsequent Pap test within 3 years. During this 10-year period, 22 million US women 18 years of age and older underwent hysterectomy, representing 21% of the population. The proportion of these women reporting a subsequent Pap test within 3 years before (68.5%) and 3 years after (69.1%) the Task Force recommendations in 1996 did not change. The authors estimate that half these women had hysterectomies that spared the cervix or were performed for cervical neoplasia, resulting in almost 10 million women being screened unnecessarily.

Essential Evidence: Medicine that Matters, Edited by David Slawson, Allen Shaughnessy, Mark Ebell, and Henry Barry.

Specific HPV strain are associated with cervical cancer risk

Clinical question

Do some oncogenic strains of HPV confer more risk of severe dysplasia or cancer than others?

Bottom line

Human papillomavirus (HPV) testing results that are positive for types 16 or 18 are associated with a 14% to 17% risk of cervical intraepithelial neoplasia 3 (CIN3) or greater over the following 10 years. Other oncogenic types are associated with a much lower risk (approximately 3%), and for women who test negative for HPV the risk is less than 1%. (LOE = 1b)

Reference

Khan MJ, Castle PE, Lorincz AT, et al. The elevated 10-year risk of cervical precancer and cancer in women with human papillomavirus (HPV) type 16 or 18 and the possible utility of type-specific HPV testing in clinical practice. J Natl Cancer Inst 2005;97:1072–1079.

Study Design

Cohort (prospective)

Funding

Unknown/not stated

Allocation

Concealed

Setting

Outpatient (any)

Synopsis

Essentially all cervical cancers are associated with HPV infection. HPV testing by Hybrid Capture 2 was performed in this cohort study of almost 21,000 women, and outcomes of CIN3 or greater within the next 10 years were determined. Women were categorized as positive for HPV16 (n = 455), positive for HPV18 (n = 154), positive for 1 of 11 other HPV oncogenic subtypes (n = 2211), or negative. Seventeen percent of women with HPV16 were given a diagnosis of CIN3 or greater over the next 10 years; 14% of those with HPV18; 3% of those with other oncogenic types; and 0.8% of those who were HPV negative. For the almost 13,000 women older than 30 years with negative cytology at baseline and a negative HPV result, only 0.5% had CIN3 or greater over the following 10 years.

Essential Evidence: Medicine that Matters, Edited by David Slawson, Allen Shaughnessy, Mark Ebell, and Henry Barry.

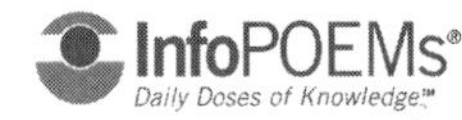

Vaccine effective against HPV

Clinical question

Is a vaccine effective against human papillomavirus strains associated with cervical cancer?

Bottom line

A bivalent vaccine against human papillomavirus (HPV) types 16 and 18 is well-tolerated and effective in reducing HPV infection and HPV-associated cytologic abnormalities. What we need now is a larger, longer-termed, adequately powered study to look at the effect of this vaccine on the development of cervical cancer. (LOE = 1b)

Reference

Harper DM, Franco EL, Wheeler C, et al. Efficacy of a bivalent L1 virus-like particle vaccine in prevention of infection with human papillomavirus types 16 and 18 in young women: a randomised controlled trial. Lancet 2004;364:1757–1765.

Study Design

Randomized controlled trial (double-blinded)

Funding

Industry

Allocation

Concealed

Setting

Population-based

Synopsis

This team of researchers randomly assigned healthy women aged 15 to 25 years with no more than 6 sexual partners and no history of condyloma or cervical cancer to receive a bivalent vaccine active against HPV serotypes 16 and 18 or placebo. They administered the vaccine or placebo at 0, 1, and 6 months. They evaluated the patients after 27 months to determine the presence of HPV infection or cytologic abnormalities. Using an intention-to-treat approach to these outcomes, the vaccine was 95% effective against persistent HPV infection and 93% effective against cytologic abnormalities associated with HPV. In the intention-to-treat analysis, the absolute reduction in new HPV infections was 6.4% (number needed to treat [NNT] = 16) and 3.5% for persistent infections (NNT = 29). Other than local injection site symptoms, there were no differences in side effects between the active and placebo vaccines.

Essential Evidence: Medicine that Matters, Edited by David Slawson, Allen Shaughnessy, Mark Ebell, and Henry Barry.

Bivalent vaccine against HPV effective for 4.5 years

Clinical question

Does a vaccine confer long-term protection against human papillomavirus strains associated with cervical cancer?

Bottom line

A bivalent vaccine against human papillomavirus (HPV) types 16 and 18 is well-tolerated and effective in reducing HPV infection and HPV-associated cytologic abnormalities for 4.5 years. (LOE = 1b)

Reference

Harper DM, Franco EL, Wheeler CM, et al, for the HPV Vaccine Study group. Sustained efficacy up to 4.5 years of a bivalent L1 virus-like particle vaccine against human papillomavirus types 16 and 18: follow-up from a randomised control trial. Lancet 2006;367:1247–1255.

Study Design

Randomized controlled trial (double-blinded)

Funding

Industry

Allocation

Concealed

Setting

Population-based

Synopsis

We previously reviewed the initial report from this study (Lancet 2004;364:1757–65) that demonstrated after 27 months that a bivalent vaccine active against HPV serotypes 16 and 18 was more effective than placebo in reducing HPV infection and HPV-associated cytologic abnormalities. In this study, the investigators provide additional follow-up on 776 of 1113 women from the original study who received all 3 doses of vaccine or placebo, and for whom treatment allocation remained double blinded. In the original study, women were eligible if they were 15 to 25 years old, had no more than 6 sexual partners and had no history of condyloma or cervical cancer. They administered the vaccine or placebo at 0, 1, and 6 months. In the intention-to-treat analysis for the subsequent follow-up period, the absolute reduction in new HPV infections was 7.4% (number needed to treat [NNT] = 14; 95% CI, 10–23). If you combine the results for events occurring during the initial study period with the results from this follow-up period, the absolute reduction is 13.7% (NNT = 8; 6–10). Furthermore, no vaccinated woman developed HPV 16/18-associated CIN1 or worse (and only 2 developed HPV 16/18-associated ASCUS) compared with 1.7% of those receiving placebo (NNT = 59; 30–182). Interestingly, this vaccine also appeared to have some cross-protection against HPV 45 and HPV 31. Additional data and analyses are needed to understand the mechanisms of cross-protection and its importance to lesion development. Finally, the vaccine was well-tolerated. A total of 14% of those vaccinated reported at least one adverse side effect compared with 22% of those receiving placebo; 3% reported at least one new onset chronic disease compared with 5% taking placebo; and 4% reported at least one serious adverse event compared with 5% taking placebo.

Essential Evidence: Medicine that Matters, Edited by David Slawson, Allen Shaughnessy, Mark Ebell, and Henry Barry.

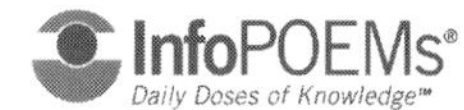

Liquid-based not better than conventional Pap

Clinical question

Is liquid-based cytology better than conventional cytology in detecting high-grade cervical disease?

Bottom line

High-quality studies fail to demonstrate that liquid-based cervical cytology is more reliable or more accurate at detecting high-grade abnormalities than conventional cytology. (LOE = 2a)

Reference

Davey E, Barratt A, Irwig L, et al. Effect of study design and quality on unsatisfactory rates, cytology classifications, and accuracy in liquid-based versus conventional cervical cytology: a systematic review. Lancet 2006;367:122–132.

Study Design

Systematic review

Funding

Government

Setting

Outpatient (any)

Synopsis

These authors searched MEDLINE and EMBASE to find studies that directly assessed liquid-based cytology and conventional cytology in cervical cancer screening. The studies had to have used a manual review of the slides rather than automated screening systems. The team also reviewed the bibliographies of included studies to find additional candidates. They didn't look for unpublished studies. Since positive results of novel technologies and interventions are more likely to be published, this raises the possibility of bias in favor of liquid-based cytology. Two reviewers independently assessed study eligibility with discrepancies resolved by consensus. Additionally, 2 reviewers independently assessed the methodologic validity of the studies. These reviewers were blinded to the study results. The 56 eligible studies included more than 1.2 million slides. The quality of the studies was generally poor and only two thirds used a gold standard. None of the studies were ideal and only 5 were considered high quality. There was no significant difference in the rate of unsatisfactory smears, especially in larger studies. Overall, the rates of cytologic abnormalities were similar; in the high-quality studies, however, conventional cytology was more likely to detect high-grade cervical lesions. If there was significant publication bias, it is more likely that this systematic review would make liquid-based cytology would look better.

Endometrial sampling adequate for diagnosing endometrial cancer

Clinical question

Is endometrial sampling a suitable substitute for D & C for the diagnosis of endometrial cancer in postmenopausal women?

Bottom line

Outpatient endometrial sampling is a highly accurate diagnostic test for endometrial cancer when compared with D & C. In the hands of the clinicians participating in the studies included in this meta-analysis, an inadequate sample could be considered a negative test result. It is uncertain whether that conclusion is generalizable to other clinicians. (LOE = 1a)

Reference

Clark TJ, Mann CH, Shah N, Khan KS, Song F, Gupta JK. Accuracy of outpatient endometrial biopsy in the diagnosis of endometrial cancer: a systematic quantitative review. Br J Obstet Gynecol 2002;109:313–321.

Study Design

Meta-analysis (other)

Setting

Various (meta-analysis)

Synopsis

This was a meta-analysis of 11 studies of endometrial sampling as diagnostic test for endometrial cancer. The methodology was top notch. Summary likelihood ratios were calculated as measures of diagnostic accuracy. Six brands of devices were represented, of which the most common was the Pipelle device (n = 7 studies). Postmenopausal women represented 79% of the populations studied. The reference (gold) standard was most often dilatation and curettage (D & C), though hysterectomy and directed biopsy were accepted in some studies. In all included studies the reference standard procedure was performed regardless of endometrial biopsy results. The biggest weakness of the group of studies was lack of reporting of blinding (9 of the 11). For adequate endometrial samples, the pooled likelihood ratios for endometrial cancer were 66.48 (95% CI, 30.04–147.13) for a positive test result and 0.14 (95% CI, 0.08–0.27) for a negative test result. The pretest probability of endometrial cancer was 6.3%. It increased to 81.7% with a positive test result, and decreased to 0.9% with a negative test result. If inadequate samples were considered as negative test results, the results were even more accurate.

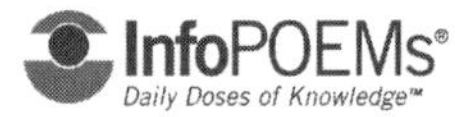

Avoid nonoxynol-9 spermicides with less than 100g per dose

Clinical question

Are any commercially available nonoxynol-9 containing spermicides more effective than others to prevent pregnancy?

Bottom line

Nonoxynol-9 spermicide preparations vary in their contraceptive effectiveness. The low-dose gel preparation with 52.5g nonoxynol-9 per dose was significantly less effective than the other preparations. In the U.S., Encare Inserts and Gynol II are among the contraceptive products containing at least 100g of nonoxynol-9. (LOE = 2b)

Reference

Raymond EG, Chen PL, Luoto J. Contraceptive effectiveness and safety of five nonoxynol-9 spermicides: a randomized trial. Obstet Gynecol 2004;103:430–439.

Study Design

Randomized controlled trial (nonblinded)

Setting

Outpatient (primary care)

Synopsis

Nonoxynol-9 spermicides are widely available over the counter. Head-to-head comparisons of contraceptive effectiveness in a randomized trial had not previously been undertaken. For this study, women were randomized (allocation concealed) to 1 of 5 nonoxynol-9 preparations: (1) 52.5g gel; (2) 100g gel; (3) 150g gel; (4) 100g film; and (5) 100g suppository. Study groups each included 295 to 300 women. Characteristics of the women were similar between groups, including age distribution, parity, education level, and intention to have children in the future. The proportion of women who relied on spermicide exclusively as contraception was similar between groups (46%–52%). Loss to follow-up was also similar between groups (20%–25%). Pregnancy rates in 6 months for typical use were 22%, 15%, 14%, 12%, and 10% respectively. (Typical use was defined as relying primarily on spermicide for contraception.) Only the lowest dose gel (52.5g) had a pregnancy rate that was statistically different from any others. Perfect use pregnancy rates were 16%, 8%, 9%, 7%, and 5%, respectively. (Perfect use was defined as patient agreement that she used only the assigned spermicide as her method of contraception with each coitus and inserted it into the vagina before coitus as indicated by the manufacturer's instructions.) There were no differences between preparations for adverse events of vulvovaginal candidiasis, bacterial vaginosis, vulvovaginal irritation without infection, urinary tract infections, or partner side effects. The study was not large enough to determine whether the 4% to 5% greater pregnancy rates between the higher dose gels, film, and suppository was real.

Metformin increases fertility in PCOS

Clinical question

Is metformin (Glucophage, Metforal) more effective than clomiphene (Clomid, Serophene) for improving fertility in nonobese women with polycystic ovary syndrome?

Bottom line

In nonobese women with polycystic ovary syndrome, metformin is more effective than clomiphene for improving the rate of conception. (LOE = 1b)

Reference

Palomba S, Orio F Jr, Falbo A, et al. Prospective parallel randomized, double-blind, double-dummy controlled clinical trial comparing clomiphene citrate and metformin as the first-line treatment for ovulation induction in nonobese anovulatory women with polycystic ovary syndrome. J Clin Endocrinol Metab 2005;90:4068–4074.

Study Design

Randomized controlled trial (double-blinded)

Funding

Unknown/not stated

Allocation

Concealed

Setting

Outpatient (any)

Synopsis

Metformin (Glucophage, Metforal) and clomiphene (Clomid, Serophene) have each been used to increase fertility in women with polycystic ovary syndrome: This is the first study to evaluate them head-to-head. One hundred women between the ages of 20 and 34 years with a body mass index of less than 30 were randomly assigned (masked allocation) to receive metformin 850 mg twice daily or clomiphene 150 mg 3 times daily. Each patient also received placebos of the opposite drug. Before starting the medications, the patients received a progesterone challenge, and medication was then started on the third day of progesterone-induced menstruation. The main outcome, pregnancy rate, was assessed via intention to treat. Five patients receiving metformin and 3 receiving clomiphene dropped out and weren't included in the analysis. At the end of 6 months of treatment, 31 patients (69%) taking metformin became pregnant compared with 16 (34%) taking clomiphene. If all the patients lost to follow-up in the clomiphene group became pregnant and none of those taking metformin did, the pregnancy rate would still be significantly higher with metformin. We would need to treat 3 women with metformin instead of clomiphene for 6 months for 1 additional woman to become pregnant (95% CI, 1.9–6.9). The rate of side effects was similar in each group (approximately 20%) and 1 patient in each group dropped out because of side effects.

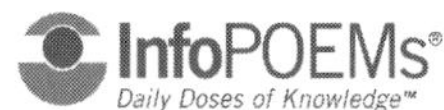

HRT with estrogen alone increases stroke, decreases fractures

Clinical question

Is hormone replacement therapy with estrogen alone beneficial for postmenopausal women with hysterectomy?

Bottom line

Estrogen replacement therapy in postmenopausal women with hysterectomy increases the risk of stroke, has no effect on cardiovascular disease, prevents hip and vertebral fracture, and may or may not affect the likelihood of breast cancer-related deaths. On the basis of both the estrogen-progestin and estrogen-alone arms of the Women's Health Initiative study, it appears prudent to use hormone replacement therapy in postmenopausal women only for significant menopausal symptoms at the smallest effective dose for the shortest possible time. Treatment for up to 4 or 5 years early in menopause appears to offer the greatest amount of osteoporosis and fracture prevention. Don't forget to recommend high-dose vitamin D and calcium. (LOE = 1b)

Reference

Women's Health Initiative Steering Committee. Effects of conjugated equine estrogen in postmenopausal women with hysterectomy. The Women's Health Initiative randomized controlled trial. JAMA 2004;291:1701–1712.

Study Design

Randomized controlled trial (double-blinded)

Setting

Outpatient (any)

Synopsis

The Women's Health Initiative estrogen plus progestin trial was stopped early when women in the treatment group were found to be at an increased risk of coronary events, stroke, breast cancer, and pulmonary embolism. Benefits of the therapy included a reduced risk of hip fracture and colon cancer. This paper summarizes the results from the estrogen-alone trial of 10,739 healthy women with hysterectomy, aged 50 to 79 years, who were randomly assigned in a double-blind fashion (concealed allocation) to receive either 0.625 mg per day of conjugated equine estrogen or placebo. Outcomes were assigned by individuals blinded to treatment group assignment. Follow-up for an average of 6.8 years was complete for 98% of participants. Using intention-to-treat analysis, estrogen alone compared with placebo increased the risk of stroke (hazard ratio (HR) = 1.39; 95% CI, 1.10–1.77; number needed to treat to harm = 12/10,000 person-years), but had no significant effect on the risk of pulmonary embolus, coronary heart disease, colorectal cancer, or all-cause mortality. Benefits of estrogen alone included a reduced risk of hip fracture (HR = 0.61; 95% CI, 0.41–0.91; number needed to treat = 6/10,000 person-years) and total fractures (HR = 0.70; 95% CI, 0.63–0.79). The risk of breast cancer in women using estrogen alone was lower (23%), but not significantly (HR = 0.77; 95% CI, 0.59–1.01). The power of the study to determine a 20% difference between the 2 groups was less than 80%. A high degree of noncompliance with estrogen (more than 50% by the seventh year) further reduced the power and may underestimate the true harms and benefits of treatment. The mean age of women in the trial was 63 years, so the results may not apply to women treated early in menopause.

Essential Evidence: Medicine that Matters, Edited by David Slawson, Allen Shaughnessy, Mark Ebell, and Henry Barry.

Clonidine, gabapentin, and some SSRIs effective for hot flashes

Clinical question

Which nonhormonal therapies are effective in the management of menopausal hot flashes?

Bottom line

Evidence supports the nonhormonal treatment of menopausal hot flashes with paroxetine (Paxil), clonidine (Catapres), gabapentin (Neurontin), and soy isoflavone extract. The overall effect size of all nonhormonal treatments is less than that of estrogen. Treatment should be individualized according to symptom severity and risk profiles. (LOE = 1a–)

Reference

Nelson HD, Vesco KK, Haney E, et al. Nonhormonal therapies for menopausal hot flashes. Systematic review and meta-analysis. JAMA 2006;295:2057–2071.

Study Design

Meta-analysis (randomized controlled trials)

Funding

Unknown/not stated

Setting

Various (meta-analysis)

Synopsis

Recent concerns about adverse effects of hormonal therapy has increased interest in alternative treatments of menopausal hot flashes. These investigators thoroughly searched MEDLINE, The Cochrane Registry, other large databases, reference lists of recent systematic reviews and relevant articles, and they consulted experts. To be included, studies must be English-language randomized double-blind placebo-controlled trials evaluating the treatment of menopausal hot flashes with nonhormonal interventions. Two reviewers independently rated the quality of trials; disagreements were resolved by consensus agreement with a third reviewer. Formal assessment found no evidence of publication bias. A total of 43 trials met inclusion criteria, including 10 trials of antidepressants, 10 of clonidine, 6 of other prescribed medications, and 17 of isoflavone extracts. Among various antidepressants, high-quality studies supported only the efficacy of paroxetine (Paxil). Of the 10 trials comparing clonidine with placebo, only 3 met criteria for fair quality. Four of the 10 trials reported a reduced hot flash frequency with clonidine compared with placebo and 6 found no difference, with the overall meta-analysis reporting a small benefit. The efficacy of clonidine is strongest in women taking tamoxifen for breast cancer. Two fair-quality trials of gabapentin (Neurontin) reported significantly reduced hot flash frequency compared with placebo. Only 1 of 6 trials of red clover isoflavones reported reduced hot flash frequency compared with placebo. Soy isoflavones were compared with placebo in 11 trials, mostly of poor quality. Although the results were heterogeneous, overall results showed that soy isoflavone extract was significantly better than placebo.

Essential Evidence: Medicine that Matters, Edited by David Slawson, Allen Shaughnessy, Mark Ebell, and Henry Barry.

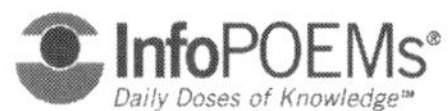

Black cohosh ineffective for vasomotor symptoms

Clinical question

Do soy, black cohosh, or a naturopathic multibotanical provide greater relief from vasomotor symptoms than placebo in menopausal or perimenopausal women?

Bottom line

Neither soy, black cohosh, or a naturopathic multibotanical was effective in decreasing the duration or severity of vasomotor symptoms. These results are similar to other research findings. (LOE = 1b)

Reference

Newton KM, Reed SD, LaCroix AZ, Grothaus LC, Ehrlich K, Guiltinan J. Treatment of vasomotor symptoms of menopause with black cohosh, multibotanicals, soy, hormone therapy, or placebo. Ann Intern Med 2006;145:869–879.

Study Design

Randomized controlled trial (double-blinded)

Funding

Government

Allocation

Concealed

Setting

Outpatient (any)

Synopsis

Women in this US study were members of a managed care organization and were recruited by mail. The 351 women were perimenopausal or menopausal and had at least 2 menopausal symptoms daily, with at least 6 moderate to severe symptoms over a 2-week period. The women were randomly assigned, using concealed allocation, to receive 1 of the following treatments daily for 1 year: black cohosh 160 mg (Cimipure); a multibotanical frequently used by naturopaths (Progyne) containing black cohosh and 9 other products; the same multibotanical with dietary soy counseling; conjugated estrogens 0.625 mg; or placebo. Analysis was by intention to treat. Vasomotor symptoms per day, symptom intensity, or scores on the Wiklund Vasomotor Symptom Subscale did not differ between herbal interventions and placebo at 3, 6, or 12 months or on average over all follow-up points. However, symptom intensity was significantly worse for patients treated with the multibotanical plus soy diet at 1 year ($P = .016$). This small study was designed to find a effect of herbs halfway between the expected effects of hormone and placebo therapy, and small changes in symptoms conceivably could have been missed. However, none of the treatments approached the effectiveness of estrogen therapy.

Essential Evidence: Medicine that Matters, Edited by David Slawson, Allen Shaughnessy, Mark Ebell, and Henry Barry.

Acupuncture ineffective for hot flashes

Clinical question
Is acupuncture an effective treatment for perimenopausal and postmenopausal hot flashes?

Bottom line
Acupuncture is not an effective treatment for menopausal hot flashes. (LOE = 1b)

Reference
Vincent A, Barton DL, Mandrekar JN, et al. Acupuncture for hot flashes: randomized, sham-controlled clinical study. Menopause 2007;14:45–52.

Study Design
Randomized controlled trial (single-blinded)

Funding
Foundation

Allocation
Uncertain

Setting
Outpatient (specialty)

Synopsis
In this single-blinded study, 103 perimenopausal and postmenopausal women aged 45 years to 59 years were randomized to acupuncture or sham procedure twice weekly for 5 weeks. Perimenopausal status was defined as menstrual irregularity or amenorrhea for at least 3 months, and postmenopausal status as amenorrhea for at least 12 months. Women were eligible if they reported at least 5 hot flashes daily and were not taking estrogen, soy, progesterone, vitamin E, black cohosh, gabapentin, or antidepressants used for treating hot flashes. Other exclusion criteria were the use of coumadin, certain skin disorders, the presence of a pacemaker or prosthetic joint, diabetic neuropathy, and active chemotherapy. A single acupuncturist with more than 5000 hours experience provided the treatments. Women used a daily diary to note the number of hot flashes and the severity of each (from 1 [mild] to 3 [severe]). The sum of the severity scores for each hot flash provided a daily hot flash score. The authors used survival curve statistics with an intention-to-treat analysis, and performed an appropriate power analysis. There were no differences between groups at baseline, 6 weeks, or 12 weeks.

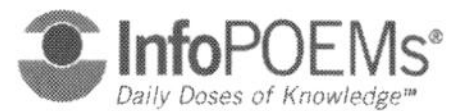

HRT increases risk of stress, urge urinary incontinence

Clinical question

Can hormone replacement therapy decrease the risk of urinary incontinence in postmenopausal women?

Bottom line

Despite what we learned about the beneficial effects of menopausal hormone therapy on reversing urethral and bladder mucosal atrophy, postmenopausal women using either estrogen alone or estrogen plus progestin are at an increased risk of both stress and urge urinary incontinence. (LOE = 1b)

Reference

Hendrix SL, Cochrane BB, Nygaard IE, et al. Effects of estrogen with and without progestin on urinary incontinence. JAMA 2005;293:935–948.

Study Design

Randomized controlled trial (double-blinded)

Funding

Government

Allocation

Concealed

Setting

Outpatient (any)

Synopsis

As predicted, more spin-off studies are coming from the Women's Health Initiative (WHI) multicenter clinical trial of hormone therapy in postmenopausal women. These investigators randomized 27,347 postmenopausal women aged 50 to 79 years to active treatment (estrogen alone or estrogen plus progestin) or placebo. The randomization (concealed allocation assignment) was based on hysterectomy status. Outcomes were assessed by individuals blinded to treatment group assignment. Follow-up was available at 1 year for 96% of the women. Using intention-to-treat analysis, menopausal hormone replacement therapy with estrogen alone or estrogen plus progestin increased the risk for both urge urinary incontinence (14% vs 13%; number needed to treat to harm [NNTH] = 100) and stress urinary incontinence (17% vs 9%; NNTH = 13; 95% CI, 10–15) compared with placebo, respectively.

Essential Evidence: Medicine that Matters, Edited by David Slawson, Allen Shaughnessy, Mark Ebell, and Henry Barry.

Weekly fluconazole reduces recurrent candidiasis, though costly

Clinical question

Is prophylactic oral fluconazole a safe and effective way to prevent the recurrence of vulvovaginal candidiasis?

Bottom line

A weekly oral dose of 150 mg fluconazole reduces the risk of recurrent vulvovaginal candidiasis. We need a study comparing the efficacy and acceptability of this expensive therapy with the treatment of symptomatic recurrences only or with prophylactic use of vaginal antimycotics, particularly since fluconazole is associated with a number of important drug interactions. (LOE = 1b)

Reference

Sobel JD, Wiesenfeld HC, Martens M, et al. Maintenance fluconazole therapy for recurrent vulvovaginal candidiasis. N Engl J Med 2004;351:876–883.

Study Design	Funding	Allocation	Setting
Randomized controlled trial (double-blinded)	Industry	Uncertain	Outpatient (any)

Synopsis

In this study, the investigators identified and enrolled 427 women who presented with an episode of vulvovaginal candidiasis and a history of at least 4 such episodes in the previous year. The women were given 3 oral doses of fluconazole (Diflucan) 150 mg at 3-day intervals and were re-examined after 2 weeks. Patients were excluded if they had a negative fungal yeast culture at the time of enrollment (n = 26), or if they dropped out (n = 5), were lost to follow-up (n = 3), suffered adverse effects (n = 4), violated the study protocol (n = 7), or were not clinically cured by the initial open-label treatment (n = 9). Thus, the investigators selected a group of women who definitely had a vulvovaginal yeast infection, were compliant, and whose yeast infection responded well to fluconazole. The remaining 373 women were randomly assigned to receive either oral fluconazole 150 mg once weekly or matching placebo for 6 months, followed by a 6-month untreated observation phase. They were evaluated monthly during the first 6 months and at months 9 and 12. Results are only reported for the efficacy analysis, but the authors assure us that they were similar for the intention-to-treat analysis. The treated women had fewer recurrences during the 6 months they received weekly treatment. The difference was relatively small in the first month after the initial open-label treatment (3.6% vs 14.9%) and increased gradually until the sixth month (9.2% vs 64.1%; $P < 0.001$; absolute risk reduction = 54.9%; number needed to treat = 2). However, the benefit waned once the drug was discontinued. During the second (untreated) 6-month period, more episodes of vulvovaginal candidiasis were seen in patients who had previously taken fluconazole than in women in the control group. The median time to symptomatic recurrence was 10.2 months for fluconazole and 4 months for placebo. Treatment was generally well tolerated, although it is important to keep in mind that azoles are potent CYP3A inhibitors, and a recent report (N Engl J Med 2004; 351:1089–96) reminds us that their use with erythromycin is associated with a significant increase in the risk of sudden cardiac death.

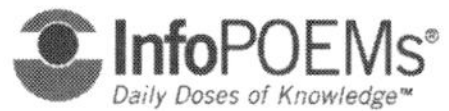

Lactobacillus doesn't prevent post-antibiotic vaginitis

Clinical question

Can lactobacillus preparations, whether given orally, vaginally, or both, prevent post-antibiotic vaginal candidiasis?

Bottom line

Lactobacillus, whether given orally, vaginally, or both, had no effect on the development of culture-proven vaginal candidiasis. Lactobacillus probiotics have been shown effective, however, in decreasing antibiotic-associated diarrhea (Aliment Pharmacol Ther 2002; 16:1461–67). (LOE = 1b)

Reference

Pirotta M, Gunn J, Chondros P, et al. Effect of lactobacillus in preventing post-antibiotic vulvovaginal candidiasis: a randomised controlled trial. BMJ 2004;329:548–551.

Study Design

Randomized controlled trial (double-blinded)

Allocation

Concealed

Setting

Outpatient (primary care)

Synopsis

Probiotics, commensal microorganisms given to antagonize the activity of pathogenic microorganisms, have been used to replace bacterial flora wiped out by antibiotics with the aim of preventing antibiotic-associated diarrhea or vaginal candidiasis. The investigators of this study evaluated the role of products containing Lactobacillus spp. to prevent vaginal candidiasis in 278 nonpregnant women who required a short course of antibiotics for a nongynecological infection. The actual antibiotics were not specified. The women were randomly assigned, using concealed allocation, to receive an oral powder containing Lactobacillus spp (Lactobac), a vaginal pessary containing Lactobacillus (Femilac), both treatments, or placebo. The women took the powder twice daily 20 minutes before meals and used one pessary at night for 10 nights during the 6-day course of antibiotics and for 4 days after. Viability of the lactobacilli was confirmed. Candida was cultured in 23% of women, a rate consistent with other research. There was no difference in the rate of vaginal candidiasis in women receiving one or both forms of probiotic or placebo. The study was stopped early because of lack of benefit.

Essential Evidence: Medicine that Matters, Edited by David Slawson, Allen Shaughnessy, Mark Ebell, and Henry Barry.

Anemia not prevented by iron in infants

Clinical question

Does prophylactic administration of iron prevent the development of anemia in infants?

Bottom line

Routine iron supplementation in infants, starting at 6 months of age, does not affect the prevalence of anemia when it is evaluated at the 9-month visit. Anemia in the infants in this study was related to maternal anemia during pregnancy, which was present in 43% of the mothers in this sample; the children were likely anemic since birth. (LOE = 1b)

Reference

Geltman PL, Meyers AF, Mehta SD, et al. Daily multivitamins with iron to prevent anemia in high-risk infants: a randomized clinical trial. Pediatrics 2004;114:86–93.

Study Design

Randomized controlled trial (double-blinded)

Setting

Outpatient (primary care)

Synopsis

The investigators of this study enrolled 376 healthy, full-term infants at their 6-month well visit. Approximately 90% of mothers received supplemental nutrition vouchers through the Special Supplemental Nutrition Program for Women, Infants, and Children, and 43% of the mothers were anemic during pregnancy. Iron status of the infants was not determined at this time. The children were randomized (allocation concealed) to receive a multivitamin with or without 10 mg of elemental iron for 3 months. Approximately 74% of the children were available 3 months to 6 months later for follow-up. At this visit, 84% of the children were either anemic (21% of total) or possibly iron deficient (defined by the number of indices, other than hemoglobin, that were abnormal). There was no statistical difference in the proportion of the children in either group who developed anemia, nor were there any differences in any specific anemia measure. The presence of anemia at ages 9 to 12 months was correlated with maternal anemia during pregnancy. The results were similar when including all patients, whether or not they were fully adherent to therapy (intention-to-treat analysis), or when analyzing only children who received iron daily. Since the children may have been anemic at the start of the study, another interpretation may be that 10 mg of iron is not sufficient to replete iron in anemic children.

Essential Evidence: Medicine that Matters, Edited by David Slawson, Allen Shaughnessy, Mark Ebell, and Henry Barry.

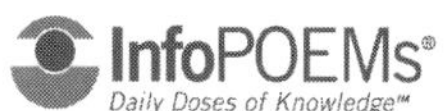

Anemia doesn't predict iron deficiency among toddlers

Clinical question

Does screening toddlers for anemia identify those with iron deficiency?

Bottom line

We cannot feel assured that a young child doesn't have iron deficiency if they show a normal hemoglobin level, and we can't be sure that he or she has iron deficiency anemia if the hemoglobin level is low. Screening for iron deficiency in toddlers by checking serum hemoglobin misses most children with a deficiency, and most of the children with anemia do not have an iron deficiency. (LOE = 1b)

Reference

White KC. Anemia is a poor predictor of iron deficiency among toddlers in the United States: For heme the bell tolls. Pediatrics 2005;115:315–320.

Study Design

Cohort (prospective)

Funding

Government

Setting

Population-based

Synopsis

An insufficent level of iron (which is used in more than 200 enzymes in the body) is associated with developmental disabilities in young children. Measuring serum hemoglobin as an indicator of anemia is used to screen for iron deficiency in young children. The author of this study evaluated the correlation between anemia and iron deficiency by examining the findings of the National Health and Nutrition Survey (NHANES) conducted between 1988 and 1994. The NHANES is a stratified population sample performed across the United States. The survey included 1289 toddlers between the ages of 12 and 35 months, and all of these children underwent complete blood counts, as well as measures of iron stores: ferritin, transferrin saturation, and free erythrocyte protoporphyrin. Iron deficiency, identified in 10.9% of the children studied, was defined as at least 2 of the iron indices being below normal. Anemia was defined as a hemoglobin level of less than 11.0 g/dL. There was little relation in this sample between the presence of iron deficiency and anemia. Children with iron deficiency had an average hemoglobin level of 11.5 g/dL, which, although statistically lower than the average 12.1 g/dL in nondeficient toddlers, was still above the cutoff for anemia. Only 28% (95% CI, 20–38) of toddlers with low hemoglobin actually had iron deficiency. The ability of anemia to rule out iron deficiency was also low: the sensitivity of the test was only 30% (95% CI, 20–40). In other words, for every 100 toddlers studied, 9 will have anemia, and 9 will have iron deficiency, but only 3 of the children with iron deficiency will be anemic and only 3 of the children with anemia will be iron deficient; not a great overlap. Similar results have been shown in data from New Zealand, Britain, and Europe (see the Discussion section of this study).

Essential Evidence: Medicine that Matters, Edited by David Slawson, Allen Shaughnessy, Mark Ebell, and Henry Barry.

Repeated blood testing causes anemia

Clinical question

Does phlebotomy contribute to changes in hemoglobin and hemotocrit levels in hospitalized patients?

Bottom line

The typical patient admitted for a 6-day admission will have 75 mL of blood drawn and this will drop his or her hemoglobin by 0.79 g/dL (7.9 g/L) and hematocrit by 2.1 percentage points. As a result, 1 in 6 patients will become anemic as a result of blood draws. (LOE = 2b)

Reference

Thavendiranathan P, Bagai A, Ebidia A, Detsky AS, Choudhry NK. Do blood tests cause anemia in hospitalized patients? J Gen Intern Med 2005;20:520–524.

Study Design

Cohort (retrospective)

Funding

Self-funded or unfunded

Setting

Inpatient (ward only)

Synopsis

The researchers conducting this study evaluated 404 patients hospitalized and cared for on an internal medicine service in Canada. The researchers identified all 989 admissions over a 6-month period, excluding any patients from analysis who had illnesses or were on medications that could possibly affect hemoglobin/hematocrit (H/H) levels or who did not have at least 2 H/H values during the admission. Blood volume during phlebotomy was determined by establishing the volume of blood obtained during a typical phlebotomy in the hospital and then by counting the number and types of blood tubes collected during hospitalization. The researchers also roughly accounted for hydration status in patients by evaluating the ratio of creatinine to blood urea nitrogen and calculating osmolality. The typical patient had approximately 75 mL of blood drawn over an average 5.6 days of hospitalization. On average, hemoglobin levels changed by 0.79 g/dL (7.9 g/L) during hospitalization (from 12.5 g/dL to 11.8 g/dL, 125.6 g/L to 117.6 g/L) and hematocrit levels changed an average of 2.1 percentage points ($P < .001$). During hospitalization, 1 in 6 (15.8%) patients became anemic and and 1 in 7 (13.9%) had some workup for anemia, such as iron studies or a fecal occult blood test. After controlling for a number of variables, including length of hospitalization, age, and hydration status, volume of phlebotomy was still associated with decreases in H/H. As a rough estimate, every routine laboratory test requiring 10 mL of blood will change hemoglobin levels by 0.07 g/dL (0.7 g/L) and hematocrit levels by 0.19 percentage points.

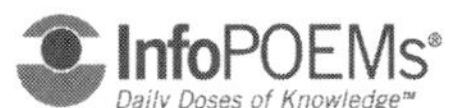

Oral as good as IM vitamin B12 replacement

Clinical question

Is oral vitamin B12 replacement as effective as intramuscular replacement?

Bottom line

Based on 2 small studies, both oral and intramuscular (IM) vitamin B12 replacement increase serum B12 levels and improve neurological outcomes. Oral vitamin B12 replacement should be considered for patients with documented deficiency. It is available over the counter in 1000 mcg and 2000 mcg doses in the United States. (LOE = 2a)

Reference

Butler CC, Vidal-Alaball J, Cannings-John R, et al. Oral vitamin B12 versus intramuscular vitamin B12 for vitamin B12 deficiency: a systemic review of randomized controlled trials. Fam Pract 2006;23:279–285.

Study Design

Meta-analysis (randomized controlled trials)

Funding

Unknown/not stated

Setting

Various (meta-analysis)

Synopsis

Although many US physicians still give vitamin B12 via IM injection, oral administration may be just as effective. In fact, in Canada and Sweden, most patients receive oral vitamin B12 if they suffer from deficiency. These authors searched for studies that randomly compared oral with IM vitamin B12 for patients with B12 deficiency; studies of vitamin B12 to prevent heart disease, treat folate deficiency, or in patients with renal disease were excluded. Only 2 studies with a total of 108 patients met the inclusion criteria; the follow-up periods were from 2 to 4 months. Neither study was blinded or used intention-to-treat analysis. The first study found greater B12 levels in the oral replacement group than in the IM group (643 vs 306 pg/mL at 2 months, and 1005 vs 325 pg/mL at 4 months). The oral dose was 2000 mcg per day. Neurologic improvement was similar between groups (4 of 15 who received IM B12 and 4 of 18 who received oral B12). The second study found improvements in the vitamin B12 level for both oral and IM groups, but did not analyze which was more effective.

Essential Evidence: Medicine that Matters, Edited by David Slawson, Allen Shaughnessy, Mark Ebell, and Henry Barry.

LMWH better than warfarin in preventing recurrent DVT in cancer patients

Clinical question

In patients with cancer and venous thromboembolism, is low-molecular-weight heparin more effective than warfarin in the prevention of recurrent emboli?

Bottom line

For every 13 cancer patients with an episode of venous thromboembolism (VTE) who receive 6 months of a low-molecular-weight heparin (dalteparin) instead of warfarin, there is 1 fewer recurrent episode of VTE. (LOE = 1b)

Reference

Lee AY, Levine MN, Baker RI, et al. Low-molecular-weight heparin versus a coumarin for the prevention of recurrent venous thromboembolism in patients with cancer. N Engl J Med 2003;349:146–153.

Study Design

Randomized controlled trial (single-blinded)

Setting

Outpatient (any)

Synopsis

Patients with cancer who have an episode of VTE, either deep vein thrombosis (DVT) or pulmonary embolism (PE), have an approximately 15% risk of recurrence during a 6-month follow-up period, even if treated appropriately with warfarin. All patients in this trial were given dalteparin in a dose of 200 IU/kg for 5 to 7 days. The 338 patients randomized to oral anticoagulation received a vitamin K antagonist (usually warfarin) for the remainder of the 6 months, adjusted to maintain the INR between 2.0 and 3.0. The 338 patients randomized (allocation concealed) to low-molecular-weight heparin received dalterparin in a dose of 200 IU/kg given once daily for the remainder of the first month, and then 150 IU/kg given once daily for the following 5 months. Groups were similar at baseline, with a mean age of 62 years, and 78% had metastatic disease. Approximately two thirds had a DVT alone, and one third had a PE with or without DVT. Patients were contacted at 2-week intervals during the 6-month follow-up period, and any suspected episodes of DVT or PE were investigated. At the end of the follow-up period, there were 14 DVTs, 8 nonfatal Pes, and 5 fatal PEs in the dalteparin group and 37 DVTs, 9 nonfatal PEs, and 7 fatal PEs in the oral anticoagulant group. The overall risk of VTE was significantly lower in the dalteparin group (8.0% vs 15.8%; P = .002, number needed to treat = 13). Major bleeding was more likely in the dalteparin group (19 vs 14 episodes), but this difference was not statistically significant. There was no difference in mortality between the groups (39% vs 41%; P = .53). The major limitation of the study was the failure to blind patients and physicians, although outcome adjudicators were masked to treatment assignment.

Essential Evidence: Medicine that Matters, Edited by David Slawson, Allen Shaughnessy, Mark Ebell, and Henry Barry.

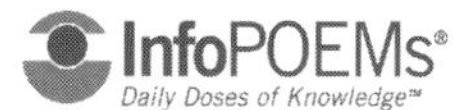

Testing for prothrombotic defects not necessary after first DVT

Clinical question

What risk factors predict recurrence after a first venous thrombotic event?

Bottom line

The risk of recurrence after a first venous thrombotic event (VTE) is increased in men, patients whose initial event is idiopathic, and women using oral contraceptives after the initial VTE. This study found no increased risk for recurrence in patients with prothrombotic abnormalities. Testing for prothrombotic abnormalities should be considered only in patients with a recurrent VTE. (LOE = 1b–)

Reference

Christiansen SC, Cannegieter SC, Koster T, Vandenbroucke JP, Rosendaal FR. Thrombophilia, clinical factors, and recurrent venous thrombotic events. JAMA 2005;293:2352–2361.

Study Design

Cohort (prospective)

Funding

Self-funded or unfunded

Setting

Inpatient (any location) with outpatient follow-up

Synopsis

The potential usefulness of screening for thrombophilia to prevent recurrence after a venous VTE is unknown. These investigators prospectively followed up 474 consecutive 18- to 70-year-old patients treated for a first confirmed VTE at participating hospitals and clinics in the Netherlands. Patients with a known malignancy were excluded. Complete follow-up occurred for 94% of the patients for an average of 7.3 years. Patients and clinicians were not blinded to outcome assessments. Recurrence of thrombotic events occurred in 90 patients, with the highest incidence during the first 2 years. Recurrence risk was statistically increased in men, patients whose initial event was idiopathic rather than provoked, and in women who used oral contraceptives after the initial VTE. There was no significant increased risk in patients with elevated levels of any prothrombotic abnormalities.

Essential Evidence: Medicine that Matters, Edited by David Slawson, Allen Shaughnessy, Mark Ebell, and Henry Barry.

Management of antiphospholipid antibody syndrome

Clinical question

What is the optimal management of antiphospholipid antibody syndrome?

Bottom line

Patients who test positive for antiphospholipid antibodies are at an increased risk of thrombotic events. Similarly afflicted pregnant women are at an increased risk of fetal loss. Moderate-intensity anticoagulation with warfarin (target international normalized ratio (INR) = 2.0–3.0) prevents recurrent venous thrombosis. The optimal management of other thrombotic aspects of patients with antiphospholipid antibodies remains uncertain. (LOE = 1a–)

Reference

Lim W, Crowther MA, Eikelboom JW. Management of antiphospholipid antibody syndrome. A systematic review. JAMA 2006;295:1050–1057.

Study Design

Systematic review

Funding

Self-funded or unfunded

Setting

Various (meta-analysis)

Synopsis

Antiphospholipid antibodies are associated with an increased risk of thrombotic events and pregnancy morbidity. To fully evaluate this risk and potential treatments, the investigators systematically searched MEDLINE, the Cochrane Library, and reference lists from significant articles for randomized trials and cohort studies reporting on patients with antiphospholipid antibodies. The risk of developing a new thrombosis in otherwise healthy patients with antiphospholipid antibodies without prior thrombotic events is low (<1% per year). Among other patients with antiphospholipid antibodies, the risk of a new thrombotic event is moderately increased in women with recurrent fetal loss without prior thrombosis (up to 10% per year), and highest in patients with a history of venous thrombosis who have discontinued anticoagulant drugs within 6 months (>10% per year). Moderate-intensity anticoagulation (target INR = 2.0–3.0) significantly reduces the risk of recurrent thrombosis; no additional benefit is gained with high-intensity anticoagulation (target INR = >3.0). Evidence is lacking to make clear recommendations for patients with antiphospholipid antibodies without prior thrombosis, recurrent thrombosis despite anticoagulation, treatment of arterial thrombosis, and treatment of women with recurrent fetal loss.

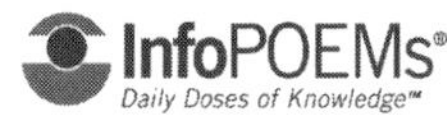

Oral rotavirus vaccines safe and effective

Clinical question
Is an oral vaccine safe and effective for the prevention of a rotavirus infection in young children?

Bottom line
Oral vaccines have been developed that are safe and effective for the prevention of rotavirus in young children. This will be particularly useful in third world countries where this disease is a major cause of infant mortality. (LOE = 1b)

Reference
Ruiz-Palacios GM, Perez-Schael I, Velazquez FR, et al, for the Human Rotavirus Vaccine Study Group. Safety and efficacy of an attenuated vaccine against severe rotavirus gastroenteritis. N Engl J Med 2006;354:11–22.

Study Design
Randomized controlled trial (double-blinded)

Funding
Industry

Allocation
Uncertain

Setting
Population-based

Synopsis
The first vaccine for rotavirus (Rotashield) was withdrawn from the market because in rare cases it caused intussusception. This study evaluated a live attenuated vaccine (Rotarix) given in 2 oral doses 1 to 2 months apart, with the first dose given to patients between the ages of 6 weeks and 13 weeks. The study randomized more than 62,000 infants to the vaccine or placebo in Finland and in 11 South American and Central American countries. Allocation concealment and randomization procedures are not clearly described by the authors. The entire group was followed up for a median of 100 days to assess the safety of the vaccine, and a subgroup of 20,169 infants was followed up for 9 to 10 months to evaluate efficacy. There was no significant difference between groups in the likelihood of intussusception (9 in the vaccine group and 16 in the placebo group). Regarding efficacy, the risk of severe gastroenteritis of any cause (defined using a standard symptoms scale) was reduced from 52 to 31 episodes per 1000 infants per year (number needed to treat [NNT] = 48; 95% CI, 26–303) and the number of diarrhea-related hospitalizations was reduced from 42 to 25 episodes per 1000 infants per year (NNT = 56; 29–486). Both of these differences were statistically significant. A second study in the same issue of the journal reported similar findings for a second oral vaccine given in 3 doses called Rotateq (N Engl J Med 2006;354:23–33).

Essential Evidence: Medicine that Matters, Edited by David Slawson, Allen Shaughnessy, Mark Ebell, and Henry Barry.

Acellular pertussis vaccine 63% to 92% effective

Clinical question
Is an acellular pertussis vaccine safe and effective for adults and adolescents?

Bottom line
An acellular pertussis vaccine reduces the risk of pertussis in adults and is well tolerated. (LOE = 1b)

Reference
Ward JI, Cherry JD, Chang SJ, et al, for the APERT Study Group. Efficacy of an acellular pertussis vaccine among adolescents and adults. N Engl J Med 2005;353:1555–1563.

Study Design
Randomized controlled trial (double-blinded)

Funding
Industry + govt

Allocation
Uncertain

Setting
Outpatient (any)

Synopsis
Pertussis in adults is on the rise. In this study, 2781 healthy adults were randomized to 3 component acellular pertussis vaccine (GlaxoSmithKline) or heaptitis A vaccine (Havrix) as a placebo. Groups were balanced at the start of the study, analysis was by intention to treat, and outcomes were blindly assessed. Patients were followed up for a median of 22 months. The researchers called the participants every 2 weeks to ascertain any episode of cough illness lasting more than 5 days, of which there were a total of 2672. Pertussis was defined 4 ways; the strictest required a positive culture, polymerase chain reaction (PCR), or stringent serologic evidence of infection. Approximately 80% of participants completed the study, with the bulk of withdrawals occurring during the final 6 months. Using the strictest case definition, there were 9 cases of pertussis in the control group and 1 in the vaccinated group (92% adjusted vaccine efficacy). With the least strict definition of pertussis infection the vaccine efficacy declined to 63%. It is interesting to note that there were 1047 cough illnesses lasting more than 3 weeks in the 2781 participants (1 for every 5 person-years) and 310 lasting more than 6 weeks (1 for every 16 person-years). Only a tiny minority of these episodes were caused by pertussis (5.7% of those coughing more than 8 weeks), and there were actually more episodes of cough in the pertussis group (1388 vs 1284), although the authors state that this was not statistically significant. There was no difference between groups in the likelihood of serious adverse events.

Essential Evidence: Medicine that Matters, Edited by David Slawson, Allen Shaughnessy, Mark Ebell, and Henry Barry.

InfoPOEMs® Daily Doses of Knowledge™

Vaccine exposure does not increase risk of infectious disease hospitalization

Clinical question

Does exposure to multiple-antigen vaccine or aggregated vaccine increase the risk of infectious disease hospitalization?

Bottom line

There is no evidence for an increased risk of infectious-disease hospitalizations in children receiving multiple-antigen vaccines or aggregated vaccine exposure. (LOE = 1b)

Reference

Hviid A, Wohlfahrt J, Stellfeld M, Melbye M. Childhood vaccination and nontargeted infectious disease hospitalization. JAMA 2005;294:699–705.

Study Design

Cohort (prospective)

Funding

Government

Setting

Population-based

Synopsis

Many clinicians and laypersons are concerned that exposure to multiple-antigen vaccines and/ or cumulative vaccine causes immune dysfunction secondary to an "overload" mechanism, resulting in an increased risk of subsequent infectious disease. The investigators monitored all children born in Denmark from January 1, 1990, through December 31, 2001. Individuals living in Denmark are given a unique identification number at birth allowing accurate linkage to information on childhood vaccinations, infectious disease hospitalizations, and potential confounding factors. Vaccines given during this time included the Haemophilus influenza type b (Hib), diphtheria-tetanus-inactivated pertussis, inactivated poliovirus, live attenuated oral polio virus, and mumps-measles-rubella. The effect of vaccination was evaluated in 3 different periods: within 14 days, 14 days through 3 months, and more than 3 months after vaccination. Appropriate statistical analyses accounted for potential confounders including sex, place of birth, birth weight, mother's age at birth, and month of birth. In the 805,206 children born during the study period, the investigators identified 84,317 cases of infectious disease hospitalization. Adequate follow-up occurred for more than 98% of the children. The only adverse association occurred between exposure to the Hib vaccine and subsequent hospitalization for acute upper respiratory tract infection (URI) more than 3 months after exposure (relative risk = 1.05; 95% CI, 1.01–1.08; number needed to treat to harm = 31,250; 19,531–156,250). Given that the authors tested 42 possible associations, it's likely they would find a significant difference in one of them by chance alone. In addition, there was no temporal or dose response relationship between Hib vaccination and hospitalization for URI, arguing against a causal relationship. No association was found between cumulative vaccine exposure and infectious diseases.

Essential Evidence: Medicine that Matters, Edited by David Slawson, Allen Shaughnessy, Mark Ebell, and Henry Barry.

Antibacterial household products don't reduce infectious symptoms

Clinical question
Does the use of antibacterial household products reduce symptoms of infectious disease?

Bottom line
The use of antibacterial household products did not reduce infectious disease symptoms in this urban Hispanic population of households, all of which included preschool children. (LOE = 1b)

Reference
Larson EL, Lin SX, Gomez-Pichardo C, Della-Latta P. Effect of antibacterial home cleaning and handwashing products on infectious disease symptoms. Ann Intern Med 2004;140:321–329.

Study Design
Randomized controlled trial (double-blinded)

Allocation
Concealed

Setting
Population-based

Synopsis
The effect of antibacterial products on infectious disease symptoms has not been previously studied despite their widespread use. This rigorously designed randomized double-blind study included 238 urban households of at least 3 persons, at least one of whom was a preschool child. Each household received products with or without antibacterial ingredients to use for 48 weeks. Analysis was by intention to treat. The antibacterial products were a general spray cleaner with a quaternary ammonium compound for use on hard surfaces, a handwashing product with triclosan, and a laundry detergent with oxygenated bleach. Households were surveyed weekly for infectious disease symptoms including vomiting, diarrhea, fever, cough, runny nose, skin infections, and conjunctivitis. During a total of 2737 household-months there were no differences between the 2 groups for the presence of any infectious disease symptom (33% vs 32%), specific infectious disease symptoms, or the number of infectious disease symptoms.

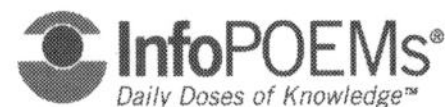

Cephalosporins often safe in PCN-allergic patients

Clinical question

What is the evidence regarding the use of cephalosporins in patients with penicillin allergy?

Bottom line

The risk of cross-reactivity between penicillin and cephalosporins has been overestimated for second- and third-generation drugs. It is only a significant risk in first-generation cephalosporins that have a similar side chain to penicillin (cephalothin, cephalexin, cefadroxil, and cefazolin). With appropriate monitoring physicians could consider using second- and third-generation cephalosporins in these patients. (LOE = 2a)

Reference

Pichichero ME. Cephalosporins can be prescribed safely for penicillin-allergic patients. J Fam Pract 2006;55:106–112.

Study Design

Systematic review

Funding

Unknown/not stated

Setting

Various (meta-analysis)

Synopsis

The author did a comprehensive search of MEDLINE and EMBASE to identify the 101 articles that were used as the basis for this systematic review. The overall rate of rash is approximately 2%. Anaphylaxis is very rare, with a risk between 0.1% and 0.0001%. Physicians often worry about cross-reactivity between penicillins and cephalosporins, but this only seems to apply to first-generation cephalosporins such as cephalothin, cephaloridine, cephalexin, cefadroxil, or cefazolin. No increase in the risk of an allergic reaction is seen in second- and third-generation cephalosporins, including cefprozil, cefuroxime, ceftazidime, cefpodoxime, and ceftriaxone. The author speculates that this is because of similar side chains in the chemical structure between penicillins and first-generation (but not second- or third-generation) cephalosporins. Patients with a previous IgE mediated reaction to penicillin (eg, wheezing, angioedema, urticaria, laryngeal edema, or anaphylaxis) should not use first-generation cephalosporins but may be able to safely take second- and third-generation cephalosporins.

Essential Evidence: Medicine that Matters, Edited by David Slawson, Allen Shaughnessy, Mark Ebell, and Henry Barry.

Prescribing antibiotics does not save time

Clinical question

Does prescribing antibiotics for viral infections save time?

Bottom line

Prescribing antibiotics for respiratory infections in children does not improve patient satisfaction and, as shown in this study, doesn't save time. Of course, as you know, antibiotic prescribing also doesn't affect the duration or severity of these viral illnesses. (LOE = 2c)

Reference

Coco A, Mainous AG. Relation of time spent in an encounter with the use of antibiotics in pediatric office visits for viral respiratory infections. Arch Pediatr Adolesc Med 2005;159:1145–1149.

Study Design

Cross-sectional

Funding

Foundation

Setting

Outpatient (primary care)

Synopsis

"If I don't give antibiotics, they won't be satisfied." "If I don't give antibiotics, they will change doctors." "If I don't give antibiotics, I will have to waste time explaining why." These are only a smattering of the excuses physicians use to justify bad practice. In this study, the authors used the National Ambulatory Medical Care Survey to evaluate the duration of visits for children presenting with colds or bronchitis. The survey, completed by physicians and office staff, includes an item labeled "time spent with a physician." The mean duration of the visits during which antibiotics were prescribed was 14.24 minutes; the mean duration of the visits when antibiotics were not prescribed was 14.18. Other studies have demonstrated that patient demand, patient satisfaction, and the likelihood of switching physicians are not affected by the receipt of an antibiotic. About the only thing prescribing antibiotics does is increase the likelihood of subsequent drug-seeking behaviors.

Essential Evidence: Medicine that Matters, Edited by David Slawson, Allen Shaughnessy, Mark Ebell, and Henry Barry.

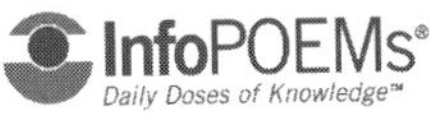

Delayed prescription for AOM reduces unnecessary antibiotics

Clinical question

Will asking parents to delay filling a prescription for the treatment of acute otitis media reduce unnecessary antibiotic use?

Bottom line

A wait-and-see approach of asking parents of children given a diagnosis of acute otitis media (AOM) in the emergency department to delay filling a prescription significantly reduces unnecessary antibiotic use. Parents of children in the delayed group reported otalgia slightly, if any, more often than the parents of children in the standard group. All parents received explicit instructions to provide both ibuprofen and otic analgesic drops to their children. Children in the standard treatment group were more likely to have diarrhea. (LOE = 1b)

Reference

Spiro DM, Tay KY, Arnold DH, Dziura JD, Baker MD, Shapiro ED. Wait-and-see prescription for the treatment of acute otitis media: a randomized controlled trial. JAMA 2006;296:1235–1241.

Study Design

Randomized controlled trial (single-blinded)

Funding

Foundation

Allocation

Concealed

Setting

Emergency department

Synopsis

Previous studies evaluating the effects of asking parents to delay filling antibiotic prescriptions for children with AOM excluded children with high fever. These investigators enrolled 283 consecutive children, aged 6 months to 12 years, seen in an emergency department who were given a diagnosis of AOM. Exclusion criteria included: another bacterial infection, such as pneumonia; "toxic" appearance; immunocompromization; myringotomy tubes or perforated tympanic membrane; or antibiotic use within 7 days. Parents of children with AOM randomly received (concealed allocation assignment) verbal and written instructions "not to fill the antibiotic prescription unless your child either is not better or is worse 48 hours (2 days) after today's visit" (intervention group) or to "fill the antibiotic prescription and give the antibiotic to your child after today's visit" (standard group). Amoxicillin was prescribed for most patients. All subjects also received ibuprofen and otic analgesic drops (containing antipyrene and benzocaine) in standard doses. Individuals blinded to treatment group assignment assessed outcomes at 4 to 6 days, 11 to 14 days, and 30 to 40 days after enrollment. In addition, a research assistant called pharmacies 4 days after enrollment to confirm whether prescriptions were filled. Follow-up occurred for more than 94% of participants. Using intention-to-treat analysis, prescriptions were filled significantly less often for children in the wait-and-see group versus the standard group (62% vs 13%). The difference was also significant in the subgroup of children younger than 2 years of age (47% wait-and-see vs 5% standard). Verification of whether prescriptions were actually filled was assessed for 28% of the study population; the pharmacy confirmed parental report in almost all instances. Otalgia occurred for a slightly greater period (0.4 days) in the wait-and-see group, but the overall rate of otalgia after 4 days was similar in both groups. Unscheduled follow-up visits were similar in both groups. No serious adverse events occurred in either treatment group, but parents in the standard group reported significantly more diarrhea in their children (23% vs 8%; number needed to treat to harm = 7).

Essential Evidence: Medicine that Matters, Edited by David Slawson, Allen Shaughnessy, Mark Ebell, and Henry Barry.

Delayed prescriptions for URIs reduce antibiotic use

Clinical question

Do delayed prescriptions reduce antibiotic use in upper respiratory tract infections?

Bottom line

Delayed prescriptions for upper respiratory tract infections reduces the use of antibiotics; patient satisfaction, however, may be worse. (LOE = 1a−)

Reference

Arroll B, Kenealy T, Kerse N. Do delayed prescriptions reduce antibiotic use in respiratory tract infections? A systematic review. Br J Gen Pract 2003;53:871–877.

Study Design

Systematic review

Setting

Outpatient (primary care)

Synopsis

For this systematic review, the authors included controlled trials of studies in which the intervention was a delayed prescription compared with an immediate prescription for patients with upper respiratory tract infections. They searched several databases (MEDLINE, Embase, Cochrane) and searched for unpublished studies. Two of the authors independently assessed the quality of the trials (randomization, concealment of allocation, co-interventions, losses to follow-up, and so forth). Disagreements among the reviewers were resolved by discussion and consensus. The authors were only able to find 5 controlled trials, 4 of which were randomized. All the randomized controlled trials had Jadad scores above 3, indicating reasonable to good quality. Since the authors found significant heterogeneity among the studies, they refrained from pooling the data. However, each study demonstrated significant reduction in the rate of antibiotic use. In 2 of the studies, however, patient satisfaction was significantly worse, and in 3 studies the symptoms were worse among those receiving a delayed prescription.

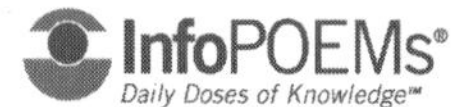

Flu shots are effective in elderly

Clinical question
Are flu shots effective in preventing influenza and influenza-like illness?

Bottom line
Flu shots prevent influenza and influenza-like illness in the elderly. (LOE = 1a–)

Reference
Jefferson T, Rivetti D, Rivetti A, Rudin M, Di Pietrantonj C, Demicheli V. Efficacy and effectiveness of influenza vaccines in elderly people: a systematic review. Lancet 2005;366:1165–1174.

Study Design
Systematic review

Funding
Foundation

Setting
Various (meta-analysis)

Synopsis
The authors systematically searched multiple databases looking for controlled studies (randomized controlled trials, cohort studies, case-control studies) of flu shots in the elderly. They don't describe searching for unpublished studies. The authors included nonrandomized studies "to enhance the relevance to public-health decision-making." It seems curious to include highly confounded studies for this stated purpose. Two reviewers independently applied inclusion criteria and 3 independently extracted the data. They identified 5 randomized controlled trials, 49 cohort studies, and 10 case-control studies. The overall effect was small. Flu shots were associated with 23% relative reduction in influenza-like illness and no reduction in confirmed influenza. Among nursing home patients, though, the vaccine reduced death due to influenza or pneumonia by 42%. If you only look at the randomized controlled trials, 2 studies with 2047 patients had an overall efficacy of 43% for preventing influenza-like illness and 3 studies with 2217 patients had an overall efficacy of 58% for preventing influenza.

Essential Evidence: Medicine that Matters, Edited by David Slawson, Allen Shaughnessy, Mark Ebell, and Henry Barry.

Useful signs and symptoms for diagnosis of influenza

Clinical question

How accurate is the history and physical examination in the diagnosis of influenza?

Bottom line

Three signs or symptoms are most useful to rule-in influenza: rigors, fever and onset of symptoms less than 3 days prior to office visit, and sweating. Four symptoms are helpful at ruling out influenza: absence of systemic symptoms, absence of coughing, no difficulty coping with daily activities, and not needing to be confined to bed. (LOE = 2b)

Reference

Ebell MH, White LL, Casault T. A systematic review of the history and physical examination to diagnose influenza. J Am Board Fam Pract 2004;17:1–5.

Study Design

Systematic review

Setting

Various (meta-analysis)

Synopsis

Evidence on the accuracy of the history and physical examination (HPE) in the diagnosis of influenza has not been systematically reviewed. The authors searched MEDLINE, bibliographies of identified studies, the Database of Abstracts of Reviews of Effectiveness, and contacted experts for articles reporting information on the accuracy of the HPE in the diagnosis of influenza A and B. Two investigators separately reviewed all abstracts of identified studies, and a consensus approach was used to determine which articles were included in the review. Included articles were cohort studies (following patients identified at the initial time of illness) that used a reference laboratory test as the gold standard for the diagnosis of influenza. Although not specifically stated, it is likely that physicians performing the HPE were unaware of the results of the reference standard. From an initial group of 97 studies, only 7 met the inclusion criteria. Results were pooled for the diagnosis of either influenza A or B. Three signs or symptoms were most useful to help rule-in influenza: rigors (positive likelihood ratio [LR+] = 7.2); fever and onset of symptoms less than 3 days before office visit (LR+ = 4.0); and sweating (LR+ = 3.0). Symptoms that were helpful in ruling out influenza were: no systemic symptoms (negative likelihood ratio [LR−] = 0.36); absence of coughing (LR− = 0.38); being able to cope with daily activities (LR− = 0.39); and not needing to be confined to bed (LR− = 0.50).

Essential Evidence: Medicine that Matters, Edited by David Slawson, Allen Shaughnessy, Mark Ebell, and Henry Barry.

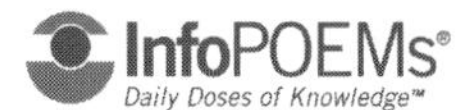

Steroids provide brief relief of pain in mononucleosis

Clinical question

Does dexamethasone reduce throat pain in acute mononucleosis?

Bottom line

Dexamethasone provides improvement in throat pain in children with acute mononucleosis but the effect lasts less than 24 hours. (LOE = 1b−)

Reference

Roy M, Bailey B, Amre DK, et al. Dexamethasone for the treatment of sore throat in children with suspected infectious mononucleosis: a randomized, double-blind, placebo-controlled, clinical trial. Arch Pediatr Adolesc Med 2004;158:250–254.

Study Design

Randomized controlled trial (double-blinded)

Setting

Emergency department

Synopsis

The investigators enrolled children between the ages of 8 and 18 years with suspected mononucleosis in this small study. The 40 children were randomly assigned (masked allocation) to receive a single oral dose of dexamethasone (0.3 mg/kg, maximum 15 mg) or a matched placebo. Pain was measured using a 100-mm visual analog scale, with a 20 mm or greater difference chosen as the main outcome. Pain was assessed 12, 24, 48, and 72 hours after treatment, and then one final time on day 7. Analysis was by intention to treat. To assess the quality of blinding, the investigators tried to guess whether participants received dexamethasone or placebo after patients completed the pain scale (they couldn't). At the 12-hour assessment, 12 of 20 in the dexamethasone group improved (at least 20 mm on the scale) compared with 5 of 19 taking placebo (number needed to treat = 4; P = .03). At 24 hours, half the patients treated with dexamethasone (11/20) had pain relief compared with one third (6/20) taking placebo. The study did not have sufficient power to detect whether this difference was real or not. Assessments after the first 24 hours were virtually identical.

Essential Evidence: Medicine that Matters, Edited by David Slawson, Allen Shaughnessy, Mark Ebell, and Henry Barry.

ACE inhibitors beneficial in diabetics

Clinical question

Are ACE inhibitors or angiotensin receptor blockers beneficial in patients with diabetes who have microalbuminuria or macroalbuminuria?

Bottom line

Treatment with an angiotensin converting enzyme inhibitor, but not angiotensin receptor blockers, delay mortality in patients with diabetes who also have microalbuminuria (and pre-existing heart disease) or frank albuminuria. This benefit occurs regardless of whether patients were also hypertensive. Angiotensin receptor blockers have been demonstrated to prevent a decline in renal function and decrease the likelihood of end-stage renal disease in high-risk patients. This analysis does not provide good evidence that screening for and treating microalbuminuria in patients with diabetes but without heart disease is effective. (LOE = 1a)

Reference

Strippoli GF, Craig M, Deeks JJ, Schena FP, Craig JC. Effects of angiotensin converting enzyme inhibitors and angiotensin II receptor antagonists on mortality and renal outcomes in diabetic nephropathy: systematic review. BMJ 2004;329:828. Epub 2004 Sep 30.

Study Design	Funding	Setting
Meta-analysis (randomized controlled trials)	Government	Outpatient (any)

Synopsis

Angiotensin converting enzyme inhibitors (ACE inhibitors) and angiotensin II receptor blockers (ARBs) are recommended for use in patients with diabetes with either microalbuminuria or frank albuminuria, regardless of blood pressure status. This meta-analysis summarized the current data on the effectiveness of these drugs in preventing overall mortality and end-stage renal disease, reducing the likelihood of a decline in renal function, and, less important, the progression from microalbuminuria to frank albuminuria. The investigators searched several databases using Cochrane Collaboration search strategies. Study selection, data extraction, and quality assessment were performed in the usual manner. They ended up with 43 randomized studies enrolling 7545 patients. Most of the research compares an ACE inhibitor with placebo in patients with microalbuminuria and pre-existing heart disease (the Micro-HOPE study). Treatment with an ACE inhibitor decreases overall mortality (8.50% vs 12.12%). The number needed to treat is 44 for approximately 4.5 years, though the range is very large (95% CI, 24.2–938). ARBs, studied on similar numbers of patients but for shorter time periods, have not shown any effect on mortality. ACE inhibitors do not decrease the development of end-stage renal disease, although the rate was low to begin with (4.3%) in the studied patients. ARBs have been demonstrated to have an effect in patients at high risk (19.3%) of developing end-stage renal disease. Similarly, ARBs but not ACE inhibitors have been demonstrated to have an effect on progression of renal disease as measured by the doubling of serum creatinine. Both types of drugs decrease the number of patients with microalbuminuria who progress to macroalbuminuria, although the significance of this outcome is not known. There is not enough research that directly compares the 2 types of drugs to provide guidance regarding which is better.

Essential Evidence: Medicine that Matters, Edited by David Slawson, Allen Shaughnessy, Mark Ebell, and Henry Barry.

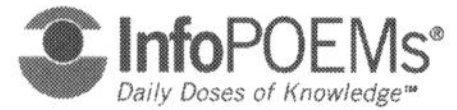

ARB no better than ACEI for prevention of nephropathy progression

Clinical question

Are angiotensin receptor blockers as good as angiotensin-converting enzyme inhibitors at preventing the progression of nephropathy?

Bottom line

Enalapril (Vasotec) was at least as effective as telmisartan (Micardis) and showed a trend toward greater benefit in preventing decline in glomerular filtration rate. Although this study measured a disease-oriented end point, its results are consistent with the body of literature that supports the less expensive angiotensin-converting enzyme (ACE) inhibitors as the drug of choice over angiotensin receptor blockers (ARBs). (LOE = 1b)

Reference

Barnett AH, Bain SC, Bouter P, et al. Angiotensin-receptor blockade versus converting-enzyme inhibition in Type 2 diabetes and nephropathy. N Engl J Med 2004;351:1952–1961.

Study Design

Randomized controlled trial (double-blinded)

Funding

Industry

Allocation

Uncertain

Setting

Outpatient (any)

Synopsis

This study is what we call a DOE (disease-oriented evidence) since it measured progression of nephropathy instead of the patient-oriented outcome of renal failure or need for dialysis. However, the results are worth knowing about because we so often hear of the potential DOE-related advantages of ARBs over the older, less expensive, and less often promoted ACE inhibitors. In this study 250 diabetic subjects with mild to moderate hypertension and evidence of early nephropathy (urinary albumin excretion rate between 11 and 999 mcg/minute and a serum creatinine less than 1.6 mg/dL) were randomized to receive either telmisartan 40 mg per day or enalapril 10 mg per day. If tolerated, the dose was increased to 80 mg and 20 mg respectively after one month. Blood pressure medicines other than an ACE inhibitor or ARB could be added at the discretion of the treating physician to control blood pressure. The primary outcome was the glomerular filtration rate. There was a high dropout rate, and the last observation was appropriately carried forward for the analysis. The results for only those patients with complete data were also reported. In both cases, there was almost no difference in glomerular filtration rate for the first 2 years, with a trend toward greater benefit for enalapril that almost became significant at 4 years and declined slightly at 5 years.

Essential Evidence: Medicine that Matters, Edited by David Slawson, Allen Shaughnessy, Mark Ebell, and Henry Barry.

Meat, seafood, and little dairy are risk factors for gout

Clinical question

Which dietary factors are associated with the development of gout?

Bottom line

There is a small but significant association between incidence of gout and increased consumption of meat and seafood or decreased consumption of dairy. It is not clear whether modifying diet in this way for patients with known gout will reduce the number of recurrences. (LOE = 2b)

Reference

Choi HK, Atkinson K, Karlson EW, Willett W, Curhan G. Purine-rich foods, dairy and protein intake, and the risk of gout in men. N Engl J Med 2004;350:1093–1103.

Study Design

Cohort (prospective)

Setting

Population-based

Synopsis

Patients with gout are generally advised to avoid purine-rich foods such as meat, seafood, oatmeal, and some vegetables (peas, beans, lentils, spinach, mushrooms, and cauliflower). However, this recommendation is based more on a theory than on actual evidence of an association. In this study, 49,932 men aged 40 to 75 years without gout completed a food frequency questionnaire at baseline (1986); it was updated in 1990 and 1994. The men were followed up prospectively every 2 years for 12 years. If they reported a new diagnosis of gout by a physician, that diagnosis was confirmed by a supplemememental survey using standard diagnostic criteria. A total of 730 new cases of gout were diagnosed during the study period. The primary outcome was the multivariate relative risk (RR) of gout between the highest and lowest quintiles of intake of a particular type of food. The risk of gout was increased among patients eating more meat (RR = 1.41; 95% CI, 1.07–1.86) and more seafood (RR = 1.51; 95% CI, 1.17–1.95), and decreased among those consuming more dairy products (RR = 0.56; 95% CI, 0.42–0.74). The absolute number of additional cases is relatively small, though. For example, the number of new cases of gout per person year was 124/100,000 in the lowest meat consumption group and 167/100,000 in the highest, a difference of only 1 additional case per 2325 patient years. There was no association between gout and either purine-rich vegetables, high body mass index, total protein intake, or alcohol intake.

Essential Evidence: Medicine that Matters, Edited by David Slawson, Allen Shaughnessy, Mark Ebell, and Henry Barry.

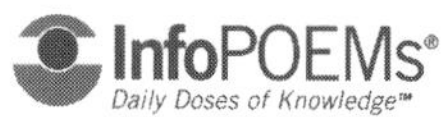

Febuxostat = allopurinol for gout prophylaxis

Clinical question

Is febuxostat more effective than allopurinol for the prevention of gout flares?

Bottom line

Febuxostat is better than allopurinol at lowering uric acid levels but no better at preventing gout flares. Despite assurances from the authors, the 4 deaths in this study should give us some pause, as should the greater number of drop-outs in the febuxostat groups and the almost surely higher cost if the drug is approved. (LOE = 1b)

Reference

Becker MA, Schumacher HR, Wortmann RL, et al. Febuxostat compared with allopurinol in patients with hyperuricemia and gout. N Engl J Med 2005;353:2450–2461.

Study Design	Funding	Allocation
Randomized controlled trial (double-blinded)	Industry	Concealed

Setting

Outpatient (specialty)

Synopsis

Like allopurinol, febuxostat is a xanthine oxidase inhibitor. This study enrolled 762 patients who met the standard criteria for gout and who had a serum urate concentration of 8.0 mg/dL (480 umol/L) or higher. The patients were randomized to either febuxostat 80 mg per day, febuxostat 120 mg per day, or allopurinol 300 mg per day. Each drug was given as a single daily dose; randomization and allocation concealment were appropriate, and groups were balanced at the start of the study. Analysis was by intention to treat. Because xanthine oxidase inhibitors cause an initial increase in attacks of gout, patients were given prophylaxis with colchicine 0.6 mg once daily or naproxen sodium 250 mg twice daily during the first 8 weeks of the study. Febuxostat in both doses was more effective at helping patients achieve a serum urate level of less than 6.0 mg/dL (53% for 80 mg dose, 62% for 120 mg dose, and 21% for allopurinol). This is a disease-oriented outcome, though – what really matters is whether the new and presumably more expensive drug is better at preventing gouty flare-ups. Unfortunately, it was not. During weeks 9 through 52 of the study, 64% of those receiving 80 mg febuxostat, 70% receiving 120 mg febuxostat, and 64% of those receiving allopurinol had at least one gouty flare. During the initial 8 weeks, presumably because of its more pronounced effect on uric acid levels, more patients receiving the higher dose of febuxostat had a flare-up (36% vs 21% for allopurinol; $P < .001$; number needed to treat to harm = 7; 95% CI, 4–13). The percentage reduction in the tophus area was greater in the febuxostat groups but not significantly so. There was no difference between groups regarding serious or treatment-related adverse events. There were 4 deaths in the 2 febuxostat groups (heart failure, retroperitoneal bleeding in an anticoagulated patient, metastatic colon cancer, and cardiac arrest) and none in the allopurinol group, but the investigators did not feel that any of the deaths were related to the study drug. There were also more drop-outs in the febuxostat groups than in the allopurinol group (88 and 98 vs 66), including more due to adverse events (16 and 23 vs 8).

Essential Evidence: Medicine that Matters, Edited by David Slawson, Allen Shaughnessy, Mark Ebell, and Henry Barry.

Low-dose dopamine ineffective for acute renal failure

Clinical question
Is low-dose dopamine effective in preserving renal function or preventing mortality in patients with or at risk for acute renal failure?

Bottom line
Low-dose (or renal-dose) dopamine causes short-term – 1 day – improvements in measures of renal function but does not improve outcomes in patients with or at risk for acute renal failure. Though urine output improves on the first day of therapy, the use of low-dose dopamine does not result in decreased mortality or the need for dialysis. (LOE = 1a–)

Reference
Friedrich JO, Adhikari N, Herridge MS, Beyene J. Meta-analysis: low-dose dopamine increases urine output but does not prevent renal dysfunction or death. Ann Intern Med 2005;142:510–524.

Study Design
Meta-analysis (randomized controlled trials)

Funding
Self-funded or unfunded

Setting
Various (meta-analysis)

Synopsis
Low-dose dopamine (1–3 mcg/kg/min), often called renal-dose dopamine, is used to treat oliguria or renal dysfunction because it increases renal blood flow and promotes sodium excretion. This meta-analysis combined the results of 61 randomized or quasi-randomized controlled studies of low-dose dopamine evaluating a total of 3359 patients. To find these studies (in any language), 2 authors independently searched several databases that use specific inclusion criteria, reference lists of retrieved publications, and review articles. Two reviewers then independently screened the studies and extracted data, which is standard practice in meta-analysis. They also evaluated the validity of each article and contacted 49 of the authors to obtain additional information. In the studies, dopamine was used to preserve renal function in patients who had undergone surgery, in patients with renal dysfunction due to intravenous contrast dye, in neonates, and in critically ill patients with other causes of acute decline in renal function. The median dose of dopamine in the studies was 2.5 mcg/kg/min infused for a median of 31 hours, and all but 8 of the studies used a dose of less than 3 mcg/kg/min. There was no heterogeneity among the studies with regard to the patient-oriented outcomes and no evidence of publication bias. Overall, dopamine had no effect on mortality or the need for renal replacement therapy. There was no benefit shown in any specific subgroup, including neonates. Analysis by dose found no benefit with either lower or higher doses. Urine output, on average, was increased on the first day of therapy by approximately 25% but was no longer significantly better on days 2 or 3. Similarly, serum creatinine levels decreased on day 1 but were no longer statistically different on days 2 or 3. Adverse effects, where measured, did not increase with dopamine.

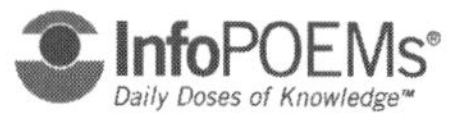

Furosemide doesn't prevent acute renal failure

Clinical question

Is furosemide (frusemide) effective in treating or preventing acute renal failure in adults?

Bottom line

In-hospital mortality is not affected by the use of high-dose furosemide to treat or prevent acute renal failure, and furosemide increases the hospital length of stay. (LOE = 1a)

Reference

Ho KM, Sheridan DJ. Meta-analysis of frusemide to prevent or treat acute renal failure. BMJ 2006;333:406–407.

Study Design

Meta-analysis (randomized controlled trials)

Funding

Self-funded or unfunded

Setting

Inpatient (ICU only)

Synopsis

The rationale behind loop diuretic use in acute renal failure is the better prognosis of nonoliguric renal failure as compared with oliguric renal failure; artificially maintaining urine production with a diuretic seems, therefore, to make sense. These researchers combined the results of 9 randomized controlled trials enrolling a total of 849 patients. The studies were found through a search of 3 databases and checking the reference lists of retrieved articles. Two researchers independently selected the studies and abstracted the data. The quality of the study was low (Jadad score = 2.6 of 5). Doses of furosemide varied among the studies and included continuous infusion or single bolus doses. Doses ranged from 600 to 3400 mg daily for treatment. In-hospital mortality was approximately 32% and was not different between groups treated with furosemide or placebo to prevent or treat acute renal failure. Furosemide use to prevent acute renal failure increased the length of hospital stay by an average 3.57 days (95% CI, 0.03–7.12; P = .049). The need for dialysis was heterogeneous across studies but was not affected by the use of furosemide. The authors report a possibility of publication bias in which small studies showing a benefit of furosemide have not been published.

Essential Evidence: Medicine that Matters, Edited by David Slawson, Allen Shaughnessy, Mark Ebell, and Henry Barry.

Treating negative dipstick dysuria decreases symptoms

Clinical question

In women with dysuria and frequency but a negative dipstick test result for nitrites and leukocytes, do antibiotics decrease symptoms?

Bottom line

No infection, no antibiotic, right? Maybe not. In women with dysuria and frequency but a negative urine dipstick result for nitrites and leukocytes, 3 of 4 women will respond to antibiotic treatment as compared with 1 of 4 taking placebo. The negative dipstick result correlated with culture 92% of the time. These results imply that some women have microbial infections that are not identified by dipstick or culture. Or, perhaps, the antibiotic is doing something other than killing bacteria. (LOE = 1b)

Reference

Richards D, Toop L, Chambers S, Fletcher L. Response to antibiotics of women with symptoms of urinary tract infection but negative dipstick urine test results: double blind randomised controlled trial. BMJ 2005;331:143–146.

Study Design

Randomized controlled trial (double-blinded)

Funding

Government

Allocation

Concealed

Setting

Outpatient (primary care)

Synopsis

The authors invited women between the ages of 16 years and 50 years to participate in this study if they presented to their New Zealand general practitioner with a history of dysuria and frequency but with a midstream urine specimen that was negative for nitrites and leukocytes using a standard urine dipstick. As a check on the validity of the dipstick, urine specimens were also cultured, though the results were not known until after the treatment and assessment had been completed. The 59 participants were randomized to receive, using concealed allocation, either placebo or trimethoprim 300 mg daily for 3 days. At the end of treatment, 76% of the women treated with antibiotic had resolution of dysuria, as compared with 26% of women who were treated with placebo (P = .0005). By 7 days, 90% of treated women had resolution of dysuria as compared with 59% of women receiving placebo (P = .02). One additional patient had resolution of symptoms by 7 days for every 4 women who received treatment instead of placebo (number needed to treat = 4; 95% CI, 1.9–14.1). Urinary frequency was unaffected by treatment. It's not that the dipstick failed to diagnose infection: Culture of dipstick-negative urine grew organisms in only 5 of 59 women; therefore, the negative predictive value of the dipstick was 92%.

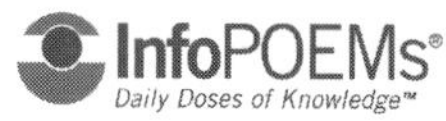

Immediate- and extended-release ciprofloxacin similar for UTI

Clinical question

Does a single dose of extended-release ciprofloxacin improve outcomes for women with uncomplicated urinary tract infection?

Bottom line

A single dose of an extended-release version of ciprofloxacin (Cipro XR) is as effective as the immediate-release version taken twice daily for 3 days. The tiny reduction in the likelihood of gastrointestinal adverse effects (number needed to treat (NNT) = 60–80) is likely to be heavily promoted, and must be balanced against the higher cost of this formulation. As we are given more such options, it is important to remember the key elements in choosing a drug: its safety, tolerability, efficacy, price, and simplicity. Although extended-release ciprofloxacin is simpler, it is no more effective and will almost certainly cost more. (LOE = 1b)

Reference

Fourcroy JL, Berner B, Chiang YK, Cramer M, Rowe L, Shore N. Efficacy and safety of a novel once-daily extended-release ciprofloxacin tablet formulation for treatment of uncomplicated urinary tract infection in women. Antimicrob Agents Chemother 2005;49:4137–4143.

Study Design

Randomized controlled trial (double-blinded)

Funding

Industry

Allocation

Concealed

Setting

Outpatient (any)

Synopsis

Although 3 days of trimethoprim-sulfamethoxazole is the recommended first-line therapy for uncomplicated urinary tract infection (UTI), ciprofloxacin is a treatment option when resistance to trimethoprim-sulfamethoxazole is greater than 20%. The critical problem with ciprofloxacin is that it is available in generic form, so manufacturers are working hard to create innovative delivery systems that can be sold under patent. In this study, the authors compared an extended-release version of ciprofloxacin 500 mg (Proquin XR) given once with the immediate-release formulation of ciprofloxacin 250 mg given twice a day for 3 days. Of 1027 nonpregnant adult women with an uncomplicated UTI, only the 540 with a positive urine culture for an organism susceptible to ciprofloxacin were included in the modified intention-to-treat analysis. Most UTIs (81%) were caused by E. coli. There was no difference between groups regarding microbiologic or clinical cure rates (86% for both groups). There was a slight reduction in the likelihood of nausea or diarrhea (NNT = 60 for nausea; NNT = 80 for diarrhea).

Essential Evidence: Medicine that Matters, Edited by David Slawson, Allen Shaughnessy, Mark Ebell, and Henry Barry.

Acupuncture effective for chronic back pain

Clinical question

Is acupuncture effective in treating acute or chronic low back pain?

Bottom line

Acupuncture is an effective treatment for decreasing pain in patients with chronic low back pain. It doesn't seem to be a placebo effect; acupuncture produces a significantly greater effect on pain than sham acupuncture. There is not enough research to allow a conclusion for the treatment of acute low back pain. (LOE = 1a)

Reference

Manheimer E, White A, Berman B, Forys K, Ernst E. Meta-analysis: Acupuncture for low back pain. Ann Intern Med 2005;142:651–663.

Study Design

Meta-analysis (randomized controlled trials)

Funding

Industry + govt

Setting

Various (meta-analysis)

Synopsis

Acupuncture is becoming more common in Western medicine, with many traditionally trained physicians crosstrained in its use. This meta-analysis assembled 22 randomized controlled trials comparing acupuncture with no treatment, sham acupuncture, or another active treatment such as massage or analgesics in the treatment of chronic low back pain. Sham acupuncture is used to convince patients they are receiving acupuncture and consists of inserting acupuncture needles either superficially or at inappropriate sites, or by using the acupuncture needle tube or other blunt device to provide pressure without actual penetration. The studies (in any language) were identified by searching 7 databases, contacting experts, handsearching a Japanese acupuncture journal, and using previous review articles. Two authors independently selected the studies and abstracted the data. Results of sham-controlled studies were homogeneous. One study of the 5 studies that compared acupuncture with no additional therapy produced heterogeneous results favoring no treatment as compared with acupuncture. Publication bias could not be assessed. For patients with chronic low back pain, lasting at least 3 months, acupuncture was more effective than sham acupuncture, sham transcutaneous nerve stimulation (TENS), and no treatment for short-term pain relief. It was not significantly better or worse than massage, medication therapy, or actual TENS treatment, and was significantly less effective than spinal manipulation. It provided long-term pain relief as compared with sham TENS or no treatment but was not different from sham acupuncture or active TENS. There is not enough data on the effectiveness of acupuncture for acute back pain to provide a conclusion. Three studies evaluated the use of acupuncture in the treatment of antenatal low back pain; all 3 studies found a benefit, though their results could not be combined.

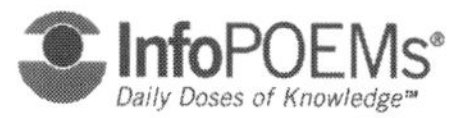

Surgery better than no surgery for spinal stenosis

Clinical question

In adults with spinal stenosis, is surgical treatment more effective than nonsurgical treatment?

Bottom line

Most patients with lumbar spinal stenosis treated surgically and nonsurgically improve over time. However, patients treated surgically have greater improvement in pain. There are no meaningful differences in disability or in walking capacity. (LOE = 2b)

Reference

Malmivaara A, Slatis P, Heliovaara M, et al, for the Finnish Lumbar Spinal Research Group. Surgical or nonoperative treatment for lumbar spinal stenosis? a randomized controlled trial. Spine 2007;32:1–8.

Study Design

Randomized controlled trial (nonblinded)

Funding

Government

Allocation

Concealed

Setting

Inpatient (any location) with outpatient follow-up

Synopsis

In this unblinded study from Finland, 94 adults with at least 6 months of symptoms due to lumbar spinal stenosis were randomly assigned to receive surgery or nonsurgical treatment. The researchers excluded patients with progressive neurologic deficits, with prior surgery, with severe or minimal symptoms, who were poor surgical candidates, and who had other conditions explaining their symptoms. The researchers evaluated the patients 6 months, 12 months, and 24 months after enrollment using intention-to-treat analysis. At the end of the study, approximately 15% of the patients had dropped out. Patients in both groups improved over the course of the study. Although disability scores were more likely to improve in patients treated surgically, the 7.8-point difference on a 100-point scale is not clinically meaningful. However, improvements in pain scores in the patients treated with surgery were clinically better. Finally, there was no significant difference between the groups in self-reported walking ability.

Essential Evidence: Medicine that Matters, Edited by David Slawson, Allen Shaughnessy, Mark Ebell, and Henry Barry.

Acupuncture better than sham treatment for neck pain

Clinical question

Is acupuncture more effective than sham treatments for patients with neck pain?

Bottom line

If this systematic review identified all the relevant literature, there is moderate evidence that acupuncture is more effective than some sham treatments or inactive therapies in relieving neck pain at the end of treatment and at 3 months of follow up. The overall quality of the research, however, is poor. (LOE = 1a–)

Reference

Trinh K, Graham N, Gross A, et al. Acupuncture for neck disorders. Spine 2007;32:236–243.

Study Design

Meta-analysis (other)

Funding

Self-funded or unfunded

Setting

Outpatient (any)

Synopsis

The authors of this Cochrane review searched multiple databases looking for trials (randomized and quasi-randomized) of acupuncture compared with sham acupuncture or other inactive treatment in the treatment of adults with neck pain. The authors do not describe looking for unpublished studies. At least 2 authors independently assessed articles for inclusion and extracted the data. Additionally, at least 2 authors independently assessed the methodologic quality of the included studies. In each of these quality steps, they used a consensus process to reconcile discrepancies. Finally, they also rated the overall strength of evidence. Overall, most of the studies were of poor quality and did not have enough power to detect modest differences in treatment effect. In general, the authors found modest evidence that acupuncture was effective in reducing pain. Of the 10 small trials (with a total 661 patients) included, only 4 were of high quality. One underpowered study found no difference between acupuncture and sham electro-acupuncture. The remaining trials were fairly consistent in finding some benefit with acupuncture (range of numbers needed to treat from the studies = 2–17). The authors don't address this, but it is possible that publication bias in favor of studies with positive results will not reflect what we are likely to see in the real world.

Essential Evidence: Medicine that Matters, Edited by David Slawson, Allen Shaughnessy, Mark Ebell, and Henry Barry.

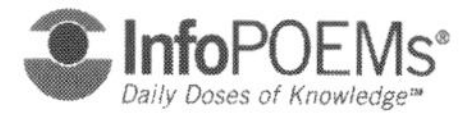

Useful treatments for fibromyalgia syndrome

Clinical question

What treatment modalities are most effective for fibromyalgia syndrome?

Bottom line

Treatments for fibromyalgia syndrome with the strongest evidence for efficacy include amitriptyline (Elavil), cyclobenzaprine (Flexeril), exercise, cognitive behavioral therapy, patient education, and multidisciplinary therapy. (LOE = 1a–)

Reference

Goldenberg DL, Burchhardt C, Crofford L. Management of fibromyalgia syndrome. JAMA 2004;292:2388–2395.

Study Design

Meta-analysis (other)

Funding

Foundation

Setting

Various (meta-analysis)

Synopsis

The optimal method for treating fibromyalgia syndrome is unclear. The investigators thoroughly searched multiple sources including MEDLINE, EMBASE, Science Citation Index, and the Cochrane Collaboration, for trials evaluating the effectiveness of treatment for fibromyalgia syndrome. A total of 505 articles were reviewed and classified according to their level of evidence. The authors don't state whether the articles were reviewed independently and do not discuss the potential for publication bias. Evidence was ranked as strong (positive results from a meta-analysis or consistent results from more than one randomized controlled trial [RCT]), moderate (positive results from one RCT or mostly positive results from multiple RCTs or consistently positive results from non-RCT studies), or weak (positive results from descriptive and case studies, inconsistent results from RCTs, or both). Strong evidence for efficacy was found for treatment with amitriptyline (Elavil), cyclobenzaprine (Flexeril), exercise, cognitive behavioral therapy, and patient education. Modest evidence for efficacy was found for tramadol (Ultram), various selective serotonin reuptake inhibitors, acupuncture, hypnotherapy, and biofeedback. Weak evidence for efficacy was found for growth hormone therapy, SAM (S-adenosyl-methionine), chiropractic and massage therapy, electrotherapy, and ultrasound. No evidence of any evaluation or effectiveness was found for steroids, nonsteroidal anti-inflammatory drugs, melatonin, benzodiazepine hypnotics, or trigger point injections.

Essential Evidence: Medicine that Matters, Edited by David Slawson, Allen Shaughnessy, Mark Ebell, and Henry Barry.

Acupuncture ineffective for fibromyalgia

Clinical question

Is standardized acupuncture effective in decreasing symptoms in patients with fibromyalgia?

Bottom line

A standardized acupuncture protocol was no better than sham acupuncture in relieving pain or improving other symptoms in patients with significant fibromyalgia symptoms. Patients in all groups reported slightly better scores. Acupuncture is just one aspect of traditional Chinese medicine, however, and this fairly artificial study does not help us understand if this approach is effective. (LOE = 1b)

Reference

Assefi NP, Sherman KJ, Jacobsen C, Goldberg J, Smith WR, Buchwald D. A randomized clinical trial of acupuncture compared with sham acupuncture in fibromyalgia. Ann Intern Med 2005;143:10–19.

Study Design

Randomized controlled trial (double-blinded)

Funding

Government

Allocation

Concealed

Setting

Outpatient (any)

Synopsis

The researchers recruited by advertisement 100 people with a diagnosis of fibromyalgia, who had a global pain score of 4 or more (average = 7) on a visual analog scale of 0 (no pain) to 10 (worst pain ever), and who agreed to maintain current treatment during the study. Using concealed allocation, the patients were randomized to receive either traditional Chinese Medicine acupuncture according to a standardized (ie, not individualized) protocol (n = 25) or 1 of 3 sham acupuncture treatments (n = 25 patients each) administered by 8 practitioners. The participants were treated twice weekly for 12 weeks with acupuncture only. The study, in its attempt to maintain consistency of the acupuncture treatment, resulted in artificial treatment, since acupuncture is just one aspect of traditional Chinese medicine and the clinician usually adjusts treatment to the specific patients. Using intention-to-treat analysis, no differences were found in any outcome; pain intensity and fatigue intensity improved similarly in all 4 groups, as did sleep quality and overall well-being. Scores of general health status, as measured by the Short Form 36-item Health Survey, did not change in any of the 4 groups.

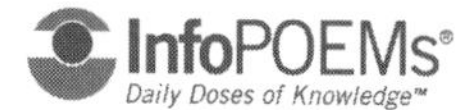

Acetaminophen = celecoxib in DJD

Clinical question

Are celecoxib and paracetamol equivalent in providing pain relief in patients with degenerative joint disease?

Bottom line

In this short-term study emphasizing individual response, acetaminophen and celecoxib (Celebrex) are virtually indistinguishable in improving pain, stiffness, and function in patients with clinically diagnosed degenerative joint disease (DJD). Since acetaminophen is less expensive and has fewer safety concerns, it should be the drug of first choice. (LOE = 1b)

Reference

Yelland MJ, Nikles CJ, McNairn N, Del Mar CB, Schluter PJ, Brown RM. Celecoxib compared with sustained-release paracetamol for osteoarthritis: a series of n-of-1 trials. Rheumatology 2007;46:135–140.

Study Design

Cross-over trial (randomized)

Funding

Industry + govt

Allocation

Uncertain

Setting

Outpatient (primary care)

Synopsis

Randomized trials suffer from limited applicability to patients we see in the real world. The best research design to determine the most effective intervention for a specific patient is the N-of-1 trial. These use methods as rigorous as a clinical trial, yet we rarely see them published. In this paper, patients with a clinical diagnosis of DJD for at least 1 month, and who were candidates for long-term therapy received sustained-release either paracetamol (acetaminophen; 1.3 grams 3 times daily), celecoxib (200 mg daily or 200 mg twice daily), or placebo. These drugs were administered in 2-week cycles and the order of medication was randomly assigned. Furthermore, the appearance of each medication was masked to ensure blinding. The main outcomes were pain, stiffness, and functional limitation (each on a 10-point scale), and medication preference and adverse effects. The main assessments were made during the second week of each treatment period to minimize the potential of the effects of any drug carrying over into the subsequent treatment period. At the time the study was stopped (because of celecoxib safety concerns), 41 patients had completed each study period. Most patients were unable to detect differences in pain (59%), stiffness (54%), function (63%), medication preference (68%) or side effects (61%). A few patients had detectable differences in pain (10 of 12 favored celecoxib), stiffness (12 of 14 favored celecoxib), and function (2 of 2 favored celecoxib). In spite of this 33 patients (80%) failed to identify these differences in terms of overall symptom relief.

Essential Evidence: Medicine that Matters, Edited by David Slawson, Allen Shaughnessy, Mark Ebell, and Henry Barry.

Knee taping useful for osteoarthritis pain

Clinical question

Does knee taping decrease pain and disability in patients with knee osteoarthritis?

Bottom line

Rigid taping by physical therapists, applied above the knee and, when necessary, below the knee, significantly decreased pain and disability, which lasted 3 weeks after taping was stopped. (LOE = 1b)

Reference

Hinman RS, Crossley KM, McConnell J, Bennell KL. Efficacy of knee tape in the management of osteoarthritis of the knee: blinded randomised controlled trial. BMJ 2003;327:135–138.

Study Design

Randomized controlled trial (single-blinded)

Setting

Outpatient (any)

Synopsis

The investigators investigated the American College of Rheumatology's (ACR) recommendation of knee taping for patients with osteoarthritis of the knee. Eighty-seven volunteers, at least 50 years old, who met ACR criteria for osteoarthritis of the knee were randomized (using concealed allocation) to receive no intervention, active taping, or sham taping. The tape was applied by physical therapists. The taping consisted of rigid strapping tape and hypoallergenic undertape and was applied above the knee to provide medial glide, medial tilt, and anteroposterior tilt to the patella. Additional taping was done, if necessary, to unload either the infrapatellar fat pad or the pes anserinus. Tape was applied weekly for 3 weeks and the study was continued for an additional 3 weeks. Pain, as measured on an 11-point, 10-cm scale, was significantly improved as compared with no taping or sham taping. Pain on movement decreased from 5.7 to 3.6 (out of 10) with the therapeutic taping. Results were similar for pain reported during most painful activity, Western Ontario and McMaster Universities osteoarthritis index, restriction of activity, and physical functioning. The benefits were maintained for 3 weeks after stopping treatment.

Essential Evidence: Medicine that Matters, Edited by David Slawson, Allen Shaughnessy, Mark Ebell, and Henry Barry.

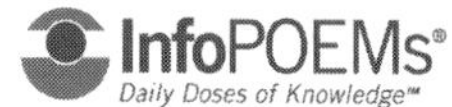

Tai chi improves symptoms of osteoarthritis

Clinical question

Can a specifically designed tai chi exercise program improve symptoms and physical functioning in women with osteoarthritis?

Bottom line

A specifically designed tai chi program for older women with osteoarthritis decreased pain and joint stiffness and improved physical functioning, balance, and abdominal muscle strength in the women who continued the exercises. The results may be a bit inflated because the researchers evaluating the outcomes may have known which patients had received treatment. (LOE = 1b–)

Reference

Song R, Lee EO, Lam P, Bae SC. Effects of tai chi exercise on pain, balance, muscle strength, and perceived difficulties in physical functioning in older women with osteoarthritis: a randomized clinical trial. J Rheumatol 2003;30:2039–2044.

Study Design

Randomized controlled trial (nonblinded)

Setting

Outpatient (specialty)

Synopsis

Tai chi is a martial art that involves slow, continuous, and gentle motions including isometric exercise, relaxation, stretching, and correct body posturing. A series of 12 Sun-style tai chi exercises have been developed to meet the specific needs of patients with arthritis. Patients in this study were older women in South Korea with radiologic and clinical evidence of osteoarthritis (OA) who were not in an exercise program. The investigators started with 72 women, but only 43 women completed the 12 weeks of the study. Approximately half the patients completing the study considered themselves to be in poor or very poor health. The average body mass index iof the women was 25. They were randomly assigned (using concealed allocation) to regular care without exercise or tai chi training. The tai chi group members participated in classes 3 times a week for the first 2 weeks, followed by weekly classes supplemented with twice weekly home exercise for 20 minutes for the next 10 weeks. The analysis only included the 43 women who completed all 12 weeks of the study. Using the Korean version of the Western Ontario and McMaster Universities Osteoarthritis Index, joint pain, stiffness, and physical functioning all were significantly different in the exercise group. Balance on one foot was significantly increased (by 7 seconds vs −1 seconds; $P < .05$) as was abdominal muscle strength (an increase of 2 sit-ups vs 0; $P < .05$). Muscle strength and endurance, flexibility, and weight were not affected. A concern: The investigators evaluating the outcomes may not have been blinded to the treatment the patients received.

Essential Evidence: Medicine that Matters, Edited by David Slawson, Allen Shaughnessy, Mark Ebell, and Henry Barry.

Acupuncture effective for OA of the knee

Clinical question

Is acupuncture effective in decreasing pain and improving function in patients with osteoarthritis of the knee?

Bottom line

Acupuncture, as compared with sham acupuncture treatment or no treatment, decreases pain scores by an average of 40% and improves function similarly in patients who stick with it. The acupuncture used in this study was based on the Traditional Chinese Medicine meridian theory and was used for the entire 6 months of the study. (LOE = 1b)

Reference

Berman BM, Lao L, Langenberg P, Lee WL, Gilpin AM, Hochberg MC. Effectiveness of acupuncture as adjunctive therapy in osteoarthritis of the knee: a randomized, controlled trial. Ann Intern Med 2004;141:901–910.

Study Design

Randomized controlled trial (double-blinded)

Funding

Government

Allocation

Concealed

Setting

Outpatient (any)

Synopsis

This is the largest and most rigorous study to date of the effect of acupuncture in the treatment of osteoarthritis. The authors enrolled 570 patients who had radiologic and clinical evidence of osteoarthritis of the knee and who had not had any intra-articular injections. The patients were assigned to 1 of 3 treatment groups: (1) "true acupuncture" based on Traditional Chinese Medicine meridian theory to treat knee joint pain; (2) a sham treatment that mimicked true acupuncture, except that the needles weren't actually inserted (the acupuncture guiding tubes were tapped at sham points, followed by affixing needles, without insertion, at these sites with adhesive tape); and (3) a control group that received 62-hour group education sessions lead by a patient education specialist, with follow-up mailed educational materials. Treatment was rendered twice a week for 8 weeks, tapering over the next month to 1 treatment per month, which was continued through the end of the study. This design addresses 2 issues that have plagued previous acupuncture research by providing a sham treatment, as well as a no-treatment group. At week 14, pain scores using the Western Ontario and McMaster University Osteoarthritis Index (WOMAC) decreased from an initial average score of 8.9 (of a possible 20) by 3.6 units (40% improvement) in the true acupuncture group compared with a 2.7 unit increase in the sham group and a 1.5 unit decrease in the education group. This change with true acupuncture was statistically significant compared with the other 2 groups. Pain scores continued to improve in all 3 groups over the course of the study, though true acupuncture scores continued to improve statistically more than the other 2 groups. Functional deficit diminished from an average 32 units (of a possible 68 at baseline) to 19 units at the end of the study, an almost 40% improvement that was statistically better than the other 2 groups. Patient global assessment scores also improved in the acupuncture group to a statistically greater extent than in either other group. Distance during the 6-minute walk and 36-Item Short-Form Health Survey scores improved more with true and sham acupuncture treatment than with education, but the results were similar between those 2 groups.

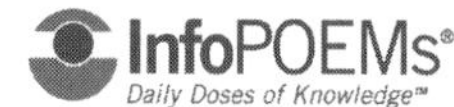

Rofecoxib increases risk of cardiovascular events

Clinical question
Does rofecoxib (Vioxx) increase the risk of cardiovascular events?

Bottom line
For every 62 patients who take rofecoxib instead of placebo for 3 years, 1 additional patient will experience a serious cardiovascular event. Remember, there is no greater symptomatic relief with COX-2 inhibitors than with older drugs; acetaminophen is a very safe alternative. The decrease in risk of serious gastrointestinal complications is marginal with COX-2 inhibitors and the cost is high. (LOE = 1b)

Reference
Bresalier RS, Sandler RS, Quan H, et al, for the Adenomatous Polyp Prevention on Vioxx (APPROVe) Trial Investigators. Cardiovascular events associated with rofecoxib in a colorectal adenoma chemoprevention trial. N Engl J Med 2005;352:1092–1102.

Study Design
Randomized controlled trial (double-blinded)

Funding
Industry

Allocation
Concealed

Setting
Outpatient (any)

Synopsis
The manufacturer of rofecoxib (Vioxx) designed this study to help include the prevention of colon polyps as an indication for the drug. Because of concerns about the safety of rofecoxib raised by earlier the studies, the Food and Drug Administration asked the researchers to also monitor cardiovascular outcomes. The authors identified 2586 adults older than 40 years who had a history of colon polyps; some patients taking aspirin were allowed into the study (ultimately, 1 in 6). After a placebo run-in period to assure that patients would be compliant, they were randomized (allocation concealed) to receive rofecoxib 25 mg or placebo once daily for up to 3 years. Groups were balanced at the start of the study, but more patients in the rofecoxib group withdrew because of adverse clinical events (16% vs 11%). Outcomes were assessed blindly and analysis was by intention to treat. The likelihood of any cardiovascular event was higher in the rofecoxib group (3.6% vs 2.0%). One additional cardiovascular event would occur in every 62 patients treated with rofecoxib for three years (95% CI 35–330). This increased was largely the result of more myocardial infarction and other cardiac events. The number of strokes was also greater in the rofecoxib group, but this difference was not statistically significant (15 vs 7). The risk of adverse events was as high or higher during the second 18-month period compared with the first. There were 10 deaths in each group.

Essential Evidence: Medicine that Matters, Edited by David Slawson, Allen Shaughnessy, Mark Ebell, and Henry Barry.

Celecoxib increases risk of cardiovascular complications

Clinical question

Does celecoxib (Celebrex) increase the risk of cardiovascular events?

Bottom line

One additional cardiovascular event or cardiovascular death occurs for every 126 patients treated for 1 year with celecoxib. There appears to be a dose response relationship. It is difficult to justify continued use of this and other coxibs, except in the most exceptional circumstances. (LOE = 1b)

Reference

Solomon SD, McMurray JJ, Pfeffer MA, et al, for the Adenoma Prevention with Celecoxib (APC) Study Investigators. Cardiovascular risk associated with celecoxib in a clinical trial for colorectal adenoma prevention. N Engl J Med 2005;352:1071–1080.

Study Design

Randomized controlled trial (double-blinded)

Funding

Industry

Allocation

Concealed

Setting

Outpatient (specialty)

Synopsis

This study was an attempt to broaden the indication of this widely used drug even further by seeing if celecoxib (Celebrex) can prevent recurrent colon polyps. When the results of a similar study of rofecoxib (Vioxx) were released to the media, the authors of this study decided to similarly analyze their existing data to look for cardiovascular complications. In this study, 2035 patients aged 32 to 88 years with a history of a single large colon adenoma or multiple adenomas were randomized (allocation concealed) to placebo, celecoxib 200 mg twice daily, or celecoxib 400 mg twice daily. Groups were balanced at the start of the study, analysis was by intention to treat, and patients were followed up for 3 years. Cardiovascular endpoints were blindly assessed and mortality data were available for all patients. Although 41% of patients were hypertensive, only 4% had a history of myocardial infarction (MI); 2% had a history of stroke; 7%, angina; and 2%, heart failure. After 2.8 to 3.1 years of follow-up, the likelihood of cardiovascular death, MI, stroke, or heart failure was 1.0% in the placebo group, 2.3% in the 200 mg group, and 3.4% in the 400 mg group. The increase in this group of outcomes between the 400 mg and placebo groups was statistically significant, with a 95% confidence interval of 1.4% to 7.8%. The difference between the 200 mg and placebo groups just missed being statistically higher with celecoxib (95% CI 0.9 to 5.5). The number needed to treat to harm for treating with 400 mg per day for 3 years is 42, or 126 per year of use.

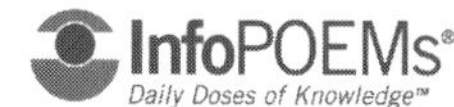

Rofecoxib, diclofenac and indomethacin increase risk of CVD

Clinical question

Which NSAIDs increase the risk of cardiovascular disease (CVD)?

Bottom line

Rofecoxib (Vioxx), diclofenac (Voltaren, Cataflam), and indomethacin (Indocin) are associated with a significant increased risk of CVD. It is likely that all NSAIDs carry some risk, but the risks may vary between medicines. Current evidence does not point to an increased risk for low dose (over the counter) ibuprofen and this remains safe to use at recommended doses. (LOE = 2a–)

Reference

McGettigan P, Henry D. Cardiovascular risk and inhibition of cyclooxygenase. A systematic review of the observational studies of selective and nonselective inhibitors of cyclooxygenase 2. JAMA 2006;296:1633–1644.

Study Design

Systematic review

Funding

Foundation

Setting

Various (meta-analysis)

Synopsis

Recent evidence that rofecoxib (Vioxx) increases the risk of CVD has raised concern about other nonsteroidal anti-inflammatory drugs (NSAIDs). These investigators searched multiple databases including MEDLINE, EMBASE, the Cochrane Library, abstracts of scientific meetings and bibliographies of relevant studies for reports on cardiovascular events and NSAID use. Of 7086 potentially eligible titles, 17 case-control including 86,193 cases and 6 cohort studies including 75,520 users met study criteria. Most exclusions were a result of reports not providing sufficient information on study outcomes or the drugs of interest. The mean age of study participants was rarely less than 55 years, and in most cases was grater than 60 years. Two individuals independently extracted data and assessed study quality with disagreements resolved by consensus. Individual studies underwent assessment using a standardized instrument. All studies scored well (7–8 points in total from a possible 9). As expected, rofecoxib use significantly increased the risk of CVD, with risk being highest with doses in excess of 25 mg/day. Diclofenac (Voltaren, Cataflam) and indomethacin (Indocin) were also associated with a significantly increased risk of CVD. Data on meloxicam (Mobic) came from 3 trials, only one of which showed a statistically significant elevated risk. Authors of the article state that these data do not allow definite conclusions about the risk of meloxicam. Celecoxib (Celebrex), naproxen, piroxicam and inbuprofen exposure did not increase CVD risk. Stay tuned, however, as more studies are forthcoming shortly. In a related study in the same journal (Zhang J, Ding E, Song Y. JAMA;296:1619–32), only rofecoxib was associated with a significant increased risk of renal events and heart arrhythmia. Celecoxib (Celebrex) was significantly associated with a reduced risk of renal dysfunction.

Essential Evidence: Medicine that Matters, Edited by David Slawson, Allen Shaughnessy, Mark Ebell, and Henry Barry.

Rofecoxib cardiovascular risks known in 2000

Clinical question

When were the risks of rofecoxib (Vioxx) well established?

Bottom line

If anyone had been minding the store and looking at the cumulative data as they became available, rofecoxib would have been associated with an increased cardiovascular risk by the end of 2000. United States government agencies and other watch dogs failed to recognize the risk. Clinicians need to be wary about the selective reporting of harms and benefits of new drugs. (LOE = 1a)

Reference

Juni P, Nartey L, Reichenbach S, et al. Risk of cardiovascular events and rofecoxib: cumulative meta-analysis. Lancet 2004;364:2021–2029.

Study Design

Meta-analysis (other)

Funding

Government

Setting

Various (meta-analysis)

Synopsis

Rofecoxib (Vioxx) was removed from the market under a hailstorm of controversy. The manufacturer apparently decided to remove it on the basis of a single small trial. Among the controversial issues was whether the manufacturer covered up known harms and manipulated the release of data to provide a favorable outlook, and whether the manufacturer inappropriately created demand by skewing the information reported to the public. These authors searched the Cochrane Controlled Trials Register and several other databases (including MEDLINE, EMBASE, and CINAHL), examined citations of key papers in the Science Citation Index, searched conference proceedings, screened reference lists of relevant papers, contacted experts, and reviewed the proceedings of the Food and Drug Administration advisory panels. They were in search of all randomized clinical trials comparing rofecoxib with another anti-inflammatory drug or placebo. Since they found no large-scale comparisons with other drugs, they also identified observational studies. Two people independently extracted the data using an explicit approach. Two other researchers independently checked the data. The researchers evaluated 2 key quality issues in the clinical trials: concealed allocation and independent external review of serious adverse events. Finally, they analyzed the study data using standard meta-analytic methods (also on a cumulative basis). For this latter evaluation, they included cardiovascular safety data in the year they first became available. The authors found 18 placebo-controlled trials (including more than 25,000 patients; all trials sponsored by the manufacturer) and 11 observational studies. If all the data had been evaluated systematically on an ongoing basis, the cumulative risk of acute myocardial infarction would have become significant by the end of 2000.

Essential Evidence: Medicine that Matters, Edited by David Slawson, Allen Shaughnessy, Mark Ebell, and Henry Barry.

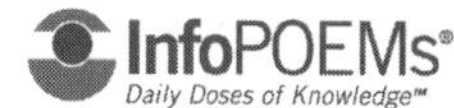

Arthroscopy ineffective for osteoarthritis of knee

Clinical question

Does arthroscopic surgery improve outcomes for patients with osteoarthritis of the knee?

Bottom line

Arthroscopy is not effective for the treatment of osteoarthritis. The procedure may still have a role in the repair of meniscal and ligamentous injuries, unless we find out that it is ineffective here too. (LOE = 1b)

Reference

Moseley JB, O'Malley K, Petersen NJ, et al. A controlled trial of arthroscopic surgery for osteoarthritis of the knee. N Engl J Med 2002;347:81–88.

Study Design

Randomized controlled trial (double-blinded)

Setting

Inpatient (any location) with outpatient follow-up

Synopsis

This is one of the few studies in the literature to properly evaluate a surgical procedure. Patients (n = 180) with osteoarthritis of the knee, moderate pain, no recent arthroscopy, and no suspected ligament or meniscal problems were randomly assigned to either arthroscopy with lavage only, arthroscopy with lavage and debridement, or "sham arthroscopy." During the sham procedure, patients were mildly sedated, and the surgical team manipulated the knee, made small superficial incisions, and even made all of the noises that they would normally make during surgery. Patients were followed for 2 years by properly blinded study personnel, and patients were not able to guess their treatment assignment. Allocation was properly concealed, and groups were similar at baseline. Interestingly, all groups experienced an immediate improvement of 6 to 12 points on the 100-point Knee-Specific Pain Scale. Pain gradually increased in all groups over time, but never returned to baseline levels, and at the end of the study period all groups had a similar degree of improvement in pain. A test of physical functioning (length of time for patients to walk 100 feet and then climb up and down a flight of stairs as quickly as possible) found a slight worsening immediately after arthroscopy but no long-term difference between groups.

Essential Evidence: Medicine that Matters, Edited by David Slawson, Allen Shaughnessy, Mark Ebell, and Henry Barry.

Obesity does not effect 5-year knee replacement outcomes

Clinical question

Do obese patients undergoing knee replacement have more long-term complications than patients who are not obese?

Bottom line

In this study, obese patients undergoing primary knee arthroplasty had comparable long-term outcomes with nonobese patients. (LOE = 1b–)

Reference

Amin AK, Patton JT, Cook RE, Brenkel IJ. Does obesity influence the clinical outcome at five years following total knee replacement for osteoarthritis? J Bone Joint Surg Br 2006;88:335–340.

Study Design	Funding	Setting
Cohort (prospective)	Unknown/not stated	Outpatient (specialty)

Synopsis

In spite of conflicting data, obesity has been blamed for everything from premature mortality to halitosis. In this study, the researchers enrolled 370 consecutive patients who had a primary knee arthroplasty for degenerative joint disease and evaluated them sequentially for up to 5 years with 92% having complete follow-up. In addition to baseline data, the researchers prospectively assessed knee pain, function, radiographic changes, and complications (perioperative mortality, wound infection, deep vein thrombosis, and repeat surgery). The authors don't describe how the patients were originally referred or whether the outcomes were assessed blindly. They didn't include functional data on 37 patients who died before completing 5 years of follow up, but the outcome data were used. Using a body mass index (BMI) of 30 kg/m^2 as a cutoff, 158 nonobese patients (181 knees) and 125 obese patients (147 knees) underwent surgery. A total of 54% of the nonobese patients were men; only 41% of the obese patients were men. The baseline levels of function were comparable in the obese and nonobese patients. At the end of 5 years, there were no significant differences in knee pain or function between the obese and nonobese patients. Additionally, the rate of complications was not significantly different between nonobese and obese patients (wound infection = 3.7% vs 4.9%; deep vein thrombosis = 0.5% vs 1.2%; mortality = 0.5% vs 0; repeat surgery = 1.4% vs 2.5%. The authors similarly compared nonobese to obese women and patients weighing over and under 100 kg and found no differences in in the outcomes of those subcategories, either. Only 6 patients in the study were morbidly obese (BMI > 40 kg/m^2). Interestingly, all of these patients did well and had no complications. A cautionary note: BMI is an unreliable measure of obesity in fit patients. My orthopedic colleagues would tell me that the reason the obese patients did well in this study is because the surgeons selected good protoplasm. My methodologically driven colleagues would demand a randomized controlled trial to confirm this.

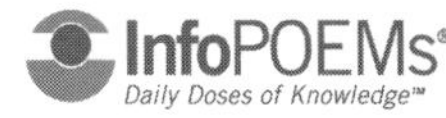

Monthly vitamin D prevents fractures

Clinical question

Can vitamin D, given every 4 months, prevent fractures in men and women?

Bottom line

In this preliminary study, taking vitamin D once every 4 months, without additional calcium, lead to a decrease in osteoporotic fractures in older people, primarily women. The dose is big – 100,000 units, which works out to be a little more than 800 IU daily. This daily dose, along with calcium supplementation, has been shown to decrease fractures (N Engl J Med 1997; 337:670–76). A lower dose – 400 IU per day – does not work. Unfortunately, this is the dose that usually is used in comparative trials with other drugs. (LOE = 1b)

Reference

Trivedi DP, Doll R, Khaw KT. Effect of four monthly oral vitamin D3 (cholecalciferol) supplementation on fractures and mortality in men and women living in the community: randomised double blind controlled trial. BMJ 2003;326:469–472.

Study Design

Randomized controlled trial (double-blinded)

Setting

Outpatient (primary care)

Synopsis

The investigators enrolled 2686 men and women who were 65 to 85 years old, living at home, and not taking vitamin D. Only 649 of the enrollees were women. Allocation to treatment assignment may not have been concealed from the enrolling investigator. The patients took either placebo or vitamin D3 (cholecalciferol) 100,000 IU every 4 months – a single capsule was sent by mail and patients were asked to take it immediately. The supplementation lasted 5 years. Supplemental calcium was neither given nor its use controlled. Over this period approximately 10% of the group (15% of the women and 8% of the men) experienced a fracture. Overall fracture rates were significantly less in the patients receiving vitamin D (8.8% vs 11.1%; number needed to treat [NNT] = 44). Men, on average, did not receive benefit, though women did (fracture rate = 12.9% vs 18%; NNT = 20). In the relatively small number of women, hip or vertebral fractures were not individually decreased, although the study probably was too small to find a difference if one exists. This study was designed as a pilot study, with the eventual goal of enrolling 20,000 men and women. Unfortunately, because of lack of funding, the larger study will not be completed. Seems no one is interested in this relatively simple and inexpensive treatment. Still, the authors were able to demonstrate a difference with a smaller amount of patients, which makes it very likely the larger study would have found a similar benefit, and may also have found a decreased hip fracture risk.

Essential Evidence: Medicine that Matters, Edited by David Slawson, Allen Shaughnessy, Mark Ebell, and Henry Barry.

Calcium/vitamin D effective for prevention of first fracture

Clinical question

Does supplementation with vitamin D and calcium prevent a first hip fracture or nonvertebral fracture in older people?

Bottom line

Supplementation with calcium 1000 mg and vitamin D3 800 IU daily decreases the likelihood that older people will experience a first hip fracture or other nonvertebral fracture. The dose of calcium is lower than the 1500 mg daily that is recommended and usually used; the vitamin D dose is higher than the dose usually used in comparison studies with other drugs. These results conflict with 2 large studies in patients at high risk or with a previous osteoporotic fracture for whom these doses did not decrease the rate of fracture (BMJ 2005; 330:1003–06 and Lancet 2005; 365:1621–28). (LOE = 1a)

Reference

Bischoff-Ferrari HA, Willett WC, Wong JB, Giovannucci E, Dietrich T, Dawson-Hughes B. Fracture prevention with vitamin D supplementation. A meta-analysis of randomized controlled trials. JAMA 2005;293:2257–2264.

Study Design

Meta-analysis (randomized controlled trials)

Funding

Foundation

Setting

Outpatient (any)

Synopsis

This meta-analysis combined the results of randomized controlled trials evaluating the role of the combination of calcium and vitamin D3. The researchers searched 3 databases for studies evaluating the effect of the combination on hip fractures or nonvertebral fractures, searched reference lists and meeting abstracts, and contacted experts. The researchers did not comment on the quality of the studies other than to note that treatment allocation was masked and all but one used an intention-to-treat analysis. Two researchers independently extracted the data from the 7 studies, which enrolled a total of 9820 people with an average age of 79 years. Patients lived in the community, in housing for the elderly or in nursing homes, and the majority were women. Hip fracture occurred in a high proportion of patients: 7.3%. The researchers found heterogeneity among the trial results, which was resolved when they separated the studies by dose of vitamin D. Vitamin D 400 IU per day did not prevent fractures. Vitamin D doses of 700 IU to 800 IU per day resulted in a significant decrease in hip fractures (5.8% vs 7.7%), translating into 1 fewer hip fracture for every 50 patients treated for 2 years (number needed to treat = 50; 95% CI, 34–109). Similarly, the nonvertebral fracture rate was decreased only by the higher dose, with a number needed to treat of 28 (19–49) for at least 1 year.

Essential Evidence: Medicine that Matters, Edited by David Slawson, Allen Shaughnessy, Mark Ebell, and Henry Barry.

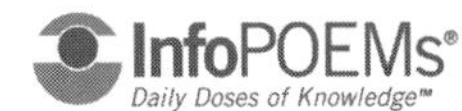

Calcium/vitamin D not effective for secondary prevention of fracture (RECORD)

Clinical question

In older people who have already experienced an osteoporosis-related fracture, does vitamin D, calcium, or the combination prevent secondary fractures?

Bottom line

The combination of calcium 1000 mg and vitamin D3 800 IU was ineffective in preventing fractures in 2 studies enrolling a total of more than 8500 participants, almost all of whom were female and at least 70 years old and either had a previous osteoporotic fracture or were at high risk. The dose of calcium is lower than the 1500 mg commonly recommended and used. These results conflict with a meta-analysis that found that the combination therapy reduced fracture rate, including hip fracture, in older patients who have not had a previous hip or nonvertebral fracture (JAMA 2005; 293:2257–64). (LOE = 1b)

Reference

Grant AM, Avenell A, Campbell MK, et al, for the RECORD Trial Group. Oral vitamin D3 and calcium for secondary prevention of low-trauma fractures in elderly people (Randomised Evaluation Of Calcium OR vitamin D, RECORD): a randomised placebo-controlled trial. Lancet 2005;365:1621–1628. Porthouse J, Cockayne S, King C, et al. Randomised controlled trial of supplementation with calcium and cholecalciferol (vitamin D3) for prevention of fractures in primary care. BMJ 2005;330:1003–1006.

Study Design	Funding	Allocation	Setting
Randomized controlled trial (double-blinded)	Other	Concealed	Population-based

Synopsis

Two studies, both conducted in the United Kingdom, studied the effect of calcium and vitamin D. In the first study, the researchers recruited 5292 participants following treatment for a fracture. Most (85%) were white women, all were at least 70 years old and ambulatory, and all had a previous osteoporotic fracture. Using concealed allocation, the researchers randomly assigned patients to receive 800 IU daily oral vitamin D3, 1000 mg calcium, the combination of both, or placebo. The patients took their assigned treatment for at least 2 years. Overall, new fractures occurred in 13.0% of the participants; hip fracture, the more clinically relevant outcome, occurred in 3.4% of participants. Compliance was not good in the study; by 2 years only half the patients were still taking their assigned treatment, and the 2 groups taking calcium had significantly higher noncompliance, with only 42% still taking their assigned treatment at 2 years. Neither calcium supplementation, vitamin D, nor the combination was effective in decreasing the rate of overall fractures or hip fractures. Compliant patients also did not have lower fracture rates, though the number of patients (508) taking both vitamin D and calcium may not have been large enough to find a difference, if one existed. In the second study, the researchers surveyed general practices across England to find women 70 years or older who had either a previous fracture or at least one risk factor. The 3314 women were randomized, using concealed allocation, to receive either placebo or the combination of calcium 1000 mg and vitamin D3 800 IU. Over a median follow-up of slightly more than 2 years, 4.3% of women experienced a fracture, and 0.7% experienced a hip fracture. Similar to the first study, there was no difference in fracture rates or hip fracture rates with treatment, either overall or in patients who were compliant.

1000 mg calcium/400 IU vit D not very effective for fracture prevention (WHI)

Clinical question

Does supplementation with 1000 mg calcium and 400 IU vitamin D reduce the risk of fracture in healthy women?

Bottom line

The ability of a small dose of calcium and vitamin D to prevent fractures in healthy community-dwelling women is modest at best. This study used a relatively low dose of vitamin D (less than the 700 IU to 800 IU found most beneficial in previous studies), and the patients were generally at low risk of fracture. Perhaps that explains the discordance of these findings with the bulk of the literature on this topic. (LOE = 1b)

Reference

Jackson RD, LaCroix AZ, Gass M, et al, for the Women's Health Initiative Investigators. Calcium plus vitamin D supplementation and the risk of fractures. N Engl J Med 2006;354:669–683.

Study Design	Funding	Allocation
Randomized controlled trial (double-blinded)	Government	Uncertain

Setting

Population-based

Synopsis

A previous meta-analysis limited to studies in which women received more than 400 IU of vitamin D found a significant 37% reduction in vertebral fractures (Endocr Rev 2002;23:560–69). In this substudy of the Women's Health Initiative, 36,282 women were randomized to receive either 1000 mg calcium and 400 IU vitamin D per day or placebo. The study had 85% power to detect an 18% decrease in hip fractures and 99% power to detect an 18% decrease in total fractures. The primary outcome was the number of hip fractures and a secondary outcome was total fractures. Fractures of the ribs, sternum, skull, face, fingers, toes, and cervical vertebrae did not contribute toward the total fracture number. The groups were balanced at the start of the study, analysis was by intention to treat, and the number of patients who dropped out or were lost to follow-up was modest (approximately 500 in each group). After a mean of 7 years, there was a nonsignificant trend toward fewer hip fractures (0.14% vs 0.16% per year; hazard ratio [HR] = 0.88; 95% CI, 0.72–1.08) and a similar nonsignificant trend toward fewer total fractures (1.64% vs 1.70%). The authors did quite a bit of data-dredging (ie, post-hoc subgroup analyses) and found that if there was any benefit, it was among older women and women who fell less often. Women who were adherent to the calcium and vitamin D regimen also had fewer hip fractures (relative risk = 0.71; 95% CI, 0.52–0.97). The total intake of calcium and vitamin D from diet and supplements varied considerably, with no clear trend toward greater benefit in women ingesting more of either substance. Interestingly, all-cause mortality was lower in the supplement group, although this didn't quite reach statistical significance (HR = 0.91; 95% CI, 0.83–1.01). Not surprisingly, women in the supplement group had 17% more kidney stones. A subgroup also had regular bone mineral density measurements, which showed greater preservation of bone density among women taking the supplements.

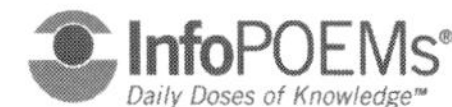

HRT with estrogen alone increases stroke, decreases fractures

Clinical question

Is hormone replacement therapy with estrogen alone beneficial for postmenopausal women with hysterectomy?

Bottom line

Estrogen replacement therapy in postmenopausal women with hysterectomy increases the risk of stroke, has no effect on cardiovascular disease, prevents hip and vertebral fracture, and may or may not affect the likelihood of breast cancer-related deaths. On the basis of both the estrogen-progestin and estrogen-alone arms of the Women's Health Initiative study, it appears prudent to use hormone replacement therapy in postmenopausal women only for significant menopausal symptoms at the smallest effective dose for the shortest possible time. Treatment for up to 4 or 5 years early in menopause appears to offer the greatest amount of osteoporosis and fracture prevention. Don't forget to recommend high-dose vitamin D and calcium. (LOE = 1b)

Reference

Women's Health Initiative Steering Committee. Effects of conjugated equine estrogen in postmenopausal women with hysterectomy. The Women's Health Initiative randomized controlled trial. JAMA 2004;291:1701–1712.

Study Design

Randomized controlled trial (double-blinded)

Setting

Outpatient (any)

Synopsis

The Women's Health Initiative estrogen plus progestin trial was stopped early when women in the treatment group were found to be at an increased risk of coronary events, stroke, breast cancer, and pulmonary embolism. Benefits of the therapy included a reduced risk of hip fracture and colon cancer. This paper summarizes the results from the estrogen-alone trial of 10,739 healthy women with hysterectomy, aged 50 to 79 years, who were randomly assigned in a double-blind fashion (concealed allocation) to receive either 0.625 mg per day of conjugated equine estrogen or placebo. Outcomes were assigned by individuals blinded to treatment group assignment. Follow-up for an average of 6.8 years was complete for 98% of participants. Using intention-to-treat analysis, estrogen alone compared with placebo increased the risk of stroke (hazard ratio (HR) = 1.39; 95% CI, 1.10–1.77; number needed to treat to harm = 12/10,000 person-years), but had no significant effect on the risk of pulmonary embolus, coronary heart disease, colorectal cancer, or all-cause mortality. Benefits of estrogen alone included a reduced risk of hip fracture (HR = 0.61; 95% CI, 0.41–0.91; number needed to treat = 6/10,000 person-years) and total fractures (HR = 0.70; 95% CI, 0.63–0.79). The risk of breast cancer in women using estrogen alone was lower (23%), but not significantly (HR = 0.77; 95% CI, 0.59–1.01). The power of the study to determine a 20% difference between the 2 groups was less than 80%. A high degree of noncompliance with estrogen (more than 50% by the seventh year) further reduced the power and may underestimate the true harms and benefits of treatment. The mean age of women in the trial was 63 years, so the results may not apply to women treated early in menopause.

Essential Evidence: Medicine that Matters, Edited by David Slawson, Allen Shaughnessy, Mark Ebell, and Henry Barry.

Long-term PPI use increases hip fracture risk

Clinical question

Does the long-term use of proton pump inhibitors (PPIs) increase the risk of hip fracture?

Bottom line

Long-term use (greater than one year) of proton pump inhibitors (PPIs) is associated with an increased risk of hip fracture in adults over age 50 years. Risk is also higher among individuals taking higher doses of PPIs and increases with duration of use. Appropriate use, dose, and duration of therapy should be carefully assessed on an individual basis. (LOE = 3b)

Reference

Yang YX, Lewis JD, Epstein S, Metz DC. Long-term proton pump inhibitor therapy and risk of hip fracture. JAMA 2006;296:2947–2953.

Study Design

Case-control

Funding

Industry + govt

Setting

Population-based

Synopsis

Significant hypochlorhydria as a result of proton pump inhibitor (PPI) therapy may cause calcium malabsorption, resulting in a higher risk of bone fractures. These investigators analyzed data obtained from the United Kingdom General Practice Research Database relating to prescription use and subsequent diagnoses and hospitalizations for hip fracture. Previous studies validate information obtained in this manner from the same source. Cases consisted of individuals older than 50 years of age with first occurrence of hip fracture at least 1 year after the beginning of their standard follow-up period. Up to 10 controls were selected for each case matching for multiple variables, including sex, year of birth, and duration of follow-up. The exposure of interest was the effect of cumulative duration of PPI therapy for up to 4 years. The authors performed a statistical analysis of the data to control for other potential confounders, including body mass index, smoking history, alcoholism, impaired mobility, atherosclerotic vascular disease, peptic ulcer disease, renal failure, among others. There were 13,556 hip fracture cases and 135,386 controls. PPI use for more than 1 year was associated with a significantly increased risk of hip fracture (adjusted Hazard Ratio = 1.44, 95% CI, 1.30–1.59; NNTH/person-years = 1266; 944–1856). The associated risk was further increased among patients taking higher doses of PPI and with increasing duration of use. Histamine 2 receptor antagonist therapy (e.g. ranitidine, cimetidine) did not significantly increase hip fracture risk.

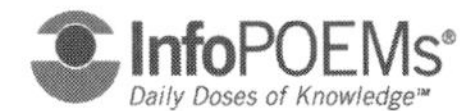

Most women quickly stop taking bisphosphonates

Clinical question

Do women continue osteoporosis therapy for a meaningful period?

Bottom line

Approximately half the women initially prescribed a bisphosphonate – daily or weekly treatment – will not be taking it after 3 months, and only 1 in 5 will be taking it after a year. Since this short duration is unlikely to provide them with meaningful benefit, the money spent on bone mineral density testing and the rest of the diagnostic work-up and follow-up, along with the cost of the initial drug therapy, is essentially wasted on 4 of 5 women diagnosed with osteoporosis. (LOE = 1b)

Reference

Downey TW, Foltz SH, Boccuzzi SJ, Omar MA, Kahler KH. Adherence and persistence associated with the pharmacologic treatment of osteoporosis in a managed care setting. South Med J 2006;99:570–575.

Study Design

Cohort (retrospective)

Funding

Industry

Setting

Population-based

Synopsis

The authors of this analysis evaluated a very large managed care drug database to determine the use patterns of patients who were prescribed drugs for osteoporosis. They evaluated adherence (the percentage of doses taken) and persistence (the use of continuous therapy) in 10,566 women. The women (average age = 64 years) were newly diagnosed with osteoporosis and had been started on a bisphosphonate and probably calcium/vitamin D, though these weren't tracked in the database. All women were continuously eligible for medical benefits coverage over the 18 months of the study. Eighty-five percent of the women were placed on a weekly dosing regimen. Women quickly stopped taking the drug therapy, with only approximately 50% of the women taking it after 3 months, and only 1 in 5 still taking the drug after 1 year. Accordingly, the women missed approximately 40% of the doses they should have taken over the course of a year. Weekly users were slightly more adherent than daily users, although the results are still poor (63% vs 54%; $P < .05$). Persistence and adherence did not vary among the 3 bisphosphonates. These results are similar to those seen in other studies.

Essential Evidence: Medicine that Matters, Edited by David Slawson, Allen Shaughnessy, Mark Ebell, and Henry Barry.

Evidence lacking for milk's benefit in children

Clinical question

Is abundant dietary calcium from dairy or other sources associated with better bone mineral density, bone mineral content, or lower fracture risk in children and young adults?

Bottom line

Although milk has a prominent place in the current recommendations for diet in children (see: www.mypyramid.com) there is a lack of convincing evidence that increased consumption of total dietary calcium generally, or dairy products specifically, provide even modest benefits for bone health in children and adolescents. (LOE = 1a)

Reference

Lanou AJ, Berkow SE, Barnard ND. Calcium, dairy products, and bone health in children and young adults: a reevaluation of the evidence. Pediatrics 2005;115:736–743.

Study Design

Systematic review

Funding

Other

Setting

Various (meta-analysis)

Synopsis

Current dietary guidelines in the U.S. recommend 2–3 cups (480 mL–720 mL) of milk daily for children. This review sought to determine whether there is sufficient evidence to support current recommendations of abundant intake of calcium in childhood to promote bone integrity, and whether milk or other dairy products are better than other calcium-containing foods or calcium supplements. Most studies were conducted with white preadolescent and adolescent girls. The review included 17 cross-sectional studies, 7 retrospective studies, 10 prospective studies, and 12 randomized controlled trials. Most studies assessed surrogate markers of bone health such as bone mineral density (BMD), bone mineral content (BMC), and calcium balance, although susceptibility to fractures was assessed in a few studies. There was no consistent evidence found for a relationship between dairy intake or total calcium intake and BMD, BMC, or fracture risk.

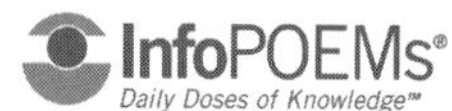

Folate and vitamin B12 lowers fracture risk after stroke

Clinical question

Is supplementation with folate and mecobalamin (vitamin B12) effective in reducing the risk of hip fractures in patients with stroke?

Bottom line

Combined supplementation with oral high dose folate and mecobalamin reduces the risk of hip fractures in elderly patients with stroke and elevated homocysteine levels. The baseline fracture rate in this population is higher than generally reported and all study subjects had low baseline serum levels of folate and vitamin B12. Since the adverse risk of treatment is minimal, it makes sense to consider supplementation at this time in similar patients. (LOE = 1b)

Reference

Sato Y, Honda Y, Iwamoto J, Kanoko T, Satoh K. Effect of folate and mecobalamin on hip fractures in patients with stroke. A randomized controlled trial. JAMA 2005;293:1082–1088.

Study Design

Randomized controlled trial (double-blinded)

Funding

Self-funded or unfunded

Allocation

Concealed

Setting

Outpatient (specialty)

Synopsis

Elevated levels of homocysteine are associated with an increased risk of stroke and osteoporotic hip fractures. Folate and mecobalamin (vitamin B12) supplementation may decrease homocysteine levels. The investigators enrolled 628 consecutive patients, 65 years or older, with residual hemiplegia at least 1 year following their first ischemic stroke. All subjects were recruited from a single Japanese hospital. Eligible subjects were randomized in a double-blind fashion (concealed allocation assignment) to receive either high dose folate (5 mg daily) and mecobalamin (1500 mcg daily) or double placebo. At baseline, all subjects had high levels of plasma homocysteine and low levels of serum cobalamin and serum folate. Follow-up was complete for 89% of the patients at 2 years. Individuals assessing outcomes were blinded to treatment group assignment. Using intention-to-treat analysis, the numbers of hip fractures per 1000 patient-years were 10 and 43 for the treatment and placebo groups, respectively (number needed to treat = 15; 95% CI, 10–31). The overall rate of fractures in the placebo group (8.6%) is higher than previously reported in a community-based elderly population with stroke (1.75%–4.65%; Sato Y, et al. Stroke 2001; 32:1673–77.). Thus, the number needed to treat for a benefit in lower risk populations may be higher than reported in this study. Adverse events attributed to folate and vitamin B12 supplementation were minimal and not clinically significant.

Essential Evidence: Medicine that Matters, Edited by David Slawson, Allen Shaughnessy, Mark Ebell, and Henry Barry.

Falls prevented in elderly by formal assessment or exercise program

Clinical question

What is the best way to prevent falls in older adults?

Bottom line

A multifactorial risk assessment and management program that includes attention to potential hazards of drug therapy is effective in decreasing the risk of falls. An exercise program also decreases the risk of falling. Simple education and inspecting the home for hazards alone were ineffective interventions. (LOE = 1a)

Reference

Chang JT, Morton SC, Rubenstein LZ, et al. Interventions for the prevention of falls in older adults: systematic review and meta-analysis of randomised clinical trials. BMJ 2004;328:680–683.

Study Design

Meta-analysis (randomized controlled trials)

Setting

Outpatient (any)

Synopsis

Falls in older adults are common and can be devastating, so it makes sense to figure out how best to prevent them. The investigators conducting this meta-analysis performed the typical broad and thorough literature search, finding 40 randomized trials comparing an intervention with usual care or a control group. Two of the authors independently reviewed and extracted information from the studies. None of the studies directly assessed the relative effectiveness of the different interventions. A multifactorial falls risk assessment and management program was the most effective. In this approach, patients at a high risk for falls, or who had already experienced a fall, underwent a systematic screening, including a review of drugs. Falls were prevented over the 6 to 18 months by the various study interventions, with 1 additional person being fall-free for every 11 people undergoing the assessment and appropriate intervention (number needed to treat [NNT] = 11). The monthly fall rate also was significantly lower: 11.8 fewer falls per 100 people per month (NNT = 16). Exercise programs were also effective: Falls were prevented in 1 patient for every 16 exercising patients (NNT = 16), and the monthly fall rate also decreased by 2.7 falls per 100 exercising patients per month. There was no difference in benefit among the different types of exercise programs. Home visits to check for environmental hazards and educational interventions such as posters or pamphlets (which were evaluated in only 2 studies) were not effective.

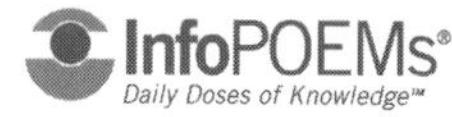

Early mobilization better for acute limb injuries

Clinical question

What is better for acute limb injuries, rest or early mobilization?

Bottom line

Early mobilization following acute limb injuries generally improves function, reduces pain and swelling, and speeds return to work and sports. With proper supervision and education it is preferred over rest for an array of injuries. Unfortunately, this report does not provide very specific guidance for specific mobilization of individual injuries. (LOE = 2a)

Reference

Nash CE, Mickan SM, Del Mar CB, Glasziou PP. Resting injured limbs delays recovery: a systematic review. J Fam Pract 2004;53:706–712.

Study Design

Systematic review

Funding

Government

Allocation

Unconcealed

Setting

Various (meta-analysis)

Synopsis

The acronym that we all learned for treatment of musculoskeletal injuries is RICES: Rest, Ice, Compression, Elevation, and Splinting. Of course, none of these therapies has been well or systematically studied. The authors of this study performed a thorough search of the literature to identify all studies of rest versus early mobilization for acute limb injuries, including fractures, strains, sprains, and other soft tissue injuries. Included were randomized controlled trials with less than 20% loss to follow-up (or an intention-to-treat analysis), that studied mostly adults, and had adequate data reporting. The authors identified 187 potential articles, of which 49 met their inclusion criteria. The quality of studies was rated on a scale from 0 to 16; most were of low quality, and the recommendations for this study are based in large part on the higher quality studies. The definition of early mobilization varied between studies and often involved comparison with splinting or immobilization. Regarding pain and swelling, 13 studies demonstrated an improvement with early mobilization and 9 showed improved patient satisfaction, while none reported an improvement with rest. The better quality studies either found no difference or favored early mobilization. Overall function scores were also more likely to be improved by early mobilization than by rest, and return to work was hastened in 13 of 14 studies of this outcome. Patient preferences, though, perhaps because of their expectations, tended to favor braces or casting following acute injuries. Cost was not studied.

Essential Evidence: Medicine that Matters, Edited by David Slawson, Allen Shaughnessy, Mark Ebell, and Henry Barry.

Nonsurgical treatment effective for carpal tunnel

Clinical question

Are nonsurgical approaches to carpal tunnel syndrome effective?

Bottom line

In this systematic review, nonsurgical treatments of carpal tunnel syndrome using injected or oral steroids provided temporary relief. Spontaneous resolution is more common than you may think: nearly 50% of patients receiving placebos improved. Long-term data on most treatments are lacking. In the few studies with long-term follow up, as many as 50% of patients had surgery during the first year after enrollment. (LOE = 1a−)

Reference

Goodyear-Smith F, Arroll B. What can family physicians offer patients with carpal tunnel syndrome other than surgery? A systematic review of nonsurgical management. Ann Fam Med 2004;2:267–273.

Study Design

Systematic review

Setting

Various (meta-analysis)

Synopsis

These authors systematically reviewed English language randomized controlled trials of nonsurgical treatments of carpal tunnel syndrome. They did an exhaustive search of the literature, including MEDLINE, EMBASE, the Cochrane Library, and the registry of controlled trials. They also hand searched references from previously retrieved articles and communicated with authors to obtain unpublished material. Each author assessed the quality of the studies using the PEDro (Physiotherapy Evidence Database) scale, which gives a total score of 10 possible points. Any disagreements were resolved by consensus. Studies had to have a score of at least 3 for inclusion. The authors ended up with 2 systematic reviews, 16 randomized controlled trials, and 1 quasi-experimental study that met their requirements. They found a fairly high rate of spontaneous resolution; nearly 50% of patients treated with placebo improved. Local steroid injection significantly improved symptoms, but 50% of the patients had surgery within 1 year. Oral steroids provide short-term improvement, but there are no long-term data. The following treatment modalities had limited data on their effectiveness (small studies, poor design, mixed or conflicting results): laser-acupuncture, exercises, ultrasound, splinting, and yoga. The authors were unable to find support for the use of nonsteroidal anti-inflammatory drugs, chiropractic manipulation, pyridoxine, diuretics, or magnets.

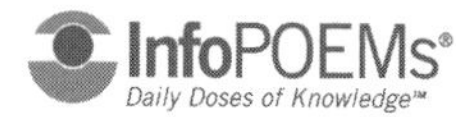

PET scan best in chronic osteomyelitis diagnosis

Clinical question

Which test is most accurate in diagnosing chronic osteomyelitis?

Bottom line

Positron emission tomography (PET) is the most accurate test to diagnose chronic osteomyelitis. (LOE = 3a)

Reference

Termaat MF, Raijmakers PG, Scholten HJ, Bakker FC, Patka P, Haarman HJ. The accuracy of diagnostic imaging for the assessment of chronic osteomyelitis: a systematic review and meta-analysis. J Bone Joint Surg Am 2005;87:2464–2471.

Study Design

Meta-analysis (randomized controlled trials)

Funding

Foundation

Setting

Various (meta-analysis)

Synopsis

This team searched MEDLINE, EMBASE, and Current Contents for studies including at least 10 adults evaluated for chronic osteomyelitis with noninvasive diagnostic tests (radiography, PET scan, leukocyte scintigraphy, bone scintigraphy, gallium scintigraphy, magnetic resonance imaging, and computerized tomography) who also then had a gold standard test (histology, culture results, or clinical follow-up). Since one of the hallmarks of a good diagnostic test is its ability to distinguish among similar conditions, it is noteworthy that they excluded studies that evaluated septic or aseptic loosening of prosthetic joints. They only included studies that provided enough detail to calculate the characteristics of the various diagnostic tests. Two reviewers independently determined study eligibility and extracted the data. Any discrepancies were settled by consensus. They also evaluated each study's methodologic quality on 6 criteria. When they found excessive variability in the data across studies, they did subgroup analyses to see if the tests perform differently in axial and peripheral skeletal infections. A total of 23 studies with 1269 patients were included. The methodologic quality was highly variable; the researchers nonetheless pooled the data for all studies. PET scanning, compared with any single test, was the most sensitive (96%) and specific (91%). This translates to a positive likelihood ratio of 10.7 (95% CI, 4.6–19.8) and a negative likelihood ratio of 0.04 (95% CI, 0.01–0.15). Some combinations of tests (bone scintigraphy + leukocyte scintigraphy; bone scintigraphy + gallium scintigraphy) had comparable sensitivity. These estimates are likely to be biased because poor-quality studies were included.

Essential Evidence: Medicine that Matters, Edited by David Slawson, Allen Shaughnessy, Mark Ebell, and Henry Barry.

Extracorporeal shock wave therapy is ineffective for tennis elbow

Clinical question

Is extracorporeal shock wave therapy effective in treating lateral epicondylitis?

Bottom line

Extracorporeal shock wave therapy is no more effective than sham therapy in treating patients with lateral epicondylitis. Other studies have also found this therapy ineffective for this condition. Those few studies that show a difference are usually small and funded by the companies that make the machines. (LOE = 1b)

Reference

Chung B, Wiley JP. Effectiveness of extracorporeal shock wave therapy in the treatment of previously untreated lateral epicondylitis: A randomized controlled trial. Am J Sports Medicine 2004;32:1660–1667.

Study Design

Randomized controlled trial (double-blinded)

Funding

Government

Allocation

Concealed

Setting

Outpatient (any)

Synopsis

These authors randomly assigned (concealed allocation) 60 patients with previously untreated lateral epicondylitis to receive extracorporeal shock wave therapy) or sham therapy. All patients were also instructed in forearm extensor stretching exercises. The main outcome of this 8-week study was "treatment success," as defined by at least a 50% reduction in elbow pain, a pain score no higher than 4 on a scale of 10, and no analgesic use in the last 2 weeks of the study. The person evaluating these outcomes was not told which treatment the patients received and the outcome was assessed via intention to treat. Twelve of the 31 patients (39%) treated with extracorporeal shock wave therapy were treatment successes compared with 9 of the 29 (23%) treated with sham therapy. The difference in success was not significant. The study was powerful enough to detect modest differences in effect if one were present.

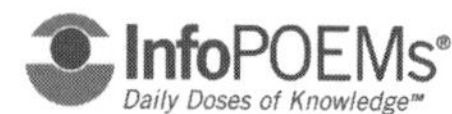

Tennis elbow: injection better short-term, worse long-term

Clinical question

Is a steroid injection or physical therapy more effective than general treatment in patients with tennis elbow?

Bottom line

Over the short-term, the injection of painful sites in patients with tennis elbow will decrease symptoms more than general nonspecific treatment or physical therapy. However, after 1 year, patients receiving physical therapy consisting of exercises and a specific method of elbow manipulation – not described in the article – will have better function and will report greater improvement than those receiving a steroid injection, primarily because of frequent recurrences following the injection. (LOE = 1b)

Reference

Bisset L, Beller E, Jull G, Brooks P, Darnell R, Vicenzino B. Mobilisation with movement and exercise, corticosteroid injection, or wait and see for tennis elbow: randomised trial. BMJ 2006;333:939.

Study Design

Randomized controlled trial (single-blinded)

Funding

Government

Allocation

Concealed

Setting

Outpatient (any)

Synopsis

The Australian researchers conducting this study enrolled 198 adults with tennis elbow symptoms for an average of 22 weeks. Patients were, on average, in their mid-40s and approximately one third were women. Approximately 57% had symptoms due to unknown causes and not due to overuse or trauma. The average pain score was 57 of a possible 100. The patients were randomly assigned, using concealed allocation, to receive 1 of 3 treatments: 10 mg triamcinolone (Aristocort) with 1% lidocaine injected to painful elbow points, repeated after 2 weeks as necessary; eight 30-minute physical therapy treatments consisting of elbow manipulation and exercises done during the session and at home; and, general nonspecific treatment of analgesics, heat, cold, and braces, as desired. Primary outcome evaluation occurred at 6 weeks and 52 weeks and consisted of global improvement, measured on a 6-point Likert-type scale from "completely recovered" to "much worse," along with pain-free grip strength and overall assessment of severity by an assessor unaware of treatment. Using an intention-to-treat analysis, at 6 weeks 78% of injected patients were "much improved" or "completely recovered" as were 65% of patients receiving physical therapy and 27% of patients not receiving specific treatment. Pain-free grip strength and assessors' evaluations were significantly better at this time in the injection group than in the other 2 groups. However, 72% of patients receiving the injections reported recurrences. At 1 year, patients receiving a steroid injection had significantly lower scores on all 3 outcomes than did those with either physical therapy or nonspecific treatment.

Essential Evidence: Medicine that Matters, Edited by David Slawson, Allen Shaughnessy, Mark Ebell, and Henry Barry.

Metoclopramide (Reglan) effective in migraine

Clinical question
In patients with acute migraine, if metoclopramide, either alone or in combination, effective in diminishing pain and nausea?

Bottom line
Parenteral metoclopramide (Reglan) 10 mg is somewhat effective when used alone and seems to add to treatment when used with other migraine treatments. Given its cost and its two-pronged effect on pain and nausea, it should be considered in patients with acute migraine (LOE = 1a)

Reference
Colman I, Brown MD, Innes GD, Grafstein TE, Rowe BH. Parenteral metoclopramide for acute migraine: meta-analysis of randomised controlled trials. BMJ 2004;329:1369–1373.

Study Design
Systematic review

Funding
Unknown/not stated

Setting
Emergency department

Synopsis
Metoclopramide (Reglan) was originally used to treat nausea due to gastric stasis associated with acute migraine as well as to enhance absorption of orally-administered drugs. Subsequent studies showed relief of pain with metoclopramide alone. This meta-analysis culled 13 randomized controlled trials from 596 potentially relevant studies identified by a search of several databases and source. These 13 studies evaluated parenteral metoclopramide, 10 mg, to treat acute migraine in adults in an acute setting: emergency departments or headache clinics. The search was thorough and included an attempt to find unpublished research. The articles were screened by two independent reviewers to determine inclusion. As compared with placebo in 5 small studies enrolling a total of 185 patients, metoclopramide produced significant reductions in headache pain, though the effect was not consistent (number needed to treat [NNT] = 4; 95% CI 2.1–95.1). In comparison with other emetics, metoclopramide was nearly as effective or as effective in reducing headache pain and nausea (the study results could not be combined. It was found, in 40 patients, to be as effective as sumatriptan (Imitrex) in the rate of complete pain resolution or significant reduction of pain or the likelihood of reduction of nausea. Combining metoclopramide with dihydroergotamine (DHE) found the combination to be more effective than dihydroergotamine alone, valproate (Depakene) alone, meperidine (Demerol)/hydroxyzine (Vistaril), Ketorolac (Toradol), and promethazine (Phenergan)/meperidine (Demerol). Drowsiness, restlessness, and dizziness were reported with the use of metoclopramide.

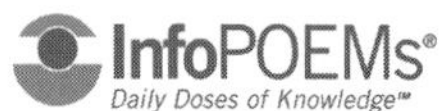

Intranasal zolmitriptan effective for cluster headaches

Clinical question

Is intranasal zolmitriptan effective in treating cluster headaches?

Bottom line

Intranasal zolmitriptan (Zomig) is more effective than placebo in treating cluster headaches. (LOE = 2b–)

Reference

Cittadini E, May A, Straube A, Evers S, Bussone G, Goadsby PJ. Effectiveness of intranasal zolmitriptan in acute cluster headache: a randomized, placebo-controlled, double-blind crossover study. Arch Neurol 2006;63:1537–1542.

Study Design

Cross-over trial (randomized)

Funding

Industry

Allocation

Uncertain

Setting

Outpatient (any)

Synopsis

Ninety-two adult patients with cluster headaches were randomly assigned to receive intranasal zolmitriptan (5 mg or 10 mg) or placebo. Each patient treated 1 moderately severe headache with 1 study drug in rotation for a total of 3 headaches each separated by at least 24 hours. The patients graded the severity of their headaches on a 5-point scale. They could use oxygen for rescue. The main outcome was resolution of the headache to no pain or mild pain. When measured 30 minutes after administration, placebo relieved headaches 23% of the time compared with 42% for 5 mg zolmitriptan (number needed to treat [NNT] = 5; 95% CI, 3–18) and 61% for 10 mg zolmitriptan (NNT = 3; 2–5). These results may be inflated because the authors only had complete data for 75% of the patients. Zolmitriptan is more effective in patients with episodic cluster headaches than in those with chronic cluster headaches. The authors report no serious adverse events in this study.

Essential Evidence: Medicine that Matters, Edited by David Slawson, Allen Shaughnessy, Mark Ebell, and Henry Barry.

Specific headache criteria useful for migraine diagnose, neuroimaging

Clinical question

What components of the history and physical are helpful in determining which patients with a headache have a migraine or need neuroimaging?

Bottom line

Useful clinical criteria from the history and physical for distinguishing migraine from tension-type headache include: nausea, photophobia, phonophobia, and exacerbation by physical activity. Combined findings useful for distinguishing migraine can be summarized by the mnemonic: POUNDing (Pulsatile quality; duration of 4 to 72 hOurs; Unilateral location; Nausea or vomiting; Disabling intensity). Patients with 4 or more of these criteria are most likely to have migraine headaches. Criteria increasing the risk of intracranial pathology include: cluster-type headache; abnormal neurologic examination result; undefined headache; headache with aura; headache aggravated by exertion or valsalva-like maneuver; and headache with vomiting. No clinical features from the history and physical are useful for significantly reducing the likelihood of intracranial pathology. (LOE = 3a)

Reference

Detsky ME, McDonald DR, Baerlocher MO, Tomlinson GA, McCrory DC, Booth CM. Does this patient with headache have a migraine or need neuroimaging? JAMA 2006;296:1274–1283.

Study Design	Funding	Setting
Diagnostic test evaluation	Unknown/not stated	Population-based

Synopsis

After a thorough search of the MEDLINE database and secondary sources including citations from relevant studies, 2 authors independently reviewed studies for inclusion and methodologic quality. Disagreements were resolved by consensus with a third author. Studies were included if they assessed the accuracy of the history and physical examination in predicting the diagnosis of migraine using criteria developed by the International Headache Society. Similar studies assessing clinical criteria predicting significant intracranial pathology in adults with nontraumatic headache were also included. From a total of 771 potential studies on migraine diagnosis, 4 studies of 1745 patients met inclusion criteria. Of these, only 1 study met Level 1 quality criteria for a diagnosis article and only 1 study included patients from the primary care setting. Eleven neuroimaging studies with 3725 patients met inclusion criteria, with only 1 study meeting Level 1 quality criteria. Statistically significant individual criteria for distinguishing migraine from tension-type headache included: nausea (positive likelihood ratio [+LR] = 19, negative likelihood ratio [−LR] = 0.19), photophobia (+LR = 5.8, −LR = 0.24), phonophobia (+LR = 5.2, −LR = 0.38), and exacerbation by physical activity (+LR = 3.7, −LR = 0.24). Criteria increasing the risk of intracranial pathology include: cluster-type headache (+LR = 11); abnormal neurologic examination result (+LR = 5.3); undefined headache (+LR = 3.8); headache with aura (+LR = 3.2); headache aggravated by exertion or valsalva-like maneuver (+LR = 2.3), and headache with vomiting (+LR = 1.8). No clinical features from the history and physical are useful for significantly reducing the likelihood of intracranial pathology.

Essential Evidence: Medicine that Matters, Edited by David Slawson, Allen Shaughnessy, Mark Ebell, and Henry Barry.

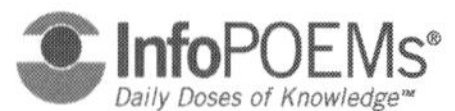

Herpes zoster vaccine safe and effective for older adults

Clinical question

Can a vaccine prevent herpes zoster and postherpetic neuralgia?

Bottom line

Herpes zoster vaccine is safe and effective for the prevention of herpes zoster and postherpetic neuralgia (PHN) in older adults. The number needed to treat is quite large on an annual basis, particularly for PHN. Even if the NNT of 1111 is linear for a 10-year period, one would have to vaccinate 111 older patients to prevent 1 case of PHN during that period. The number needed to treat to prevent a case of herpes zoster is 175. Given the strength of this vaccination and the target population, long-term follow-up studies are needed to identify any unexpected but serious complications that may appear down the road. (LOE = 1b)

Reference

Oxman MN, Levin MJ, Johnson GR, et al, for the Shingles Prevention Study Group. A vaccine to prevent herpes zoster and postherpetic neuralgia in older adults. N Engl J Med 2005;352:2271–2284.

Study Design	Funding	Allocation	Setting
Randomized controlled trial (double-blinded)	Industry + govt	Concealed	Outpatient (any)

Synopsis

Patients with herpes zoster (shingles) feel miserable, and PHN – which complicates about 10% of cases – makes them feel even worse. This study identified adults older than 60 years (47% were older than 70 years) who had either a history of varicella or were presumed to have one because they had lived in the United States for at least 30 years. A total of 59% were men, 95% were white, and they had a generally good baseline health status. Patients were randomized (allocation concealed) to either 0.5 mL of live attenuated Oka/Merck varicella-zoster virus vaccine (n = 19,270) or placebo (n = 19,276). The vaccine is 14 times stronger than the vaccine used to prevent primary varicella infection in children. Groups were balanced at baseline and analysis was by intention to treat. Patients were followed for a median of 3.1 years, and 95% of patients completed the study, which is excellent. The primary outcomes were the number of episodes of herpes zoster and PHN; cases within 30 days of vaccination and second episodes were excluded. Fewer patients in the vaccination group developed herpes zoster (11.1 vs 5.4 episodes per 1000 person-years; $P < .001$; number needed to treat [NNT] = 175 per year). Patients in the vaccinated group also had a somewhat shorter course (21 vs 24 days; $P = .03$) and were less likely to develop PHN (0.48 vs 1.38 per 1000 person-years; $P < .001$; NNT = 1111). The benefit was more pronounced in patients aged 60 years to 69 years than in older patients. Safety is an important issue in prevention studies since we are treating otherwise healthy patients. Safety was monitored in 2 ways: by patient or physician report for the entire population, and by diary entries for a subset of 6716 patients. For the entire study population, there was no difference in mortality between groups and no difference in possible vaccine-related adverse events, either during the first 42 days or for the duration of the 3-year study. For the adverse event substudy group, one or more adverse events – primarily erythema, pain, swelling or pruritus at the injection site – occurred more often during the first 42 days. As noted above, this is a higher potency vaccine; the current vaccine used for children should not be used for adults.

Essential Evidence: Medicine that Matters, Edited by David Slawson, Allen Shaughnessy, Mark Ebell, and Henry Barry.

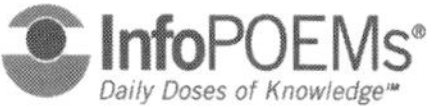

Tricyclics drug of choice for post-herpetic neuralgia

Clinical question

What are the most effective treatments for postherpetic neuralgia?

Bottom line

Tricyclics should be the drug of choice for treatment of PHN; consider gabapentin or capsaicin for treatment failures or patients who do not tolerate a tricyclic antidepressant. (LOE = 1a)

Reference

Alper BS, Lewis PR. Treatment of postherpetic neuralgia: A systematic review of the literature. J Fam Pract 2002;51:121–128.

Study Design

Systematic review

Setting

Various

Synopsis

The authors did a thorough and well-designed meta-analysis to determine the most effective treatment (not prevention) for postherpetic neuralgia (PHN). Most of the 27 trials they identified were well-designed (Jadad quality score 4 out of a possible 5). A particularly bad study (Jadad score = 1) was excluded. Because PHN is rare in patients younger than 50 years, most studies included a majority of (or exclusively) older patients. They found the best evidence to support the use of the tricylcic antidepressants amitriptyline, nortriptyline, and desipramine (number needed to treat = 2–3). Amitriptyline (Elavil) was the best studied, with a usual dose of 75 mg by mouth at bedtime. There was also evidence from a smaller number of studies to support the use of topical capsaicin (Zostrix), gabapentin (Neurontin), and controlled release oxycodone. Lidocaine patch, benzydamine cream, tramadol, and vincristine have not been well studied, while lorazepam, fluphenazine, dextromethorphan, memantine, acyclovir, and acupuncture are unlikely to be beneficial.

Essential Evidence: Medicine that Matters, Edited by David Slawson, Allen Shaughnessy, Mark Ebell, and Henry Barry.

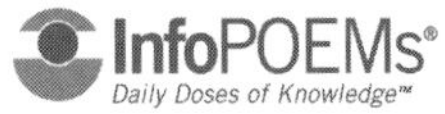

Melatonin effective for some sleep disorders

Clinical question
Is melatonin effective for insomnia and other sleep problems?

Bottom line
Melatonin in doses from 0.1 mg to 10 mg is effective in helping adults and children who have difficulty falling asleep. It is particularly helpful in patients whose circadian rhythm is permanently off kilter (delayed sleep phase syndrome). It increases sleep length, but not sleep quality, in patients who perform shift work or who have jet lag. (LOE = 1a)

Reference
Buscemi N, Vandermeer B, Hooton PR, et al. Melatonin for treatment of sleep disorders. Evidence Report/Technology Assessment No. 108. AHRQ Publication No. 05-E002-1. Rockville MD: Agency for Healthcare Research and Quality. November 2004.

Study Design
Meta-analysis (randomized controlled trials)

Funding
Government

Setting
Outpatient (any)

Synopsis
The authors of this systematic review evaluated the role of melatonin in the treatment of different types of sleep problems in different types of patients. They performed a thorough search of the literature though they limited the research to English-language publications. Potential research was screened by 2 independent reviewers and the data were abstracted by 1 reviewer and then checked for accuracy by another. They included controlled clinical trials and reviewed all studies for quality using the established Jadad criteria. In normal sleepers, melatonin had a clinically insignificant effect on the time to sleep onset (sleep onset latency) or the amount of time actually spent asleep (sleep efficiency). Melatonin in doses of 1 mg to 3 mg caused an average 12.7 minute delay in rapid eye movement onset (REM latency) as compared with placebo. In patients with simple insomnia, melatonin helped adults to fall asleep an average 10.7 minutes faster (95% CI, 3.7–17.6 min). Children had a better response, falling asleep an average 17 minutes faster. It was particularly effective in patients with delayed sleep phase syndrome, a condition in which we might say that a person's circadian rhythm is misaligned without an external cause such as jet lag or shift work. In these patients, sleep onset was an average 38.8 minutes faster (95% CI, 27.3–50.3 min). Melatonin had no effect on sleep quality, wakefulness, total sleep time, or percent time spent in REM sleep. In patients suffering from jet lag, melatonin did not decrease sleep onset latency or increase sleep efficiency, sleep quality, or the time spent in REM sleep, though it was effective in increasing the total sleep time. It had a similar effect as zolpidem (Ambien) in patients with jet lag in one study. Melatonin is not effective in patients with a secondary sleep disorder.

Essential Evidence: Medicine that Matters, Edited by David Slawson, Allen Shaughnessy, Mark Ebell, and Henry Barry.

Cognitive therapy superior to zopiclone for insomnia

Clinical question
What is the optimal management strategy for chronic insomnia: cognitive therapy or zopiclone?

Bottom line
Cognitive behavioral therapy (CBT), consisting of one 50-minute session per week for 6 weeks, is significantly more effective than zopiclone (Imovane) in the treatment of chronic insomnia in older adults. It is uncertain whether less intensive counseling offered directly by primary care clinicians is similarly effective. (LOE = 1b)

Reference
Sivertsen B, Omvik S, Pallesen S, et al. Cognitive behavioral therapy vs zopiclone for treatment of chronic primary insomnia in older adults. A randomized controlled trial. JAMA 2006;295:2851–2858.

Study Design
Randomized controlled trial (double-blinded)

Funding
Foundation

Allocation
Concealed

Setting
Outpatient (specialty)

Synopsis
Both pharmacological and psychological treatments are beneficial for patients with chronic insomnia. To directly compare these treatment approaches, the investigators identified 46 adults with a mean age 61 years who met DSM-IV criteria for chronic insomnia. Eligible patients were randomized (concealed allocation assignment) to 1 of 3 treatment groups: (1) CBT, including an individual 50-minute treatment session once a week for 6 weeks, focusing on sleep hygiene education, sleep restriction, stimulus control, cognitive therapy, and progressive relaxation techniques; (2) zopiclone therapy, 7.5 mg nightly; or (3) placebo. Individuals assessing outcomes were blinded to treatment group assignment. Follow-up occurred for 98% and 83% of subjects at 6 weeks and 6 months, respectively. Using intention-to-treat analysis, total wake time while attempting to sleep was significantly reduced in the CBT group (52%) at 6 weeks compared with 4% and 16% in the zopiclone and placebo groups. At 6 months, total wake time, sleep efficiency, and slow-wave sleep were all significantly better in the CBT group than in the other 2 groups. The percentage of patients who reached a predetermined clinically significant level of sleep efficiency of at least 85% at 6 months was significantly higher in the CBT group than in the zopiclone group (78% vs 40%; number needed to treat = 2.5; 95% CI, 1.5–14). Self-adherence to treatment remained similar in both the CBT and zopiclone group, but was significantly lower in the placebo group. Daytime sleepiness was not specifically assessed.

Essential Evidence: Medicine that Matters, Edited by David Slawson, Allen Shaughnessy, Mark Ebell, and Henry Barry.

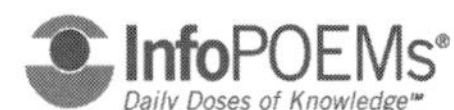

Simple maneuvers can decrease vasovagal syncope episodes

Clinical question

Can a simple counterpressure maneuver prevent vasovagal syncope in susceptible patients?

Bottom line

A simple set of maneuvers (crossing and squeezing legs, grasping a ball tightly, and arm tensing) was effective in decreasing the number of patients with presyncope who experienced a syncopal episode. The maneuvers are simple to perform and can provide an effective way for patients to decrease their number of syncopal episodes if they have prodromal symptoms or can identify triggers that might cause syncope. (LOE = 1b)

Reference

van Dijk N, Quartieri F, Blanc JJ, et al, for the PC-Trial Investigators. Effectiveness of physical counterpressure maneuvers in preventing vasovagal syncope. J Am Coll Cardiol 2006;48:1652–1657.

Study Design	Funding	Allocation
Randomized controlled trial (nonblinded)	Government	Concealed

Setting

Outpatient (specialty)

Synopsis

The authors recruited 223 patients with recurrent vasovagal syncope and recognizable prodromal symptoms. The patients, with an average age of 38 years, had at least 3 syncope episodes in the previous 2 years or at least 1 syncopal episode and 3 presyncopal episodes in the previous year. Vasovagal syncope was diagnosed using the European Society of Cardiology guidelines and included tilt-table testing. Patients all had a normal electrocardiogram result. Using concealed allocation, patients were randomized to receive either conventional therapy or training in physical counterpressure (PC). Conventional therapy consisted of an explanation of the mechanism of syncope and advice regarding lifestyle modification. PC training consisted of teaching the patients a set of maneuvers – leg crossing, handgrip, or arm tensing – to be performed in situations known to provoke syncope or when prodromal symptoms occur. Leg crossing included tensing of the leg, abdominal, and buttock muscles. Handgrip consisted of squeezing a ball or any available object using the dominant hand. Arm tensing occurred by gripping 1 hand with the other while abducting both arms. Patients were instructed to breathe normally and choose one maneuver and hold it until the symptoms disappeared or to move on to another maneuver, if necessary. Over 14 months, the number of patients reporting at least 1 presyncopal episode was similar in both groups: approximately 75%. However, patients in the PC group had fewer episodes of syncope (32% vs 51%; number needed to treat = 5; 95% CI, 3–17). Patients were instructed in the methods and then given biofeedback to gauge their blood pressure response to the maneuvers. Simply teaching the methods in the office, without this feedback, might not be as effective.

Steroid effective for vestibular neuritis, valacyclovir is not

Clinical question

Which is more effective for vestibular neuritis, valacyclovir or methylprednisolone?

Bottom line

Methylprednisolone, starting at 100 mg per day and tapering to 10 mg over 3 weeks, is an effective treatment for vestibular neuritis. Valacyclovir (Valtrex) is not effective. (LOE = 1b)

Reference

Strupp M, Zingler VC, Arbusow V, et al. Methylprednisolone, valacyclovir, or the combination for vestibular neuritis. N Engl J Med 2004;351:354–361.

Study Design

Randomized controlled trial (double-blinded)

Funding

Industry

Allocation

Concealed

Setting

Emergency department

Synopsis

Vestibular neuritis is characterized by sustained rotatory vertigo, positive Romberg's sign falling toward the affected ear, horizontal nystagmus toward the unaffected ear, and nausea. Because vestibular neuritis is thought to be a virally triggered inflammatory condition, it makes sense that antiviral drugs or steroids may be helpful. These authors identified 141 adults presenting to 2 German emergency departments with vestibular neuritis diagnosed after a detailed clinical examination. They then randomized the patients (allocation concealed) to 1 of 4 groups: placebo only, methylprednisolone (MP), valacyclovir (Valtrex), or both. MP was initially given in a dose of 100 mg each morning for 3 days and then tapered slowly to 10 mg over 3 weeks. Valacyclovir was given as 100 mg 3 times daily for 1 week. All patients were also given 150 mg pirenzepine to reduce gastric acid secretion, and antiemetics as needed, and were admitted to the hospital for at least 1 day. The 4 groups were similar at baseline, with a mean age between 46 and 52 years. Patients were followed up for 12 months. Outcomes were evaluated by assessors blinded to treatment assignment, but analysis was does not appear to have been by intention to treat. A total of 114 patients completed the study. The number of patients dropping out or lost to follow-up was similar in each group (6–8). The primary outcome was the degree of nystagmus provoked by caloric irrigation. This is relatively easy to quantify, and it's unfortunate that the researchers did not report any more global symptom measures. They found that treatment with MP was more effective than placebo, but valacyclovir was not. The number of patients with complete or nearly complete recovery of vestibular function was 8 of 30 in the placebo group, 10 of 27 in the valacyclovir group, 22 of 29 in the MP group, and 22 of 28 in the group receiving both drugs (27% for placebo vs 76% for MP; $P < .001$, number needed to treat = 2). One patient in the MP group had a bleeding gastric ulcer and several others had mood swings or dyspepsia.

Essential Evidence: Medicine that Matters, Edited by David Slawson, Allen Shaughnessy, Mark Ebell, and Henry Barry.

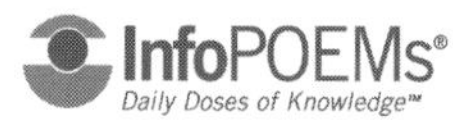

ASA prevents stroke, not MI, in women

Clinical question
Does aspirin prevent cardiovascular disease in women?

Bottom line
Aspirin reduces the risk of stroke and transient ischemic attack in women but does not reduce the risk of myocardial infarction or cardiovascular death. The reduction in strokes over 10 years (number needed to treat = 444) must be balanced against an increase in serious gastrointestinal bleeds (number needed to treat to harm = 553). No change was seen in this large, long study regarding all-cause mortality. (LOE = 1b)

Reference
Ridker PM, Cook NR, Lee IM, et al. A randomized trial of low-dose aspirin in the primary prevention of cardiovascular disease in women. N Engl J Med 2005;352:1293–1304.

Study Design
Randomized controlled trial (double-blinded)

Funding
Government

Allocation
Uncertain

Setting
Population-based

Synopsis
Most of the data on aspirin for the prevention of cardiovascular events comes from studies in men. The current study represents the largest and best evidence to date for women. Women older than 45 years without a history of coronary artery disease, cerebrovascular disease, or cancer were initially enrolled in a 3-month placebo run-in period to establish compliance with the study protocol. Those who complied throughout the run-in period (n = 39,876) were randomized (allocation not specified, but likely concealed) to receive either 100 mg aspirin every other day or matching placebo. They were followed up for a mean of 10 years, with 97% complete data on morbidity and 99% complete data on mortality. Very impressive. The mean age was 55 years, and the 10-year risk of heart disease was less than 5% in 85% of the women. Groups were balanced at the start of the study, outcomes were blindly assessed, and analysis was by intention to treat. Women taking aspirin were less likely to have a stroke (1.1% vs 1.3%; P = .04; number needed to treat [NNT] = 444 for 10 years) or transient ischemic attack (0.9% vs 1.2%; P = .01; NNT = 384 for 10 years) than women taking placebo. However, there were no differences between groups in the likelihood of myocardial infarction (0.99% for aspirin and 0.97% for placebo) or death from cardiovascular causes (0.6% vs 0.63%), any major cardiovascular event (2.4% vs 2.6%), or any cause (3.1% vs 3.2%). Gastrointestinal bleeds requiring transfusion were more common in the aspirin group (0.64% vs 0.46%; P = .02; number needed to treat to harm = 553 for 10 years). The study was powered to have an 86% chance to detect a 25% reduction in the primary outcome of any major cardiovascular event. Review of the survival curve reveals a steady but small trend in favor of aspirin regarding the primary outcome. This apparent benefit, equivalent to a 5% to 10% relative reduction in all-cause mortality, was not statistically significant despite the study's large size.

Essential Evidence: Medicine that Matters, Edited by David Slawson, Allen Shaughnessy, Mark Ebell, and Henry Barry.

ASA + dipyridamole better than ASA for cerebral ischemia (ESPRIT)

Clinical question
Is aspirin plus dipyridamole better than aspirin alone in preventing recurrent cerebral ischemia?

Bottom line
In this unblinded study, the combination of aspirin plus dipyridamole is more effective than aspirin alone in preventing death from all vascular causes, nonfatal stroke, nonfatal myocardial infarction, or major bleeding complications. However, patients taking dipyridamole are much more likely to experience headaches sufficient to stop taking it. (LOE = 2b)

Reference
The ESPRIT Study Group; Halkes PH, van Gijn J, Kappelle LJ, Koudstaal PJ, Algra A. Aspirin plus dipyridamole versus aspirin alone after cerebral ischaemia of arterial origin (ESPRIT): randomised controlled trial. Lancet 2006;367:1665–1673.

Study Design
Randomized controlled trial (nonblinded)

Funding
Government

Allocation
Concealed

Setting
Outpatient (specialty)

Synopsis
Patients referred to a participating hospital within 6 months of a transient ischemic attack or a minor ischemic stroke (grade 3 or less on the modified Rankin Scale) were randomly assigned to receive aspirin alone (average dose = 75 mg; n = 1376) or the same dose of aspirin plus dipyridamole 200 mg twice daily (average dose = 75 mg; n = 1363). The patients were evaluated every 6 months for up to 5 years, either by phone or in person. The primary outcome – a composite of death from all vascular causes, nonfatal stroke, nonfatal myocardial infarction, or major bleeding complication, blindly determined – was assessed by intention to treat. The mean length of follow-up was 3.5 years. At the end of the study period, 15.7% of patients taking aspirin alone experienced the composite outcome compared with 12.7% of patients taking aspirin and dipyridamole (number needed to treat = 34 for 3.5 years; 95% CI, 18–257). Patients taking the combination therapy, however, stopped taking it more often than those taking aspirin alone (34% vs 13%; number needed to treat to harm = 5; 4–6), mainly because of headache.

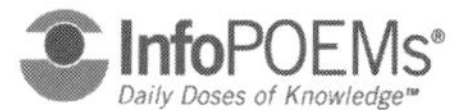

Warfarin increases mortality in intracranial arterial stenosis

Clinical question

Is warfarin better than aspirin for patients with intracranial arterial stenosis?

Bottom line

Warfarin instead of aspirin causes 1 extra death every 2 years for patients with intracranial arterial stenosis and a recent stroke or transient ischemic attack. Given the risk and cost of the imaging studies done to diagnose intracranial arterial stenosis, one has to wonder whether we should just prescribe 650 mg aspirin twice a day for these patients and leave it at that. (LOE = 1b)

Reference

Chimowitz MI, Lynn MJ, Howlett-Smith H, et al, for the Warfarin-Aspirin Symptomatic Intracranial Disease Trial Investigators. Comparison of warfarin and aspirin for symptomatic intracranial arterial stenosis. N Engl J Med 2005;352:1305–1316.

Study Design	Funding	Allocation
Randomized controlled trial (double-blinded)	Government	Concealed

Setting

Outpatient (any)

Synopsis

Retrospective studies have suggested that warfarin may be more effective than aspirin at preventing stroke in patients with intracranial arterial stenosis. However, these studies may be biased by poor ascertainment of outcomes and limited follow-up; that is, if patients who die because of warfarin complications are not identified, the drug may look better than it actually is. This study is the largest and best-to-date to address this question. The investigators enrolled adults at least 40 years of age with a transient ischemic attack or nondisabling stroke in the previous 90 days and a 50% to 99% stenosis of the internal carotid, middle cerebral, vertebral, or basilar arteries. They excluded patients with atrial fibrillation, major comorbidities, or significant stenosis of the extracranial carotid artery. The mean age of participants was 63 years, 61% were men, and 58% were white. The most common lesions was middle cerebral at 32%. Approximately 20% of patients had internal carotid, vertebral, or basilar artery lesions and 6% had multiple lesions. Half of patients had a 50% to 69% stenosis and slightly more than one third had a 70% to 99% stenosis. Patients were randomly assigned (allocation concealed) to receive either warfarin with a target international normalized ratio of 2.0 to 3.0 or aspirin in a dose of 650 mg twice daily. If patients had dyspepsia the aspirin dose could be lowered (minimum 325 mg once daily). Groups were balanced at baseline, outcomes were blindly assessed, and analysis was by intention to treat. Although the researchers planned to follow patients up for a mean of 36 months, the study was stopped prematurely by the safety committee. After a mean follow-up of 1.8 years, it was clear that patients receiving warfarin were more likely to die (9.7% vs 4.3%; P = .02; number needed to treat to harm [NNTH] = 18 for 1.8 years; 95% CI, 10–84). There were also more major hemorrhages in the warfarin group (8.3% vs 3.2%; P = .01; NNTH = 20 for 1.8 years; 11–80).

Essential Evidence: Medicine that Matters, Edited by David Slawson, Allen Shaughnessy, Mark Ebell, and Henry Barry.

Lipid-lowering prevents stroke in patients with or without CHD

Clinical question

In patients with or without heart disease, does lipid-lowering decrease stroke risk?

Bottom line

Statins produce a statistically significant 25% average reduction in the risk of experiencing either a fatal or nonfatal stroke. Other approaches to lipid lowering do not. However, before we start putting statins in the drinking water we need to realize that this reduction translates into 1 less stroke in every 2778 patients at low risk (that is, without heart disease) and 1 less stroke for every 617 patients with pre-existing heart disease. (LOE = 1a)

Reference

Briel M, Studer M, Glass TR, Bucher HC. Effects of statins on stroke prevention in patients with and without coronary heart disease: a meta-analysis of randomized controlled trials. Am J Med 2004;117:596–606.

Study Design

Meta-analysis (randomized controlled trials)

Funding

Unknown/not stated

Setting

Outpatient (any)

Synopsis

The authors of this meta-analysis set out to determine whether lipid-lowering of any type – we already know that statins work – decreases stroke likelihood in patients with or without coronary heart disease (CHD). They started by identifying all 65 randomized controlled trials comparing any intervention with placebo or usual diet, including a total of 200,607 patients. They conducted the appropriate search of 5 databases, including articles in all languages, and they also searched reference lists. Two investigators independently assessed the studies, assessed the quality of the studies, and evaluated the possible influence of the study quality on the results. As has been previously shown, treatment with a statin decreased fatal and nonfatal stroke risk by approximately 25% in patients with or without CHD (primary and secondary prevention). For patients at low risk (0.2% likelihood per year in these studies), this benefit translates into 1 less stroke for every 2778 patients treated for 1 year (95% CI, 2083–5000). For those at high risk (0.9% per year), the benefit was 1 less stroke for every 617 patients treated for 1 year (463–1111). The benefit was not quite as pronounced in the higher quality studies that used concealed allocation when enrolling patients. Treatment with other cholesterol-lowering approaches, including diet, did not have an effect on stroke risk.

Essential Evidence: Medicine that Matters, Edited by David Slawson, Allen Shaughnessy, Mark Ebell, and Henry Barry.

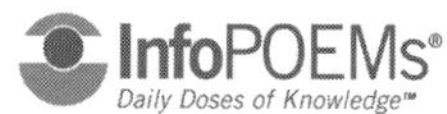

High-dose atorvastatin reduces recurrent stroke, not mortality (SPARCL)

Clinical question

Does high-dose atorvastatin improve outcomes after stroke or transient ischemic attack?

Bottom line

High-dose atorvastatin reduces the risk of recurrent stroke, but does not improve mortality rates. A reduction in the risk of transient ischemic attack (TIA) or unclassified stroke was partially offset by an increase in the risk of hemorrhagic stroke. (LOE = 1b)

Reference

Amarenco P, Bogousslavsky J, Callahan A 3rd, et al, for the Stroke Prevention by Aggressive Reduction in Cholesterol Levels (SPARCL) Investigators. High-dose atorvastatin after stroke or transient ischemic attack. N Engl J Med 2006;355:549–559.

Study Design

Randomized controlled trial (double-blinded)

Funding

Industry

Allocation

Uncertain

Setting

Inpatient (any location) with outpatient follow-up

Synopsis

In this study, patients presenting within 6 months of an ischemic or hemorrhagic stroke or TIA were randomly assigned (allocation concealment uncertain) to either atorvastatin 80 mg per day or placebo. Patients had to be ambulatory, have a Rankin scale score of less than 4 of 6, and a low-density lipoprotein cholesterol level of 100 mg/dL to 190 mg/dL (2.6 to 4.9 mmol/L). Their mean age was 63 years, 60% were male, and 69% suffered a stroke as the index event. Analysis was by intention to treat and patients were followed up for a mean of 4.9 years. Groups were balanced at the start of the study and of the 4731 patients who were randomized, a similar number in each group (2272 vs 2253) were observed through the end of the study. At the end of the study, patients who took atorvastatin were less likely to have a stroke (11.2% vs 13.1%; P = .03; number needed to treat = 53 for 5 years to prevent 1 stroke). However, there was no difference in overall mortality bewteen groups (9.1% for atorvastatin vs 8.9% for placebo; P = .77) and there was a significant increase in the risk of hemorrhagic stroke in those taking atorvastatin (1.66; 95% CI, 1.08–2.55; number needed to treat to harm = 107 for 5 years). To be fair, the study was not powered to detect a difference in mortality rate.

Essential Evidence: Medicine that Matters, Edited by David Slawson, Allen Shaughnessy, Mark Ebell, and Henry Barry.

ABCD rule predicts 7-day stroke risk in TIA

Clinical question
Can clinical factors be used in patients with transient ischemic attack to predict subsequent stroke?

Bottom line
Easy-to-assess clinical and demographic variables can be used to predict which patients with transient ischemic attacks (TIAs) are at greatest risk of stroke in the subsequent week. (LOE = 1b−)

Reference
Rothwell PM, Giles MF, Flossmann E, et al. A simple score (ABCD) to identify individuals at high early risk of stroke after transient ischaemic attack. Lancet 2005;366:29–36.

Study Design
Decision rule (validation)

Funding
Foundation + Government

Setting
Population-based

Synopsis
These authors studied more than 100,000 patients registered with 50 British family physicians. Between 1981 and 1986, all patients with a possible first TIA were referred to a study neurologist as soon after the event as possible. The neurologist agreed with the initial diagnosis approximately half the time. A study nurse re-evaluated these patients 1 month after the initial neurologist evaluation. Among 209 patients with a first TIA, 18 had a stroke within 1 week. These patients were used to develop a predictive model that the authors then tested prospectively on another group of 190 patients with TIAs. This validation group came from more than 90,000 patients registered with 63 British family physicians and were evaluated in a manner similar as the first group. Twenty of these patients had a stroke in the 7 days after TIA. Finally, the authors also tested how well the predictive model worked when used by non-neurologists on a less rigorously studied group of patients with TIAs. In the predictive model, called ABCD (for Age, Blood pressure, Clinical factors, and Duration), patients are given points as follows: 60 years or older (1 point); systolic blood pressure greater than 140 mm Hg and/or diastolic blood pressure greater than or equal to 90 mm Hg (1 point); unilateral weakness (2 points), speech disturbance without weakness (1 point); and duration of symptoms of 60 minutes or more (2 points), 10 minutes to 59 minutes (1 point), less than 10 minutes (0 points). In the validation group, 19 of the 20 patients who later had a stroke had a score of 5 or more. In the group assessed by non-neurologists, no patient with a score lower than 4 had a stroke.

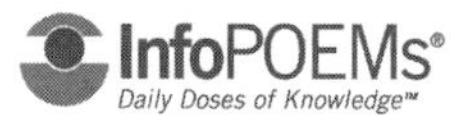

ABCD rule predicts 7- and 30-day stroke risk in patients with TIA

Clinical question

Do clinical factors reliably predict which patients with transient ischemic attacks will experience a stroke in the next 30 days?

Bottom line

The ABCD score, determined by using clinical factors previously tested on other populations, appears to reliably predict the risk of stroke in the 30 days following hospitalization for transient ischemic attack (TIA). It may not have the same validity in patients not admitted to the hospital. (LOE = 1b)

Reference

Tsivgoulis G, Spengos K, Manta P, et al. Validation of the ABCD score in identifying individuals at high early risk of stroke after a transient ischemic attack: a hospital-based case series study. Stroke 2006;37:2892–2897.

Study Design

Decision rule (validation)

Funding

Unknown/not stated

Setting

Inpatient (any location) with outpatient follow-up

Synopsis

These authors retrospectively studied 226 consecutive patients hospitalized with TIA. They compared the outcome predicted by the ABCD score with the real outcome. To determine the ABCD (for Age, Blood pressure, Clinical factors, and Duration) score, points are given as follows: 60 years or older (1 point); systolic blood pressure greater than 140 mm Hg and/or diastolic blood pressure greater than or equal to 90 mm Hg (1 point); unilateral weakness (2 points), speech disturbance without weakness (1 point); and a duration of symptoms of 60 minutes or more (2 points), of 10 minutes to 59 minutes (1 point), of less than 10 minutes (0 points). The researchers calculating the ABCD score were unaware of the real outcome. Within 30 days of the index TIA, 22 (9.7%) patients had a subsequent stroke. The ABCD score was highly correlated with the risk of stroke: ABCD score 7-day stroke risk (95% CI) 30-day stroke risk (95% CI)2 or less 0 03 1.7% (0%–5.1%) 3.5% (0%–8.2%)4 7.6% (1.2%–14%) 7.6% (1.2%–14%)5 19.1% (7.8%–30.4%) 21.3% (10.4%–33%)6 18.8% (0%–37.9%) 31.3% (8.6%–54%). There is one limitation to this generally well-done study: The ABCD model was developed in an outpatient setting to predict risk for all TIA patients. This study only addresses its application to hospitalized patients.

Essential Evidence: Medicine that Matters, Edited by David Slawson, Allen Shaughnessy, Mark Ebell, and Henry Barry.

Eight clinical findings distinguish stroke from stroke mimics

Clinical question

Can clinical factors detectable at the bedside help distinguish stroke from stroke mimics?

Bottom line

In this study, 31% of patients with suspected stroke actually had a stroke mimic. Eight clinical factors helped distinguish these patients from those with stroke. (LOE = 2b)

Reference

Hand PJ, Kwan J, Lindley RI, Dennis MS, Wardlaw JM. Distinguishing between stroke and mimic at the bedside: the brain attack study. Stroke 2006;37:769–775.

Study Design

Cross-sectional

Funding

Government

Setting

Inpatient (any location)

Synopsis

As many as 1 in 3 patients presenting with acute onset of focal neurologic deficits have not had a stroke. This is an important factor in the controversy surrounding the use of thrombolytics in acute ischemic infarct. In this study, the researchers enrolled more than 300 consecutive patients presenting to an urban teaching hospital with a possible stroke. One of 4 physicians with at least 5 years experience performed a standardized bedside assessment of all patients. The final diagnosis of stroke was made by a consensus panel of stroke experts who reviewed the clinical details, imaging studies, and "other relevant investigations." The final diagnoses was stroke in 69% and mimic in 31%. Eight clinical variables independently predicted the final diagnosis. Cognitive impairment and abnormal signs in other systems suggested a stroke mimic. Having an exact time of onset, definite focal symptoms, and abnormal vascular findings; the presence of neurological signs; and being able to lateralize the signs to the left or right side of the brain, and being able to determine a clinical stroke subclassification suggested a stroke. The authors don't provide enough data to be able to calculate the sensitivity, specificity, or likelihood ratios for these factors.

Essential Evidence: Medicine that Matters, Edited by David Slawson, Allen Shaughnessy, Mark Ebell, and Henry Barry.

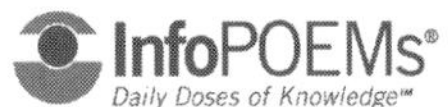

Noninvasive carotid imaging can replace invasive imaging

Clinical question

Can noninvasive imaging replace invasive testing in patients with suspected carotid artery disease?

Bottom line

Noninvasive testing, especially contrast-enhanced magnetic resonance angiography (CEMRA), compares very favorably with invasive angiography. Since noninvasive testing appears to be less accurate in patients with less severe stenosis, a reasonable strategy might begin with CEMRA. If CEMRA demonstrates a greater than 70% stenosis, the diagnosis is settled. If the stenosis appears to be less than 70%, invasive angiography might be considered. Of course, this diagnostic approach needs formal evaluation. (LOE = 1a−)

Reference

Wardlaw JM, Chappell FM, Best JJ, Wartolowska K, Berry E; NHS Research and Development Health Technology Assessment Carotid Stenosis Imaging Group. Non-invasive imaging compared with intra-arterial angiography in the diagnosis of symptomatic carotid stenosis: a meta-analysis. Lancet 2006;367:1503–1512.

Study Design

Systematic review

Funding

Government

Setting

Various (meta-analysis)

Synopsis

Two members of this research team searched MEDLINE and EMBASE and hand-searched several journals to identify 41 prospective studies of at least 20 patients with suspected carotid artery disease who underwent 1 or more noninvasive test and invasive angiography. Any disagreements were settled by discussion with a third reviewer. Similarly, 2 reviewers extracted the data and discrepancies were arbitrated by a third reviewer. The identified studies included a total of 2541 patients. Overall, CEMRA generally performed best, although computed tomographic angiography, magnetic resonance angiography, and Doppler ultrasound also performed well. The authors found some variability in test performance, mainly due to differences in accuracy on the basis of the degree of stenosis. Nonetheless, depending on the degree of stenosis, CEMRA provided the most diagnostic information (positive likelihood ratio ranged from 13 to 26 and negative likelihood ratio from 0.04 to 0.24). Generally speaking, the noninvasive tests were not as accurate in patients with moderate stenosis (50%–69%). Since this group also has a narrow surgical risk-benefit margin, diagnostic certainty is critical. Finally, CEMRA results may be biased because of small study sizes and, as a new technology, the potential for reporting overly positive studies. Stay tuned.

Essential Evidence: Medicine that Matters, Edited by David Slawson, Allen Shaughnessy, Mark Ebell, and Henry Barry.

Three percent of TIA patients have a stroke within 30 days (BASIC)

Clinical question

What is the risk of stroke after a transient ischemic attack?

Bottom line

The rate of stroke following a transient ischemic attack was approximately 3% within 30 days and approximately 7% within 1 year. We have all been taught that a transient ischemic attack is a harbinger of bad things and thus we should urgently work up these patients and initiate aggressive risk modification. Although this study can't address these issues, it suggests that perhaps we don't need to panic. (LOE = 1b–)

Reference

Lisabeth LD, Ireland JK, Risser JMH, et al. Stroke risk after transient ischemic attack in a population-based setting. Stroke 2004;35:1842–1846.

Study Design

Cohort (prospective)

Setting

Population-based

Synopsis

This study took place in a unique setting – an isolated county in southeast Texas that has approximately 50% Mexican American and 50% non-Hispanic white residents. The authors studied 612 patients with a transient ischemic attack (TIA) diagnosed according to the World Health Organization criteria. The diagnosis was independently validated by board-certified neurologists. To minimize misclassification, the research team revalidated 10% of the cases and adjudicated discrepancies. Furthermore, they required that neurologists maintain a discrepancy rate of less than 1% when cases are revalidated or face retraining. The authors tracked patients over time by examining admission and emergency department logs of all area hospitals, and contacting a random sample of outpatient primary care physicians, nursing homes, and neurologists. They reported the rate of stroke during the year after the TIA: 2 days (1.64%), 7 days (1.97%), 30 days (3.15%), 90 days (4.03%), and 12 months (7.27%). Other studies have reported significantly higher rates of events: more than 4% at 30 days (Lovett JK, et al. Stroke 2003; 34:e138–40) and as high as 14.5% per year (Hill MD, et al. Neurology 2004 8; 62:2015–20.)

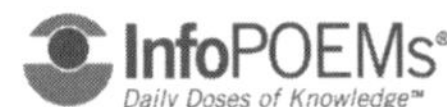

Endarterectomy best within 2 weeks of stroke or TIA

Clinical question

What factors are associated with favorable carotid endarterectomy outcomes?

Bottom line

Patients older than 75 years, men, and those who have carotid endarterectomy within 2 weeks of a cerebrovascular event have better outcomes following endarterectomy. (LOE = 1b)

Reference

Rothwell PM, Eliasziw M, Gutnikov SA, et al. Endarterectomy for symptomatic carotid stenosis in relation to clinical subgroups and timing of surgery. Lancet 2004;363:915–924

Study Design

Other

Setting

Inpatient (any location) with outpatient follow-up

Synopsis

These authors pooled the data from 2 randomized controlled trials of carotid endarterectomy. These studies represent 95% of patients ever randomized to endarterectomy versus medical treatment for symptomatic carotid stenosis. In this pooled analysis, the authors examined several specific subgroups, including sex, age, time from most recent cerebrovascular event, severity of event, diabetes, plaque characteristics, and the presence of contralateral carotid occlusion. All data were analyzed via intention to treat. The studies included 5893 patients and had a mean follow-up of 66 months. Men and patients older than 75 years had better outcomes. Those who had surgery more than 2 weeks after their event had worse outcomes. The degree of stenosis, as seen in the primary studies, was an important modifier. For those with more than 50% stenosis, the numbers needed to treat to prevent 1 ipsilateral stroke in 5 years were: 9 for men; 36 for women; 5 for patients older than 75 years; 18 for those younger than 65 years; 5 for those patients randomized within 2 weeks of their cerebrovascular event; and 125 for those randomized beyond 12 weeks.

Essential Evidence: Medicine that Matters, Edited by David Slawson, Allen Shaughnessy, Mark Ebell, and Henry Barry.

Carotid stent inferior to carotid endarterectomy

Clinical question
Is stenting a safe and effective alternative to carotid endarterectomy in patients with symptomatic carotid stenosis?

Bottom line
Carotid stenting as currently practiced should be abandoned. It significantly increases the risk of stroke in patients with symptomatic carotid stenosis. (LOE = 1b)

Reference
Mas JL, Chatellier G, Beyssen B, et al, for the EVA-3S Investigators. Endarterectomy versus stenting in patients with symptomatic severe carotid stenosis. N Engl J Med 2006;355:1660–1671.

Study Design
Randomized controlled trial (nonblinded)

Funding
Government

Allocation
Concealed

Setting
Inpatient (any location) with outpatient follow-up

Synopsis
It makes sense that carotid stenting, a less invasive procedure, might be safer than carotid endarterectomy (CE). However, several smaller previous clinical trials have not found an advantage to stenting over CE. This French study included 520 adults with a recent transient ischemic attack (TIA) or nondisabling stroke and a 60% to 99% stenosis in the symptomatic carotid artery. Patients with significant disability, uncontrolled hypertension or diabetes, unstable angina, history of bleeding, or severe proximal or intracranial lesions worse than the cervical lesion were excluded. Allocation to groups was concealed, but the patients and neurologists doing outcome assessment were not blinded. The events committee that assessed stroke, death, and other outcomes was blinded. The goal of the analysis was to determine "noninferiority" at 30 days, but the study was stopped prematurely because of significantly worse outcomes than expected in the stent group. Groups were balanced at the start of the study, analysis was by intention to treat, and the mean age of participants was 70 years. Approximately half had a history of ischemic stroke, and one third had a history of TIA. Only 4% of patients in the stent group had more than 1 stent placed. At 30 days, the risk of nonfatal stroke was much higher in the stent group (8.8% vs 2.7%; number needed to treat to harm [NNTH] = 16; 95% CI, 10–47), although the risk of death was similar (1.2% in the CE group vs 0.8% in the stent group). At 6 months, the risk of any stroke or death was 6.1% in the CE group and 11.7% in the stent group (NNTH = 18; 9–143).

Essential Evidence: Medicine that Matters, Edited by David Slawson, Allen Shaughnessy, Mark Ebell, and Henry Barry.

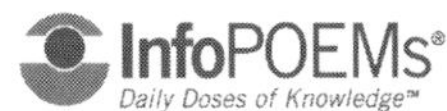

PEG tubes worsen quality of life in stroke (FOOD)

Clinical question

Do percutaneous endoscopic gastrostomy tubes improve outcomes in stroke patients with dysphagia?

Bottom line

In this underpowered study of patients with acute ischemic stroke and dysphagia, early use of enteral tube feeding achieved no better (or worse) outcomes than avoiding it. Using percutaneous endoscopic gastrostomy tubes produced a nonsignificant reduction in mortality, but significantly increased the number of patients having poor outcomes 6 months after the stroke. (LOE = 1b–)

Reference

Dennis MS, Lewis SC, Warlow C; FOOD Trial Collaboration. Effect of timing and method of enteral tube feeding for dysphagic stroke patients (FOOD): a multicentre randomised controlled trial. Lancet 2005;365:764–772.

Study Design

Randomized controlled trial (single-blinded)

Funding

Government

Allocation

Concealed

Setting

Inpatient (any location) with outpatient follow-up

Synopsis

This paper is a report of 2 FOOD (Feed Or Ordinary Diet) trials that shared the same protocols. In this report, any dysphagic patient admitted with a recent ischemic stroke whose physician was uncertain of the best approach to feeding was eligible. In the first FOOD trial (early vs avoid), the patients were randomly assigned (concealed allocation) to start enteral tube feeding as soon as possible (n = 429) or to avoid any enteral tube feeding for at least 7 days (n = 430). In the second trial (percutaneous endoscopic gastrostomy vs nasogastric feeding, or PEG vs NG), patients were randomized (concealed allocation) to enteral feeding via PEG tube (n = 162) or NG tube (n = 159) within 3 days of enrollment. The duration of feeding was not predetermined, but was based on practicality and the patients' condition. The main outcomes, assessed by intention to treat, were death or a poor outcome after 6 months of follow-up (defined as a modified Rankin score of 4 or 5). The research staff evaluating the outcomes were unaware of how the patients were fed. The researchers lost only 1 patient to follow-up. By the end of the study, nearly half of all patients died. In the early vs avoid trial, mortality and poor outcomes were not significantly affected, although ending the study early severely reduced the sample size thereby potentially missing meaningful differences. In the PEG vs NG trial, mortality was also not significantly affected, although there was an absolute increase in the number of patients having a poor outcome (number needed to treat to harm = 13; 95% CI, 6.4 – infinity; P = .05; lower confidence level for adjusted risk ratio = 0).

Essential Evidence: Medicine that Matters, Edited by David Slawson, Allen Shaughnessy, Mark Ebell, and Henry Barry.

Fetal pulse oximetry does not reduce operative delivery

Clinical question

Does the additional information provided by fetal pulse oximetry reduce operative deliveries when fetal heart rate pattern in labor is nonreassuring?

Bottom line

The addition of fetal pulse oximetry (FPO) in the presence of a nonreassuring fetal heart tracing reduced the rate of operative delivery for the indication of nonreassuring fetal status, but failed to decrease either the total cesarean delivery rate or operative vaginal delivery rate. (LOE = 1b)

Reference

East CE, Brennecke SP, King JF, Chan FY, Colditz PB, and the FOREMOST Study Group. The effect of intrapartum fetal oximetry, in the presence of a nonreassuring fetal heart rate pattern, on operative delivery rates: a multicenter, randomized, controlled trial (the FOREMOST trial). Am J Obstet Gynecol 2006;194:606.e1–16.

Study Design

Randomized controlled trial (nonblinded)

Funding

Government

Allocation

Concealed

Setting

Inpatient (ward only)

Synopsis

In this Australian randomized controlled study at 4 centers there were almost 55,000 births screened over a 5-year period. Of 2400 eligible women 601 were enrolled and randomized to FPO as an addition to continuous tococardiography (CTG) or CTG only. Each center had midwives specifically trained to place the FPO sensor in the maternal vagina. An FPO reading of 30% or more was considered normal. A fetal heart rate of less than 70 beats per minute for more than 7 minutes was considered ominous and an indication for immediate delivery regardless of FPO reading. In approximately 2% of cases the midwife was unable to place the FPO sensor. The cesarean delivery rate for nonreassuring fetal status was 14% in the FPO group and 20% in the CTG-only group, which was statistically significant. However, there was in increase of similar magnitude in cesarean deliveries for other indications, principally failure to progress. The overall cesarean delivery rate did not differ between groups (46% vs 48%). Results for operative delivery were similar. The rate of spontaneous vaginal delivery did not differ between groups (27% vs 29%).

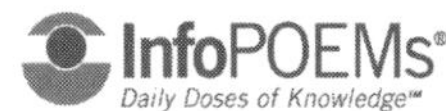

Suction before delivery of shoulders doesn't prevent meconium aspiration

Clinical question

Does suction of the oropharynx and nasopharynx before delivery of the shoulders of infants with meconium-stained amniotic fluid prevent meconium aspiration syndrome?

Bottom line

Oropharyngeal and nasopharyngeal suctioning of neonates before delivery of the shoulders does not prevent meconium aspiration syndrome. (LOE = 1b)

Reference

Vain NE, Szyld EG, Prudent LM, Wiswell TE, Aguilar AM, Vivas NI. Oropharyngeal and nasopharyngeal suctioning of meconium-stained neonates before delivery of their shoulders: multicentre, randomised controlled trial. Lancet 2004;364:597–602.

Study Design

Randomized controlled trial (nonblinded)

Allocation

Concealed

Setting

Inpatient (ward only)

Synopsis

Nasopharyngeal and oropharyngeal suction before delivery of the shoulders of infants with meconium-stained amniotic fluid is a routine practice in the United States. The benefit of this practice has not been demonstrated. In this randomized study, women in labor with a gestation of at least 37 weeks and meconium-stained amniotic fluid were randomized to oropharyngeal and nasopharyngeal suction of the neonate before delivery of the shoulders (n = 1263) or no suction (n = 1251). Delivery could be vaginal or cesarean. The study took place in 11 hospitals in Argentina and 1 in the United States. Half the hospitals served low-income populations and half served upper income populations. The need for tracheal suctioning was based on American Academy of Pediatrics recommendations. Characteristics such as cesarean deliveries and abnormal fetal heart tracings were not different between groups. Suction was with a catheter to wall suction. The study was large enough to detect a 3% absolute difference in the incidence of meconium aspiration syndrome. There were 87 neonates in the suction group that did not get suction and 26 in the no suction group who were suctioned. Allocation was concealed and analysis was by intention to treat. Although women and obstetrical attendants were not blinded, outcome assessors were blinded to treatment assignment. The incidence of meconium aspiration syndrome was 4% in each group. Mechanical ventilation was used in 2% of the suction group and 1% of the no suction group. Nine perinatal deaths occurred in the suctioned group, of which 4 were due to respiratory failure. Four deaths occurred in the no suction group, of which 2 were due to respiratory failure. There was no difference between groups in rates of endotracheal intubation, suction, and positive pressure ventilation in the delivery room (8% vs 9%).

Essential Evidence: Medicine that Matters, Edited by David Slawson, Allen Shaughnessy, Mark Ebell, and Henry Barry.

VBAC with prior vaginal delivery safer than cesarean

Clinical question
Is vaginal birth after cesarean or elective repeat cesarean delivery safer in women with a prior vaginal delivery?

Bottom line
This study provides evidence for considering separately each distinct population of candidates for vaginal birth after cesarean (VBAC). Women with a previous history of vaginal delivery are at lower risk of complications during VBAC than during elective cesarean delivery, whereas women who have never given birth vaginally do not share this decreased risk. (LOE = 2b)

Reference
Cahill AG, Stamilio DM, Odibo AO, et al. Is vaginal birth after cesarean (VBAC) or elective repeat cesarean safer in women with a prior vaginal delivery? Am J Obstet Gynecol 2006;195:1143–1147.

Study Design
Cohort (retrospective)

Funding
Government

Allocation
Concealed

Setting
Inpatient (ward only)

Synopsis
In this retrospective cohort study, the authors reviewed the medical records of 6619 women from 17 institutions in the United States with both prior vaginal delivery and prior cesarean delivery. Women were excluded if they had a history of hysterotomy other than a low transverse incision, fetal anomalies, breech presentation, or multiple gestation of higher order than twins. The majority of women (5091) chose trial of labor, and 92% had successful VBAC. Among the 1578 women who underwent elective repeat cesarean, there were more women with a history of more than one uterine incision, preterm delivery, hypertensive disorders, and pre-existing or gestational diabetes. A composite outcome of severe maternal morbidity including uterine rupture, uterine artery laceration, and bowel and bladder injuries was less frequent in the VBAC group than the cesarean group (1.07% vs 1.33%; adjusted odds ratio = 0.32; 95% CI, 0.14–0.72). Postpartum fever and transfusions were also significantly less frequent in the trial of labor group than in the cesarean group (fever = 7% vs 19%, tranfusions = 0.4% vs 2.1%, respectively). Uterine rupture occurred in 0.4% of women undergoing trial of labor, which did not differ significantly from the rate among women choosing elective cesarean (0.06%). Neonatal outcomes were not assessed.

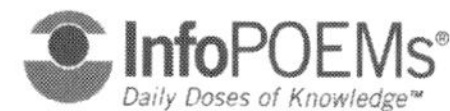

Risk-based screening for GDM effective

Clinical question

Is risk-based screening a sensitive approach to the diagnosis of gestational diabetes mellitus?

Bottom line

A simple risk assessment was effective as an initial screening approach for gestational diabetes mellitus (GDM) in this Danish population. Almost two thirds of the women in the study did not have any of the 5 risk factors and would not require blood testing. Since many women find the commonly used screening approach (universal 1-hour glucose tolerance test [GTT] followed by a 3-hour GTT for women with positive results) unpleasant and time consuming, this kind of risk-based approach deserves further study in other populations. (LOE = 1b–)

Reference

Jensen DM, Molsted-Pedersen L, Beck-Nielsen H, Westergaard JG, Ovesen P, Damm P. Screening for gestational diabetes mellitus by a model based on risk indicators: a prospective study. Am J Obstet Gynecol 2003;189:1383–1388.

Study Design

Decision rule (validation)

Setting

Population-based

Synopsis

Screening for GDM with a 50 g, 1-hour GTT is considered by many to be the standard of care despite a US Preventive Services Task force grade of I; that is, there is insufficient evidence to recommend it. In many European countries, diagnostic testing for GDM is done only in women considered at risk for GDM. These Danish authors sought to validate a simple initial screening approach using 5 risk factors: (1) glucosuria level on dipstick urine testing of 2+ or more; (2) GDM in a previous pregnancy; (3) body mass index of at least 27 kg/m2; (4) family history of diabetes in parents, siblings, grandparents, or children; and (5) previous delivery of a macrosomic infant with birth weight of at least 4500 g. Diagnostic testing with a 2-hour GTT was performed for women with any risk factor. This consisted of a fasting glucose followed by a 75 g oral glucose load and blood draw 2 hours later. Diagnosis of GDM was based on a fasting glucose level of at least 111 mg/dL or a 2-hour glucose level higher than 164 mg/dL. Of 5235 pregnant women, 3337 (64%) did not have any risk factors. Twenty-five percent of the low-risk women voluntarily underwent the 2-hour test at 28 to 32 weeks' gestation; 6 tested positive (<1%). The main weakness of the study is possible selection bias due to the low participation rate among the low-risk women. However, the authors made a fairly good case that low-risk women who agreed to be tested were not different from women who were not tested.

Steroids effective for hyperemesis gravidarum

Clinical question

In pregnant women hospitalized for intractable hyperemesis gravidarum, is high-dose hydrocortisone more effective than metoclopramide in reducing the rate of vomiting?

Bottom line

Intravenous hydrocortisone 300 mg daily will decrease the episodes of vomiting in women hospitalized with hyperemesis of pregnancy to an extent similar or greater than that of metoclopramide (Reglan). Unfortunately, the authors did not analyze the number of women who had a complete resolution of vomiting. (LOE = 1b)

Reference

Bondok RS, El Sharnouby NM, Eid HE, Abd Elmaksoud AM. Pulsed steroid therapy is an effective treatment for intractable hyperemesis gravidarum. Crit Care Med 2006;34:2781–2783.

Study Design

Randomized controlled trial (double-blinded)

Funding

Unknown/not stated

Allocation

Concealed

Setting

Inpatient (ICU only)

Synopsis

Although the mechanism of action is not known, steroids have been used informally for the treatment of hyperemesis since they were first produced. These Egyptian researchers enrolled 40 women with hyperemesis gravidarum, defined as severe persistent vomiting, ketonuria, and weight loss of greater than 5% of prepregnancy weight requiring intensive care. All women were at 16 weeks' or less gestation. Using concealed allocation, the women were randomized to receive either hydrocortisone or metoclopramide for 1 week. Hydocortisone was given intravenously each day in doses of 300 mg for 3 days, 200 mg for 2 days, and 100 mg for 2 days, with normal saline given for 2 doses daily to preserve blinding. Metoclopramide was also given intravenously, 10 mg 3 times daily for 1 week. Vomiting episodes decreased in both groups, from an average of approximately 9 episodes per day at the start of the study to approximately 0.5 episodes per woman in the steroid group and 2 episodes per day in the metoclopramide group. The authors did not report the number of women with complete cessation of vomiting. Over the subsequent 2 weeks, 6 of the 20 women treated with metoclopramide, but none treated with hydrocortisone, were readmitted for recurrence.

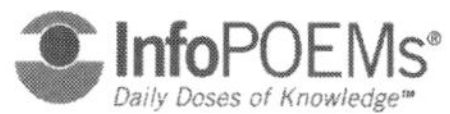

Immersion exercise reduces leg edema in pregnancy

Clinical question
Does immersion exercise reduce dependent edema in pregnant women?

Bottom line
Water immersion exercise is an option for managing leg edema in otherwise uncomplicated pregnancies. (LOE = 2b)

Reference
Hartmann S, Huch R. Response of pregnancy leg edema to a single immersion exercise session. Acta Obstet Gynecol Scand 2005;84:1150–1153.

Study Design
Cohort (prospective)

Funding
Unknown/not stated

Setting
Outpatient (specialty)

Synopsis
Dependent edema is common in pregnancy. In this study 9 women with marked edema and otherwise uncomplicated pregnancies participated in a 45-minute immersion exercise session in water. Lower leg volumes were measured before and after the session, including the foot and 10 cm of the lower leg. Mean volume decreased by 112 mL on the left leg and 84 mL on the right leg (P = .007). The women also had a subjective impression of reduction in edema. The authors did not report the duration of the effect or other patient-oriented outcomes.

Aspirin = enoxaparin for prevention of recurrent miscarriage

Clinical question

How do aspirin and enoxaparin compare for the prevention of unexplained recurrent miscarriage?

Bottom line

Daily treatment with aspirin or enoxaparin (Lovenox) each results in a high live birth rate for women with history of unexplained recurrent miscarriages. The lack of a control group is an important limitation of this study. (LOE = 1b–)

Reference

Dolitzky M, Inbal A, Segal Y, Weiss A, et al. A randomized study of thromboprophylaxis in women with unexplained consecutive recurrent miscarriages. Fertil Steril 2006;86:362–366.

Study Design

Randomized controlled trial (nonblinded)

Funding

Industry

Allocation

Concealed

Setting

Outpatient (specialty)

Synopsis

This study enrolled women (n = 104) with history of at least 3 consecutive miscarriages. The authors excluded women whose miscarriages had known causes, including cardiovascular disease, thromboembolism, and abnormal results of any of the following; karyotype of either parent, glucose tolerance test, toxoplasmosis serology, hysterosalpingogram or hysteroscopy, thyroid function, serum prolactin, antinuclear antibodies, antiphospholipid antibodies, and hereditary thrombophilias. Women were randomized to either 100 mg aspirin daily, or 40 mg enoxaparin subcutaneously daily. The study was not blinded, but allocation was concealed and analyses was by intention to treat. Live births occurred in 84% of women taking aspirin and 82% of women taking enoxaparin (NS). There were no differences in preterm births or infant Apgar scores. There was 1 infant with growth retardation in the enoxaparin group. There were 3 women with preeclampsia, all in the aspirin group. There was 1 case of infant testicular torsion and 1 infant with hypoglycemia and convulsions, both in the aspirin group. The study was too small to detect statistical differences in any of these outcomes. The was no placebo arm for this study, which the authors defended by stating that women would not want to enroll in a study in which they might be randomized to placebo. Historical control patients were cited with a 60% live birth rate after 3 consecutive miscarriages and a 40% live birth rate after 4 losses.

Essential Evidence: Medicine that Matters, Edited by David Slawson, Allen Shaughnessy, Mark Ebell, and Henry Barry.

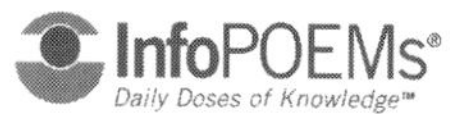

Prenatal vaginal infection screening + treating reduces preterm delivery

Clinical question

Does a program of screening asymptomatic pregnant women for vaginal infections decrease the rate of preterm delivery?

Bottom line

Routine screening of women for vaginal infections decreases the risk of preterm delivery by 43% (number needed to screen and treat = 44). This approach also decreases the number of children born weighing less than 2500 g (number needed to screen and treat = 56). This study confirms the results of an earlier nonrandomized trial (Am J Obstet Gynecol 1995; 173:157–67). Given the cost of premature birth, in both human and financial terms, it makes a lot of sense to screen for and treat all vaginal infections. (LOE = 1b)

Reference

Kiss H, Petricevic L, Husslein P. Prospective randomised controlled trial of an infection screening programme to reduce the rate of preterm delivery. BMJ 2004;329:371–374.

Study Design

Randomized controlled trial (nonblinded)

Allocation

Concealed

Setting

Outpatient (primary care)

Synopsis

In this study, 25 Austrian obstetricians enrolled pregnant women in their early second trimester to be screened for bacterial vaginosis, vaginal candidiasis, or Trichomonas vaginalis. Of the 4155 who were screened, abnormal flora were identified in 21%, with approximately 60% of these identified flora being candida and 33% being bacterial vaginosis. Trichomonas was only identified in 3 women. All women with positive smears were randomized to receive treatment, with follow-up swabbing and retreatment if necessary, or to a control group whose obstetricians were not given the vaginal smear results and who did not order treatment. Analysis was by intention to treat, meaning that the women in the treatment group were evaluated whether or not they actually received treatment for a positive result (rate not provided). The rate of spontaneous preterm birth, defined as less than 37 weeks', was 3.0% in the screen-and-treat women and 5.3% in the unscreened women (absolute risk reduction = 2.3%; 95% CI, 1.2%–3.6%). One preterm birth was avoided for every 44 women who were screened compared with those who had not been screened and treated (number needed to screen and treat = 43.5; 95% CI, 24.4–58.8). In addition, the number of preterm infants weighing less than 2500 g was also significantly lower: 1.7% vs. 3.5% (number needed to screen and treat = 56). Screening and treatment should be expanded beyond just bacterial vaginosis.

Essential Evidence: Medicine that Matters, Edited by David Slawson, Allen Shaughnessy, Mark Ebell, and Henry Barry.

Oral clindamycin for BV prevents prematurity

Clinical question

Does treatment with oral clindamycin for bacterial vaginosis before 22 weeks' gestation lead to decreased premature births and late miscarriages?

Bottom line

Women with asymptomatic BV who were treated with oral clindamycin before 22 weeks' gestation had fewer second trimester miscarriages and preterm births with a NNT of 10. The study was not large enough to show a difference in neonatal admissions to intensive care units. The gram stain screening method and generic antibiotic treatment are simple and inexpensive. The potential here for getting a big bang for a buck in our use of healthcare dollars is very attractive. Previous studies using metronidazole and treatment at later gestational age have not found screening to be beneficial. This study needs to be replicated in a larger trial before introducing widespread screening for BV in pregnancy. (LOE = 1b)

Reference

Ugwumadu A, Manyonda I, Reid F, Hay P. Effect of early oral clindamycin on late miscarriage and preterm delivery in asymptomatic women with abnormal vaginal flora and bacterial vaginosis: a randomised trial. Lancet 2003;361:983–988.

Study Design

Randomized controlled trial (double-blinded)

Setting

Outpatient (specialty)

Synopsis

Previous studies of screening for bacterial vaginosis (BV) in pregnancy performed the screening late in the second trimester and treated BV with metronidazole. In this study, a general population of 6120 asymptomatic pregnant women in the United Kingdom was screened for BV using gram stain and Nugent scoring (0–10). There were 494 (8.1%) BV-positive women with a Nugent score higher than 3 who were randomized (allocation concealed) to oral clindamycin 300 mg twice a day for 5 days (n = 249) or placebo (n = 245). By chance the treated group had a history of fewer miscarriages (26% vs. 34%), but not fewer preterm deliveries (10% vs. 9%). Spontaneous preterm deliveries between 24 and 37 weeks' gestation were 11 of 244 (5%) in the treated group versus 28 of 241 (12%) in the placebo group, and late miscarriages between 13 and 24 weeks' were 2 of 244 (1%) compared with 10 of 241 (4%) (P = .001 for the combined end point; number needed to treat [NNT] = 10). The number needed to screen to prevent one preterm birth or late miscarriage was approximately 120. There were no differences in mean birthweight, low birthweight, stillbirths, or mean gestational age at delivery. There was a trend to increased gastrointestinal side effects in the treated group (7% vs. 3%; P = .10). Admissions to neonatal intensive care were 8% in the clindamycin group compared with 10% in the placebo group (P = .41), which would be clinically significant if the study had been large enough to demonstrate a statistically significant difference.

Essential Evidence: Medicine that Matters, Edited by David Slawson, Allen Shaughnessy, Mark Ebell, and Henry Barry.

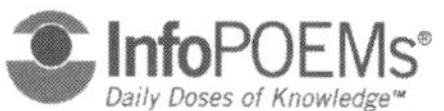

Restricted diet improves parental perception of hyperactive behavior

Clinical question

Does a diet that restricts food coloring and preservatives improve hyperactive behaviors in 3 year olds?

Bottom line

This study raises an interesting conundrum. Placing 3-year-old children on a diet that restricts food coloring and preservatives has no effect on hyperactive behaviors as observed by trained evaluators. However, the parents, who live with these kids for the remaining 23 hours of the day, report improvements in hyperactivity. There was no difference in results whether the child was hyperactive or atopic. (LOE = 2b)

Reference

Bateman B, Warner JO, Hutchinson E, et al. The effects of a double-blind, placebo-controlled, artificial food colourings and benzoate preservative challenge on hyperactivity in a general population sample of preschool children. Arch Dis Child 2004;89:506–511.

Study Design

Cross-over trial (randomized)

Setting

Outpatient (primary care)

Synopsis

These authors evaluated the effects of a restricted diet on 397 3-year-old children who were classified as hyperactive (HA) or not (HA-) and atopic (AT) or not (AT-), resulting in a 2x2 design. The study was split into 2 1-week treatment periods separated by 1-week washout periods. The children were to remain on a diet free of artificial coloring and benzoate preservatives for the entire 4 weeks. During the first week, the children were randomly assigned to receive a daily drink free of artificial coloring and sodium benzoate or an artificially colored and preserved drink identical in appearance. The children then were switched to the opposite drink during the second treatment period. Adults were unable to distinguish the taste of these beverages and the families and study personnel were all blinded to the specific treatment. Only 70% of the patients enrolled finished the study; 61 never started the study and 59 dropped out. Fifteen of the 59 parents who withdrew their child from the study did so because of behavioral changes. Nine of these withdrawals occurred during an active week and 6 during a placebo week. At the end of the study the parents were equally divided into those who did or did not correctly identify the drink order. Based on the parents ratings, their children were calmer during the week when no artificial coloring and preservatives were given. The trained observers, however, detected no significant differences during any of the treatment periods.

Essential Evidence: Medicine that Matters, Edited by David Slawson, Allen Shaughnessy, Mark Ebell, and Henry Barry.

Stimulants similarly effective for ADHD

Clinical question

Which drug therapy is more effective in children with attention-deficit hyperactivity disorder?

Bottom line

Stimulants have the best evidence of effectiveness in the treatment of children with attention-deficit hyperactivity disorder. The research does not give us a clear-cut choice among the stimulants or their formulations, so an empirical, trial-and-error approach is needed. Antidepressants may not be as effective. Behavioral therapy may add benefit to drug therapy, but is less effective than drug therapy when used alone. The role of atomoxetine (Strattera) is unclear because of few comparative studies or long-term studies. (LOE = 1a)

Reference

Brown RT, Amler RW, Freeman WS, et al. Treatment of attention-deficit/hyperactivity disorder: overview of the evidence. Pediatrics 2005;115:e749–e757.

Study Design

Systematic review

Funding

Other

Setting

Various (meta-analysis)

Synopsis

This report is from the American Academy of Pediatrics' Committee on Quality Improvement Subcommittee on Attention-Deficit/Hyperactivity Disorder. It is based on three evidence reviews performed by the McMaster Evidence-Based Practice Center, the Canadian Coordinating Office for Health Technology Assessment, the Multimodal Treatment Study for Children with ADHD, and the mysterious "supplemental reviews conducted by the subcommittee." The McMaster review seems to be the foundation for the report and is a well-described systematic review. Most of the results currently available are from short-term studies that compared the major stimulants used for attention-deficit hyperactivity disorder. Since the definition of what constitutes "improvement" varies among patients and research studies, study results could not be combined. Studies were not able to show, on average, a difference in treatment between methylphenidate (Ritalin), dextroamphetamine or its individual isomers, and pemoline (Cylert), or a difference in any formulations of the same drug. Similarly, there is no difference in the likelihood of adverse effects, though the studies are small. Studies of the antidepressants desipramine and imipramine compared with placebo show heterogeneous results. Nonpharmacologic intervention was not as effective as drug therapy, though behavioral therapy enhanced drug therapy in the Multimodal Treatment Study. Regarding the nonstimulant atomoxetine (Strattera), in a short-term study it is as effective as methylphenidate, with similar side effect profiles, causing similar appetite suppression and initial weight loss. It doesn't worsen insomnia but can cause daytime drowsiness and increase blood pressure in some adults and children. Atomexetine has a slow onset of action, taking up to 1 week to begin working, but seems to last longer throughout the day when it does work. Atomoxetine has been associated with an increased likelihood of suicidal ideation (0.4% vs 0.0% with placebo), according to the Food and Drug Administration (http://www.fda.gov/cder/drug/infopage/atomoxetine/default.htm).

Essential Evidence: Medicine that Matters, Edited by David Slawson, Allen Shaughnessy, Mark Ebell, and Henry Barry.

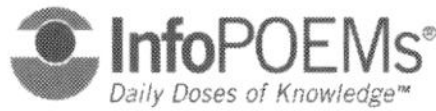

Responders to atomoxetine do well with lower doses

Clinical question

Can the dose of atomoxetine be lowered in children who respond to recommended doses?

Bottom line

In children who respond to the typical dose of atomoxetine (Strattera), a lowered dose of 0.5 mg per kg per day is similarly effective in maintaining scores on a validated measurement scale. (LOE = 1b)

Reference

Newcorn JH, Michelson D, Kratochvil C, Allen AJ, Ruff DD, Moore RJ, for the Atomoxetine Low-dose Study Group. Low-dose atomoxetine for maintenance treatment of attention-deficit/hyperactivity disorder. Pediatrics 2006;118:1701–1706.

Study Design

Randomized controlled trial (double-blinded)

Funding

Industry

Allocation

Uncertain

Setting

Outpatient (primary care)

Synopsis

The researchers conducting this study had previously conducted a study of the use of atomoxetine in children meeting the diagnostic criteria for attention-deficit/hyperactivity disorder (ADHD). The 229 children in this prior study who responded to full doses of atomoxetine, 1.2 mg per kg per day, were randomly assigned (concealed allocation uncertain) to continue their previously effective dose or to continue treatment at a dose of 0.5 mg/kg/day. The doses were only adjusted for weight changes over the 8 months of the study. The children had an average age of 10.5 years and had the combined subtype of ADHD; the majority were male. The primary measure was the Attention-Deficit/Hyperactivity Disorder Rating Scale-IV-Parent Version, an interviewer administered and scored list of 18 items. Relapse, defined as a return to 90% of baseline score, occurred over the course of the study in approximately 2.7% of children in each group. A similar percentage of children in each group also had scores that no longer met the criterion for response, but did not meet the relapse criterion (23% in the low-dose group vs 17% in the same-dose group; P = NS).

Essential Evidence: Medicine that Matters, Edited by David Slawson, Allen Shaughnessy, Mark Ebell, and Henry Barry.

Newer antipsychotics similar to older agents (CATIE)

Clinical question

Are newer antipsychotics safer and more effective than older agents?

Bottom line

There are few differences among newer antipsychotics and few differences between newer agents and perphenazine, an older agent. Olanzapine seems to offer somewhat greater effectiveness, but is less well tolerated and can produce some adverse changes to physiologic end points. All the newer antipsychotics are also much more expensive, which is a concern for this vulnerable group of patients. Based on its similar efficacy and better-than-expected tolerability, perphenazine at a dose of up to 20 mg per day should remain a treatment option for psychosis. (LOE = 1b)

Reference

Lieberman JA, Stroup TS, McEvoy JP, et al, for the Clinical Antipsychotic Trials of Intervention Effectiveness (CATIE) Investigators. Effectiveness of antipsychotic drugs in patients with chronic schizophrenia. N Engl J Med 2005;353:1209–1223.

Study Design	Funding	Allocation
Randomized controlled trial (double-blinded)	Industry + govt	Uncertain

Setting

Outpatient (any)

Synopsis

Although they are widely used, the evidence is incomplete and inconsistent that newer antipsychotic agents are more effective than older agents in clinically important ways. In this study, 1493 adults with schizophrenia at 57 US clinical sites were randomly assigned to 1 of the following agents: olanzapine (Zyprexa) 7.5 mg; quetiapine (Seroquel) 200 mg; risperidone (Risperdal) 1.5 mg; ziprasidone (Geodon) 40 mg; or the older antipsychotic perphenazine (Trilafon) 8 mg. The final dosing range was between 1 and 4 capsules daily depending on the patient's response. The mean doses were as follows: olanzapine 20 mg; quetiapine 543 mg; risperidone 4 mg; ziprasidone 113 mg; and perphenazine 21 mg. Thus, the typical dose was between 2 and 3 capsules per day. Patients had a mean age of 41 years, approximately 75% were men, and approximately 33% were African American. Patients who had previously required clozapine or who had experienced extrapyramidal side effects in the past were excluded. The primary outcome was the percentage of patients who discontinued the medication during the 18-month study period, which was distressingly high for all 5 medications: 64% for olanzapine; 75% for perphenazine; 82% for quetiapine; 74% for risperidone; and 79% for ziprasidone. Discontinuation for lack of efficacy was also somewhat less common in the olanzapine group (15% vs 24%–28%). However, olanzapine was also discontinued more often because of intolerability (19% vs 10%–16%; the rest of the patients who discontinued medication did so either by mutual agreement between patient and physician or did not give a reason. Olanzapine also caused greater increases in weight, glucose levels, and lipid levels than the other agents, which are disease-oriented outcomes of uncertain clinical significance. Patients were slightly more likely to discontinue perphenazine because of extrapyramidal side effects (8% vs 2%–4%), but this difference may have been smaller than expected because of the relatively low dose of perphenazine used in the study.

Essential Evidence: Medicine that Matters, Edited by David Slawson, Allen Shaughnessy, Mark Ebell, and Henry Barry.

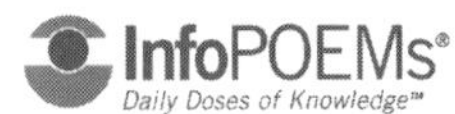

Atypical antipsychotics minimally effective, poorly tolerated in Alzheimer's disease

Clinical question

Are the newer atypical antipsychotics effective in patients with Alzheimer's disease?

Bottom line

Atypical antipsychotics are minimally, if at all, effective for patients with Alzheimer's disease (AD), and they have significant adverse effects. They should not be routinely used for the treatment of psychosis, agitation, or aggression in these patients. (LOE = 1b)

Reference

Schneider LS, Tariot PN, Dagerman KS, et al, with the CATIE-AD Study Group. Effectiveness of atypical antipsychotic drugs in patients with Alzheimer's disease. N Engl J Med 2006;355:1525–1538.

Study Design	Funding	Allocation	Setting
Randomized controlled trial (double-blinded)	Government	Uncertain	Outpatient (any)

Synopsis

Although atypical antipsychotics are widely used in the treatment of psychosis, agitation, and aggression in patients with AD, clinical trials to date have been of limited duration and have not adequately addressed the tolerability of the drugs. In addition, there are new concerns regarding the safety of these drugs, with recent studies* finding an increased risk of death (relative risk = 1.6–1.7). In this study, the authors identified 421 outpatients with probable AD, a Mini-Mental State score between 5 and 26, and delusions, hallucinations, aggression, or agitation. They were randomized in a 2:2:2:3 ratio to olanzapine (Zyprexa, 2.5 mg or 5.0 mg), quetiapine (Seroquel, 25 mg or 50 mg), risperidone (Risperdal, 0.5 mg or 1.0 mg), or placebo. Whether to use the smaller or larger dose of each drug was determined by the study physicians, who were blinded to treatment assignment. They chose an unidentified small or large pill from an envelope, then adjusted the dose on the basis of patient response. Patients were followed up for up to 3 years; the primary outcomes were the time to discontinuation of the study drug and the degree of improvement on the Clinical Global Impression of Change (CGIC) scale at week 12. Groups were balanced at the start of the study and analysis was by intention to treat. The patients' mean Mini-Mental State score was 15, their average age was 78 years, 56% were women, and 18% were African-American. The average final doses of each drug were olanzapine 5.5 mg, quetiapine 56 mg, and risperidone 1.0 mg. The mean time to discontinuation was between 5.3 weeks and 8.1 weeks for the 4 groups, with no significant difference between groups. The atypical antipsychotics were more likely to be discontinued because of adverse effects (16%–24% vs 5% for placebo), while placebo was more likely to be discontinued because of lack of efficacy (70% vs 39%–53% vs 70% for active drugs). There was no significant difference between groups regarding the response as measured by the CGIC scale at 12 weeks (21% for placebo vs 26%–32% for active drugs). Adverse effects occurring more frequently in patients receiving an active drug included parkinsonism or extrapyramidal signs (olanzapine and risperidone), sedation and weight increase (all 3 active drugs), and confusion (olanzapine and risperidone). *http://www.fda.gov/cder/drug/advisory/antipsychotics.htm

Essential Evidence: Medicine that Matters, Edited by David Slawson, Allen Shaughnessy, Mark Ebell, and Henry Barry.

Older, newer antipsychotics both increase mortality in elderly

Clinical question

Are conventional antipsychotic agents safer than atypical agents in elderly patients?

Bottom line

It seems reasonable to conclude that conventional and atypical antipsychotic agents are both associated with an increased risk of death in elderly patients. The limitations of this study do not allow us to confidently conclude that older agents are less safe than newer agents, though. (LOE = 2b)

Reference

Wang PS, Schneeweiss S, Avorn J, et al. Risk of death in elderly users of conventional vs. atypical antipsychotic medications. N Engl J Med 2005;353:2335–2341.

Study Design

Cohort (retrospective)

Funding

Government

Setting

Population-based

Synopsis

A recent public health advisory (www.fda.gov/cder/drug/advisory/antipsychotics.htm) warned that there is a two-fold increase in the risk of death among demented elderly patients when given atypical antipsychotic agents, such as aripiprazole (Abilify), clozapine (Clozaril), olanzapine (Zyprexa), quetiapine (Seroquel), risperidone (Risperdal), and ziprasidone (Geodon). Researchers performed this federally sponsored study to determine whether conventional agents (eg, haloperidol, thiothixene, loxapine) carry a similar risk. They identified patients older than 65 years who had filled a first prescription for any antipsychotic agent between 1994 and 2003. Mortality data came from the Medicare Death Master File, and they used administrative data sets to establish comorbidities, hospitalizations, nursing home residence, and use of other medications. They identified a total of 9142 patients using a conventional antipsychotic and 13,748 using an atypical agent. These groups were quite different: Patients taking conventional antipsychotics were more likely to have heart disease or cancer, but were less likely to have other mood disorders or take other psychotropic medications. In the unadjusted analysis, there were more deaths among users of conventional agents (17.9% vs 14.6%; $P < .001$; number needed to treat to harm = 30; 95% CI, 23–43). This corresponds to an unadjusted hazard ratio of 1.51 (95% CI, 1.43–1.59). After adjusting for comorbidities, the relative risk was somewhat lower but still statistically significant (1.37; 95% CI, 1.27–1.49). The risk was greatest in the first 40 days after beginning therapy, in nondemented patients, and in patients taking a higher-than-median dose of the conventional antipsychotic medication.

Essential Evidence: Medicine that Matters, Edited by David Slawson, Allen Shaughnessy, Mark Ebell, and Henry Barry.

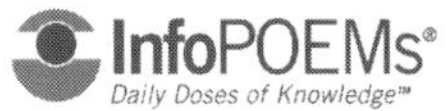

Variable support for CAM therapies for anxiety

Clinical question

Which complementary and alternative medicines are effective in the treatment of anxiety disorders?

Bottom line

The majority of complementary and alternative medicines lack valid evidence of effectiveness in the treatment of anxiety disorders. Some supporting evidence was found for inositol, acupuncture, massage (only in children), autogenic therapy, bibliotherapy, dance/movement therapy, exercise, meditation, music, and relaxation therapy. Many common herbal and homoeopathy treatments lack any evidence of effectiveness. (LOE = 2a)

Reference

Jorm AF, Christensen H, Griffiths KM, Parslow RA, Rodgers B, Blewitt KA. Effectiveness of complementary and self-help treatments for anxiety disorders. Med J Aust 2004;181:S29–S46.

Study Design

Systematic review

Funding

Government

Setting

Various (meta-analysis)

Synopsis

Anxiety disorders are estimated to affect 5% to 15% of patients each year. Less than one fifth of these people consult a health professional and many report using various self-help methods. The investigators searched PubMed, PsychLit and the Cochrane Registry of Controlled Trials (CRCT) to review the effectiveness of complementary and alternative treatments on anxiety. Articles were included if they reported treatment of individuals selected as having an anxiety disorder. Independent studies were assessed for validity using standard criteria. No mention is made whether the search for, and evaluation of, the articles was done independently by more than one person, and there is no discussion of possible publication bias. Very limited, if any, evidence of effectiveness was found for the following treatments: Bach flower essences, berocca, ginger, gotu kola, homeopathy, lemongrass leaves, licorice, magnesium, passion flower, St. John's wort, valerian, vitamin C, aromatherapy, hydrotherapy, humor, prayer, yoga, caffeine reduction, nicotine avoidance, and a carbohydrate-rich/protein-poor diet. Limited evidence was found for effectiveness for inositol, acupuncture, massage (only in children), autogenic therapy, bibliotherapy, dance/movement therapy, exercise, meditation, music, and relaxation therapy. Kava and 5-hydroxyl-L-tryptophan were effective but not recommended because of the risk of severe side effects (liver toxicity and eosinophilia-myalgia syndrome, respectively).

Essential Evidence: Medicine that Matters, Edited by David Slawson, Allen Shaughnessy, Mark Ebell, and Henry Barry.

Work stress has no meaningful effect on blood pressure

Clinical question

Does work stress increase blood pressure?

Bottom line

Work stress has no meaningful effect on blood pressure. (LOE = 1b)

Reference

Guimont C, Brisson C, Dagenais GR, et al. Effects of job strain on blood pressure: a prospective study of male and female white-collar workers. Am J Public Health 2006;96:1436–1443.

Study Design

Cohort (prospective)

Funding

Foundation

Setting

Population-based

Synopsis

"I don't need medication; my blood pressure is only high because of my stressful job." How should you respond? This team of researchers observed more than 6000 white-collar workers (men and women) for 7.5 years (84% follow-up). They excluded anyone with known cardiovascular disease and hypertension at baseline. The participants completed a series of scales to assess job stress and other psychological demands of work. Additionally, the study team assessed each participant's vital signs, body mass index, tobacco use, exercise patterns, and so forth. Women had no difference in their blood pressure whether exposed to stress at baseline or at follow-up, or at both, or neither. Men who experienced no work stress at baseline or at follow-up also showed no change in blood pressure. The excited authors, however, point out a graded response: Stress levels present only at baseline were less important than stress levels only at follow-up, and when men's stress levels were present at both baseline and at follow-up, the systolic blood pressure increased a whopping 1.8 mm Hg. This is a perfect example of how researchers can confuse and mislead us with statistics. Yes, the difference was statistically significant, but the clinical difference was trivial.

Essential Evidence: Medicine that Matters, Edited by David Slawson, Allen Shaughnessy, Mark Ebell, and Henry Barry.

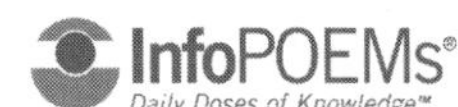

Antioxidants do not prevent dementia

Clinical question

Are antioxidants associated with a decreased risk of Alzheimer's disease?

Bottom line

In this study and in at least one other cohort study (Engelhart MJ. JAMA 2002; 287:3223–29), antioxidant consumption in the elderly was not associated with protection against developing dementia. At least one randomized controlled trial (Sano M. NEJM 1997; 336:1216–22) demonstrated that vitamin E may slow the progression of moderately severe Alzheimer's disease. (LOE = 2b)

Reference

Luchingser JA, Tang MX, Shea S, Mayeaux R. Antioxidant vitamin intake and risk of Alzheimer disease. Arch Neurol 2003;60:203–208.

Study Design

Cohort (prospective)

Setting

Outpatient (any)

Synopsis

In this cohort study, patients completed diaries of diet and vitamin supplementation (vitamin C, vitamin E, carotene). The researchers evaluated the patients at baseline and only included those who were free of dementia. After an average of 4 years of follow-up of 980 patients, they compared antioxidant consumption with subsequent development of dementia using standardized criteria. A total of 242 of these patients developed Alzheimer's disease. After adjusting for educational level and other covariates that might affect cognition, they found no association between antioxidant use and the development of dementia. Some limitations of this study include the role of recall bias since patients had to report on their dietary intake from the previous year. For those of us who can't recall what we had for breakfast (or even if we ate breakfast), this would be a major challenge.

Essential Evidence: Medicine that Matters, Edited by David Slawson, Allen Shaughnessy, Mark Ebell, and Henry Barry.

Lowering homocysteine with B vitamins doesn't improve cognition

Clinical question
Does supplementation to reduce homocysteine levels with folate, vitamin B12, and vitamin B6 have a beneficial effect on cognition in older adults?

Bottom line
There is no evidence from this well-designed study that vitamin supplementation to lower homocysteine levels has any beneficial effect on cognition. Although cognition actually appeared to worsen with the use of vitamins in one of the tests, this may be a spurious finding given the large number of comparisons made by the researchers. (LOE = 1b)

Reference
McMahon JA, Green TJ, Skeaff CM, Knight RG, Mann JI, Williams SM. A controlled trial of homocysteine lowering and cognitive performance. N Engl J Med 2006;354:2764–2772.

Study Design
Randomized controlled trial (double-blinded)

Funding
Government

Allocation
Concealed

Setting
Population-based

Synopsis
Observational studies have found an association between higher levels of serum homocysteine and Alzheimer's disease and cognitive impairment. However, it is not clear whether this association is causal, or whether lowering homocysteine levels improves cognition. In this trial, community-dwelling healthy adults older than 65 years with a plasma homocysteine level of at least 13 micromoles per liter were recruited. The authors excluded those with impaired renal function, with known cognitive impairment, who were taking folate or B vitamins, or who were taking medications that might interfere with folate metabolism. After an extensive battery of baseline cognitive tests, patients were randomly assigned to receive either 1000 mcg folate, 500 mcg vitamin B12 (cobalamin), and 10 mg vitamin B6 (pyridoxine) daily or matching placebo. The 276 patients underwent cognitive testing after 1 and 2 years; of 138 who began the study in each group, 126 in the placebo group and 127 in the treatment group had data available for analysis. The mean age of participants was 73 years and 44% were female (37% in the vitamin group, 52% in the placebo group; P = .02). The vitamins had the expected effect on homocysteine levels, reducing them approximately 16 to 12 micromoles per liter in the treatment group during the 2-year study. The homocysteine levels did not change in the placebo group. There was no improvement on cognition. In fact, the average score on the Wechsler Paragraph Recall test was worse in the vitamin group, although this difference disappeared after adjustment for sex and education. The vitamin group also did worse on the Reitan Trail Making Test, a difference that persisted after adjustment for sex and education.

Essential Evidence: Medicine that Matters, Edited by David Slawson, Allen Shaughnessy, Mark Ebell, and Henry Barry.

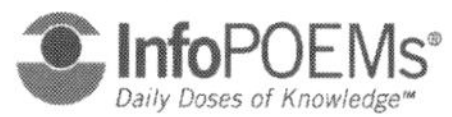

Reasoning training slows age-related functional decline

Clinical question

Can cognitive training for older adults slow functional decline resulting in less difficulty with activities of daily living?

Bottom line

Reasoning training (in this study, practicing strategies for finding patterns in letter series or word series) results in a slower decline of age-related functional ability as assessed by self-reported instrumental activities of daily living (IADLs) at 5 years of follow up. (LOE = 2b)

Reference

Willis SL, Tennstedt SL, Marsiske M, et al, for the ACTIVE Study Group. Long-term effects of cognitive training on everyday functional outcomes in older adults. JAMA 2006;296:2805–2814.

Study Design

Randomized controlled trial (single-blinded)

Funding

Government

Allocation

Concealed

Setting

Population-based

Synopsis

These investigators enrolled into their study 2832 persons, aged 64 years or older, living independently with good baseline functional and cognitive status. Patients randomly received (allocation assignment concealed) 1 of 4 interventions: 10-sessions of cognitive training for memory, reasoning, or speed of processing, or no contact (the control group). Memory training consisted of teaching mnemonic strategies for remembering material such as word lists or texts; reasoning training involved teaching strategies for finding patterns in letter series or word series; and speed of processing training consisted of improving visual search and attention skills by following objects on a computer screen. Booster training was offered at 11 months and 33 months after initial training, but only 60% of patients fully participated. Measurement of functional outcomes occurred through self-ratings of difficulties with IADLs. Assessments by individuals blinded to treatment group assignment occurred at baseline and annually for a total of 5 years. Complete follow-up occurred for only 67% of patients at 5 years. Using intention-to-treat analysis, only individuals receiving reasoning training reported significantly less difficulty in performing IADLs than control patients. No significant additional benefit occurred as a result of booster training. The effects of the training on self-reported IADL function could reflect self-report bias so the need for a placebo control group in future studies is important.

Essential Evidence: Medicine that Matters, Edited by David Slawson, Allen Shaughnessy, Mark Ebell, and Henry Barry.

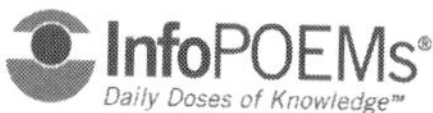

Statins not associated with decreased dementia

Clinical question

Are statins associated with a decreased risk of developing dementia?

Bottom line

In this prospective study, patients older than 65 years old taking statins developed dementia at the same rate as those not using statins. (LOE = 2b)

Reference

Rea TD, Breitner JC, Psaty BM, et al. Statin use and the risk of incident dementia: the Cardiovascular Health Study. Arch Neurol 2005;62:1047–1051.

Study Design

Cohort (prospective)

Funding

Government

Setting

Population-based

Synopsis

Several case-control studies have suggested that statin use is associated with a lower risk of developing dementia. Since these kinds of studies suffer from many limitations, they are among the weakest designs from which causal inferences can be drawn. These authors "kick it up a notch" and annually evaluated almost 2800 patients older than 65 years who didn't have dementia. They don't tell us if the evaluators knew whether the patients used statins. The authors also don't tell us the number of patients who took statins. The researchers followed the patients for a median of 5 years and they had more than 13,000 person-years in the group of patients receiving no lipid-lowering drugs, nearly 1300 person-years in those taking statins, and approximately 500 person-years in a group receiving nonstatin lipid lowering drugs. Overall, approximately 30% of the patients developed dementia. After taking other factors associated with dementia into account, the incidence of dementia among statin users was the same as for those not using statins.

Essential Evidence: Medicine that Matters, Edited by David Slawson, Allen Shaughnessy, Mark Ebell, and Henry Barry.

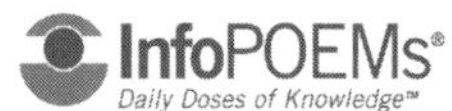

Vitamin E, donepezil ineffective for mild cognitive impairment

Clinical question

Does Vitamin E or donepezil (Aricept) prevent progression from mild cognitive impairment to Alzheimer's disease?

Bottom line

Vitamin E does not slow progression of mild cognitive impairment to full-fledged Alzheimer's disease. Donepezil provides an early benefit that is gone by 3 years. A secondary analysis found that donepezil appeared more beneficial for patients with the apolipoprotein E4 (APOE) gene. This finding requires prospective confirmation before we begin to test all patients with mild cognitive impairment for APOE and use it to guide therapy. (LOE = 1b)

Reference

Petersen RC, Thomas RG, Grundman M, et al. Vitamin E and donepezil for the treatment of mild cognitive impairment. N Engl J Med 2005;352:2379–2388.

Study Design

Randomized controlled trial (double-blinded)

Funding

Industry + govt

Allocation

Concealed

Setting

Outpatient (any)

Synopsis

Mild cognitive impairment (MCI) is an intermediate stage between normal cognition and Alzheimer's disease often characterized by deficits of memory. In this study, researchers identified 769 patients with MCI, defined as impaired memory on standardized tests, a Mini Mental State (MMS) test score between 24 and 30, and age 55 years to 90 years. These patients were randomly assigned to receiver either 2000 IU vitamin E, 10 mg donepezil (Aricept), or placebo daily; all patients received a multivitamin containing 15 IU vitamin E. MMS scores, age, and APOE gene status was considered when patients were allocated to treatment groups, but appears to have been concealed from the investigators. Analysis was by intention to treat and outcomes were blindly assessed. At the end of the 3-year study, 212 of the 769 patients who began the study had progressed to Alzheimer's disease (a rate of 16% per year). Taking vitamin E or donepezil did not have any effect on the likelihood of progression to Alzheimer's at 3 years. There was a decreased risk of progression to Alzheimer's in the donepezil group at 12 months compared with placebo (14.7% vs 6.3%; P = .04; number needed to treat [NNT] = 12), but this did not persist at 36 months. There was also no significant difference in MMS scores or other measures of cognition at 3 years. Patients with the APOE gene were much more likely to progress to Alzheimer's disease, and if you only consider that group, then the benefit of donepezil persists for the full 3 years of the study.

Essential Evidence: Medicine that Matters, Edited by David Slawson, Allen Shaughnessy, Mark Ebell, and Henry Barry.

Drug therapy minimally effective for neuropsych symptoms of dementia

Clinical question

How useful are the various pharmacologic agents in the management of neuropsychiatric symptoms of dementia?

Bottom line

Pharmacologic agents are minimally, if at all, effective in managing the neuropsychiatric symptoms of dementia. The atypical antipsychotics olanzapine (Zyprexa) and risperidone (Risperdal) are the most effective, but these agents may increase the risk of stroke. The decision to use any of these drugs must be made on the basis of individual circumstances. (LOE = 1a–)

Reference

Sink KM, Holden KF, Yaffe K. Pharmacological treatment of neuropsychiatric symptoms of dementia. A review of the evidence. JAMA 2005; 293:596–608.

Study Design	Funding	Setting
Systematic review	Government	Various (guideline)

Synopsis

Neuropsychiatric symptoms of dementia, such as agitation, aggression, delusions, hallucinations, and wandering, increase caregiver stress and an increased risk of hospitalization and nursing home placement. To evaluate the value of various pharmacologic agents in treating these symptoms, the investigators systematically reviewed the English-language literature using MEDLINE, the Cochrane Database of Systematic Reviews, and a manual search of relevant bibliographies. They included only double-blind placebo-controlled randomized trials or meta-analyses of drug trials of patients with dementia with measured outcomes including neuropsychiatric symptoms. Two authors independently evaluated the quality of each trial and a third author served as the final arbitrator when consensus was not reached. From an initial 78 articles reviewed, only 25 randomized controlled trials and 4 meta-analyses met the inclusion criteria. The investigators do not discuss the possibility of publication bias but report informally on the homogeneity of the results. The atypical antipsychotics, including olanzapine (Zyprexa) and risperidone (Risperdal), showed modest benefit in reducing agitation/aggression, hallucinations, and delusions. However, the atypical antipsychotics may increase the risk of stroke. There is no clear evidence that typical antipsychotics, such as haloperidol (Haldol), thioridazine (Mellaril), thiothixene (Navane), and chlorpromazine (Thorazine) were useful for treating any neuropsychiatric symptoms. Haloperidol may be slightly useful for reducing aggression, but the adverse effects may outweigh the benefits. There is no evidence that one typical antipsychotic is more efficacious than any other. Trials investigating the use of serotonergic antidepressants reported no efficacy for treating neuropsychiatric symptoms other than depression, with the exception of one industry sponsored trial of citalopram (Celexa) which reported a 10-point reduction (out of 168 points) in agitation compared with placebo. Mood stabilizers (eg, valproate [Depakote] and carbamazepine [Tegretol]) were ineffective. The available evidence on cholinesterase inhibitors (eg, galantamine [Reminyl], donepezil [Aricept], rivastigmine [Exelon]) shows a small benefit (summary estimate of 1.72-point improvement vs placebo on a scale of 0 to 120). Most of the statistically significant difference was driven by 2 studies on a drug never approved for use by the FDA in the United States because of toxicities. Memantine (Namenda) may be of some benefit, but the evidence is mixed and unlikely to be clinically significant.

Essential Evidence: Medicine that Matters, Edited by David Slawson, Allen Shaughnessy, Mark Ebell, and Henry Barry.

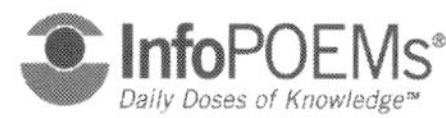

Minimal effect of cholinesterase inhibitors for Alzheimer's

Clinical question

Are cholinesterase inhibitors effective in patients with Alzheimer's disease?

Bottom line

The evidence supporting the effectiveness of cholinesterase inhibitors is based on exceedingly small effects found in poorly analyzed studies. Studies of Alzheimer's drugs need to be carefully scrutinized for methodologic errors that inflate the appearance of benefit. (LOE = 1a)

Reference

Kaduszkiewicz H, Zimmermann T, Beck-Bornholdt HP, van den Bussche H. Cholinesterase inhibitors for patients with Alzheimer's disease: systematic review of randomised trials. BMJ 2005;331:321–327.

Study Design

Meta-analysis (randomized controlled trials)

Funding

Self-funded or unfunded

Setting

Various (meta-analysis)

Synopsis

Three treatments for Alzheimer's disease work by inhibiting cholinesterase: donepezil (Aricept), rivastigmine (Exelon), and galantamine (Razadyne). The authors of this meta-analysis combined the results of 22 randomized controlled trials evaluating the drugs' effects on clinical outcomes. The research was identified by searching 3 databases for research in any language. Three researchers independently selected studies on the basis of predetermined criteria. The quality of the studies was poor for many of these studies; the most common problem was that the results were not analyzed by intention to treat, the lack of which tends to inflate evidence of benefit. Most studies used the standard evaluation tool, the Alzheimer's Disease Assessment Scale–cognitive subscale, which uses scores ranging from 0 (no impairment) to 70 (very severe impairment). For all 3 drugs, the differences between the treatment groups and placebo groups was a minimal 1.5 points to 3.9 points. In 12 trials, effectiveness was also measured using the Clinician's Interview Base on Impression of Change; these scores were not significantly different between treatment and placebo groups. One study that used a measure of cognitive decline showed an average 5 months delay with donepezil compared with placebo before a clinically evident functional decline was seen.

Essential Evidence: Medicine that Matters, Edited by David Slawson, Allen Shaughnessy, Mark Ebell, and Henry Barry.

Haloperidol shortens duration, intensity but not frequency of post-op delirium

Clinical Question
Does perioperative haloperidol (Haldol) prevent delirium in elderly patients undergoing hip surgery?

Bottom Line
Low-dose haloperidol was no more effective than placebo in preventing delirium in elderly patients undergoing hip surgery. However, when delirium occurred, it was milder and shorter in patients receiving haloperidol. Furthermore, haloperidol shortened the hospital length of stay among patients who became delirious. (LOE = 1b–)

Reference
Kalisvaart KJ, de Jonghe JF, Bogaards MJ, et al. Haloperidol prophylaxis for elderly hip-surgery patients at risk for delirium: a randomized placebo-controlled study. J Am Geriatr Soc 2005;53:1658–66.

Study Design
Randomized controlled trial (double-blinded)

Funding
Self-funded or unfunded

Allocation
Concealed

Setting
Inpatient (any location)

Synopsis
In this study, the researchers randomly assigned 430 patients older than 70 years who were admitted for acute or elective hip surgery to receive 1.5 mg haloperidol or placebo daily until 3 days after surgery. To be eligible, the patients had to be at increased risk of delirium by having at least 1 of the following: corrected visual acuity worse than 20/70; an APACHE II score of 16 or higher; a Mini-Mental State Examination score of 24 or lower; or a blood urea nitrogen to creatinine ratio of 18 or higher. Patients who were delirious at admission were ineligible to participate in this study. The main outcome, development of delirium, was assessed via intention to treat. The rate of delirium was similar in both groups (15.1% vs 16.5%, respectively; P = NS). Although the rate was similar, when patients became delirious, the delirium was slightly less severe (5-point difference on a 45-point rating scale) and had shorter duration (5.4 vs 11.8 days; $P < .001$) in the patients taking haloperidol. Additionally, among patients who became delirious, those taking haloperidol had shorter hospital stays by 5.5 days ($P < .001$). A total of 5% of the patients taking haloperidol and 11% taking placebo were lost to follow-up. It is possible that this could significantly influence the results.

Essential Evidence: Medicine that Matters, Edited by David Slawson, Allen Shaughnessy, Mark Ebell, and Henry Barry.

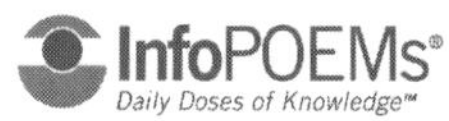

Small increased risk of death with atypical antipsychotics for dementia

Clinical question

Do atypical antipsychotic drugs increase the risk of death for patients with dementia?

Bottom line

The use of atypical antipsychotic drugs for even short periods (less than 8 to 12 weeks) is associated with a significantly increased risk of death. Antipsychotic drugs should be used only in individual situations of an identifiable risk of harm and when alternate therapies have failed. (LOE = 1a)

Reference

Schneider LS, Dagerman KS, Insel P. Risk of death with atypical antipsychotic drug treatment for dementia. Meta-analysis of randomized placebo-controlled trials. JAMA 2005;294:1934–1943.

Study Design

Meta-analysis (randomized controlled trials)

Funding

Government

Setting

Various (meta-analysis)

Synopsis

Antipsychotic drugs are commonly used to treat neuropsychiatric symptoms of depression, including aggression, agitation, and delusions. Newer atypical antipsychotic drugs, including risperidone (Risperdal), olanzapine (Zyprexa), quetiapine (Seroquel), and aripiprazole (Abilify), have generally replaced first-generation antipsychotic drugs, including haloperidol (Haldol) and thioridazine (Mellaril). However, controversy exists regarding the risk of increased mortality associated with the use of these drugs in elderly patients with dementia. The investigators thoroughly searched MEDLINE, the Cochrane Controlled Trials Register, conference programs and proceedings, and pharmaceutical manufacturer databases to identify randomized controlled double-blind trials comparing orally administered antipsychotics with placebo in elderly patients with dementia. One individual abstracted all data and another checked the results. Both investigators reviewed data discrepancies to ensure accuracy. Fifteen trials fulfilled inclusion criteria: a total of 3353 patients were randomized to active drugs and l757 to placebo. Most of the patients had Alzheimer disease (87%) and were women (70%). Follow-up occurred for an average of 8 to 12 weeks. A total of 118 deaths occurred in the atypical antipsychotic drug groups compared with 40 in the placebo groups (3.5% vs 2.3%; number needed to treat to harm = 100; 95% CI, 53–1000). Results were similar (homogenous) across the various trials. A sensitivity analysis did not find evidence for differential risk for individual drugs (including the first-generation antipsychotics) severity of symptoms, or diagnosis. A formal analysis found no evidence of publication bias.

Essential Evidence: Medicine that Matters, Edited by David Slawson, Allen Shaughnessy, Mark Ebell, and Henry Barry.

Older, newer antipsychotics both increase mortality in elderly

Clinical question

Are conventional antipsychotic agents safer than atypical agents in elderly patients?

Bottom line

It seems reasonable to conclude that conventional and atypical antipsychotic agents are both associated with an increased risk of death in elderly patients. The limitations of this study do not allow us to confidently conclude that older agents are less safe than newer agents, though. (LOE = 2b)

Reference

Wang PS, Schneeweiss S, Avorn J, et al. Risk of death in elderly users of conventional vs. atypical antipsychotic medications. N Engl J Med 2005;353:2335–2341.

Study Design

Cohort (retrospective)

Funding

Government

Setting

Population-based

Synopsis

A recent public health advisory (www.fda.gov/cder/drug/advisory/antipsychotics.htm) warned that there is a two-fold increase in the risk of death among demented elderly patients when given atypical antipsychotic agents, such as aripiprazole (Abilify), clozapine (Clozaril), olanzapine (Zyprexa), quetiapine (Seroquel), risperidone (Risperdal), and ziprasidone (Geodon). Researchers performed this federally sponsored study to determine whether conventional agents (eg, haloperidol, thiothixene, loxapine) carry a similar risk. They identified patients older than 65 years who had filled a first prescription for any antipsychotic agent between 1994 and 2003. Mortality data came from the Medicare Death Master File, and they used administrative data sets to establish comorbidities, hospitalizations, nursing home residence, and use of other medications. They identified a total of 9142 patients using a conventional antipsychotic and 13,748 using an atypical agent. These groups were quite different: Patients taking conventional antipsychotics were more likely to have heart disease or cancer, but were less likely to have other mood disorders or take other psychotropic medications. In the unadjusted analysis, there were more deaths among users of conventional agents (17.9% vs 14.6%; $P < .001$; number needed to treat to harm = 30; 95% CI, 23–43). This corresponds to an unadjusted hazard ratio of 1.51 (95% CI, 1.43–1.59). After adjusting for comorbidities, the relative risk was somewhat lower but still statistically significant (1.37; 95% CI, 1.27–1.49). The risk was greatest in the first 40 days after beginning therapy, in nondemented patients, and in patients taking a higher-than-median dose of the conventional antipsychotic medication.

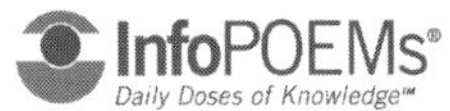

Two question screening for depression effective

Clinical question

Can asking two questions identify patients in general practice who are or aren?t depressed?

Bottom line

Two questions were very good at ruling out patients with depression and identifying most of those who were depressed in general practices in New Zealand. The questions: During the past month have you often been bothered by feeling down, depressed, or hopeless?; and, During the past month have you often been bothered by little interest or pleasure in doing things? Answering yes to at least one of the questions identified most patients with depression (as well as many who weren't), whereas answering no to both questions effectively ruled out depression. (LOE = 1b)

Reference

Arroll B, Khin N, Kerse N. Screening for depression in primary care with two verbally asked questions: cross sectional study. BMJ 2003;327:1144–1146.

Study Design

Diagnostic test evaluation

Setting

Outpatient (primary care)

Synopsis

Identifying patients with depression in primary care has been recommended by various groups, although the tools to do so may be too long and time consuming for the typical practice. The researchers enrolled 421 consecutive patients from 15 general practices in New Zealand who were not taking psychotropic drugs, and they evaluated the use of 2 questions. These 2 questions were asked by the clinician: (1) During the past month have you often been bothered by feeling down, depressed, or hopeless?; and (2) During the past month have you often been bothered by little interest or pleasure in doing things? To evaluate the usefulness of these questions, patients were then asked to complete a computerized diagnostic interview for mood (which has been compared with clinical assessment of depression). Approximately 18% of the patients eventually were given a diagnosis of depression. Answering no to both questions virtually eliminated the likelihood of depression (negative predictive value = 99.7%). Answering yes to either question identified most patients with depression (sensitivity = 97%; 95% CI, 83%–99%), although it falsely identified many patients (positive predictive value = 18%).

No difference among new antidepressants

Clinical question

Which of the newer antidepressants is safer and more effective?

Bottom line

When it comes to the new, nontricyclic antidepressants, the medical literature does not give us any clear guidance as to which one is more effective, of faster onset, safer, or better tolerated. Sexual side effects are lower with bupropion and nausea seems to occur more often with venlafaxine. Other research has shown these new drugs to be no more effective or better tolerated than tricyclic antidepressants. For now, start your patient on your favorite antidepressant, with the realization that most patients will need to switch to another drug at least once. (LOE = 1a)

Reference

Hansen RA, Gartlehner G, Lohr KN, Gaynes BN, Carey TS. Efficacy and safety of second-generation antidepressants in the treatment of major depressive disorder. Ann Intern Med 2005;143:415–426.

Study Design	Funding	Setting
Meta-analysis (randomized controlled trials)	Government	Various (meta-analysis)

Synopsis

The researchers who performed this systematic review and meta-analysis of the safety, tolerability, and effectiveness of the newer antidepressants used 6 databases to find all randomized controlled studies of one antidepressant versus another of at least 12 weeks duration. They also searched reference lists of review articles, contacted pharmaceutical manufacturers and tried, unsuccessfully, to obtain unpublished data filed with the Food and Drug Administration. Two researchers independently reviewed the articles for eligibility, and the data were abstracted from the selected studies by trained reviewers, which were then evaluated by another researcher. The 46 studies, 85% of which were sponsored by a pharmaceutical company, were of variable quality The quality of most of the effectiveness studies (21 of 22) was fair, and one study was rated as good. Twenty of these trials found no difference between the 2 antidepressants they evaluated. Two trials found a difference in at least one outcome: escitalopram (Lexapro) produced improved depression scores versus citoprolam (Celexa) in one study but not another, and paroxetine (Paxil) was found to be more effective than fluoxetine (Prozac) in 1 of 8 studies comparing the 2 drugs. In the meta-analysis, combining the results of 6 studies found no difference between fluoxetine and paroxetine. Sertraline (Zoloft), in 5 studies of a total of 1190 patients, was slightly more effective than fluoxetine (relative benefit = 1.1; 95% CI, 1.01–1.20). Venlafaxine (Effexor) was also slightly more effective than fluoxetine in 6 studies of more than 1300 patients (relative benefit = 1.12; 95% CI, 1.02–1.23). Faster onset of action was not identified consistently for any specific drug. Similarly, quality of life was not significantly different with any of the drugs. The overall incidence of adverse effects and discontinuation rates was similar among the antidepressants, although specific adverse effects were significantly different. Nausea and vomiting rates were consistently higher for venlafaxine than for other antidepressants. Sexual side effects were less frequent with bupropion (Wellbutrin) than with sertraline and fluoxetine, and were more frequent with paroxetine, sertraline, and mirtazapine (Remeron). Weight gain was not systematically compared but seemed to be highest in the patients receiving mirtazapine and lowest in those receiving fluoxetine.

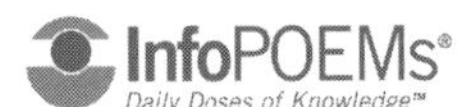

Alternative medications are similarly effective for depression treatment failures (STAR*D)

Clinical question

What is the best drug for patients who do not respond to a selective serotonin reuptake inhibitor?

Bottom line

Bupropion SR, sertraline, and venlafaxine XR are equally effective at inducing remission or response in patients with persistent symptoms of depression despite initial treatment with citalopram (Celexa). Most patients will not go into remission, though, and this study lacked a placebo control group. (LOE = 1b)

Reference

Rush AJ, Trivedi MH, Wisniewski SR, et al, for the STAR*D Study Team. Bupropion-SR, sertraline, or venlafaxine-XR after failure of SSRIs for depression. N Engl J Med 2006;354:1231–1242.

Study Design

Randomized controlled trial (nonblinded)

Funding

Government

Allocation

Uncertain

Setting

Outpatient (any)

Synopsis

The Sequenced Treatment Alternatives to Relieve Depression (STAR*D) trial was a complex study that began by treating 2876 depressed patients given citalopram in an average dose of 40 mg per day. Approximately one third of patients went into remission (no symptoms) and approximately half showed a response (at least a 50% reduction in symptoms). Those who did not respond (n = 1439) were invited to enroll in the second phase of the trial, reported here. Treatment options for patients who failed the initial course of citalopram included switching drugs (out of class to bupropion SR, within class to sertraline, or to the "dual-action" agent venlafaxine XR), switching to cognitive therapy, or augmenting by adding bupropion SR, buspirone, or cognitive therapy. Maximal doses were 400 mg daily for bupropion SR, 200 mg daily for sertraline, and 375 mg daily for venlafaxine XR. Patients could opt out of certain treatment options; for example, they could limit their randomization to only augmentation options or only switch options. Only 21 patients agreed to randomization to any of the 7 treatment options. The 3 different switch option groups had between 238 and 250 patients and they were followed up for up to 14 weeks. Their average age was 42 years, 59% were women, and 18% were African American. Most had recurrent depression with a mean of 7 previous episodes. Within the switch options, the response and remission rates as measured by the Hamilton Rating Scale for Depression (HRSD) and the Quick Inventory of Depressive Symptomatology were similar (HRSD remission rates of 21% for bupropion SR, 18% for sertraline, and 25% for venlafaxine XR). Adverse effects were generally similar between groups. A major limitation of this study was the absence of a placebo control group. Given the relapsing, remitting nature of depression it is likely that some patients would have gone into remission without any therapy at all. Not enough patients chose to be randomized to both switch and augmentation options to allow us to compare them.

Essential Evidence: Medicine that Matters, Edited by David Slawson, Allen Shaughnessy, Mark Ebell, and Henry Barry.

Suicide rates equal regardless of antidepressant type

Clinical question

Are suicide rates higher in depressed patients treated with tricyclic antidepressants instead of selective serotonin reuptake inhibitors?

Bottom line

Patients with depression were no more likely to successfully commit suicide while taking any particular class of antidepressants. Specifically, rates of successful suicide were not increased by treatment with tricyclic antidepressants. Fear of an increased risk of suicide should not be a reason to choose one type of antidepressant class over another. (LOE = 2b)

Reference

Khan, A, Khan S, Kolts R, Brown WA. Suicide rates in clinical trials of SSRIs, other antidepressants and placebo: analysis of FDA reports. Am J Psychiatry 2003;160:790–792.

Study Design

Cohort (retrospective)

Setting

Population-based

Synopsis

Many clinicians prefer prescribing selective serotonin reuptake inhibitors (SSRIs) for patients with depression to minimize the risk of suicide. By analyzing the FDA database of all reported adverse drug events, the authors compared completed (successful) suicide rates in patients treated with SSRIs (fluoxetine, sertraline, paroxetine, citalopram, fluvoxamine) and those treated with "other" antidepressants (nefazodone, mirtazapine, buproprion, venlafaxine, imipramine, amitriptyline, maprotiline, trazodone, mianserin, and dothiepin). Of 48,277 patients participating in clinical trials, 77 committed suicide. Based on patient-exposure years, similar suicide rates were seen among those randomized to an SSRI (0.59%; 95% CI, 0.31%–0.87%), a standard comparison antidepressant (0.76%; 95% CI, 0.49%–1.03%), and placebo (0.45%; 95% CI, 0.01%–0.89%). The authors speculate that the low suicide rate in patients treated with placebo is due to a short period of treatment with placebo in these clinical trials. No clear differences in the method of suicide were observed for patients treated with any of the drug classes. Participants in the studies may not represent a routine clinical sample of patients with depression. Subjects were mild to moderately depressed outpatients without suicidal ideations, co-morbid psychiatric or medical illnesses, or substance abuse disorders. The length of participation in these studies is shorter than what patients receive in clinical practice.

Essential Evidence: Medicine that Matters, Edited by David Slawson, Allen Shaughnessy, Mark Ebell, and Henry Barry.

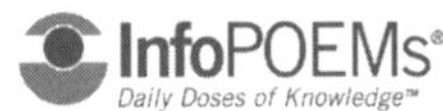

Antidepressant drugs increase suicidal behavior in children

Clinical question

Are antidepressant medications associated with an increased risk of suicidal behavior in children?

Bottom line

The use of antidepressant medications in children is associated with an increased risk of suicidal ideation and suicide-related behaviors. It is uncertain what overall effect antidepressant medications have on the morbidity and mortality of treated children. Close monitoring of patients using these medications regarding the risk of suicidality is recommended. (LOE = 1a–)

Reference

Hammad TA, Laughren T, Racoosin J. Suicidality in pediatric patients treated with antidepressant drugs. Arch Gen Psychiatry 2006;63:332–339.

Study Design

Meta-analysis (randomized controlled trials)

Funding

Government

Setting

Various (meta-analysis)

Synopsis

Concern exists about the potential for antidepressant medications to raise the risk of suicide in children and adolescents. The investigators pooled data from all 24 placebo-controlled trials comprising 4582 patients submitted to the Food and Drug Administration by various drug manufacturers. It is likely that this search method found most, if not all, clinical trials reporting safety information. Studied drugs included fluoxetine (Prozac), sertraline (Zoloft), paroxetine (Paxil), fluvoxamine (Luvox), citalopram (Celexa), bupropion (Wellbutrin), venlafaxine (Effexor), nefazodone, and mirtazapine (Remeron). Sixteen trials studied patients with major depressive disorder, and the remaining 8 studied obsessive-compulsive disorder, generalized anxiety disorder, attention-deficit/hyperactivity disorder, and social anxiety disorder. Events included either increased suicidal ideation or suicidal behavior. None of the trials reported a completed suicide. Trial durations ranged from 4 weeks to 16 weeks, so long-term risk is not included in this analysis. Individuals blinded to treatment group assignment evaluated adverse events potentially representing suicidal-related events. The selection process resulted in 130 unique patients with a suicidal-related event. The overall relative risk increase for suicidality for selective serotonin reuptake inhibitors in depression trials was 1.66 (95% CI, 1.02–2.68; number needed to treat to harm [NNTH] = 54, 21–1786) and for all drugs across all indications was 1.95 (95% CI, 1.28–2.98; NNTH = 38, 18–128). Venlafaxine (Effexor) was the only individual drug with a statistically significant increased risk of suicidality. There were no suicidal-related events reported for nefazodone and bupropion.

Essential Evidence: Medicine that Matters, Edited by David Slawson, Allen Shaughnessy, Mark Ebell, and Henry Barry.

Newer antidepressants increase suicidality in youths

Clinical question
Do newer antidepressants increase suicidality in children and adolescents aged 8 years to 18 years?

Bottom line
Newer-generation antidepressants increase suicide-related events in patients aged 8 years to 18 years. (LOE = 1a–)

Reference
Dubicka B, Hadley S, Roberts C. Suicidal behavior in youths with depression treated with new-generation antidepressants. Br J Psychiatry 2006;189:393–398.

Study Design
Meta-analysis (randomized controlled trials)

Funding
Unknown/not stated

Setting
Various (meta-analysis)

Synopsis
In this meta-analysis of 15 published and unpublished trials, the authors sought to define the risk of suicidality attributable to newer-generation antidepressants in children and adolescents aged 8 years to 18 years. All trials were 8 weeks to 12 weeks long and compared a newer-generation antidepressant with placebo. The antidepressants in the studies included fluoxetine, sertraline, paroxetine, citalopram, venlafaxine, and mirtazapine. Older antidepressants, such as tricyclics, were not considered. The majority of studies excluded subjects at high risk for suicide, by various definitions. The main outcome was the combined end point of suicide-related events, defined as self-harm, suicide attempt, or suicidal thoughts. This occurred in 4.8% of subjects receiving antidepressants and 3.0% of those receiving placebo (number needed to treat to harm = 57; 95% CI, 31–363). There were no completed suicides in any of the studies. When elements of the combined outcome were considered separately, differences between drug and placebo did not reach statistical significance. However, not all studies reported these outcomes separately. Data were insufficient to compare individual antidepressants.

Essential Evidence: Medicine that Matters, Edited by David Slawson, Allen Shaughnessy, Mark Ebell, and Henry Barry.

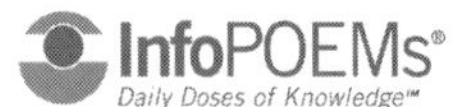

Light therapy as effective as fluoxetine for seasonal affective disorder

Clinical question

Is light therapy an acceptable alternative to antidepressants for patients with seasonal affective disorder?

Bottom line

Light therapy and fluoxetine (Prozac) are equally effective treatment options for patients with seasonal affective disorder (SAD). Patient preference and an individual assessment of risks and benefits should guide treatment selection. (LOE = 1b)

Reference

Lam RW, Levitt AJ, Levitan RD, et al. The CAN-SAD Study: A randomized controlled trial of the effectiveness of light therapy and fluoxetine in patients with winter seasonal affective disorder. Am J Psychiatry 2006;163:805–812.

Study Design

Randomized controlled trial (double-blinded)

Funding

Industry + govt

Allocation

Concealed

Setting

Outpatient (specialty)

Synopsis

Both light therapy and antidepressants are effective in the treatment of SAD, but few studies have directly compared the 2 treatments. These investigators identified 96 adults (mean age = 42 years) meeting DSM-IV criteria for major depressive disorder with a seasonal (winter) pattern with scores greater than 23 on the 24-item Hamilton Depression Rating Scale (HAM-D). Subjects were randomized in double-blind fashion (concealed allocation assignment) to 8 weeks of treatment with either 10,000-lux light treatment plus placebo or 100-lux light treatment (placebo light) plus fluoxetine 20 mg per day. Light treatment occurred for 30 minutes as soon as possible after awakening, between 7:00 AM and 8:00 AM. Individuals blinded to treatment group assignment assessed outcomes using the HAM-D. A significant clinical response included a 50% or greater reduction from baseline in HAM-D scores. Follow-up occurred for 96% of subjects for 8 weeks. Using intention-to-treat analysis, there were no significant differences between the light and fluoxetine treatment groups in clinical response rates (67% for both conditions) or remission rates (50% vs 54%, respectively). There were also no significant differences in either outcome noted between the 2 treatment groups for a subset of severely depressed patients. The placebo light, although dim, may have some clinical effect, possibly by accentuating the benefit of fluoxetine. More fluoxetine-treated patients complained of agitation, sleep disturbance, and palpitations. However, treatment emergent adverse event rates and drop-out rates were similar in both groups.

Essential Evidence: Medicine that Matters, Edited by David Slawson, Allen Shaughnessy, Mark Ebell, and Henry Barry.

Smoking cessation 6–8 weeks before surgery reduces complications

Clinical question

Is it worth trying to get smokers to quit before elective surgery?

Bottom line

Among smokers awaiting elective hip or knee replacement, participating in a weekly nurse-led smoking cessation program prevents postoperative complications. Only three patients need to go through the program to prevent one complication. (LOE = 1b)

Reference

Moller AM, Villebro N, Pedersen T, Tonneson H. Effect of preoperative smoking intervention on postoperative complications: a randomised clinical trial. Lancet 2002;359:114–117.

Study Design

Randomized controlled trial (single-blinded)

Setting

Outpatient (specialty)

Synopsis

These authors studied smokers in three Danish hospitals who were scheduled for elective hip or knee replacement. Six to eight weeks before the surgery, they randomly assigned (masked allocation) the smokers to a smoking intervention (n = 60) or control (n = 60). The intervention consisted of weekly meetings with a nurse who developed a personalized smoking cessation and free nicotine-replacement program. They strongly encouraged the patients to quit smoking, but the patients also had the option of reducing tobacco consumption by 50%. The investigators used an intention-to-treat analysis and the investigator who assessed complications was unaware of which group the patient was assigned to. Several patients in each group didn't go through with the surgery. Of the patients who went through with their surgery, 10/56 (18%) in the intervention group had a complication compared with 27/52 (52%) of the controls. We don't have any information about the severity of complications. Neither group had anybody kick off. While the largest difference was in the rate of wound infections, the study was underpowered to see significant differences in infrequent events like cardiac complications. There was no difference in hospital length of stay. They also looked at the treatment actually received and found that the benefit was noted primarily in those who actually quit rather than some other unanticipated aspect of the program.

Essential Evidence: Medicine that Matters, Edited by David Slawson, Allen Shaughnessy, Mark Ebell, and Henry Barry.

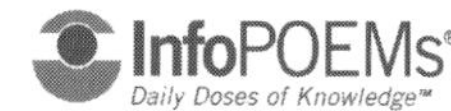

12 weeks of varenicline is effective for smoking cessation

Clinical question

Is varenicline more effective than bupropion and placebo for smoking cessation?

Bottom line

Varenicline therapy for 12 weeks is more effective than placebo at maintaining smoking abstinence at 52 weeks. Varenicline is marginally more effective than bupropion SR. Reported success rates are likely to be higher than real-world settings. (LOE = 1b)

Reference

Gonzales D, Rennard SI, Nides M, et al, for the Varenicline Phase 3 Study Group. Varenicline, an a4b2 nicotinic acetylcholine receptor partial agonist, vs sustained-release bupropion and placebo for smoking cessation. A randomized controlled trial. JAMA 2006;296:47–55.

Study Design	Funding	Allocation
Randomized controlled trial (double-blinded)	Industry	Concealed

Setting

Population-based

Synopsis

Varenicline is a nicotinic acetylcholine receptor partial agonist that may reduce the reinforcing effects of nicotine for maintaining smoking behavior. The investigators randomized 1025 healthy adult smokers, aged 18 years to 75 years, to receive varenicline (titrated to 1 mg twice daily), bupropion SR (titrated to 150 mg twice daily), or matching placebo for 12 weeks. All subjects received brief counseling and a self-help booklet. Participants who completed the initial 12-week treatment continued in a nondrug follow-up phase for 52 weeks. Smoking cessation was determined by patient self-report and an exhaled carbon monoxide measurement. Slightly more than half of patients, regardless of treatment, completed the study, but continuous abstinence rates at 52 weeks were significantly higher for varenicline vs placebo (21.9% vs 8.4%; number needed to treat [NNT] = 7; 95% CI, 4–15). The difference in quit rates at 52 weeks between varenicline and bupropion (21.9% vs 16.1%) was not statistically significant. Be aware that the method for calculating the cumulative abstinence rate gives an inflated overall estimate. Adverse events were similar for both groups: nausea was the most common adverse event associated with varenicline. Mean weight gain and drop-out rates due to adverse events occurred similarly among all 3 groups. An identically designed study in the same issue (JAMA 2006;296:56–63) found similar results, except that the difference in abstinence rates at 52 weeks between varenicline and bupropion SR was statistically significant (23.0% vs 14.6%; NNT = 12, 6–43). In a third study reported in the same issue (JAMA 2006;296:64–71) smokers who achieved abstinence at the end of 12 weeks of varenicline treatment and were then randomized to an additional 12 weeks of varenicline (instead of placebo) showed a significantly higher continuous abstinence rate at 52 weeks of follow-up (43.6% vs 36.9%; NNT = 14, 8–73). None of the subjects enrolled in any of the 3 trials had a history of previous bupropion therapy, so success rates for varenicline in patients who have failed bupropion therapy are unknown.

Essential Evidence: Medicine that Matters, Edited by David Slawson, Allen Shaughnessy, Mark Ebell, and Henry Barry.

6 weeks of varenicline is also effective for smoking cessation

Clinical question

Is varenicline effective for inducing and maintaining smoking cessation?

Bottom line

Approximately 1 in 7 highly motivated patients will not be smoking 1 year after taking varenicline (Chantix) 1 mg twice daily for 6 weeks. Lower doses did not work. Side effects will be common and will not be tolerated by some patients. (LOE = 1b−)

Reference

Nides M, Oncken C, Gonzales D, et al. Smoking cessation with varenicline, a selective alpha-4-beta-2 nicotinic receptor partial agonist: results from a 7-week, randomized, placebo- and bupropion-controlled trial with 1-year follow-up. Arch Intern Med 2006;166:1561–1568.

Study Design

Randomized controlled trial (double-blinded)

Funding

Industry

Allocation

Uncertain

Setting

Outpatient (any)

Synopsis

This US study enrolled 626 adults smokers who volunteered for the study. The patients were long-term smokers averaging 1 pack per day for 25 years. Recruitment methods were not described, but it's likely the patients responded to an advertisement and were highly motivated to quit. The patients were randomized to receive 0.3 mg, 1 mg, or 2 mg daily of varenicline, bupropion 300 mg daily, or placebo. Treatment with varenicline lasted 6 weeks and bupropion treatment was for 7 weeks. Unlike the commercially available product, which titrates dosage from a low initial dose to the full dosage, patients were started directly on their assigned dosages. Patients received weekly counseling for 10 minutes and an information booklet. Four-week continuous quit rates were determined by self-report via a diary and were confirmed by measuring inhaled carbon monoxide. Analysis was by intention to treat, with dropouts considered to be still smoking. One year following the start of the study, 14% of subjects receiving varenicline 1 mg twice daily were still not smoking, only 6% of patients receiving bupropion were still not smoking, and 5% of those receiving placebo were still not smoking. Approximately half the subjects receiving varenicline 1 mg twice daily reported nausea at some point in treatment, 35% reported headache, and 24% reported abnormal dreams. One in 3 patients did not complete the 6 weeks of treatment, with approximately 60% of those who dropped out doing so because of adverse effects.

Essential Evidence: Medicine that Matters, Edited by David Slawson, Allen Shaughnessy, Mark Ebell, and Henry Barry.

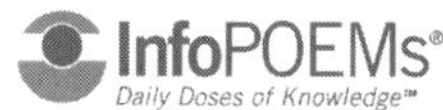

Educational programs effective for young asthmatics

Clinical question

Do educational programs for the self-management of asthma affect outcomes in children and adolescents?

Bottom line

Teaching children and adolescents how to manage their asthma improves their feeling of self-efficacy, improves lung function, decreases the number of days lost from school and the number of days with restricted activity, and decreases emergency visits. These were formal, multiple-session programs. Teaching methods focusing on individualized responses to changes in peak flow measurements had the strongest effects. (LOE = 1a)

Reference

Guevara JP, Wolf FM, Grum CM, Clark NM. Effects of educational interventions for self-management of asthma in children and adolescents: systematic review and meta-analysis. BMJ 2003;326:1308–1312.

Study Design

Meta-analysis (randomized controlled trials)

Setting

Outpatient (any)

Synopsis

An earlier meta-analysis (from 1992) of self-management education found no affect on children or adolescents; the analysis was based, however, on relatively few studies, and may not have had enough power to show a difference if one was truly there. The authors of the current meta-analysis searched several databases and identifed 32 randomized controlled trials enrolling a total of 3706 patients. They did a thorough job of searching the literature, including in their analysis articles published in any language. Their criterion for quality analysis was whether the investigators enrolling patients into the studies were unaware of the group to which the patients would be assigned (ie, concealed allocation); only 38% of the studies had a thorough description of this concealed allocation to treatment group and 10% clearly did not conceal allocation. However, results were similar when the high-quality studies were separately analyzed from lower-quality studies. The educational programs were diverse, and targeted children, adolescents, or both. These were not 2-minute this-what-you-do-with-your-peak-flow-meter lectures, but instead most of them used multiple sessions and focused on symptom-based strategies. In the 4 studies that evaluated it, the programs were associated with a moderate effect on lung function (standardized mean difference = 0.50; 95% CI, 0.25–0.75), translating into an approximately 10% increase in peak expiratory flow rate. Absences from school, night dusturbances, and the number of days with restricted activities were fewer in the children receiving the education, and children with moderate to severe asthma, as expected, experienced a greater effect. Children receiving the education reported a moderate improvement in their control of asthma. Visits to emergency departments were fewer in the educated patients, though hospitalization rate was not affected.

Bed and pillow covers ineffective for asthma

Clinical question

Do impermeable bed and pillow covers reduce asthma symptoms in mite-sensitive patients?

Bottom line

Impermeable bed, pillow, and quilt covers do not improve symptoms or reduce medication use in adult asthmatics. Other studies have suggested some benefit in asthmatic children, so we shouldn't necessarily abandon this intervention in younger patients. (LOE = 1b)

Reference

Woodcock A, Forster L, Matthews E, et al. Control of exposure to mite allergen and allergen-impermeable bed covers for adults with asthma. N Engl J Med 2003;349:225–236.

Study Design

Randomized controlled trial (double-blinded)

Setting

Outpatient (primary care)

Synopsis

Although it makes sense that patients with asthma who are also allergic to dust mites would benefit from reducing their exposure to the little creatures, evidence that impermeable bed and pillow covers actually make a difference is limited and largely comes from small, poorly designed studies. In this much larger study, patients aged 18 to 50 years who were taking inhaled steroids for a diagnosis of asthma and using rescue inhalers at least once a day were recuited from 154 English general practices. Their sensitivity to dust mites was measured at the beginning of the study, but the results were not disclosed to the patient or their physician. Of 1746 eligible patients, 1431 started a 1 month run-in phase, and 1150 were randomized (allocation concealed) to receive either impermeable or standard cotton-polyester mattress, pillow, and quilt covers. Symptoms, peak flows, and rescue inhaler use were recorded in a diary during the run-in period, and those who were compliant (those who completed the diary for 14 of 28 days) were invited to participate in the rest of the trial. Patients were seen every 3 months for 6 months, and then were asked to reduce the dose of inhaled corticosteroids during the second half of the year-long study, during which time they were more closely monitored. Mite sensitivity was documented in 366 patients in each group. At the end of the study period there was no significant difference among the mite-sensitive patients between treatment and control groups in peak flow, symptom scores, exacerbations, days of work missed, and use of beta-agonists. There was also no difference between groups regarding the average reduction in steroid dose during the second half of the study, or the percentage of patients who could stop taking inhaled steroids altogether. This study was powered to detect a difference of 20 liters per minute in peak flow, and a 50% increase in the proportion of patients who discontinued inhaled steroids. Although we aren't told if it was adequately powered to detect a clinically meaningful difference in symptom scores, it seems likely that given the number of patients it was.

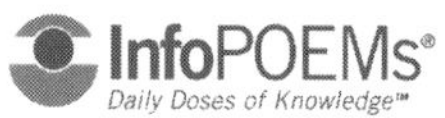

Exhaled nitric oxide and sputum analysis useful for asthma diagnosis

Clinical question

Which tests are better for diagnosing asthma: spirometry, peak flow measurements, exhaled nitric oxide, or sputum analysis?

Bottom line

Exhaled nitric oxide concentration and sputum eosinophilia show promise in establishing a diagnosis of asthma. Since the gold standard for diagnosing asthma isn't very golden, additional studies are needed to determine just how good these tests really are. (LOE = 2b)

Reference

Smith AD, Cowan JO, Filsell S, et al. Diagnosing asthma: comparisons between exhaled nitric oxide measurements and conventional tests. Am J Respir Crit Care Med 2004;169:473–478.

Study Design

Cross-sectional

Setting

Outpatient (specialty)

Synopsis

This study included 47 consecutive patients aged between 8 and 75 years referred by their family physicians for testing for possible asthma. All patients received a standard battery of questions and a fixed sequence of diagnostic tests. After the final visit, a diagnosis of asthma was made according to American Thoracic Society clinical criteria, plus a positive result for bronchial hyper-reactivity (a provocative dose of hypertonic saline resulting in a 15% fall in FEV1 of less than 20 mL) or a positive response to bronchodilator (an increase in FEV1 of 12% or greater from baseline 15 minutes after inhaled albuterol). All patients also had measurements of exhaled nitric oxide (ENO) and assessment of sputum eosinophilia. All tests were conducted in a blinded and independent fashion. The authors constructed receiver operator characteristic curves to compare the diagnostic accuracy of each test with the gold standard. Seventeen patients (36%) were diagnosed with asthma: 1 severe, 4 moderately severe, 12 mild. Peak flow measurements and FEV1 had poor sensitivity (<35%) but were very specific (93%–100%). A FEV1/FVC ratio of <70% was 35% sensitive and 100% specific; a ratio of <80% showed better sensitivity (47%) at the expense of worse specificity (80%). The presence of more than 3% eosinophils in the sputum was 86% sensitive and 88% specific, although only 40 of the patients were able to provide a sample. ENO concentration exceeding 20 parts per billion was 88% sensitive and 79% specific. The main limitations of this study include the small sample, the limited spectrum of severity, and the low proportion of smokers (42 of 47 were nonsmokers, the remaining 5 were ex-smokers). If supported with additional studies, ENO and sputum eosinophil concentration may replace conventional testing. Since ENO is relatively quick and simple to perform, it may eventually become the preferred test.

Essential Evidence: Medicine that Matters, Edited by David Slawson, Allen Shaughnessy, Mark Ebell, and Henry Barry.

Intermittent = continuous therapy for mild persistent asthma

Clinical question

Does continuous therapy with anti-inflammatory drugs improve outcomes for patients with mild persistent asthma?

Bottom line

Intermittent therapy, as measured by the outcomes that matter, is as effective as continuous therapy with oral zafirlukast or inhaled budesonide for patients with very mild but persistent asthma. Note that patients had a clear plan of action for when symptoms flared up: Begin inhaled budesonide in the "yellow zone," when symptoms initially worsen, and add prednisone 0.5 mg/kg if symptoms enter the "red zone," when breathlessness is present at rest or with activities of daily living. (LOE = 1b)

Reference

Boushey HA, Sorkness CA, King TS, et al, for the National Heart, Lung, and Blood Institute's Asthma Clinical Research Network. Daily versus as-needed corticosteroids for mild persistent asthma. N Engl J Med 2005;352:1519–1528.

Study Design	Funding	Allocation
Randomized controlled trial (double-blinded)	Government	Uncertain

Setting

Outpatient (any)

Synopsis

One of the things that primary care physicians are frequently criticized for is a failure to treat asthma patients as intensively as is recommended by some guidelines. For example, adults with mild persistent asthma (self-treatment with beta-agonist more than 2 days per week, nighttime awakenings related to asthma more than 2 days per month, or variability in the peak expiratory flow of 20% to 30%) should be taking chronic anti-inflammatory medications based on current National Heart, Lung, and Blood Institute guidelines. Or should they? After an active run-in period, adults with this severity of asthma were randomized (allocation uncertain) to receive either 200 mcg of inhaled budesonide (Pulmicort) twice daily, 20 mg of oral zafirlukast (Accolate) twice daily, or matching placebo. All groups could use rescue therapy with budesonide, as needed, according to a symptom guide, as well as inhaled albuterol (salbutamol). They were followed up for 1 year with a variety of symptoms scores and physiologic measures. Follow-up was good, with 199 of 225 patients completing the study. After 1 year, patients in the placebo group (intermittent therapy only) performed slightly worse on a number of outcome measures, such as exhaled nitric oxide levels and the percentage of eosinophils in the sputum. There was no difference regarding the primary outcome of morning peak expiratory flow. If you understand the difference between patient- and disease-oriented outcomes, you should say to yourself, "Who cares?" More important, there was no clinically significant difference in the number of courses of budesonide or asthma control scores (0.1 to 0.2 on a 6-point scale), and no difference in quality of life scores.

Essential Evidence: Medicine that Matters, Edited by David Slawson, Allen Shaughnessy, Mark Ebell, and Henry Barry.

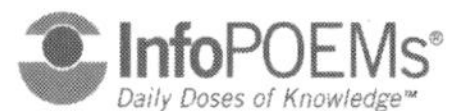

Salmeterol + fluticasone better than fluticasone for asthma (GOAL)

Clinical question

Is guideline-driven care of asthmatic patients using stepwise increases in salmeterol-fluticasone more effective than using fluticasone alone?

Bottom line

Asthmatic patients treated with stepwise increases in salmeterol/fluticasone (Seretide, Advair) are more likely to achieve total control or be well controlled at the end of 12 weeks and at the end of 1 year than patients using fluticasone (Flixotide, Flovent) alone. (LOE = 1b)

Reference

Bateman ED, Boushey HA, Bousquet J, et al. Can guideline-defined asthma control be achieved? The Gaining Optimal Asthma ControL Study. Am J Respir Crit Care Med 2004;170:836–844.

Study Design	Funding	Allocation
Randomized controlled trial (double-blinded)	Industry	Uncertain

Setting

Outpatient (any)

Synopsis

This year-long study involved 3421 patients between 12 and 80 years of age who had at least a 6-month history of asthma, had fewer than 10 pack-years of tobacco use, and hadn't used oral or long-acting beta-agonists for the 2 weeks prior to enrollment. The study began with a 4-week run-in period during which patients continued to use their usual treatment. Patients without 2 well-controlled weeks were randomized (concealment of allocation not described) to receive salmeterol/fluticasone or fluticasone propionate alone. Each treatment group was also stratified according to their use of inhaled corticosteroids for the 6 months before enrollment: no inhaled corticosteroid; 500 mcg or less of beclomethasone dipropionate; or 500 mcg to 1000 mcg of beclomethasone dipropionate daily (or equivalent). In this phase, doses of medication were increased until asthma was totally controlled or until maximum doses of medication was used: salmeterol/fluticasone, 50/500 mcg twice a day; fluticasone, 500 mcg twice a day. The patients were then maintained on the dose needed to achieve total control (or the maximum dose) for the rest of the year.Total asthma control was defined as 7 of 8 weeks of no daytime symptoms; no use of rescue medications; a morning peak expiratory flow of at least 80% of predicted; and no night-time awakenings, no exacerbations, no emergency room visits, and no medication adverse events. Well-controlled asthma was similarly defined, except as follows: no more than 2 days with a symptom score higher than 1, and the use of rescue medication on no more than 2 days and no more than 4 doses per week. These definitions came from the Global Initiative for Asthma and the National Institutes of Health. The primary study objective, assessed via intention to treat, was to determine the proportion of patients who achieved well-controlled asthma. Total control was significantly more likely to be achieved across all strata: 31% versus 19% of patients at the end of the dose escalation phases, and 41% versus 28% at one year for salmeterol/fluticasone and fluticasone, respecitively. Additionally, patients receiving the combination had 0.07 to 0.27 fewer exacerbations per year. A concern of this study, however, is that the guidelines call for an automatic dose escalation of products manufactured by the study sponsor to achieve total asthma control.

Essential Evidence: Medicine that Matters, Edited by David Slawson, Allen Shaughnessy, Mark Ebell, and Henry Barry.

Don't double steroid dose in deteriorating asthma

Clinical question

Does doubling the dose of inhaled steroids help patients with deteriorating asthma control?

Bottom line

A commonly recommended strategy of doubling the dose of inhaled steroids in patients with deteriorating asthma control does little to improve symptoms or peak flow, or to prevent the use of oral rescue prednisolone. (LOE = 2b)

Reference

Harrison TW, Oborne J, Newton S, Tattersfield AE. Doubling the dose of inhaled corticosteroid to prevent asthma exacerbations: randomised controlled trial. Lancet 2004;363:271–275.

Study Design

Randomized controlled trial (nonblinded)

Setting

Outpatient (primary care)

Synopsis

These researchers recruited asthmatic patients 16 years and older who used inhaled corticosteroids (100 to 2000 mcg per day) on a regular basis. To be included, the patients had to have taken oral corticosteroids or doubled their dose of inhaled corticosteroid temporarily in the previous 12 months to treat or prevent an exacerbation. All patients completed a 2-week run-in to assess their baseline (using morning peak flow measurements and symptom diaries). Those patients with unstable asthma during this run-in had an additional 2 week run-in. All patients were instructed to continue their usual treatment. In addition to their usual treatment, patients were randomized (masked central allocation) to receive an additional inhaler: placebo (n = 198) or active inhaler (n = 192). The active inhaler was formulated to deliver double the steroid dose the patient used at enrollment. The patients were instructed to use the study inhaler for 14-days if the morning peak flow fell by 15% or if the daytime symptom score increased by 1 point. Finally, all patients were provided oral prednisolone (30 mg per day for 10 days) for rescue when the peak flow dropped below 40% of the mean run-in value. The main outcome for this study, analyzed by intention to treat, was the use of rescue prednisolone. Approximately 9% of the randomized patients dropped out of the study. Among the patients randomized to placebo, 97 actually felt the need to use it and 24 ultimately used prednisolone. Among those in the active inhaler group, 110 used it and 22 ultimately used prednisolone. In other words, there was no real difference between groups in the use of rescue prednisolone. Additionally, there were no differences in peak flow measurements or symptom scores between the 2 groups. The study had almost 90% power to detect a 40% decrease in rescue prednisolone use.

Essential Evidence: Medicine that Matters, Edited by David Slawson, Allen Shaughnessy, Mark Ebell, and Henry Barry.

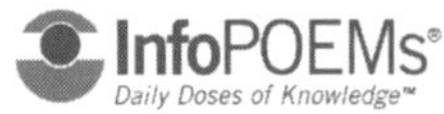

Long-term budesonide does not effect adrenal function in children

Clinical question

Does the use of chronic inhaled corticosteroids affect adrenal function in children?

Bottom line

A nagging worry about using inhaled corticosteroids in children has been relieved. In a study of more than 3 years, continuous use of budesonide (Pulmicort) had no effect on serum cortisol levels or cortisol response to adrenocorticotrophic hormone administration. (LOE = 1b)

Reference

Bacharier LB, Raissy HH, Wilson L, et al. Long-term effect of budesonide on hypothalamic-pituitary-adrenal axis function in children with mild to moderate asthma. Pediatrics 2004;113:1693–1699.

Study Design

Randomized controlled trial (nonblinded)

Setting

Outpatient (primary care)

Synopsis

Uncontrolled (eg, cross-sectional or retrospective) studies have suggested that chronic inhaled corticosteroid use in children may effect hypothalamic-pituitary-adrenal axis function. These authors evaluated this effect in 63 children with mild to moderate asthma who received standard doses of budesonide (400 mcg/day; n = 18) or either nedocromil (Tilade) or placebo (n = 45) for 36 months. At the time of enrollment children were approximately 9 years old. Serum cortisol levels and response to adrenocorticotrophic hormone (ACTH) stimulation were measured at baseline and at 12 and 36 months. At both measurements, response to ACTH stimulation was similar between the children receiving budesonide and those receiving nedocromil or placebo. Urinary excretion of cortisol over 24 hours was also not affected overall, although it was statistically lower (P = .05) if supplemental inhaled corticosteroid was used in the 4 months preceding the 36-month visit. Two caveats: (1) these 63 children may not be representative of all children with mild to moderate asthma, and (2) the analysis was by intention to treat, instead of by using only the children who had demonstrated continuous use of budesonide. Noncompliance with treatment might also be responsible for the lack of effect.

Essential Evidence: Medicine that Matters, Edited by David Slawson, Allen Shaughnessy, Mark Ebell, and Henry Barry.

Procalcitonin test can reduce antibiotic use in COPD

Clinical question

Can the procalcitonin level be used to safely guide the use of antibiotics in patients with a chronic obstructive pulmonary disease exacerbation?

Bottom line

Procalcitonin can be used to guide the use of antibiotics in patients with exacerbation of chronic obstructive pulmonary disease (COPD). Antibiotics are optional for those with a procalcitonin level between 0.1 mcg/L and 0.25 mcg/L and are recommended if the procalcitonin level of greater than 0.25 mcg/L. (LOE = 1b)

Reference

Stolz D, Christ-Crain M, Bingisser R, et al. Antibiotic treatment of exacerbations of COPD: a randomized, controlled trial comparing procalcitonin-guidance with standard therapy. Chest 2007;131:9–19.

Study Design	Funding	Allocation
Randomized controlled trial (double-blinded)	Industry	Uncertain

Setting

Emergency department

Synopsis

Procalcitonin is a biomarker that is elevated in patients with bacterial infection, but not in those with viral infection or other types of inflammation. A previous study (Lancet 2004; 363:600–07) showed that a new, more accurate assay can identify patients with lower respiratory tract infection who are unlkely to benefit from antibiotics. In this study, the researchers identified 226 adults older than 40 years who met standard criteria for an exacerbation of their COPD. All patients had a procalcitonin level drawn. Patients were then randomized into a usual care group or a group that also gave the treating physicians access to the procalcitonin level. A level less than 0.1 mcg/L was reported as absence of bacterial infection with no antibiotic recommended; a level between 0.1 and 0.25 mcg/L was reported as possible bacterial infection with antibiotic use optional; and a level greater than 0.25 mcg/L was interpreted as bacterial infection with antibiotic use recommended. Clinical success or failure was assessed between 2 weeks and 3 weeks after discharge by clinicians blinded to group assignment. Patients were also contacted 6 months after discharge for a clinical assessment. Of the 226 patients initially randomized, 11 in the procalcitonin group and 7 in the standard treatment group were removed from the study because they did not meet criteria for COPD on the basis of inpatient spirometry. Follow-up was excellent up to 6 months for the remainder of patients. Having access to the procalcitonin test result significantly reduced both antibiotic prescriptions during the index hopitalization (40% vs 72%; $P < .001$) without any difference in the number of days to the next exacerbation (76 days for each group) or the number of exacerbations or hospitalizations in the next 6 months. Interestingly, there was no association between procalcitonin levels and the presence of purulent sputum or abnormal sputum cultures. Only 10 patients developed pneumonia, too small a number to draw any conclusions about the effect of procalcitonin guidance on increasing or decreasing the likelihood of pneumonia. There was no significant difference between groups at any point regarding lung function, symptoms, functional status, or hospital length of stay.

Essential Evidence: Medicine that Matters, Edited by David Slawson, Allen Shaughnessy, Mark Ebell, and Henry Barry.

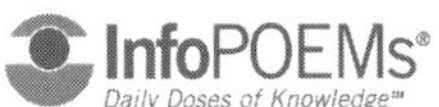

Corticosteroids benefit patients with moderate to severe COPD

Clinical question

Are inhaled corticosteroids effective in patients with chronic obstructive pulmonary disease?

Bottom line

Inhaled corticosteroids prevent exacerbations in patients with moderate to severe chronic obstructive pulmonary disease (COPD). The benefit is minor, however, and steroids don't prevent exacerbations in patients with mild COPD. The prevention of exacerbations with steroids must be balanced against the higher rate of fractures and glaucoma. (LOE = 1a−)

Reference

Gartlehner G, Hansen RA, Carson SS, Lohr KN. Efficacy and safety of inhaled corticosteroids in patients with COPD: a systematic review and meta-analysis of health outcomes. Ann Fam Med 2006;4:253–262.

Study Design

Meta-analysis (randomized controlled trials)

Funding

Foundation

Setting

Outpatient (any)

Synopsis

These authors systematically reviewed several databases looking for double-blind randomized controlled trials of at least 6 months' duration in which outpatients with COPD were treated with inhaled corticosteroids or placebo. They also reviewed observational studies, but only to evaluate adverse effects. The authors don't report looking for unpublished studies. Two reviewers independently evaluated whether studies were eligible for inclusion. Additionally, the researchers evaluated the quality of the studies and excluded poor-quality studies. The authors note the lack of a standard definition of an exacerbation as a limitation of the literature. Most studies defined an exacerbation as an episode that required oral or parenteral corticosteroids, antibiotics, emergency department visits, or hospitalizations because of increased respiratory tract symptoms. Ultimately, these authors included 12 randomized controlled trials with 5618 patients. Patients receiving inhaled corticosteroids had a 33% relative reduction in exacerbations. Although the authors don't report the absolute rate, they report that one would need to treat 12 patients with inhaled corticosteroids for 17.7 months to prevent one exacerbation. In patients with mild COPD, inhaled steroids were no more effective than placebo in preventing exacerbations. Overall, they found no significant mortality difference (2.9% of those taking placebo; 2.5% of those taking inhaled steroids). Inhaled corticosteroids are well tolerated. The pooled discontinuation rates didn't differ significantly among the groups. Finally, observational studies demonstrated higher rates of fractures and glaucoma in high-dose users.

Essential Evidence: Medicine that Matters, Edited by David Slawson, Allen Shaughnessy, Mark Ebell, and Henry Barry.

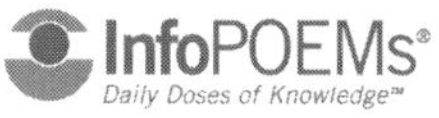

Anticholinergics are better than beta-agonists in COPD treatment

Clinical question

In patients with chronic obstructive pulmonary disease, do anticholinergics provide better benefit than beta-2 agonists?

Bottom line

Anticholinergic treatment in patients with chronic obstructive pulmonary disease (COPD) produces better results than treatment with a beta-2 agonist. Studies comparing anticholinergic treatment with placebo have shown a greater decrease in the number of exacerbations. Studies comparing beta-2 agonist treatment with placebo have shown less benefit. In direct comparison with each other, there were 2.5 more exacerbations for every 100 patients treated with a beta-2 agonist instead of an anticholinergic. (LOE = 1a)

Reference

Salpeter SR, Buckley NS, Salpeter EE. Meta-analysis: anticholinergics, but not beta-agonists, reduce severe exacerbations and respiratory mortality in COPD. J Gen Intern Med 2006;21:1011–1019.

Study Design

Meta-analysis (randomized controlled trials)

Funding

Self-funded or unfunded

Setting

Various (meta-analysis)

Synopsis

The authors conducting this meta-analysis searched 3 databases to identify a total of 22 randomized controlled studies comparing a beta-2 agonist or an anticholinergic with placebo or with each other in patients with COPD. Seven trials compared anticholinergics with placebo, 13 compared beta-2 agonists with placebo, and 7 trials compared beta-2 agonists with anticholinergics. The researchers excluded 9 studies from analysis because they did not report at least one exacerbation, hospitalization, or death. The researchers did not explain their method for selecting the studies for inclusion. Two reviewers independently assessed the validity of the studies and abstracted the data for analysis. Study results were homogeneous across the studies. There was no evidence of publication bias.The studies enrolled a total of 15,276 patients for an average duration of 20 months (range = 3–60 months). More than half the patients in these studies were also treated with a corticosteroid. As compared with placebo, anticholinergic treatment with ipratropium (Atrovent) or tiotropium (Spiriva) resulted in 4 fewer exacerbations per 100 patients treated for 1 year (number needed to treat [NNT] = 25.) Beta-2 agonist treatment resulted in 3 fewer exacerbations per 100 patients (NNT = 34). In direct comparison, there were twice as many exacerbations reported in the beta-2 agonist-treated group as in the anticholinergic-treated group: 5.1% vs 2.6% ($P < .001$). In other words, there were 2.5 more exacerbations for every 100 patients treated with a beta-2 agonist. In comparison with placebo, anticholinergics decreased death rates (NNT = 278), whereas beta-2 agonists increased death rates (0.76% per year; number needed to treat to harm = 131).

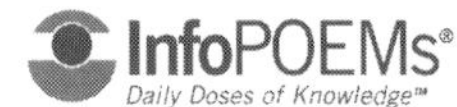

Cough suppressants ineffective in children

Clinical question

Do cough suppressants improve the sleep of children with respiratory infections, or the sleep of their parents?

Bottom line

In this single dose study, placebo worked just as well as either dextromethorphan or diphenhydramine to decrease cough frequency or severity in children. Also, the active drugs provided no additional benefit on parents' report of their own or their child's sleep. This is both bad news and good news. The bad news is that these drugs don't work any better than placebo (which, actually, was reported to work pretty well). The good news is that when parents feel the need to do something when their child has a cold all products work equally well. (LOE = 1b–)

Reference

Paul IM, Yoder KE, Crowell KR, et al. Effect of dextromethorphan, diphenhydramine, and placebo on nocturnal cough and sleep quality for coughing children and their parents. Pediatrics 2004;114:e85–e90.

Study Design

Randomized controlled trial (double-blinded)

Setting

Outpatient (primary care)

Synopsis

When a young child coughs at night, parents don't get much sleep. Although the American Academy of Pediatrics recommends against antitussives because of their lack of demonstrated benefit, these products fly off pharmacy shelves in the winter months. This study identified 100 children experiencing rhinitis and cough symptoms for 1 week or less, who didn't have asthma or allergies; in other words, children with a cold. The average age was slightly older than 4 years (range = 2–16 years). The children were randomized (allocation concealment uncertain) to receive a single dose of placebo, diphenhydramine (Diphen), or dextromethorphan (Benylin), for the single night of the study. Using a 7-point Likert scale, parents were asked to rate the effect of treatment on the child's cough frequency, as well as the effect on their own sleep and that of the child. As compared with ratings obtained for the night before the study night, parents overall reported a significant decrease in cough frequency and severity (from "somewhat" to "occasional" on the descriptive scale). The combined symptom score decreased from 19.8 to 8.9 (of a possible 30) with any treatment ($P < .01$). Parents also reported a significant improvement in both their sleep and their childrens' sleep. However, the results were not different whether the child was treated with either drug or placebo. Adverse effects were reported equally in all 3 study groups. The study had the power to find a 1-point change in scores of the 3 arms, if one truly existed.

No antibiotics necessary for lower respiratory infection

Clinical question

What is the optimal management strategy for acute uncomplicated lower respiratory tract infection?

Bottom line

After excluding patients with chronic lung disease or clinically suspected pneumonia, antibiotics provide little or no benefit for patients with cough and lower respiratory tract symptoms, including those with fever and green sputum. Regardless of treatment method, cough will last about 3 weeks for the majority of patients and for at least 1 month in 25%. Patients given an immediate prescription for an antibiotic are more likely to expect antibiotics in the future. Providing a verbal explanation about the expected course and potential complications of cough during the consultation is most likely to assure optimal patient satisfaction. (LOE = 2b)

Reference

Little P, Rumsby K, Kelly J, et al. Information leaflet and antibiotic prescribing strategies for acute lower respiratory tract infection. A randomized controlled trial. JAMA 2005;293:3029–3035.

Study Design	Funding	Allocation	Setting
Randomized controlled trial (single-blinded)	Government	Concealed	Outpatient (primary care)

Synopsis

The investigators enrolled 807 adults and children presenting to their primary care clinician with cough and at least 1 other symptom referable to the lower respiratory tract (colored sputum, chest pain, dyspnea, or wheezing). Patients with asthma, other chronic lung diseases, or suspected pneumonia were excluded. Subjects were randomly assigned to 1 of 6 groups. They received an educational leaflet on cough or no leaflet, and were then placed in 1 of 3 antibiotic groups (immediate antibiotics, no antibiotics, or delayed antibiotic). Antibiotic treatment included amoxicillin or erythromycin. The delayed prescription could be picked up from the receptionist up to 14 days later without further physician contact. Two in 3 patients reported fever and more than 40% reported production of colored sputum. Patients not blinded to treatment group assignment self-reported symptoms for 3 weeks. There was no significant difference in the duration of cough or severity of cough or other symptoms between patients receiving or not receiving antibiotics. The duration of "moderately bad symptoms" was shorter in the immediate antibiotic group, but only by 1 day. Cough lasted a mean of 12 days regardless of treatment, with 25% reporting a cough more than 17 days. Children and adults with colored sputum did not benefit more than other groups and elderly patients were less likely to benefit from antibiotics. Compared with the immediate antibiotic group, fewer patients in the delayed and control groups used antibiotics (96% vs 20% and 16%, respectively). The leaflet had no effect on any outcomes. More than 75% of patients were satisfied with not receiving an immediate prescription for an antibiotic.

Essential Evidence: Medicine that Matters, Edited by David Slawson, Allen Shaughnessy, Mark Ebell, and Henry Barry.

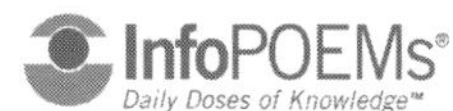

"Chest cold" instead of "bronchitis" decreases unnecessary antibiotic use

Clinical question

Will calling it a "chest cold" instead of "acute bronchitis" improve patient satisfaction and reduce inappropriate antibiotic use?

Bottom line

The use of the label "chest cold" or "viral upper respiratory infection" instead of "acute bronchitis" does not appear to affect patients' satisfaction with their diagnosis but may improve satisfaction with not receiving an antibiotic. Prospective trials are needed to confirm whether this approach will actually reduce inappropriate antibiotic use. (LOE = 2b)

Reference

Phillips TG, Hickner J. Calling acute bronchitis a chest cold may improve patient satisfaction with appropriate antibiotic use. J Am Board Fam Pract 2005;18:459–463.

Study Design

Descriptive

Funding

Foundation

Setting

Outpatient (primary care)

Synopsis

Overuse of antibiotics for acute respiratory infections is often a direct result of the pressure of patients' expectations on their personal physician. The investigators developed a written scenario representing a typical acute respiratory illness that might be called bronchitis but does not require antibiotic therapy. Patients presenting to the office for routine appointments for something other than an acute respiratory infection received both the scenario and a list of questions evaluating their satisfaction with both the diagnosis and treatment. Three different diagnostic labels – chest cold, viral upper respiratory infection, and bronchitis – correlated with a specific treatment program that excluded antibiotic treatment. Of 466 surveys offered, 459 completed forms underwent analysis; the average age of respondents was 43 years; 66% were women. Satisfaction with a diagnosis remained similar with any of the 3 diagnostic labels. However, patients with the bronchitis label reported significantly more dissatisfaction with not receiving an antibiotic (26%) than those given the label of chest cold or viral upper respiratory infection (13% and 17%, respectively) .

Essential Evidence: Medicine that Matters, Edited by David Slawson, Allen Shaughnessy, Mark Ebell, and Henry Barry.

Pelargonium effective for acute bronchitis symptoms

Clinical question

In adults with acute bronchitis symptoms of short duration, is an extract of pelargonium sidoides more effective than placebo in reducing symptoms?

Bottom line

The pelargonium sidoides extract (Umckaloabo in Germany) produced a significantly greater reduction in symptoms of acute bronchitis than placebo, and more patients were satisfied with treatment. As with all herbal products, results may be different with pelargonium products other than this extract. (LOE = 1b)

Reference

Chuchalin AG, Berman B, Lehmacher W. Treatment of acute bronchitis in adults with a pelargonium sidoides preparation (EPS 7630): a randomized, double-blind, placebo-controlled trial. Explore 2005;1:437–445.

Study Design

Randomized controlled trial (double-blinded)

Funding

Unknown/not stated

Allocation

Concealed

Setting

Outpatient (any)

Synopsis

Pelargonium sidoides is approved in several countries for the treatment of acute respiratory tract infection based on a possible antimicrobial or immune modulation action. Russian, German, and US researchers conducted this study using a root preparation available in Germany (Umckaloabo). They recruited 124 patients from outpatient clinics in Russia who'd had acute bronchitis symptoms for less than 48 hours, defined clinically and by a bronchitis severity score (BSS) greater than 4 of a possible 20 (average score = 9). The BSS rates cough, sputum, rales/rhonchi, chest pain during coughing, and dyspnea on a score from 0 to 4. Approximately 25% of the patients were current smokers and another 31% had the odd designation of "no remark or classification not possible." The patients were randomized, using concealed allocation, to receive taste- and color-matched placebo or the pelargonium extract at a dose of 1.5 mL (30 drops) 3 times daily for 8 days. The intention-to-treat analysis was performed with the statistician blinded to treatment assignment. At the end of treatment, BSS scores had decreased by an average of 7.2 points in the treatment group as compared with 4.9 points in the placebo-treated patients (absolute difference = 2.3 points; 95% CI, 1.2–3.6; $P < .001$). More than 90% of patients in the treated group had a BSS greater than 5; the rate in the placebo group was 52% ($P < .001$). Significantly more patients receiving treatment reported satisfaction than did those receiving placebo (80% vs 43%; number needed to treat = 2.7).

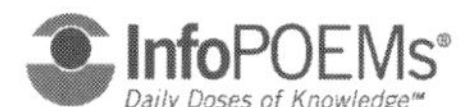

Single oral dose dexamethasone effective for even mild croup

Clinical question

Does a single oral dose of dexamethasone improve outcomes for patients with mild croup?

Bottom line

A single oral dose of dexamethasone 0.6 mg per kg improves short-term symptoms and reduces the likelihood that a child with mild croup will have to return for additional care. The dexamethasone was well tolerated, and considering the well-documented benefits of steroids in children with more severe disease, steroids in some form should be considered for most children with croup. (LOE = 1b)

Reference

Bjornson CL, Klassen TP, Williamson J, et al. A randomized trial of a single dose of oral dexamethasone for mild croup. N Engl J Med 2004;351:1306–1313.

Study Design	Funding	Allocation
Randomized controlled trial (double-blinded)	Government	Concealed

Setting

Emergency department

Synopsis

Although we know that steroids improve outcomes for children with moderate or severe croup, it isn't clear whether children with milder symptoms also benefit. Since many of our primary care patients with croup have mild symptoms, this is an important question. The authors identified children presenting with less than 72 hours of a seal-like, barking cough and a low score (2 or less) on a validated 17-point croup measure. The score assigns points for inspiratory stridor, retractions, impaired air entry, cyanosis, and impaired consciousness. Children with signs of epiglottitis, bacterial tracheitis, foreign body, chronic pulmonary disease, recent varicella, and recent steroid treatment were excluded. Children were randomly assigned (allocation concealed) to receive either 0.6 mg/kg dexamethasone or placebo, with a maximum total dose of 20 mg. The placebo was concocted to have a similar appearance and flavor to the active drug. Parents were telephoned on days 1, 2, 3, 7, and 21. The primary outcomes (based on the telephone interview) were return to a health care provider within 7 days of enrollment and continued symptoms on days 1, 2, and 3. Analysis was by intention to treat. A strength of the study was the detailed cost analysis, considering both costs to the government that pays for medical care and to the family that has to care for the child and perhaps miss work. Of the 2901 patients initially assessed for eligibility, 720 met inclusion criteria and were randomized. Follow-up was excellent (97% at three days). Children who received dexamethasone were less likely to return for care within 7 days (7.3% vs 15.3%; number needed to treat = 13). This benefit was consistent across groups, although it appeared to be greatest in younger children and those with spasmodic croup symptoms. Children receiving dexamethasone had lower croup scores on day 1, although this advantage disappeared by day 3, at which time most patients had fully recovered whether or not they were treated with steroids. Other benefits included improved sleep, reduction in parental anxiety, and reduced cost.There were no significant adverse events attributed to the dexamethasone.

Data on treating bronchiolitis severely limited

Clinical question

How effective are the various treatments for bronchiolitis?

Bottom line

In spite of the large number of studies assessing various treatments for bronchiolitis, in general the studies have been small, of poor quality, and don't assess clinically important end points. The treatments may be effective, however, just unproven. To really judge their effectiveness, we'd need large, well-designed studies that include clinically important outcomes. Until then, bronchiolitis treatment is in the "can do, but not required" category – there are few "musts" or "must nots," so don't obsess about overtreatment or undertreatment. (LOE = 1a–)

Reference

King VJ, Viswanathan M, Bordley WC, et al. Pharmacologic treatment of bronchiolitis in infants and children: a systematic review. Arch Pediatr Adolesc Med 2004;158:127–137.

Study Design

Systematic review

Setting

Various (meta-analysis)

Synopsis

The authors systematically reviewed Medline and the Cochrane Collaboration Database of Controlled Clinical Trials for randomized controlled trials published in English that assessed the effectiveness of various treatments for bronchiolitis. They used an explicit and reasonable set of search terms and did a limited search for unpublished data. The team assessed the quality of each study with disagreements adjudicated by consultation and consensus. The authors reported on 44 studies of the most commonly used agents: epinephrine, beta2-agonist bronchodilators (albuterol and salbutamol), corticosteroids, and ribavirin. They found a handful of studies evaluating inhaled helium, RSV-immunoglobulin, Chinese herbs, and so forth, but chose not to report these data in the paper. If interested, these are reported in an AHRQ Evidence Report at www.ahrq.gov/clinic/evrptfiles.htm#bronch. In general, most studies were quite small, of limited quality, looked at short-term improvement, and failed to assess clinically important outcomes. Racemic epinephrine was studied against beta2-agonists in 8 randomized controlled trials of 660 infants. Five of these studies assessed hospitalization, only 2 reported either fewer admissions or shorter stays. Most of the 13 studies of nebulized beta2-agonists had multiple treatment arms: saline placebos, unspecified placebos, ipratropium, oral agents, for example. Seven of the studies assessed hospitalization, none reported meaningful differences in rate or duration. Four studies evaluated oral corticosteroids and found no consistent effect on hospitalizations or duration of stay. Parenteral corticosteroids had no effect on clinical outcomes. In 10 randomized controlled trials of ribavirin (Copegus, Rebetol), the overall study quality was low. Of the 5 studies reporting on clinically important outcomes, 4 failed to demonstrate any effect on rate of hospitalization, length of stay, duration of illness, or use of intensive treatment. The sole study finding a benefit (on use of intensive treatment) used sterile water as the placebo. But since sterile water can induce bronchospasm, thereby making ribavirin appear more effective, this study has been criticized.

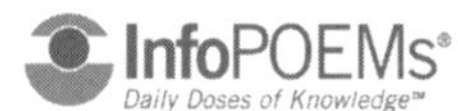

Blood cultures add little to pneumonia care

Clinical question

How useful are blood cultures in patients with community-acquired pneumonia?

Bottom line

In patients with community-acquired pneumonia, blood cultures prompted a change in antibiotic therapy in 2% of patients, but in only 0.4% of them was this change likely to have improved the patient's outcome. At a cost of approximately $60 for a pair of blood cultures at the typical American hospital, that comes to $15,200 per potentially useful change. This study provides support for the argument that routine blood cultures in patients with community-acquired pneumonia add little to their care and can be omitted in many cases. It may still be prudent to order them in cases where patients have a higher disease severity. (LOE = 2c)

Reference

Campbell SG, Marrie TJ, Anstey R, et al. The contribution of blood cultures to the clinical management of adult patients admitted to the hospital with community-acquired pneumonia. Chest 2003;123:1142–1150.

Study Design

Cohort (prospective)

Setting

Inpatient (any location)

Synopsis

While controversial, routine blood cultures for patients with community-acquired pneumonia (CAP) are still recommended by all of the major clinical practice guidelines. This is one of the largest and best designed studies of this practice, and is part of a larger clinical trial comparing strict use of a practice guideline at 9 hospitals with usual care at 10 hospitals. The authors identified 2804 patients with suspected CAP, of whom 1743 met inclusion criteria; 716 were cared for at "guideline hospitals" and 1027 at "conventional care hospitals." Patients were included if they had at least 2 signs or symptoms or CAP (fever, productive cough, chest pain, shortness of breath, or rales) and had a chest radiograph consistent with CAP. Patients with immune deficiency, those who were very ill and required direct intensive care unit admission, alcoholics, and those who were pregnant, nursing, or in renal failure were excluded. The guideline called for blood cultures before antibiotics were administered; patients in the conventional care hospitals had blood cultures at the discretion of their physician. The primary outcome was whether the use of blood cultures led to a clinically important change in management. 1022 patients were admitted to the hospital, 760 (74.4%) had blood cultures drawn, and 44 (5.7%) had a significant organism (66% strep pneumoniae, 16.3% enterobacteriacae, 11.4% staph aureus, 2.3% haemophilus influenzae). The rate of positive blood cultures did not differ between groups regardless of severity according to Fine's validated Pneumonia Severity Index (4.6%–8.0%). The really interesting part is what physicians did (or did not do) with the results. For example, physicians changed to a broader spectrum antibiotic for 9 patients during the course of the illness, but this change was only supported by blood culture results 3 times. Changes to a less expensive, narrower spectrum, or less toxic drug were more rational responses, and were supported by blood culture results 12 of 14 times. The regimen remained unchanged in 20 patients, despite the fact that in 17 of these patients the blood culture result supported a change in therapy.

Essential Evidence: Medicine that Matters, Edited by David Slawson, Allen Shaughnessy, Mark Ebell, and Henry Barry.

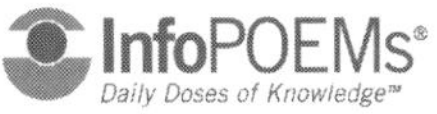

Antibiotics with atypical bacteria coverage unnecessary

Clinical question

In adults admitted for treatment of community-acquired pneumonia, is an antibiotic for atypical organisms more effective than beta-lactam-only treatment?

Bottom line

Treating community-acquired pneumonia with antibiotics effective against atypical organisms is no better and no worse than treating with a penicillin or cephalosporin alone. (LOE = 1a)

Reference

Shefet D, Robenshtok E, Paul M, Leibovici L. Empirical atypical coverage for inpatients with community-acquired pneumonia. Systematic review of randomized controlled trials. Arch Intern Med 2005;165:1992–2000.

Study Design

Meta-analysis (randomized controlled trials)

Setting

Inpatient (any location)

Synopsis

The researchers conducting this Cochrane Library meta-analysis sought to determine the benefit of empirical treatment of community-acquired pneumonia with an antibiotic regimen providing coverage of atypical pathogens (that is, Mycoplasma pneumoniae, Chlamydia pneumoniae, and Legionella pneumophila) – compared with treatment aimed primarily against Streptococcus pneumoniae, the most common pathogen. The authors searched the Cochrane Library, MEDLINE, and EMBASE for studies that directly compared these 2 types of antibiotic regimens. They also looked for additional studies in reference lists of identified studies. Two reviewers independently extracted the data from the studies. The authors found 24 studies enrolling 5015 hospitalized adults. They were unable to find any research comparing the combination of macrolide and beta-lactam antibiotics with a beta-lactam antibiotic alone. All but 1 of the studies compared a quinolone drug or macrolide drug as single therapy with a beta-lactam treatment such as amoxicillin or ceftriaxone (Rocephin). There was no difference in mortality within 30 days when comparing coverage for atypicals with coverage with a beta-lactam, either overall or for any specific drug. Clinical treatment failures were similarly the same. Study results were homogeneous and the authors found no evidence of publication bias.

Essential Evidence: Medicine that Matters, Edited by David Slawson, Allen Shaughnessy, Mark Ebell, and Henry Barry.

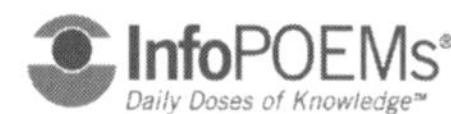

Outpatient = inpatient for low-risk patients with pneumonia

Clinical question

In low-risk patients, is outpatient treatment of pneumonia as effective as inpatient therapy?

Bottom line

This study provides good support for 2 theories in the treatment of community-acquired pneumonia: (1) Emergency physicians should calculate the Pneumonia Severity Index score for each patient; and, (2) Patients in risk classes I through III can be treated as outpatients. Patients who are sent home with a prescription and are visited by a nurse in 2 days are more satisfied with their care than inpatients and are just as likely to have a successful outcome. The Index is easy to use in calculator form on a computer, as is available in InfoRetriever. (LOE = 1b)

Reference

Carratala J, Fernandez-Sabe N, Ortega L, et al. Outpatient care compared with hospitalization for community-acquired pneumonia. Ann Intern Med 2005;142:165–172.

Study Design	Funding	Allocation
Randomized controlled trial (nonblinded)	Industry + govt	Concealed

Setting

Emergency department

Synopsis

The Pneumonia Severity Index, otherwise known as the Fine or PORT criteria, is a way to stratify patients with community-acquired pneumonia (CAP) into 5 risk classes. Patients in class I have the lowest pneumonia severity and class Vs have a 30-day mortality of 27.0%. Patients in class I should be treated as outpatients, and those in classes IV and V should be admitted; this study evaluated the role of hospitalization in patients with class II or III pneumonia. The Barcelona-based researchers enrolled 224 immunocompetent adults who received a diagnosis of CAP with no respiratory failure, complicated pleural effusions, or unstable comorbidities. The patients were randomized to be treated as inpatient or as outpatients. The patients had the usual pathogens of pneumonia, although (as is also typical) an etiology was not determined for approximately 30%. All patients received levofloxacin (Levaquin) 500 mg daily for an average 10.19 days; outpatients were treated with oral therapy and inpatients were treated with intravenous therapy and then oral therapy for an average of 10 days, although they were hospitalized for an average 5.1 days. Outpatients received one nurse visit 48 hours after discharge for assessment and received a second visit if they did not seem to be improving. The investigators used a combined endpoint of success, including: cure of pneumonia, absence of adverse drug reactions, absence of medical complications, no need for additional visits, no changes in initial treatment, and no hospital admission or death within 30 days. This outcome was achieved by 83.6% of outpatients and 80.7% of hospitalized patients. Readmission rates were similar in the 2 groups (6%–7%). Health-related quality of life scores measured at 7 and 30 days were similar in both groups. More outpatients than inpatients reported satisfaction with their overall care (91.2% vs 79.1%; P = .03).

Essential Evidence: Medicine that Matters, Edited by David Slawson, Allen Shaughnessy, Mark Ebell, and Henry Barry.

Antibiotic choice makes little difference in community-acquired pneumonia

Clinical question

In the treatment of patients with community-acquired pneumonia, is there a difference among antibiotics?

Bottom line

Strange, but true: Oral beta-lactam antibiotics – amoxicillin, amoxicillin/clavulanate (Augmentin), or a cephalosporin – are as effective in the treatment of community-acquired pneumonia as antibiotics active against atypical pathogens, even in patients infected with Mycoplasma pneumoniae or Chlamydia pneumoniae. These old standbys can be used instead of the more expensive drugs for most patients. Legionella infection still requires treatment with an antibiotic effective against atypical pathogens, but in these studies only 1.1% of the patients with nonsevere pneumonia had Legionella. These results are backed up by similar findings from clinical practice (Hedlund J, et al. Scand J Infect Dis 2002; 34:887–92). (LOE = 1a)

Reference

Mills GD, Oehley MR, Arrol B. Effectiveness of beta lactam antibiotics compared with antibiotics active against atypical pathogens in non-severe community acquired pneumonia: meta-analysis. BMJ 2005;330:456–460.

Study Design

Meta-analysis (randomized controlled trials)

Funding

Unknown/not stated

Setting

Various (meta-analysis)

Synopsis

We have to treat some patients with community-acquired pneumonia for atypical bacteria, just in case, don't we? This question was answered by the authors of this meta-analysis. They identified 18 studies comparing a beta-lactam antibiotic with an antibiotic active against the atypical pathogens Mycoplasma pneumoniae, Legionella species, and Chlamydia pneumoniae: macrolides, fluoroquinolones, or ketolides (eg, telithromycin [Ketek]). They used rigorous methods to identify the studies, searching 3 databases for articles published in any language, searching the reference lists of review articles and retrieved studies, and including unpublished research conducted by pharmaceutical companies. Two reviewers independently screened the studies for inclusion. On average, the 6749 patients in the clinical trials were younger than the typical patient with pneumonia (in most studies the average age was between 40 and 55 years) and had a better risk profile. Neither macrolides, ketolides, or fluoroquinolones were superior to beta-lactam antibiotics. When analyzed separately by type of antibiotic, neither macrolides nor fluoroquinolones were superior, either with regard to cure or mortality rates at the time specified in the study, usually end of treatment or at 10 days. The speed of response, relapse, or length of stay were not compared. Here's a surprising outcome: There was no difference between beta-lactams and the other drugs in patients who had M. pneumoniae or C. pneumoniae. The numbers of patients in these subgroups was small: 211 patients had Mycoplasma infections and 115 had Chlamydia infections. The antibiotics active against atypical pathogens were significantly better at producing clinical cures in the treatment of 75 patients with Legionella (relative risk = 0.4; 95% CI, 0.19–0.85).

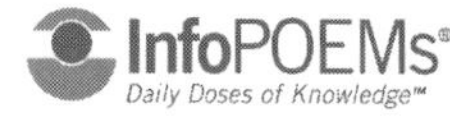

Pneumonia: 3 days of antibiotics for uncomplicated course

Clinical question

In patients hospitalized for treatment of community-acquired pneumonia, can treatment be stopped after 3 days if the patient has substantially improved?

Bottom line

Dogma successfully challenged: In patients who respond well to initial treatment, stopping antibiotic therapy after 3 days is just as effective as continuing treatment for the standard 8 days. (LOE = 1b)

Reference

el Moussaoui R, de Borgie CA, van den Broek P, et al. Effectiveness of discontinuing antibiotic treatment after three days versus eight days in mild to moderate-severe community acquired pneumonia: randomised, double blind study. BMJ 2006;332:1355–1358.

Study Design

Randomized controlled trial (double-blinded)

Funding

Industry

Allocation

Uncertain

Setting

Inpatient (any location)

Synopsis

The treatment of pneumonia for 7 days to 10 days is based on tradition, not scientific evidence. The researchers conducting this study challenged the status quo by enrolling 119 adults with mild to moderate-severe community-acquired pneumonia with a severity index score of 110 or less. On admission, all patients were started on intravenous amoxicillin, the preferred empirical treatment in the Netherlands. After 72 hours of treatment, patients who showed improvement in symptoms, had a temperature of less than 38°C, and could take oral drugs were randomized to treatment with placebo or amoxicillin 750 mg 3 times daily for 5 days. Using modified intention-to-treat analysis, after 10 days 89% of patients in both groups were clinically cured. In follow-up at 28 days, clinical cure rates were also similar between the 2 approaches, as was bacteriologic success and radiologic success. This study was designed to find a difference in success rates of at least 10%. There are a couple of notable limitations to this study. First, the patients in the short-treatment group had a median age of 54 years compared with 60 years in the 8-day group, and these younger patients may be more likely to respond to the short course, thus skewing the results. Second, the study was conducted in the Netherlands, where resistance patterns may be different than in other countries. Finally, the study was conducted in 9 hospitals over 3 years, which works out to less than 5 patients per hospital per year recruited into the study. Given the imbalance in age and this sparse representation, these patients could be highly selected and not representative of the typical patient admitted to a community hospital.

Essential Evidence: Medicine that Matters, Edited by David Slawson, Allen Shaughnessy, Mark Ebell, and Henry Barry.

Amoxicillin for 3 days effective for pediatric pneumonia

Clinical question

Is 3 days of treatment with amoxicillin as effective as 5 days of the same therapy in children with non-severe pneumonia?

Bottom line

Outpatient treatment with 3 days of amoxicillin therapy produced similar results as 5 days of treatment in children with presumed pneumonia. In both groups, treatment failures occurred in 10% of children. (LOE = 1b)

Reference

ISCAP Study Group. Three day versus five day treatment with amoxicillin for non-severe pneumonia in young children: a multicentre randomised controlled trial. BMJ 2004;328:791–794.

Study Design

Randomized controlled trial (double-blinded)

Setting

Outpatient (primary care)

Synopsis

This study enrolled more than 2100 children between the ages of 2 months and 6 years with non-severe pneumonia. The diagnostic criteria were clinical: cough, rapid respiration, or difficulty breathing not deemed to be indicative of severe pneumonia. Fever was not a criterion. Patients were randomized (using concealed allocation) to receive either 3 days or 5 days of oral amoxicillin 30 mg to 50 mg per kg per day. Treatment failure was defined as retractions (chest indrawing), convulsions, drowsiness, the inability to drink, or a cutoff respiratory rate too high or an oxygen saturation too low on day 5. In the intention-to-treat analysis cure rates were similar between the 2 groups (90%), as were relapse rates within the next 7 to 9 days (5%). Cure rates were the same whether the children had wheezes and did not vary by age. Hospitalizations were infrequent but similar in the 2 groups (2%). The study had the power to find a 5% difference in treatment failures, assuming a 12% failure rate with the longer therapy.

Essential Evidence: Medicine that Matters, Edited by David Slawson, Allen Shaughnessy, Mark Ebell, and Henry Barry.

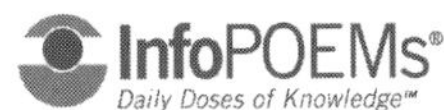

7-day levofloxacin slightly better than 1-day azithromycin for pneumonia

Clinical question

Is a single 2-gram dose of azithromycin more effective than levofloxacin in the treatment of mild-to-moderate community-acquired pneumonia?

Bottom line

Although a single dose of azithromycin in an extended-release formulation was statistically similar to 7 days of levofloxacin, resistance was more common to strep pneumoniae with azithromycin and there was a trend toward worse outcomes with azithromycin using the intention-to-treat analysis. The study was also underpowered to detect clinically important differences based on the author's sample size calculations. (LOE = 1b−)

Reference

D'Ignazio J, Camere MA, Lewis DE, Jorgensen D, Breen JD. Novel, single-dose microsphere formulation of azithromycin versus 7-day levofloxacin therapy for treatment of mild to moderate community-acquired Pneumonia in adults. Antimicrob Agents Chemother 2005;49:4035–4041.

Study Design	Funding	Allocation
Randomized controlled trial (double-blinded)	Industry	Uncertain

Setting

Outpatient (any)

Synopsis

With the coming release of azithromycin as a less expensive generic drug, an extended-release version of azithromycin (Z-Max) has been developed. This study compared a single dose of 2 grams of azithromycin extended release with levofloxacin 500 mg once daily for 7 days in patients with mild-to-moderate pneumonia. Only nonpregnant adults without serious pulmonary comorbidity were included; all had to have productive cough, at least 2 other signs or symptoms of pneumonia, and an infiltrate on their chest radiograph. The 427 patients studied came from 56 centers in 8 countries, an average of less than 8 patients per center. This raises concerns regarding the ability of the research team to monitor data collection appropriately. Results were reported for a variety of study populations; that is, all randomized, all who received at least 1 dose, all who received at least 1 dose and who actually had a pneumonia ("clinically eligible"), and all who took at least 6 days of study medication and returned for follow-up ("clinical per protocol"). The result most subject to bias is the clinical per protocol, and that is the one that the investigators highlighted in their report. They found no significant difference between groups in the clinical cure rate (89.7% for azithromycin vs 93.7 for levofloxacin; 95% CI for the difference, −9.7 to 1.7). The difference was a bit larger for the "clinically eligible" group of patients (84.6% vs 89.9%), but the authors did not, interestingly, calculate the confidence interval. Approximately half the patients had a bacterial pathogen identified: 48 with chlamydia pneumoniae, 43 with staph aureus, 35 with hemophilus parainfluenza, 28 with strep pneumoniae, 26 with hemophilus influenzae, and 28 with mycoplasma pneumoniae. One fourth of strep pneumoniae isolates were resistant to azithromycin; none were resistant to levofloxacin.

Essential Evidence: Medicine that Matters, Edited by David Slawson, Allen Shaughnessy, Mark Ebell, and Henry Barry.

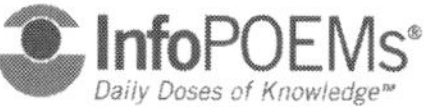

Milk intake correlates with increased risk of acne in women

Clinical question

Does milk intake increase the risk of teenage acne?

Bottom line

Whole milk and skim milk intake are associated with a slightly increased risk of teenage acne. This study design cannot, however, prove causation and we have no evidence that decreasing intake will improve acne. It is important that teenage women have an adequate intake of calcium and vitamin D to help bone growth and formation. Although a number of nondairy products with added calcium have been introduced, we should not recommend decreasing the intake of dairy products to reduce the risk or severity of acne until we have better evidence. (LOE = 2b)

Reference

Adebamowo CA, Spiegelman D, Danby FW, Frazier AL, Willett WC, Holmes MD. High school dietary dairy intake and teenage acne. J Am Acad Dermatol 2005;52:207–214.

Study Design

Cohort (retrospective)

Funding

Industry + govt

Allocation

Uncertain

Setting

Population-based

Synopsis

Most, if not all, teenagers are concerned about acne and what they can do to prevent or minimize it. These investigators analyzed data from the Nurses Health Study, a prospective cohort study of 47,355 US nurses with greater than 90% follow-up. Participants with self-reported "severe" acne (approximately 40% of the cohort) filled out a survey evaluating their food consumption between the ages of 13 years and 18 years. The diet questionnaire was validated in a small subcohort of subjects, but most participants completed it after more than 9 years had passed. Whole milk and skim milk intake were significantly associated with an increased risk of acne. The odds ratios ranged from 1.16 to 1.44. There was no significant correlation with soda, french fries, pizza, or chocolate candy. Skim milk intake was more strongly associated with an increased risk of acne than whole milk. The authors report only the body mass index and onset age of menses for the subjects, but no other demographics are noted (eg, race, birth control usage, and so forth). Possible reasons for the association include the potential of hormones in the milk and whey proteins. It is uncertain if soy milk or hormone-free milks would produce different results.

Essential Evidence: Medicine that Matters, Edited by David Slawson, Allen Shaughnessy, Mark Ebell, and Henry Barry.

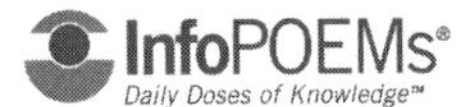

Dapsone gel effective for acne vulgaris treatment

Clinical question

Is dapsone gel 5% effective in the treatment of acne vulgaris?

Bottom line

Dapsone gel 5% (Aczone) is marginally more effective than placebo (NNT = 13, 9–23) in the treatment of acne vulgaris. At 12 weeks of treatment, less than half the patients in the treatment group received acne assessment scores of "none" or "minimal". No serious adverse events were reported, but data from follow-up longer than 3 months is forthcoming. (LOE = 1b)

Reference

Draelos ZD, Carter E, Maloney M, et al. Two randomized studies demonstrate the efficacy and safety of dapsone gel, 5% for the treatment of acne vulgaris. J Am Acad Dermatol 2007;published online 1/4/07.

Study Design

Randomized controlled trial (double-blinded)

Funding

Industry

Allocation

Concealed

Setting

Outpatient (specialty)

Synopsis

These investigators enrolled 3010 patients, aged 12 years and older, with acne vulgaris in two identically designed trials. Enrollment criteria included having at least 20 to 50 inflammatory lesions and 20 to 100 noninflammatory lesions (comedones) on the face. Exclusion criteria included severe cystic acne. In each of the two independent studies, subjects randomly applied (concealed allocation assignment) dapsone gel, 5% (Aczone) or placebo cream to the face twice daily. Individuals assessing outcomes using a validated Global Acne Assessment Score (GAAS) remained blind to treatment group assignment. Clinical success was defined as a GAAS score of "none" or "minimal". Complete follow-up occurred for 84% of patients for 12 weeks. Using intention-to-treat analysis with the last clinical observation of individual subjects carried forward, combined clinical success from both studies occurred significantly more often in patients receiving dapsone gel compared to placebo (40.5% vs 32.8%, NNT = 13, 9–23). Adverse events occurred at similar rates in both treatment groups with only a few patients (6 dapsone gel and 9 placebo gel) discontinuing treatment as a result of an adverse event. None of the adverse events related to treatment were considered serious.

Effective prevention and treatment of contact dermatitis

Clinical question

What modalities are effective in the prevention and treatment of contact dermatitis?

Bottom line

Barrier creams, high-lipid content moisturizing creams, fabric softeners, and cotton glove liners are effective for preventing irritative contact dermatitis. Rhus dermatitis can be reduced or prevented with quaternium 18 bentonite (organoclay) lotion and a topical skin protectant. The chelator diethylenetriamine pentaacetic acid is effective in preventing nickel, chrome, and copper dermatitis. Steroid preparations are effective in the treatment of both irritative and contact dermatitis. (LOE = 1a–)

Reference

Saary J, Qureshi R, Palda V, et al. A systematic review of contact dermatitis treatment and prevention. J Am Acad Dermatol 2005;53:845–855.

Study Design

Systematic review

Funding

Government

Setting

Various (meta-analysis)

Synopsis

Contact dermatitis is a common primary care disease. These investigators searched multiple databases including MEDLINE, EMBASE, the Cochrane Registry of Clinical Trials, and references of relevant articles and reviews. Two authors independently reviewed the studies for both eligibility and methodologic quality. A third author arbitrated disagreements. Only controlled trials in the English language were included. From 413 initial articles, only 49 met eligibility criteria. Of these, 12 were rated as good quality, 16 were rated as fair, and 21 were rated as poor and were not included in the final analyses. Barrier creams (eg, Dermashield, Uniderm, Dermofilm), high-lipid content moisturizing creams (eg, Keri lotion, Petrolatum, coconut oil), fabric softeners, and cotton glove liners are effective for preventing irritative contact dermatitis. Rhus dermatitis can be reduced or prevented with quaternium 18 bentonite (organoclay) lotion (Ivy Block) and a topical skin protectant. The chelator diethylenetriamine pentaacetic acid is effective in preventing nickel, chrome, and copper dermatitis (common components of jewelry). Steroid preparations are effective in the treatment of both irritative and contact dermatitis. The authors did not mention an evaluation for publication bias.

Essential Evidence: Medicine that Matters, Edited by David Slawson, Allen Shaughnessy, Mark Ebell, and Henry Barry.

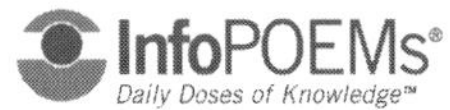

Immunosuppressives = steroids for atopic dermatitis

Clinical question

In adults or children with moderate to severe atopic dermatitis, is either tacrolimus (Protopic) or pimecrolimus (Elidel) more effective than topical corticosteroids?

Bottom line

In comparison studies to date, tacrolimus is as effective as steroids in adults and is more effective in the higher concentration (0.1%) than weak corticosteroids in children. Pimecrolimus was less effective than potent steroids in adults, and has not been studied compared with weak corticosteroids. Neither has been studied in patients with corticosteroid-resistant lesions. These are expensive alternatives to corticosteroids. The Unites States Food and Drug Administration has issued a caution linking these drugs to cancer, and does not recommend them for children younger than 2 years. (LOE = 1a)

Reference

Ashcroft DM, Dimmock P, Garside R, Stein K, Williams HC. Efficacy and tolerability of topical pimecrolimus and tacrolimus in the treatment of atopic dermatitis: meta-analysis of randomised controlled trials. BMJ 2005;330:516–525.

Study Design	Funding	Setting
Meta-analysis (randomized controlled trials)	Government	Outpatient (specialty)

Synopsis

Pimecrolimus (Elidel) and tacrolimus (Protopic) are 2 immunosuppressives used topically as alternatives for corticosteroids for the treatment of atopic dermatitis. The authors of this meta-analysis compared their effectiveness with placebo and corticosteroids by comparing the results of existing research studies. They searched for all randomized controlled trials comparing either drug with active treatment or placebo or with each other. They also searched several databases, as well as reference lists of retrieved trials. Study selection was performed independently by 2 authors, as was data extraction. They included 25 trials enrolling a total of 6897 patients. However, most of these studies compared either drug with placebo, and for most of the comparisons with active therapy we only have one study each. Both drugs are significantly more effective than placebo. In children with moderate to severe atopic dermatitis, tacrolimus was more effective than a weak corticosteroid (eg, hydrocortisone acetate) at a concentrations of 0.1% and 0.03% at 3 weeks (relative risk [RR] = 3.05; 95% CI, 2.12–4.40). In adults with moderate to severe atopic dermatitis tacrolimus at the higher concentration (0.1%) was equivalent to a high-potency corticosteroid at 3 weeks, but the 0.1% tacrolimus was significantly better than the strong corticosteroid when evaluated over 12 weeks. Pimecrolimus has not been compared with steroid treatment in children. In adults with moderate to severe disease, pimecrolimus was less effective than betamethasone valerate 0.1% (Valisone) at 3 weeks in one study of 87 patients (RR = 0.22; 95% CI, 0.09–0.54). A single study has evaluated pimecrolimus 1% versus tacrolimus 0.03% in children with moderate to severe atopic dermatitis and found equivalent response rates over 6 weeks. Dropout rates were not different between active and control groups, though burning was reported more often by patients treated with tacrolimus or pimecrolimus, which could have boosted a placebo response.

Essential Evidence: Medicine that Matters, Edited by David Slawson, Allen Shaughnessy, Mark Ebell, and Henry Barry.

Once-daily topical steroid dosing just as effective for atopic eczema

Clinical question

Is dosing topical corticosteroids more than once a day better than once-daily dosing for atopic eczema?

Bottom line

Patients should begin with once-daily dosing of topical corticosteroids for atopic eczema, increasing to twice or 3 times per day only if symptoms are not well controlled. (LOE = 1a–)

Reference

Green C, Colquitt JL, Kirby J, Davidson P. Topical corticosteroids for atopic eczema: clinical and cost effectiveness of once-daily vs. more frequent use. Br J Dermatol 2005;152:130–141.

Study Design

Meta-analysis (randomized controlled trials)

Funding

Government

Setting

Outpatient (any)

Synopsis

The authors searched the literature for randomized controlled trials (RCTs) comparing once-daily with more frequent dosing of topical corticosteroids for atopic eczema. They excluded studies of seborrheic eczema, varicose eczema, discoid eczema, and contact dermatitis. The 2 primary outcomes consistent between most studies was "at least a good response or 50% improvement" and "eczema rated as cleared or controlled." The meta-analysis was well executed with a comprehensive search, a good description of inclusion criteria, careful abstracting of data, and an appropriate analysis. Of the 10 RCTs enrolling a total of 1,819 patient, 1 studied a very potent steroid, 8 studied potent steroids, and 1 studied a moderately potent steroid. Results between studies were heterogeneous, so it was inappropriate to combine the results – which is frustrating for clinicians who want an answer, but it's good policy for a meta-analysis. Review of the individual studies shows little support for dosing more than once a day: only 1 of 7 studies showed a benefit regarding "at least a good response or 50% improvement" and only 1 of 6 regarding "eczema cleared or controlled." Most showed no difference between dosing regimens.

Essential Evidence: Medicine that Matters, Edited by David Slawson, Allen Shaughnessy, Mark Ebell, and Henry Barry.

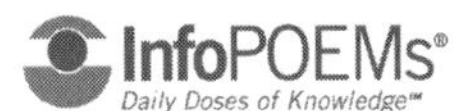

Herpes zoster vaccine safe and effective for older adults

Clinical question

Can a vaccine prevent herpes zoster and postherpetic neuralgia?

Bottom line

Herpes zoster vaccine is safe and effective for the prevention of herpes zoster and postherpetic neuralgia (PHN) in older adults. The number needed to treat is quite large on an annual basis, particularly for PHN. Even if the NNT of 1111 is linear for a 10-year period, one would have to vaccinate 111 older patients to prevent 1 case of PHN during that period. The number needed to treat to prevent a case of herpes zoster is 175. Given the strength of this vaccination and the target population, long-term follow-up studies are needed to identify any unexpected but serious complications that may appear down the road. (LOE = 1b)

Reference

Oxman MN, Levin MJ, Johnson GR, et al, for the Shingles Prevention Study Group. A vaccine to prevent herpes zoster and postherpetic neuralgia in older adults. N Engl J Med 2005;352:2271–2284.

Study Design	Funding	Allocation	Setting
Randomized controlled trial (double-blinded)	Industry + govt	Concealed	Outpatient (any)

Synopsis

Patients with herpes zoster (shingles) feel miserable, and PHN – which complicates about 10% of cases – makes them feel even worse. This study identified adults older than 60 years (47% were older than 70 years) who had either a history of varicella or were presumed to have one because they had lived in the United States for at least 30 years. A total of 59% were men, 95% were white, and they had a generally good baseline health status. Patients were randomized (allocation concealed) to either 0.5 mL of live attenuated Oka/Merck varicella-zoster virus vaccine (n=19,270) or placebo (n=19,276). The vaccine is 14 times stronger than the vaccine used to prevent primary varicella infection in children. Groups were balanced at baseline and analysis was by intention to treat. Patients were followed for a median of 3.1 years, and 95% of patients completed the study, which is excellent. The primary outcomes were the number of episodes of herpes zoster and PHN; cases within 30 days of vaccination and second episodes were excluded. Fewer patients in the vaccination group developed herpes zoster (11.1 vs 5.4 episodes per 1000 person-years; $P < .001$; number needed to treat [NNT] = 175 per year). Patients in the vaccinated group also had a somewhat shorter course (21 vs 24 days; $P = .03$) and were less likely to develop PHN (0.48 vs 1.38 per 1000 person-years; $P < .001$; NNT = 1111). The benefit was more pronounced in patients aged 60 years to 69 years than in older patients. Safety is an important issue in prevention studies since we are treating otherwise healthy patients. Safety was monitored in 2 ways: by patient or physician report for the entire population, and by diary entries for a subset of 6716 patients. For the entire study population, there was no difference in mortality between groups and no difference in possible vaccine-related adverse events, either during the first 42 days or for the duration of the 3-year study. For the adverse event substudy group, one or more adverse events – primarily erythema, pain, swelling or pruritus at the injection site – occurred more often during the first 42 days. As noted above, this is a higher potency vaccine; the current vaccine used for children should not be used for adults.

Essential Evidence: Medicine that Matters, Edited by David Slawson, Allen Shaughnessy, Mark Ebell, and Henry Barry.

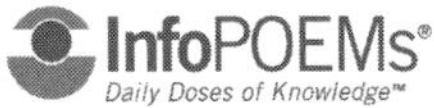

Tricyclics drug of choice for post-herpetic neuralgia

Clinical question
What are the most effective treatments for postherpetic neuralgia?

Bottom line
Tricyclics should be the drug of choice for treatment of PHN; consider gabapentin or capsaicin for treatment failures or patients who do not tolerate a tricyclic antidepressant. (LOE = 1a)

Reference
Alper BS, Lewis PR. Treatment of postherpetic neuralgia: A systematic review of the literature. J Fam Pract 2002;51:121–128.

Study Design
Systematic review

Setting
Various

Synopsis
The authors did a thorough and well-designed meta-analysis to determine the most effective treatment (not prevention) for postherpetic neuralgia (PHN). Most of the 27 trials they identified were well-designed (Jadad quality score 4 out of a possible 5). A particularly bad study (Jadad score = 1) was excluded. Because PHN is rare in patients younger than 50 years, most studies included a majority of (or exclusively) older patients. They found the best evidence to support the use of the tricylcic antidepressants amitriptyline, nortriptyline, and desipramine (number needed to treat = 2–3). Amitriptyline (Elavil) was the best studied, with a usual dose of 75 mg by mouth at bedtime. There was also evidence from a smaller number of studies to support the use of topical capsaicin (Zostrix), gabapentin (Neurontin), and controlled release oxycodone. Lidocaine patch, benzydamine cream, tramadol, and vincristine have not been well studied, while lorazepam, fluphenazine, dextromethorphan, memantine, acyclovir, and acupuncture are unlikely to be beneficial.

Essential Evidence: Medicine that Matters, Edited by David Slawson, Allen Shaughnessy, Mark Ebell, and Henry Barry.

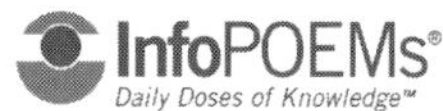

Melanoma incidence really not rising

Clinical question

Has the incidence of skin melanoma increased?

Bottom line

This study provides preliminary evidence that the incidence of melanoma is increasing not because of factors such as skin burns and ozone layer holes, but simply because more dermatologists are biopsying more lesions. In a 5-year period the incidence of melanoma increased 2.4-fold, whereas the biopsy rate over this same period increased a similar 2.5 times. (LOE = 2c)

Reference

Welch HG, Woloshin S, Schwartz LM. Skin biopsy rates and incidence of melanoma: population based ecological study. BMJ 2005;33:481–484.

Study Design

Ecologic

Funding

Government

Setting

Population-based

Synopsis

The incidence of skin melanoma is now 6 times higher than in 1950. The researchers conducting this study attempted to determine whether the true incidence is rising or whether the increase is simply due to an increased biopsy rate. Histologic diagnosis of melanoma is difficult, and several studies have shown that pathologists cannot agree on which samples are really melanoma (see: Pathology as art appreciation: melanoma diagnosis. http://www.jr2.ox.ac.uk/bandolier/band37/b37-2.html). This study compared skin biopsy rates for people older than 65 years with the incidence of melanoma over 5 years in 9 geographical areas in the United States. Over this period the number of biopsies in this age group increased 2.5-fold, from 1 in 35 people to 1 in 14 people. The incidence of melanoma increased 2.4-fold, from 1 in every 2222 people to 1 in every 925 people. Despite this increase in diagnoses, mortality due to melanoma changed little. Although these data don't prove it, they suggest that the increase in melanoma diagnoses is simply because more lesions are being biopsied that wouldn't have been biopsied in the past.

Essential Evidence: Medicine that Matters, Edited by David Slawson, Allen Shaughnessy, Mark Ebell, and Henry Barry.

Lifetime risk of mole transforming to melanoma very low

Clinical question

What is the risk that any given mole will become a melanoma?

Bottom line

Using a theoretical model and existing sources of data, the authors estimate that the lifetime risk that a mole will become melanoma in a 50-year-old man is 1 in 2000 and in a 50-year-old woman is 1 in 9000. These findings call into question the cost-effectiveness of surveillance programs and frequent excisions, especially for young or low-risk patients. (LOE = 2c)

Reference

Tsao H, Bevona C, Goggins W, Quinn T. The transformation rate of moles (melanocytic nevi) into cutaneous melanoma. Arch Dermatol 2003;139:282–288.

Study Design

Decision analysis

Setting

Population-based

Synopsis

This is an interesting question, and may be helpful as we talk to our patients about moles and melanoma. The authors took data from a variety of sources, including surveys of the number per adult of melanocytic nevi at least 2 to 3 mm in diameter and a community-based pathology database of skin biopsies. They created a theoretical model to determine the transformation rate, and stratified their findings by age. The risk that any single mole on a 30 year old will become a melanoma by age 80 was 38 in 100,000 in men and 11 in 100,000 in women. The lifetime risk of transformation to melanoma gradually increases in men from 31.6 in 100,000 in 20 year olds to 50.1 in 100,000 in 50 year olds (that is, 1 in 3000 to 1 in 2000).

0.7% of congenital melanocytic nevi become malignant

Clinical question

What is the risk that a congenital melanocytic nevus will undergo malignant transformation?

Bottom line

Less than 1% of congenital melanocytic nevi (CMN) reported in the medical literature underwent malignant transformation, although the heterogeneous nature of the studies permits only a broad estimate of risk. The true rate of malignant transformation may be lower because of selection bias inherent in smaller studies. (LOE = 2a)

Reference

Krengel S, Hauschild A, Schafer T. Melanoma risk in congenital melanocytic naevi: a systematic review. Br J Dermatol 2006;155:1–8.

Study Design

Meta-analysis (other)

Funding

Unknown/not stated

Setting

Outpatient (any)

Synopsis

Congenital melanocytic nevi (CMN) are pigmented lesions of varying size that are present at or shortly after birth. They occur in between 0.2% and 2.1% of infants, and range in size from less than 1 square centimeter to hundreds of square centimeters. Previous case series and cohort studies have provided varying estimates of the risk of malignant transformation. This systematic review identified 14 relevant articles after a comprehensive literature search. Studies with fewer than 20 patients or those with fewer than 3 years of follow-up were appropriately excluded. Eight studies were retrospective and 6 were prospective, and the mean follow-up ranged from 3.4 to nearly 24 years. Six studies had fewer than 100 patients; 2 studies were quite large, with 1008 and 3922 patients. The proportion of patients with melanoma ranged from 0% to 10.7% (6 of 56 patients in 1 small retrospective study). The age at diagnosis of melanoma ranged from birth to 57 years, with a mean age of 15 years. Overall, 49 melanomas were reported in 46 of 6571 patients (0.7%). Most (75%) arose in so-called "garment nevi," which are greater than 40 cm in diameter. Because of the higher rate in small studies, suggesting selection bias, this figure of 0.7% probably represents an upper bound. The largest, and perhaps best, population-based study found that 0.2% of all newborns were registered as having CMN, of whom only 2 (0.05%) underwent malignant transformation after a median follow-up of 10 years.

Essential Evidence: Medicine that Matters, Edited by David Slawson, Allen Shaughnessy, Mark Ebell, and Henry Barry.

Dermoscopy with validated criteria more sensitive than unaided eye

Clinical question

Does use of a dermoscope improve the accuracy of diagnosis of melanoma?

Bottom line

Dermoscopy, especially when used in conjunction with the Menzies method, is more sensitive than the unaided eye in diagnosing melanoma. This technique is not widely used in the United States and deserves further study. We don't know whether it was the validated criteria or the use of dermoscopy that made the intervention more sensitive. (LOE = 2b)

Reference

Dolianitis C, Kelly J, Wolfe R, Simpson P. Comparative performance of 4 dermoscopic algorithms by nonexperts for the diagnosis of melanocytic lesions. Arch Dermatol 2005;141:1008–1014.

Study Design

Diagnostic test evaluation

Funding

Foundation

Setting

Outpatient (any)

Synopsis

Dermoscopy, also called dermatoscopy, involves use of a low-power handheld microscope (typically 10x) used with or without oil immersion to view suspicious skin lesions (http://www.dermoscopy.org/default.asp). Previous studies have shown that in expert hands it increases the accuracy of diagnosis. In this study, 60 physicians (35 general practitioners, 10 dermatologists, and 16 dermatology trainees) were presented with unaided photos of 40 lesions and asked to use their standard clinical judgment to make a diagnosis of melanoma or nonmelanoma. They were then presented with dermascopic images of the same lesions 4 times in succession and asked to apply 4 different set of standard, validated criteria for diagnosing melanoma (the ABCD rule, the Menzies method, a 7-point checklist, and pattern analysis). They were instructed in each of these methods using a CD-ROM. Interrater reliability for key melanoma diagnostic features was fair, with kappas in the range from 0.21 to 0.56. The unaided eye using a standard photo of the lesion was 61% sensitive and 85% specific with a 73% diagnostic accuracy. The dermoscopic photo used in conjunction with each of the 4 sets of criteria were more sensitive (68% for pattern analysis, 77% for the ABCD rule, 81% for the 7-point checklist, and 85% for the Menzies method). The specificity of pattern analysis is similar to the clinical examination (85%). The specificity of all other methods ranged from 73% to 80%. In this situation, sensitivity is more important than specificity; you don't want to miss any cancers, and the biopsy is an even more specific test that will hopefully sort out the nonmalignant tumors. Note that this study does not tell us that patients diagnosed with dermoscopy live longer or better lives: it's not a POEM. Rather, it's a SMORE (Surrogate Marker Of Relevant Outcomes), if one assumes that more accurate diagnosis of melanoma leads to better outcomes.

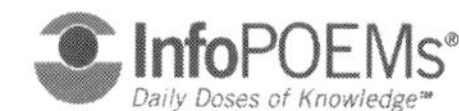

Effective methods for preventing pressure ulcers

Clinical question

Which interventions are effective for the prevention of pressure ulcers?

Bottom line

Effective strategies for preventing pressure ulcers include the use of support surfaces (mattresses, beds, and cushions), mattress overlays on operating tables, and specialized foam and sheepskin overlays. Frequent repositioning is effective, but the optimal schedule for turning is uncertain. Nutritional supplements are beneficial in patients with impaired nutrition. Simple skin moisturizers, specifically to the sacral area, are also effective. (LOE = 1a−)

Reference

Reddy M, Gill SS. Rochon PA. Preventing pressure ulcers: a systematic review. JAMA 2006;296:974–984.

Study Design

Systematic review

Funding

Government

Setting

Various (meta-analysis)

Synopsis

Multiple preventive approaches are used in the management of pressure ulcers. These authors systematically searched multiple evidence-based databases including the Cochrane Registry, bibliographies of identified articles, and scientific meeting abstracts for randomized controlled trials (RCTs) evaluating preventive measures for pressure ulcers. No language restrictions were applied. They used standard methods to critically appraise individual RCTs. The search strategy identified 763 citations, from which 59 trials meeting eligibility criteria were selected. The methodologic quality of the RCTs was generally suboptimal. Interventions were grouped into 3 categories: those addressing impairments in (1) mobility, (2) nutrition, and (3) skin health. Effective strategies for those with impaired mobility included the use of support surfaces (mattresses, beds, and cushions), mattress overlays on operating tables, and specialized foam and sheepskin overlays. Frequent repositioning is effective, but the optimal schedule for turning (every 2 vs every 4 hours) is uncertain. Nutritional supplements are beneficial in patients with impaired nutrition. Simple skin moisturizers, specifically to the sacral area, were helpful, but the incremental benefit of other specific topical agents is minimal.

Essential Evidence: Medicine that Matters, Edited by David Slawson, Allen Shaughnessy, Mark Ebell, and Henry Barry.

Duct tape seems effective for warts

Clinical question
Is duct tape effective for treating warts?

Bottom line
This small study is intriguing. While we cannot say with certainty that duct tape is better than cryotherapy for treating warts, it seems to be just as effective. (LOE = 2b−)

Reference
Focht DR, Spicer C, Fairchok MP. The efficacy of duct tape vs cryotherapy in the treatment of verruca vulgaris (the common wart). Arch Pediatr Adol Med 2002;156:971–974.

Study Design
Randomized controlled trial (single-blinded)

Setting
Outpatient (primary care)

Synopsis
Is this a great country or what?! Where else would somebody think about using duct tape for therapeutic purposes? Sixty-one patients between the ages of 3 and 22 years with warts were randomly assigned (allocation concealment not mentioned) to cryotherapy or duct tape. Cryotherapy consisted of a 10 second application of liquid nitrogen after local debridement with an emery board or a pumice stone. This was repeated every 2–3 weeks for a total of 6 treatments. The investigators gave a roll of duct tape to the other group. The duct tape was cut to the size of the wart and applied directly to it. They told the patients to remove it after 6 days, wash and then debride with an emery board or pumice stone. The patient was to re-apply the duct tape the next morning and to continue the cycle for 2 months. The patients were to remove all tape before coming in for the assessments performed by blinded evaluators. They had no follow-up for 10 patients: 4 in the group treated with duct tape, including one unfortunate soul who had a traumatic amputation of an affected toe, and 6 in the cryotherapy group. Twenty-two of the 26 patients treated with duct tape (85%) had complete resolution of the wart as compared with 15 of the 25 treated with cryotherapy (60%). There are a few problems with the study. Complete removal of all duct tape without residual glue is difficult, so the assessments may not have been truly blind. Also, the total number of patients is small enough that the missing patients could significantly alter the outcome. Finally, many of the assessments made in the group treated with duct tape were made via telephone self-report rather than direct inspection.

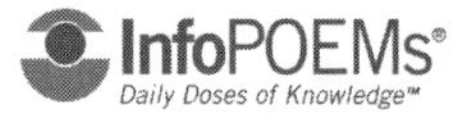

Effective treatments for rosacea

Clinical question

What treatments are effective for rosacea?

Bottom line

Effective treatments for rosacea include topical metronidazole, benzoyl peroxide 5%/erythromycin 3% gel, benzoyl peroxide 5%/clindamycin 1% gel, benzoyl peroxide alone, azelaic acid, and sodium sulfacetamide10%/sulfur 5%. Oral tetracycline was significantly better than placebo by physician assessment, but not by patient assessment. (LOE = 1a)

Reference

van Zuuren EJ, Gupta AK, Gover MD, Graber M, Hollis S. Systematic review of rosacea treatments. J Am Acad Dermatol 2006;online:Nov 3.

Study Design

Meta-analysis (randomized controlled trials)

Funding

Unknown/not stated

Setting

Various (meta-analysis)

Synopsis

These investigators thoroughly searched multiple databases – including MEDLINE, EMBASE, The Cochrane Registry of Clinical Trials, Science Citation Index, and reference lists – and consulted with experts. They also searched unpublished literature through correspondence with authors and pharmaceutical companies. Two reviewers independently performed searches and assessed articles for eligibility. Disagreement was resolved by consensus discussion. From a total of 71 possible clinical trials, the authors included 29 randomized trials meeting appropriate criteria for high quality (8) and intermediate quality (21). Fourteen trials used adequate blinding to treatment allocation and 17 used intention-to-treat analysis. Only data on outcome measures from trials on topical metronidazole, topical azelaic acid, and oral tetracycline could be pooled. The primary outcome measure, quality of life, was not assessed in any of the studies and only a few studies assessed the participant?s own opinion regarding rosacea severity. The following medications were significantly superior to placebo: topical metronidazole, benzoyl peroxide 5%/erythromycin 3% gel, benzoyl peroxide 5%/clindamycin 1% gel, benzoyl peroxide alone, azelaic acid, and sodium sulfacetamide10%/sulfur 5%. Oral tetracycline was significantly better than placebo by physician assessment, but not by patient assessment. There was no significant difference in efficacy between topical metronidazole and azelaic acid or between topical metronidazole and oral tetracycline. Rilmenidine and permethrin were not significantly better than placebo.

Essential Evidence: Medicine that Matters, Edited by David Slawson, Allen Shaughnessy, Mark Ebell, and Henry Barry.

Larger margins better in melanoma >2 mm thick

Clinical question
What is the optimal margin for excision of melanomas at least 2-mm thick?

Bottom line
There is a greater likelihood of local or regional recurrence of melanoma in patients who have a 1-cm margin compared with those who have excision with a 3-cm margin. However, the benefit in terms of disease-specific mortality is only marginally significant, and is nonsignificant for all-cause mortality. (LOE = 1b)

Reference
Thomas JM, Newton-Bishop J, A'Hern R, et al. Excision margins in high-risk malignant melanoma. N Engl J Med 2004;350:757–766.

Study Design
Randomized controlled trial (single-blinded)

Setting
Outpatient (specialty)

Synopsis
A previous study found no difference in outcomes for patients with melanoma who had excisions with 2-cm or 4-cm margins. This larger study randomized 900 patients (allocation concealed) with a melanoma at least 2-mm thick to either 1-cm or 3-cm margins. These are relatively high-risk lesions. The mean age of included patients was 57 years, and approximately half were women. Most had an initial 1-mm biopsy margin followed by later 1-cm or 3-cm excision. Patients were followed up for a median of 60 months, although no details are given on how often or in what way patients were evaluated. Outcomes were adjudicated by a central group blinded to treatment group. Groups were similar at baseline and analysis was by intention to treat. Patients with a 1-cm margin were more likely to have a locoregional recurrence at 3 years (168 vs 142; hazard ratio [HR] = 1.26; 95% CI, 1.0–1.59). There was also a trend toward a greater likelihood of death from melanoma (128 vs 105; HR = 1.24; 95% CI, 0.96–1.61). However, there was no significant difference in the likelihood of death from any cause (144 vs 137; HR = 1.07; 95% CI, 0.85–1.36).

Essential Evidence: Medicine that Matters, Edited by David Slawson, Allen Shaughnessy, Mark Ebell, and Henry Barry.

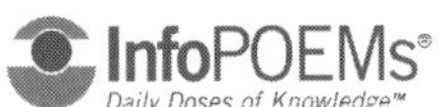

Radical prostatectomy improves outcomes in symptom-detected prostate cancer

Clinical question

What is the best treatment for moderately differentiated or well-differentiated prostate cancer?

Bottom line

Radical prostatectomy is better than watchful waiting for men with moderately differentiated or well-differentiated prostate cancer, especially (and perhaps only) in men younger than 65 years. Although these are the best data on treatment in this group to date, only 5% of the men in this study had their cancer detected by screening. Whether these data generalize to men with screening-detected prostate cancer is unclear but will likely be assumed by most clinicians and their patients. (LOE = 1b)

Reference

Bill-Axelson A, Holmberg L, Ruutu M, et al, for the Scandinavian Prostate Cancer Group Study No. 4. Radical prostatectomy versus watchful waiting in early prostate cancer. N Engl J Med 2005;352:1977–1984.

Study Design

Randomized controlled trial (single-blinded)

Funding

Government

Allocation

Concealed

Setting

Outpatient (specialty)

Synopsis

This is a 3-year follow-up study to one originally reported in 2002. The researchers randomized men with localized, well-differentiated, or moderately differentiated prostate cancer according to World Health Organization grading to either radical prostatectomy or watchful waiting. Gleason scores were 2 to 4 for 13% of the men, 5 or 6 for 48%, 7 for 23%, and 8 to 10 for 5%. The Gleason score was unknown for 11% of patients. Only 5% of cancers were detected by screening, although more than 85% had a prostate-specific antigen (PSA) level higher than 4.0 ng/mL. Allocation was concealed, outcomes were blindly assessed, and analysis was by intention to treat. The vast majority of patients, however, stayed in the group to which they were assigned. The median duration of follow-up was 8.2 years, and 10-year follow-up data were available for 222 patients. The researchers prespecified several subgroup analyses by age, Gleason score, and PSA. Overall, results became more favorable for radical prostatectomy with an increased duration of follow-up. All-cause mortality was lower in the radical prostatectomy group (27% vs 32%; P = .04; number needed to treat [NNT] = 20), as was disease-specific mortality (9.6% vs 14.9%; P = .01; NNT = 19). The likelihood of local progression and distant metastases was also lower in the treated group. Radical prostatectomy was especially beneficial in men younger than 65 years; there was little difference between watchful waiting and surgery in patients older than 65. Although there was no association between the benefit of surgery and the Gleason score, more than 70% had a Gleason score of 5 to 7. Therefore, there were too few patients with lower or higher Gleason scores to confidently assess the benefit of surgery in those groups or in men with screening-detected prostate cancer.

Essential Evidence: Medicine that Matters, Edited by David Slawson, Allen Shaughnessy, Mark Ebell, and Henry Barry.

Implantable defibrillators are not effective post-MI

Clinical question

Do implantable cardioverter-defibrillators improve outcomes in at-risk patients after myocardial infarction?

Bottom line

Implantable cardioverter-defibrillators do not reduce mortality in patients with myocardial infarction who are at high risk for ventricular arrhythmia. (LOE = 1b)

Reference

Hohnloser SH, Kuck KH, Dorian P, et al. Prophylactic use of an implantable cardioverter-defibrillator after acute myocardial infarction. N Engl J Med 2004;351:2481–2488.

Study Design

Randomized controlled trial (single-blinded)

Funding

Industry

Allocation

Concealed

Setting

Inpatient (any location) with outpatient follow-up

Synopsis

Implantable cardioverter-defibrillators (ICDs) can reduce mortality in selected patients. In this industry-sponsored study, adults with a recent myocardial infarction, a left ventricular ejection fraction less than or equal to 0.35, and either relative tachycardia (>80 beats per minute) or decreased heart rate variability were randomized to either ICD or usual care. This was an open-label trial with no attempt at sham surgery or sham ICD implantation. The primary outcomes of all-cause mortality or death due to cardiac arrhythmia were blindly assessed and analysis was by intention to treat. The groups were balanced at the beginning of the study, with 332 in the ICD group and 342 in the control group. Patients were followed up for a mean of 30 months, with a maximum follow-up of 48 months. On the bright side, patients in the ICD group experienced significantly fewer arrhythmic deaths (1.5% vs 3.5%; number needed to treat = 50; 95% CI, 27–209). On the not-so-bright side, they also experienced more nonarrhythmic deaths (6.1% vs 3.5%; number needed to treat to harm = 38; 20–150). There was no significant difference between groups regarding the most important patient-oriented outcome: all-cause mortality (7.5% for the ICD group vs 6.9% for the control group). The difference in nonarrhythmic deaths was largely caused by more cardiac nonarrhythmic deaths. The authors speculate that a group of patients with severe heart disease are "saved" from an arrhythmic death only to die from pump failure without any clinically important increase in the overall lifespan. Implantable defibrillators have been shown to be effective in patients with non-ischemic cardiomyopathy (JAMA 2004; 292:2874–79).

Essential Evidence: Medicine that Matters, Edited by David Slawson, Allen Shaughnessy, Mark Ebell, and Henry Barry.

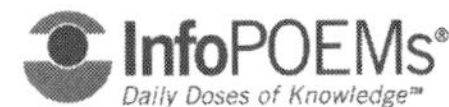

Implantable defibrillators reduce mortality in NYHA Class II heart failure

Clinical question

For patients with moderate or severe heart failure, is amiodarone or an implanatable defibrillator the best way to reduce mortality?

Bottom line

Patients with moderate to severe heart failure benefit from an implantable ICD (NNT = 14 for 4 year mortality). However, the benefit was confined to the subgroup with NYHA Class II disease in this study. Those with NYHA Class III HF did not benefit from ICD, and amiodarone actually increased mortality in that subgroup. (LOE = 1b)

Reference

Bardy GH, Kerry LL, Mark DB, et al. Amiodarone or an implantable cardioverter-defibrillator for congestive heart failure. N Engl J Med 2005;352:225–237.

Study Design

Randomized controlled trial (nonblinded)

Funding

Industry + govt

Allocation

Uncertain

Setting

Outpatient (specialty)

Synopsis

Patients with heart failure are at increased of sudden death. Could these patients benefit from an implantable cardioverter-defibrillator (ICD)? The researchers in this study recruited patients with moderate systolic heart failure (HF) defined as an ejection fraction of less than 35%. Patients were identified as having ischemic HF if they had at least one coronary artery with 75% stenosis or a history of acute myocardial infarction (AMI). Patients were randomly assigned (allocation concealment uncertain) to receive either amiodarone (median dose 300 mg daily, n = 845), placebo pill (n = 847), or a single lead ICD programmed to treat only sustained ventricular tachycardia or ventricular fibrillation (n = 829). Groups were balanced at the beginning of the study, with an average age of 60 years, 23% being women, and an average ejection fraction of 25%. Patients were followed for a mean of 45 months and the vital status (i.e. whether they were alive or dead) was known for each of the 2521 patients at the end of the study. About one-third of patients with an ICD were shocked at some point during follow-up. All-cause mortality was lower in the ICD group than in the amiodarone or placebo groups (22% vs 28% vs 29%, p = 0.007, number need to treat compared with amiodarone = 17 over four years). Patients with NYHA Class II HF had a clear benefit, while those with NYHA Class III HF did not. The authors argue that we should embrace the results for patients with NYHA Class II HF but ignore those for patients with more severe disease, since other studies in studies with different inclusion criteria showed greater absolute benefit with greater disease. The alternate view is that in patients with more severe disease, the episode of VT or VF is an indicator of worsening death and the ICD merely prolongs the inevitable for a few days or weeks. It is also noteworthy that amiodarone did not improve survival compared with placebo in patients with NYHA Class II heart failure and actually increased mortality in those with Class III HF (hazard ratio 1.44, 95% CI 1.05 to 1.97), and that there was no difference overall between patients with ischemic and non-ischemic causes of HF.

Essential Evidence: Medicine that Matters, Edited by David Slawson, Allen Shaughnessy, Mark Ebell, and Henry Barry.

Small punch biopsies don't require sutures

Clinical question
What is the best way to close (or not close) punch biopsy sites?

Bottom line
When accompanied by careful instructions regarding wound care and the use of occlusive dressings, healing of 4 mm punch biopsies by secondary intention was just as good as suturing. Blinded observers saw relatively little difference, but unblinded patients preferred suture closer of the larger 8 mm punch biopsy sites. (LOE = 1b–)

Reference
Christenson LJ, Phillips PK, Weaver AL, Otley CC. Primary closure vs second-intention treatment of skin punch biopsy sites. Arch Dermatol 2005;141:1093–1099.

Study Design
Randomized controlled trial (single-blinded)

Funding
Foundation

Allocation
Concealed

Setting
Outpatient (specialty)

Synopsis
Healthy volunteers each received 2 4-mm or 8-mm punch biopsies on their limbs or back. Their mean age was 47 years, 70% were women, and sites were evenly distributed between 4 mm and 8 mm and between the upper back, arm, and thigh. Before each biopsy the site was prepped with alcohol and injected with lidocaine 1% with epinephrine. One site was randomly chosen to be closed with a 4-0 nylon interrupted suture (one for 4-mm lesions and 2 for 8-mm lesions) or left to heal by secondary intention (gel foam was applied for hemostasis). All wounds were dressed with petroleum jelly, gauze, and a transparent occlusive (Tegaderm) dressing. After 3 days the occlusive dressings were removed, the gel foam was removed (if present), the sites cleansed, and then an occlusive dressing was reapplied. Subjects were then advised to change their dressings at least weekly. The primary outcome was the visual appearance of the site on a validated 100-point scale as assessed by 3 physicians blinded to treatment assignment (100 = best cosmetic outcome). Follow-up was good, with 77 of the 82 volunteers returning after 9 months. There was no significant difference regarding the primary outcome at 9 months, with a mean score of 57.1 for the secondary-intention closure and 58.9 for the sutured sites. Patients were asked to evaluate the lesions and were equally satisfied with each closure method for the 4-mm punches but preferred suturing to secondary closure for the 8-mm punches (53% vs 14%, with 33% having no preference; P = .007).

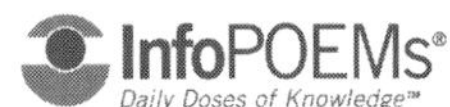

Suturing of hand lacerations not necessary

Clinical question

Do small (<2 cm) lacerations of the hand require suturing?

Bottom line

Hand lacerations less than 2 cm long without tendon, joint, fracture, or nerve complications can be dressed without suturing, with similar cosmetic results and time to resume normal activities. (LOE = 1b)

Reference

Quinn J, Cummings S, Callaham M, Sellers K. Suturing versus conservative management of lacerations of the hand: randomised controlled trial. BMJ 2002;325:299–300.

Study Design

Randomized controlled trial (single-blinded)

Setting

Emergency department

Synopsis

This study enrolled 91 consecutive patients with 95 uncomplicated lacerations of the hand (full thickness <2 cm, without tendon, joint, fracture, or nerve complications) who normally require sutures. Concealment of allocation was not reported. Patients were excluded with diabetes, if they were receiving anticoagulants or chronic steroids, or if their laceration was due to a bite. The participants were randomized to suturing or conservative treatment consisting of an antibiotic ointment and dressing. As assessed by independent, blinded doctors after three months, cosmetic appearance was similar in both groups (83 mm vs. 80 mm on a visual analog rating scale). The mean time to resume normal activities was the same in both groups (3.4 days). Pain and treatment time was less in the unsutured group.

Essential Evidence: Medicine that Matters, Edited by David Slawson, Allen Shaughnessy, Mark Ebell, and Henry Barry.

Sterile gloves not necessary for laceration repair

Clinical question

Do sterile gloves offer greater protection from wound infection than clean nonsterile gloves?

Bottom line

Infection rate in patients undergoing uncomplicated laceration repair are not different when sterile gloves, rather than simply clean gloves, are worn. (LOE = 1b)

Reference

Perelman VS, Grancis GJ, Rutledge T, et al. Sterile versus nonsterile gloves for repair of uncomplicated lacerations in the emergency department: a randomized controlled trial. Ann Emerg Med 2004;43:362–370.

Study Design

Randomized controlled trial (single-blinded)

Setting

Emergency department

Synopsis

The investigators enrolled 816 patients (81% of eligible patients) presenting to the emergency department of 3 hospitals with clean, nonbite lacerations deemed not to require antibiotic therapy. Patients were randomized to be treated by physicians who wore either sterilized latex-free gloves or standard, boxed, nonsterilized latex-free gloves to perform the repair. Allocation to group assignment did not seem to be concealed from the enrolling physician (ie, the person enrolling the patient could have known to which group the patient would be assigned, which may have affected enrollment). Patients were not aware of whether sterile or nonsterile gloves were used. The treating physicians, however, were aware of the type of gloves they were wearing, and it is possible that they were more scrupulous with cleaning if they had the nonsterile gloves. Follow-up was performed by a physician unaware of treatment assignment, with only 2% lost. Infection occurred in 6.1% of patients treated with sterile gloves and 4.4% of patients treated with nonsterile gloves, a nonsignificant difference. The study had the ability to find a 50% difference in infection rate, if one existed.

Essential Evidence: Medicine that Matters, Edited by David Slawson, Allen Shaughnessy, Mark Ebell, and Henry Barry.

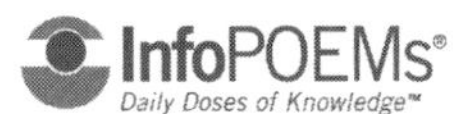

Hot water (45 C) immersion best for jellyfish, man-of-war stings

Clinical question

Is hot water (45 C) immersion more effective than ice pack application for relief of pain caused by bluebottle jellyfish stings?

Bottom line

Immediate hot water immersion (45 C) for up to 20 minutes is significantly more effective than ice pack application for pain caused by bluebottle jellyfish (Portuguese man-of-war) stings. (LOE = 1b–)

Reference

Loten C, Stokes B, Worsley D, Seymour JE, Jiang S, Isbistergk GK. A randomized controlled trial of hot water (45 C) immersion versus ice packs for pain relief in bluebottle stings. Med J Aust 2006;184:329–333.

Study Design

Randomized controlled trial (nonblinded)

Funding

Foundation

Allocation

Uncertain

Setting

Population-based

Synopsis

Bluebottle jellyfish (Portuguese man-of-war) stings can cause significant pain that usually resolves within 1 hour. Most first-aid organizations recommend the application of ice packs. To evaluate the potential effectiveness of hot water immersion (since many marine venoms are heat labile in vitro), the investigators randomized (uncertain allocation concealment) 96 patients with an apparent bluebottle sting at 2 beaches in eastern Australia to either hot water immersion or ice pack application. Accurate water temperature at 45 C was insured by using thermostatic mixing valves to prevent superficial burns. Patients self-reported pain levels at baseline and at 10 minutes and 20 minutes after the commencement of treatment using a visual analog scale (VAS) of 0 to 100. The primary outcome was a clinically important reduction in pain, defined as a change in millimeters on the VAS scale dependent on the baseline starting point (16 mm for an initial VAS between 0–33 mm; 33 mm for an initial 34–66 mm; and 48 mm for an initial 67–100 mm). One investigator microscopically evaluated adhesive tape placed over all sting sites to confirm the presence of nematocysts. Follow-up occurred for 92% of the patients at 20 minutes. Analysis was by intention to treat. At 10 minutes, 53% of the hot water group reported a clinically significant reduction in pain compared with 32% treated with an ice pack (number needed to treat [NNT] = 5; 95% CI, 3–72). At 20 minutes, 87% of the hot water group reported a clinically significant reduction in pain compared with 33% treated with an ice pack (NNT = 2; 1–3). Radiating pain also occurred significantly less with hot water and no patient suffered a burn from hot water immersion. Nematocysts were confirmed in 42 (44%) of the subjects. Hot water immersion remained significantly more effective than ice packs in an analysis of only those patients with nematocyst-confirmed stings. Itch, redness, and rash at 24 hours occurred similarly in both groups.

Essential Evidence: Medicine that Matters, Edited by David Slawson, Allen Shaughnessy, Mark Ebell, and Henry Barry.

Surgery better than no surgery for spinal stenosis

Clinical question

In adults with spinal stenosis, is surgical treatment more effective than nonsurgical treatment?

Bottom line

Most patients with lumbar spinal stenosis treated surgically and nonsurgically improve over time. However, patients treated surgically have greater improvement in pain. There are no meaningful differences in disability or in walking capacity. (LOE = 2b)

Reference

Malmivaara A, Slatis P, Heliovaara M, et al, for the Finnish Lumbar Spinal Research Group. Surgical or nonoperative treatment for lumbar spinal stenosis? a randomized controlled trial. Spine 2007;32:1–8.

Study Design

Randomized controlled trial (nonblinded)

Funding

Government

Allocation

Concealed

Setting

Inpatient (any location) with outpatient follow-up

Synopsis

In this unblinded study from Finland, 94 adults with at least 6 months of symptoms due to lumbar spinal stenosis were randomly assigned to receive surgery or nonsurgical treatment. The researchers excluded patients with progressive neurologic deficits, with prior surgery, with severe or minimal symptoms, who were poor surgical candidates, and who had other conditions explaining their symptoms. The researchers evaluated the patients 6 months, 12 months, and 24 months after enrollment using intention-to-treat analysis. At the end of the study, approximately 15% of the patients had dropped out. Patients in both groups improved over the course of the study. Although disability scores were more likely to improve in patients treated surgically, the 7.8-point difference on a 100-point scale is not clinically meaningful. However, improvements in pain scores in the patients treated with surgery were clinically better. Finally, there was no significant difference between the groups in self-reported walking ability.

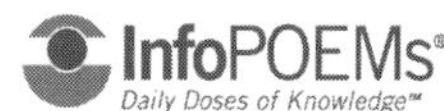

Knee taping useful for osteoarthritis pain

Clinical question

Does knee taping decrease pain and disability in patients with knee osteoarthritis?

Bottom line

Rigid taping by physical therapists, applied above the knee and, when necessary, below the knee, significantly decreased pain and disability, which lasted 3 weeks after taping was stopped. (LOE = 1b)

Reference

Hinman RS, Crossley KM, McConnell J, Bennell KL. Efficacy of knee tape in the management of osteoarthritis of the knee: blinded randomised controlled trial. BMJ 2003;327:135–138.

Study Design

Randomized controlled trial (single-blinded)

Setting

Outpatient (any)

Synopsis

The investigators investigated the American College of Rheumatology's (ACR) recommendation of knee taping for patients with osteoarthritis of the knee. Eighty-seven volunteers, at least 50 years old, who met ACR criteria for osteoarthritis of the knee were randomized (using concealed allocation) to receive no intervention, active taping, or sham taping. The tape was applied by physical therapists. The taping consisted of rigid strapping tape and hypoallergenic undertape and was applied above the knee to provide medial glide, medial tilt, and anteroposterior tilt to the patella. Additional taping was done, if necessary, to unload either the infrapatellar fat pad or the pes anserinus. Tape was applied weekly for 3 weeks and the study was continued for an additional 3 weeks. Pain, as measured on an 11-point, 10-cm scale, was significantly improved as compared with no taping or sham taping. Pain on movement decreased from 5.7 to 3.6 (out of 10) with the therapeutic taping. Results were similar for pain reported during most painful activity, Western Ontario and McMaster Universities osteoarthritis index, restriction of activity, and physical functioning. The benefits were maintained for 3 weeks after stopping treatment.

Essential Evidence: Medicine that Matters, Edited by David Slawson, Allen Shaughnessy, Mark Ebell, and Henry Barry.

Arthroscopy ineffective for osteoarthritis of knee

Clinical question

Does arthroscopic surgery improve outcomes for patients with osteoarthritis of the knee?

Bottom line

Arthroscopy is not effective for the treatment of osteoarthritis. The procedure may still have a role in the repair of meniscal and ligamentous injuries, unless we find out that it is ineffective here too. (LOE = 1b)

Reference

Moseley JB, O'Malley K, Petersen NJ, et al. A controlled trial of arthroscopic surgery for osteoarthritis of the knee. N Engl J Med 2002;347:81–88.

Study Design

Randomized controlled trial (double-blinded)

Setting

Inpatient (any location) with outpatient follow-up

Synopsis

This is one of the few studies in the literature to properly evaluate a surgical procedure. Patients (n = 180) with osteoarthritis of the knee, moderate pain, no recent arthroscopy, and no suspected ligament or meniscal problems were randomly assigned to either arthroscopy with lavage only, arthroscopy with lavage and debridement, or "sham arthroscopy." During the sham procedure, patients were mildly sedated, and the surgical team manipulated the knee, made small superficial incisions, and even made all of the noises that they would normally make during surgery. Patients were followed for 2 years by properly blinded study personnel, and patients were not able to guess their treatment assignment. Allocation was properly concealed, and groups were similar at baseline. Interestingly, all groups experienced an immediate improvement of 6 to 12 points on the 100-point Knee-Specific Pain Scale. Pain gradually increased in all groups over time, but never returned to baseline levels, and at the end of the study period all groups had a similar degree of improvement in pain. A test of physical functioning (length of time for patients to walk 100 feet and then climb up and down a flight of stairs as quickly as possible) found a slight worsening immediately after arthroscopy but no long-term difference between groups.

Essential Evidence: Medicine that Matters, Edited by David Slawson, Allen Shaughnessy, Mark Ebell, and Henry Barry.

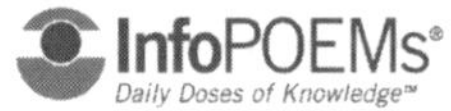

Extracorporeal shock wave therapy is ineffective for tennis elbow

Clinical question

Is extracorporeal shock wave therapy effective in treating lateral epicondylitis?

Bottom line

Extracorporeal shock wave therapy is no more effective than sham therapy in treating patients with lateral epicondylitis. Other studies have also found this therapy ineffective for this condition. Those few studies that show a difference are usually small and funded by the companies that make the machines. (LOE = 1b)

Reference

Chung B, Wiley JP. Effectiveness of extracorporeal shock wave therapy in the treatment of previously untreated lateral epicondylitis: A randomized controlled trial. Am J Sports Medicine 2004;32:1660–1667.

Study Design

Randomized controlled trial (double-blinded)

Funding

Government

Allocation

Concealed

Setting

Outpatient (any)

Synopsis

These authors randomly assigned (concealed allocation) 60 patients with previously untreated lateral epicondylitis to receive extracorporeal shock wave therapy) or sham therapy. All patients were also instructed in forearm extensor stretching exercises. The main outcome of this 8-week study was "treatment success," as defined by at least a 50% reduction in elbow pain, a pain score no higher than 4 on a scale of 10, and no analgesic use in the last 2 weeks of the study. The person evaluating these outcomes was not told which treatment the patients received and the outcome was assessed via intention to treat. Twelve of the 31 patients (39%) treated with extracorporeal shock wave therapy were treatment successes compared with 9 of the 29 (23%) treated with sham therapy. The difference in success was not significant. The study was powerful enough to detect modest differences in effect if one were present.

Essential Evidence: Medicine that Matters, Edited by David Slawson, Allen Shaughnessy, Mark Ebell, and Henry Barry.

Tennis elbow: injection better short-term, worse long-term

Clinical question

Is a steroid injection or physical therapy more effective than general treatment in patients with tennis elbow?

Bottom line

Over the short-term, the injection of painful sites in patients with tennis elbow will decrease symptoms more than general nonspecific treatment or physical therapy. However, after 1 year, patients receiving physical therapy consisting of exercises and a specific method of elbow manipulation – not described in the article – will have better function and will report greater improvement than those receiving a steroid injection, primarily because of frequent recurrences following the injection. (LOE = 1b)

Reference

Bisset L, Beller E, Jull G, Brooks P, Darnell R, Vicenzino B. Mobilisation with movement and exercise, corticosteroid injection, or wait and see for tennis elbow: randomised trial. BMJ 2006;333:939.

Study Design

Randomized controlled trial (single-blinded)

Funding

Government

Allocation

Concealed

Setting

Outpatient (any)

Synopsis

The Australian researchers conducting this study enrolled 198 adults with tennis elbow symptoms for an average of 22 weeks. Patients were, on average, in their mid-40s and approximately one third were women. Approximately 57% had symptoms due to unknown causes and not due to overuse or trauma. The average pain score was 57 of a possible 100. The patients were randomly assigned, using concealed allocation, to receive 1 of 3 treatments: 10 mg triamcinolone (Aristocort) with 1% lidocaine injected to painful elbow points, repeated after 2 weeks as necessary; eight 30-minute physical therapy treatments consisting of elbow manipulation and exercises done during the session and at home; and, general nonspecific treatment of analgesics, heat, cold, and braces, as desired. Primary outcome evaluation occurred at 6 weeks and 52 weeks and consisted of global improvement, measured on a 6-point Likert-type scale from "completely recovered" to "much worse," along with pain-free grip strength and overall assessment of severity by an assessor unaware of treatment. Using an intention-to-treat analysis, at 6 weeks 78% of injected patients were "much improved" or "completely recovered" as were 65% of patients receiving physical therapy and 27% of patients not receiving specific treatment. Pain-free grip strength and assessors' evaluations were significantly better at this time in the injection group than in the other 2 groups. However, 72% of patients receiving the injections reported recurrences. At 1 year, patients receiving a steroid injection had significantly lower scores on all 3 outcomes than did those with either physical therapy or nonspecific treatment.

Essential Evidence: Medicine that Matters, Edited by David Slawson, Allen Shaughnessy, Mark Ebell, and Henry Barry.

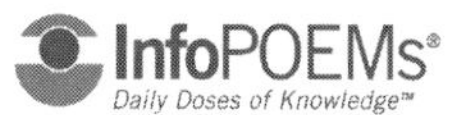

Tubes marginally effective in otitis media with effusion

Clinical question

Are ventilation tubes effective in managing children with otitis media with effusion?

Bottom line

Compared with watchful waiting, inserting pressure-equalizing tubes improves hearing in children with otitis media with effusion over the short term. Outcomes within 18 months, however, are the same. The tubes have no effect on language development. Watchful waiting is a reasonable option in most of these children. (LOE = 1a)

Reference

Rovers MM, Black N, Browning GG, Maw R, Zielhuis GA, Haggard MP. Grommets in otitis media with effusion: an individual patient data meta-analysis. Arch Dis Child 2005;90:480–485.

Study Design

Meta-analysis (randomized controlled trials)

Funding

Government

Setting

Various (meta-analysis)

Synopsis

This research team systematically reviewed several databases (including PubMed and Cochrane) looking for randomized controlled trials of ventilation tubes for children with otitis media with effusion. Ultimately, they included only the 7 studies (including a total of 1234 children) that were randomized to "a high standard" (ie, concealed allocation). They contacted the authors of the studies to get the individual patient data. After pooling all these data, the researchers looked at 3 outcomes: duration of the effusion, hearing, and language development. Since each of the studies had slightly different intermediate (6 and 9 months) and final (12 and 18 months) follow-up periods, the authors simply aggregated them. Children with tubes had a shorter duration of effusions (19.7 weeks vs 37 weeks; P = .001) than the control patients. At 6 months of follow-up, the mean hearing level was 26.6 dB in the children with tubes compared with 31.1 dB in the control group (P = .001). However, by the time of the final follow-up 12 months to 18 months later, there were no differences in hearing. Finally, the tubes had no effect on language development. The authors suggest that children attending daycare and/or those with worse hearing loss at baseline may benefit more from tubes, but this conclusion requires further study.

Essential Evidence: Medicine that Matters, Edited by David Slawson, Allen Shaughnessy, Mark Ebell, and Henry Barry.

Early tympanostomy tubes do not improve outcomes after 3 or more years

Clinical question
Does early insertion of tympanostomy tubes improve important clinical outcomes more than delayed insertion?

Bottom line
Early insertion of tympanostomy tubes does not improve long-term clinical outcomes of importance (speech acquisition and hearing) in children with persistent otitis media with effusion. Delaying 6 months for bilateral effusion and 9 months for unilateral effusion before revisiting the decision to insert tubes is the preferred approach to management, since it results in fewer procedures with equivalent outcomes. (LOE = 1b)

Reference
Paradise JL, Campbell TF, Dollaghan CA, et al. Developmental outcomes after early or delayed insertion of tympanostomy tubes. N Engl J Med 2005;353:576–586.

Study Design
Randomized controlled trial (single-blinded)

Funding
Industry + govt

Allocation
Concealed

Setting
Outpatient (any)

Synopsis
The initial report of this study's results found that early insertion of tympanostomy tubes in children with persistent otitis media with effusion did not improve outcomes at 3 years of age over delaying up to 9 months (see: Delaying tymp tubes doesn't worsen outcomes in effusion. N Engl J Med 2005;344:1179–87). In brief, children were enrolled before 2 months of age and underwent pneumatic otoscopy monthly until 3 years of age. If they had a persistent otitis media with effusion – defined as 90 days of bilateral effusion, 135 of unilateral effusion, or at least 67% of 180- and 270-day periods for bilateral and unilateral effusion in children with intermittent effusion – they were randomized to either immediate insertion of tympanostomy tubes or delaying 6 months to 9 months and only inserting tubes at that time if the effusion persisted. Outcome assessors were blinded to treatment assignment and allocation was concealed. At the end of the study, 85% in the early treatment group had received tubes, compared with only 41% in the delayed insertion group. Of course, the children who received immediate tubes could hear and speak better, right? Although that would make perfect sense, it is not what happened in this carefully done follow-up study that reports outcomes at 6 years of age. There was no difference between groups in tests of intelligence, speech complexity, hearing, auditory processing, behavior, or parental stress. With approximately 200 children in each group, the study had adequate statistical power to detect clinically meaningful differences if they existed.

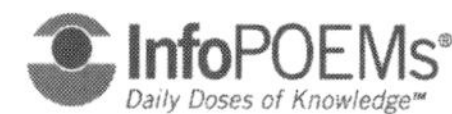

Prompt tympanostomy tube insertion doesn't improve 9 year outcomes

Clinical question

Does the delayed insertion of tympanostomy tubes impair the long-term outcomes in children with persistent middle-ear effusion?

Bottom line

Delayed tympanostomy tube insertion successfully helps many children avoid tubes and does not result in any developmental or other impairment. (LOE = 1b)

Reference

Paradise JL, Feldman HM, Campbell TF, et al. Tympanostomy tubes and developmental outcomes at 9 to 11 years of age. N Engl J Med 2007;356:248–261.

Study Design

Randomized controlled trial (single-blinded)

Funding

Government

Allocation

Concealed

Setting

Outpatient (any)

Synopsis

Many parents and clinicians still believe that there is a significant risk of permanent harm if tympanostomy tubes are not promptly inserted for children with persistent middle-ear effusion. In this study, which is a follow-up to a previously published POEM (N Engl J Med 2005;353:576), 429 children between the ages of 2 months and 3 years with middle-ear effusion for at least 90 days (bilateral) or 135 days (unilateral) were randomized to receive either prompt or delayed tympanostomy tube insertion. The delay was 6 months for bilateral effusion and 9 months for unilateral effusion. Allocation was concealed, groups were balanced at the start of the study, and analysis was by intention to treat. The researchers did an excellent job of following up: 195 of 216 in the early treatment group and 196 of 213 in the delayed treatment group underwent developmental testing between the ages of 9 years and 11 years. At the time of this final evaluation, 86% in the early treatment group had received tympanostomy tubes compared with only 49% in the delayed treatment group. There was no differences between groups in the results of a broad range of tests including evaluation of hearing, reading, oral fluency, auditory processing, phonological processing, behavior, or intelligence. There was also no difference between these groups and a group of children with ear problems that weren't bad enough to qualify them for the study.

Beta-blockade reduces cardiac events in major noncardiac surgery

Clinical question

Are β-blockers administered perioperatively useful for reducing the risk of adverse cardiac events in major noncardiac surgery?

Bottom line

Perioperative β-blockade may be beneficial in reducing the risk of cardiac-related morbidity and mortality in patients undergoing major noncardiac surgery. (LOE = 2a)

Reference

Auerbach AD, Goldman L. B-blockers and reduction of cardiac events in noncardiac surgery. Scientific review. JAMA 2002;287:1435–1444.

Study Design

Systematic review

Setting

Various (meta-analysis)

Synopsis

The authors performed a minimally adequate search of English-language studies using MEDLINE and reference lists from relevant articles since 1980 to identify studies analyzing the impact of perioperative β-blockade on cardiac events and mortality after major noncardiac surgery. A more thorough search could have been performed using the Cochrane Registry of Controlled Trials and other databases. No quality scoring of the individual trials was performed. A total of 5 separate randomized controlled trials were identified. The effect of B-blockade titrated before the induction of anesthesia to a target heart rate of 70 was effective in reducing myocardial ischemia (number needed to treat [NNT] = 2.5–6.7) and both cardiac or all-cause mortality (NNT = 3.2–8.3). The most marked effect was in patients at high risk (as assessed by both a history of previous coronary artery disease and presurgical cardiac stress testing). Because of differences in treatment protocols, the authors were unable to give specific suggestions on optimal duration of therapy after surgery.

Essential Evidence: Medicine that Matters, Edited by David Slawson, Allen Shaughnessy, Mark Ebell, and Henry Barry.

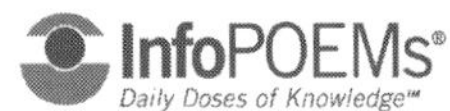

High-risk but not low-risk patients benefit from perioperative beta-blockade

Clinical question

Which patients benefit from perioperative beta-blockade?

Bottom line

Patients undergoing major surgery who are at high risk of complications – those with heart disease, cerebrovascular disease, diabetes, or renal insufficiency – benefit from perioperative beta-blockade. Low-risk patients (except perhaps those with hypertension and those undergoing high-risk surgery) do not. However, given the possible harms of suddenly discontinuing beta-blockers, those who are already taking them should continue doing so, even if they are at low-risk. (LOE = 2b)

Reference

Lindenauer PK, Pekow P, Wang K, Mamidi DK, Gutierrez B, Benjamin EM. Perioperative beta-blocker therapy and mortality after major noncardiac surgery. N Engl J Med 2005;353:349–361.

Study Design	Funding	Setting
Cohort (retrospective)	Unknown/not stated	Inpatient (any location)

Synopsis

Although initial studies looked very promising for perioperative beta-blockade (POBB) as a way to reduce perioperative mortality, not all studies have found benefit. The degree of risk appears to be an important factor. In this retrospective cohort study, the authors identified patients undergoing major noncardiac surgery who had no contraindications to beta-blockers and who either received one during the first 2 days of hospitalization (n = 122,338) or who did not (n = 541,297). Patients were more likely to receive POBB if they were white, were undergoing vascular surgery, had higher perioperative risk, were at a teaching hospital, an urban hospital, a larger hospital, or a hospital in the northeast United States. Perioperative risk was measured by assigning 1 point each for high-risk surgery, ischemic heart disease, cerebrovascular disease, renal insufficiency, and diabetes mellitus. A propensity score was calculated using logistic regression that predicted the probability that a patient would receive POBB according to patient and hospital characteristics. This score was then used to match patients who did and did not receive POBB, and logistic regression followed to evaluate the independent effect of POBB on the risk of in-hospital death. Logistic regression was also used to evaluate the independent effect of POBB on the risk of in-hospital death using the entire study cohort. In both cases, there was slight harm for very low-risk patients with a risk score of 0 (odds ratio [OR] = 1.43; 95% CI, 1.29–1.58 using the propensity score matched cohort). However, there was increasing benefit as the risk score increased: OR 1.13 for risk score = 1; 0.9 for risk score = 2; 0.71 for risk score = 3; and 0.57 for risk score = 4. Using data from the entire cohort the number needed to treat (NNT) was 33 for the highest-risk patients and 62 for those with a risk score of 3. Among very low-risk patients (those with a risk score of 0), those with hypertension benefited slightly (NNT = 2349), and among low risk patients with a score of 1, only those undergoing high-risk surgery benefited at all (NNT = 864). The study was limited by a number of important factors, most notably lack of randomization, retrospective data collection, and failure to distinguish between chronic beta-blocker use and beta-blockers initiated at the time of surgery.

Essential Evidence: Medicine that Matters, Edited by David Slawson, Allen Shaughnessy, Mark Ebell, and Henry Barry.

Smoking cessation 6–8 weeks before surgery reduces complications

Clinical question

Is it worth trying to get smokers to quit before elective surgery?

Bottom line

Among smokers awaiting elective hip or knee replacement, participating in a weekly nurse-led smoking cessation program prevents postoperative complications. Only three patients need to go through the program to prevent one complication. (LOE = 1b)

Reference

Moller AM, Villebro N, Pedersen T, Tonneson H. Effect of preoperative smoking intervention on postoperative complications: a randomised clinical trial. Lancet 2002;359:114–117.

Study Design

Randomized controlled trial (single-blinded)

Setting

Outpatient (specialty)

Synopsis

These authors studied smokers in three Danish hospitals who were scheduled for elective hip or knee replacement. Six to eight weeks before the surgery, they randomly assigned (masked allocation) the smokers to a smoking intervention (n = 60) or control (n = 60). The intervention consisted of weekly meetings with a nurse who developed a personalized smoking cessation and free nicotine-replacement program. They strongly encouraged the patients to quit smoking, but the patients also had the option of reducing tobacco consumption by 50%. The investigators used an intention-to-treat analysis and the investigator who assessed complications was unaware of which group the patient was assigned to. Several patients in each group didn't go through with the surgery. Of the patients who went through with their surgery, 10/56 (18%) in the intervention group had a complication compared with 27/52 (52%) of the controls. We don't have any information about the severity of complications. Neither group had anybody kick off. While the largest difference was in the rate of wound infections, the study was underpowered to see significant differences in infrequent events like cardiac complications. There was no difference in hospital length of stay. They also looked at the treatment actually received and found that the benefit was noted primarily in those who actually quit rather than some other unanticipated aspect of the program.

Essential Evidence: Medicine that Matters, Edited by David Slawson, Allen Shaughnessy, Mark Ebell, and Henry Barry.

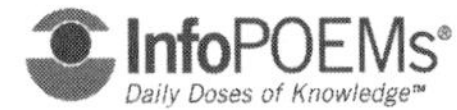

Better outcomes with CABG than PCI with stent for 2,3 vessel disease

Clinical question

Which is the better treatment for multivessel coronary disease: bypass surgery or stenting?

Bottom line

Coronary artery bypass grafting (CABG) is associated with lower long-term mortality than percutaneous coronary interventions (PCI) with stenting for most anatomic groups in patients with multivessel disease, and a lower risk of requiring revascularization in the 3 years following intervention. Of course, this was an observational study and the groups were quite different at baseline, so we must be cautious about drawing firm treatment conclusions, even with appropriate statistical adjustments. Stenting is less invasive and is associated with lower unadjusted in-hospital mortality, so it remains a good option for many patients. (LOE = 2b)

Reference

Hannan EL, Racz MJ, Walford G, et al. Long-term outcomes of coronary-artery bypass grafting versus stent implantation. N Engl J Med 2005;352:2174–2183.

Study Design

Cohort (prospective)

Funding

Unknown/not stated

Setting

Inpatient (any location) with outpatient follow-up

Synopsis

Randomized trials comparing PCI with CABG were done before stenting was widely used. This analysis used data from 2 New York cardiac registries, 1 for PCI and 1 for CABG. Data were collected for all patients undergoing CABG or PCI with stent placement for at least 1 lesion between 1997 and 2000. All patients had at least a 70% stenosis in 2 of the main coronary arteries. Patients with left main disease or myocardial infarction within 24 hours of the procedure were excluded. The groups were quite different: Patients in the CABG group were older (67 vs 65 years), more likely to be male (70.9% vs 68.6%), more likely to be white (89.2% vs 87%), and more likely to have a decreased ejection fraction. The researchers were unable to determine how many patients were lost to follow-up. The analysis first identified factors that were associated with the risk of death and adjusted for these factors in a multivariate analysis. Separate analyses were done for the different anatomical combinations of 2-vessel and 3-vessel disease. Patients were followed up for a mean of 706 days in the CABG group and 585 days in the stent group. The adjusted hazard ratio for death after CABG compared with the risk for stent was between 0.64 and 0.76 for the 5 different types of 2- and 3-vessel disease. The benefit was generally greater for patients with diabetes (hazard ratio = 0.59–0.71). There was no difference between outcomes for CABG or stent for patients with 2-vessel disease not including the proximal left anterior descending (LAD) artery and decreased ejection fraction. The benefit was greatest for patients with 3-vessel disease involving the LAD artery. Patients undergoing stent were much more likely to require revascularization with CABG (7.8% vs 0.3%) or subsequent PCI (27.3% vs 4.6%). Not surprisingly, unadjusted inpatient mortality was higher in the CABG group (1.75% vs 0.68%).

Essential Evidence: Medicine that Matters, Edited by David Slawson, Allen Shaughnessy, Mark Ebell, and Henry Barry.

Routine invasive strategy may be preferred for ACS

Clinical question

Is a routine or selective invasive strategy more effective in the treatment of acute coronary syndrome?

Bottom line

High-risk patients with unstable angina or non-ST-segment elevation myocardial infarction (NSTEMI) and positive cardiac biomarkers benefit from immediate coronary angiography and revascularization when appropriate. Similar patients with negative cardiac biomarkers appear to do as well with initial pharmacologic treatment, reserving angiography and revascularization for those with evidence of ongoing ischemia. (LOE = 1a–)

Reference

Mehta SR, Cannon CP, Fox KA, et al. Routine vs selective invasive strategies in patients with acute coronary syndrome. A collaborative meta-analysis of randomized trials. JAMA 2005;293:2908–2917.

Study Design	Funding	Setting
Meta-analysis (randomized controlled trials)	Government	Various (meta-analysis)

Synopsis

Optimal treatment for patients with unstable angina or NSTEMI remains controversial. The investigators comprehensively searched MEDLINE, the Cochrane Registry of Controlled Trials, abstracts from major cardiology meetings, and cross-references from original articles and reviews for relevant trials comparing benefits and risks of routine versus selective invasive treatment strategies. A routine invasive strategy was defined as all patients with unstable angina or NSTEMI undergoing immediate coronary angiography followed by revascularization when appropriate. A selective invasive strategy was defined as all patients being initially treated pharmacologically, followed by angiography and revascularization only for those with persistent symptoms or evidence of ongoing ischemia. Only randomized trials with adequate concealment and follow-up were included in the review. Two individuals independently assessed the individual trials and extracted pertinent data. Of 84 initially identified articles, only 7 involving 9208 patients met inclusion criteria. Follow-up occurred for a mean of 17 months. Mortality was significantly increased during the initial hospitalization in the routine invasive strategy group (1.8% vs 1.1% in the selective invasive strategy group), but after discharge the routine strategy was associated with a significantly lower mortality (3.8% vs 4.9%). Overall, the composite outcome of death or recurrent myocardial infarction was lower in patients in the routine group than in the selective group (12.2% vs 14.4%; number needed to treat = 45; 95% CI, 28–119). Higher risk patients with elevated cardiac biomarkers (eg, troponin and creatine kinase levels) at baseline benefited the most from the routine invasive strategy, but there was no benefit to the routine strategy for patients with negative biomarkers. There was some heterogeneity in the outcomes of the various trials, but the authors speculate that it's related to the concurrent use of other medications in some, but not all, trials. Trials published after 1999 demonstrated the most benefit to routine invasive strategy, suggesting a positive impact of improved treatment protocols.

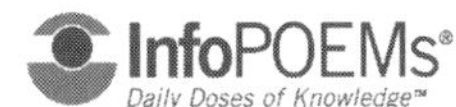

In ACS, 5 years of invasive tx decreases MI but not all cause mortality (FRISC-II)

Clinical question

Are the long-term outcomes of invasive intervention better than those for medical management in the face of acute coronary syndromes?

Bottom line

In this study of patients with non-ST-elevation acute coronary syndromes, patients treated invasively had fewer subsequent myocardial infarctions after 5 years than patients treated medically. The benefits are seen mainly in men, nonsmokers, and patients with at least 2 risk factors. (LOE = 1b)

Reference

Lagerqvist B, Husted S, Kontny F, et al, for the Fast Revascularisation during InStability in Coronary artery disease (FRISC-II) Investigators. 5-year outcomes in the FRISC-II randomised trial of an invasive versus a non-invasive strategy in non-ST-elevation acute coronary syndrome: a follow-up study. Lancet 2006;368:998–1004.

Study Design

Randomized controlled trial (nonblinded)

Funding

Industry + govt

Allocation

Concealed

Setting

Inpatient (any location) with outpatient follow-up

Synopsis

The FRISC-II was a randomized trial designed to study the effects of invasive intervention or medical management of patients with acute coronary syndromes. This study reports the 5-year follow up on more than 99% of the original participants. The patients were eligible if they had less than 48 hours of chest pain with signs of myocardial ischemia or non-ST-elevation myocardial infarction. All patients received aspirin and dalteparin for at least 5 days. Those in the intervention group received aspirin and dalteparin every day until their revascularization; their last dose was the evening before the procedure. Patients also received beta-blockers unless contraindicated. During the first 24 months, the study team directly contacted patients. After this, the data for vital status were obtained from national population registries and the national registries of cause of death. The researchers used intention-to-treat analysis to analyze the outcomes. At the end of 5 years, there was no difference in all-cause morality (9.7% in the group managed invasively; 10.1% in the group managed medically). However, the patients managed invasively had fewer myocardial infarctions (12.9% vs 17.7%; number needed to treat = 21; 95% CI, 13–56). The benefit was seen mainly in men, nonsmokers, and patients with 2 or more risk factors.

Essential Evidence: Medicine that Matters, Edited by David Slawson, Allen Shaughnessy, Mark Ebell, and Henry Barry.

CABG not helpful before AAA or peripheral vascular surgery

Clinical question
In patients with significant, stable coronary disease, is coronary artery revascularization helpful before major vascular surgery?

Bottom line
Patients with significant, stable coronary artery disease do not benefit from revascularization before major peripheral vascular surgery. (LOE = 1b)

Reference
McFalls EO, Ward HB, Moritz TE, et al. Coronary-artery revascularization before elective major vascular surgery. N Engl J Med 2004;351:2795–2804.

Study Design
Randomized controlled trial (nonblinded)

Funding
Government

Allocation
Concealed

Setting
Inpatient (any location) with outpatient follow-up

Synopsis
Do you put patients through a risky procedure to make a second risky procedure safer? Tough question, when that first procedure may reduce long-term mortality. Patients undergoing either repair of an expanding abdominal aortic aneurysm or peripheral vascular surgery underwent angiography if they were felt to be at high risk for cardiovascular complications based standard guidelines. If one or more coronary arteries had a 70% stenosis they were randomized to either revascularization (59% got angioplasty, 41% coronary artery bypass graft) or no revascularization. Of 5859 patients initially enrolled, 1654 were not at high risk, 1025 required urgent surgery, 626 had prior revascularization, 731 had a severe coexisting illness, 633 were already in another study or declined to participate, and 680 were excluded for various other reasons. That left 510 for randomization; groups were balanced at the start of the study, and allocation to groups was concealed. Patients were followed for up to 6 years; the mean follow-up was 2.8 years. There were not surprisingly more deaths before surgery in the revascularization group (10 vs 1), no difference in the 30 days after the peripheral vascular surgery or AAA repair (7 vs 8), and no difference in long-term all-cause mortality (22% in the revascularization group vs 23% in the no revascularization group). The outcomes were the same for intention to treat and per protocol analyses.

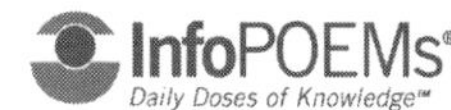

EVAR worse than open repair of AAA (EVAR Trial 1)

Clinical question

Is open repair better than endovascular repair for patients with abdominal aortic aneurysms?

Bottom line

Endovascular aneurysm repair (EVAR) offers no real advantage over traditional open repair in medically fit patients with abdominal aortic aneurysms. (LOE = 1b–)

Reference

EVAR trial participants. Endovascular aneurysm repair versus open repair in patients with abdominal aortic aneurysm (EVAR trial 1): randomised controlled trial. Lancet 2005;365:2179–2186.

Study Design

Randomized controlled trial (nonblinded)

Funding

Government

Allocation

Concealed

Setting

Inpatient (any location) with outpatient follow-up

Synopsis

In this multicenter study, patients 60 and older with abdominal aortic aneurysms at least 5.5 cm in diameter were randomly assigned (masked central allocation) to endovascular aneurysm repair (EVAR; n = 543) or traditional open repair (n = 539). The patients had to be "medically fit" for surgery. After repair of the aneurysm, the researchers evaluated the patients at 1, 3, and 12 months, and then yearly thereafter. While the study was unblinded, it is pretty hard to fudge the main outcome, all-cause mortality, assessed via intention to treat. The study was designed to be able to detect a 5% difference in all-cause mortality. The median duration of follow up was 2.9 years and only 5 patients were lost to follow up (2 in the EVAR group and 3 in the open repair group). The all-cause mortality rate was about 28% in each group. While there was a 3% absolute reduction in aneurysm-specific mortality in the first 30 days after EVAR (1.7% vs. 4.7%), EVAR cost more, didn't improve health-related quality of life, increased post-operative complications and increased the need for repeat procedures. So other than that, Mrs. Lincoln, how was the play?

Essential Evidence: Medicine that Matters, Edited by David Slawson, Allen Shaughnessy, Mark Ebell, and Henry Barry.

Bypass = angioplasty for severe leg ischemia, but costs more (BASIL)

Clinical question

Is bypass better than angioplasty in patients with severe ischemic disease of the legs?

Bottom line

Patients with advanced peripheral vascular disease who undergo either bypass surgery or balloon angioplasty have comparable amputation-free survival. Even though patients initially treated with angioplasty had a higher rate of re-intervention, the medical costs during the first year after treatment were one third higher in patients treated surgically. (LOE = 1b–)

Reference

Adam DJ, Beard JD, Cleveland T, et al, for the BASIL trial participants. Bypass versus angioplasty in severe ischaemia of the leg (BASIL): multicentre, randomised controlled trial. Lancet 2005;366:1925–1934.

Study Design

Randomized controlled trial (nonblinded)

Funding

Government

Allocation

Concealed

Setting

Inpatient (any location) with outpatient follow-up

Synopsis

Patients with severe peripheral vascular disease of a lower limb, defined as rest pain, ischemic ulcer, or gangrene, were randomly assigned (concealed allocation) to initial treatment with bypass surgery or balloon angioplasty (with no stents). To be eligible, the patients had to have confirmed infra-inguinal disease. Approximately one third of the patients presenting with severe disease were eligible to participate. The main outcomes were analyzed by intention to treat. Although this was an unblinded study, the outcomes, other than quality of life, are relatively free from measurement bias. However, decision-making about re-intervention and hospital resource use could have been influenced by any biases held by the performing surgeons. The researchers continued to follow each patient until the main end point (death or amputation) was reached. The study was designed to have 90% power to detect a 15% difference in 3-year amputation-free survival. Approximately two thirds of the patients were older than 70 years, nearly 80% were current or former smokers, and 40% had diabetes. Only 2% of the patients were lost to follow-up after randomization. Among the 228 patients initially managed surgically, 30 eventually died and 20 had an amputation; among the 224 initially treated with angioplasty, 28 died and 25 had an amputation. The patients treated with angioplasty had a significantly higher rate of re-intervention (26% vs 18%). The hospital costs during the first year after randomization for the patients treated surgically were approximately one third higher than the costs for the patients initially treated with angioplasty. In a post hoc analysis, patients treated with surgery seemed to do better after 2 years; the number of events after 2 years was small, though. Since post hoc analyses are fraught with problems, they should only be used to generate hypotheses.

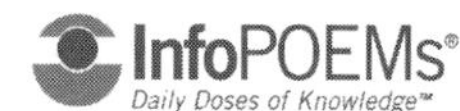

Endarterectomy best within 2 weeks of stroke or TIA

Clinical question

What factors are associated with favorable carotid endarterectomy outcomes?

Bottom line

Patients older than 75 years, men, and those who have carotid endarterectomy within 2 weeks of a cerebrovascular event have better outcomes following endarterectomy. (LOE = 1b)

Reference

Rothwell PM, Eliasziw M, Gutnikov SA, et al. Endarterectomy for symptomatic carotid stenosis in relation to clinical subgroups and timing of surgery. Lancet 2004;363:915–924.

Study Design

Other

Setting

Inpatient (any location) with outpatient follow-up

Synopsis

These authors pooled the data from 2 randomized controlled trials of carotid endarterectomy. These studies represent 95% of patients ever randomized to endarterectomy versus medical treatment for symptomatic carotid stenosis. In this pooled analysis, the authors examined several specific subgroups, including sex, age, time from most recent cerebrovascular event, severity of event, diabetes, plaque characteristics, and the presence of contralateral carotid occlusion. All data were analyzed via intention to treat. The studies included 5893 patients and had a mean follow-up of 66 months. Men and patients older than 75 years had better outcomes. Those who had surgery more than 2 weeks after their event had worse outcomes. The degree of stenosis, as seen in the primary studies, was an important modifier. For those with more than 50% stenosis, the numbers needed to treat to prevent 1 ipsilateral stroke in 5 years were: 9 for men; 36 for women; 5 for patients older than 75 years; 18 for those younger than 65 years; 5 for those patients randomized within 2 weeks of their cerebrovascular event; and 125 for those randomized beyond 12 weeks.

Essential Evidence: Medicine that Matters, Edited by David Slawson, Allen Shaughnessy, Mark Ebell, and Henry Barry.

Carotid stent inferior to carotid endarterectomy

Clinical question

Is stenting a safe and effective alternative to carotid endarterectomy in patients with symptomatic carotid stenosis?

Bottom line

Carotid stenting as currently practiced should be abandoned. It significantly increases the risk of stroke in patients with symptomatic carotid stenosis. (LOE = 1b)

Reference

Mas JL, Chatellier G, Beyssen B, et al, for the EVA-3S Investigators. Endarterectomy versus stenting in patients with symptomatic severe carotid stenosis. N Engl J Med 2006;355:1660–1671.

Study Design

Randomized controlled trial (nonblinded)

Funding

Government

Allocation

Concealed

Setting

Inpatient (any location) with outpatient follow-up

Synopsis

It makes sense that carotid stenting, a less invasive procedure, might be safer than carotid endarterectomy (CE). However, several smaller previous clinical trials have not found an advantage to stenting over CE. This French study included 520 adults with a recent transient ischemic attack (TIA) or nondisabling stroke and a 60% to 99% stenosis in the symptomatic carotid artery. Patients with significant disability, uncontrolled hypertension or diabetes, unstable angina, history of bleeding, or severe proximal or intracranial lesions worse than the cervical lesion were excluded. Allocation to groups was concealed, but the patients and neurologists doing outcome assessment were not blinded. The events committee that assessed stroke, death, and other outcomes was blinded. The goal of the analysis was to determine "noninferiority" at 30 days, but the study was stopped prematurely because of significantly worse outcomes than expected in the stent group. Groups were balanced at the start of the study, analysis was by intention to treat, and the mean age of participants was 70 years. Approximately half had a history of ischemic stroke, and one third had a history of TIA. Only 4% of patients in the stent group had more than 1 stent placed. At 30 days, the risk of nonfatal stroke was much higher in the stent group (8.8% vs 2.7%; number needed to treat to harm [NNTH] = 16; 95% CI, 10–47), although the risk of death was similar (1.2% in the CE group vs 0.8% in the stent group). At 6 months, the risk of any stroke or death was 6.1% in the CE group and 11.7% in the stent group (NNTH = 18; 9–143).

Essential Evidence: Medicine that Matters, Edited by David Slawson, Allen Shaughnessy, Mark Ebell, and Henry Barry.

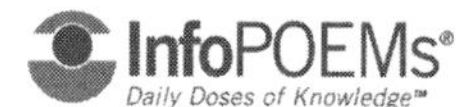

Routine use of vena cava filters doesn't reduce mortality

Clinical question

Does routine use of vena cava filters improve outcomes in patients with venous thromboembolism?

Bottom line

In a fairly high-risk group of patients with venous thromboembolism (VTE), vena cava filters reduce the risk of pulmonary embolism (PE), increase the risk of deep vein thrombosis (DVT), and do not alter the risk of death. However, this group was not typical of the group that is usually given these filters in clinical practice. (LOE = 1b)

Reference

PREPIC Study Group. Eight-year follow-up of patients with permanent vena cava filters in the prevention of pulmonary embolism. Circulation 2005;112:416–422.

Study Design

Randomized controlled trial (nonblinded)

Funding

Government

Setting

Inpatient (any location) with outpatient follow-up

Synopsis

Patients with acute proximal DVT with or without PE were randomized to permanent vena cava filter or usual treatment. All received warfarin for at least 3 months. Approximately one third were anticoagulated for only 3 months, one third for the entire 8-year follow-up period, and one third for an intermediate duration. The mean age of the 400 participants was 72 years, 95% were men, 36% had a PE, and 35% had a history of previous VTE. Although the study group is probably of higher-than-average risk among all patients with VTE, it is important to note that vena cava filters are generally only recommended for patients who have recurrent VTE despite adequate anticoagulation or those who cannot tolerate anticoagulation. Groups were balanced at the start of the study and analysis was by intention to treat. Patients and their physicians were aware of treatment assignment, but outcomes were adjudicated by a group blinded to treatment assignment. After 8 years, outcome data were available for all but 1 patient. Patients receiving a filter were less likely to have a PE (6.2% vs 15.1%; P = .008; number needed to treat = 11), but more likely to have a DVT (36% vs 27%; number needed to treat to harm = 11). There was no difference in the likelihood of post-thrombotic syndrome or death (50% in both groups).

Essential Evidence: Medicine that Matters, Edited by David Slawson, Allen Shaughnessy, Mark Ebell, and Henry Barry.

School-based violence prevention programs not proved

Clinical question

Are school-based violence prevention programs directed at high risk kids effective?

Bottom line

The studies included in this meta-analysis demonstrate modest reductions in aggressive behaviors, but that there is a need for larger, high quality studies. This is analogous to the studies of the DARE program: sounds good, doesn't work. (LOE = 1a–)

Reference

Mytton JA, DiGuiseppi, Gough DA, et al. School-based violence prevention programs: systematic review of secondary prevention programs. Arch Pediatr Adolesc Med 2002;156:752–762.

Study Design

Meta-analysis of randomized controlled trials

Setting

Other

Synopsis

The authors searched numerous databases and made a reasonable effort to locate unpublished randomized controlled studies of school-based violence prevention programs directed at children who had previously been identified as being at risk for aggressive behaviors. Two investigators independently extracted the data and when important elements were missing from the study, they contacted the authors. Unfortunately, they did not explicitly assess the quality of the studies. They ended up with 28 studies with 2096 children that met their criteria. None of them reported any data on violent injuries. While the studies demonstrated a 36% relative reduction in aggressive behaviors, there was significant and worrisome variation among the studies. They also found that larger studies found the least effect and that small studies showing harm or no benefit were lacking, suggesting that publication bias exists. That means that these small "negative" studies may have been rejected, creating a bias in the literature toward studies that show an effect.

Essential Evidence: Medicine that Matters, Edited by David Slawson, Allen Shaughnessy, Mark Ebell, and Henry Barry.

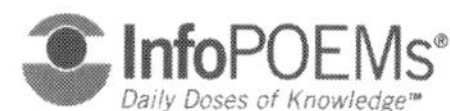

Risk scoring system predicts mortality in pediatric ICU

Clinical question

Can mortality in pediatric ICU patients be predicted using an easy scoring system?

Bottom line

Scoring systems can effectively predict mortality in children admitted to the ICU. The PIM, a point-of-care score, is easier to administer. (LOE = 1b)

Reference

Tibby SM, Taylor D, Festa M, et al. A comparison of three scoring systems for mortality risk among retrieved intensive care patients. Arch Dis Child 2002:87:421–425.

Study Design

Cohort (prospective)

Setting

Inpatient (ICU only)

Synopsis

These authors compared three different risk scoring systems in 928 critically ill children admitted to ICU. Two of the scoring systems, pre-ICU PRISM and PIM, use clinical data collected before admission to the ICU while the PRISM II also includes data from the first 24 hours after ICU admission. They were able to get complete scoring for only 24% using the pre-ICU PRISM, 88% for the PIM, and 60% using PRISM II. The authors calculated the area under the receiver operator characteristic curve (AUROCC) to determine which system was better at predicting mortality. All three systems performed reasonably well with AURROC between 0.83 and 0.87. They found, however, that all of the systems were not as good at predicting those at medium risk. The PIM was better in children with respiratory diseases.

Essential Evidence: Medicine that Matters, Edited by David Slawson, Allen Shaughnessy, Mark Ebell, and Henry Barry.

Parent satisfaction okay with no treatment of AOM

Clinical question

Are parents whose children do not receive treatment for acute otitis media less satisfied with their child's care?

Bottom line

Parents don't seem to mind if their children are not treated with antibiotics. In this study comparing no treatment to immediate antibiotic treatment of acute otitis media, parent satisfaction scores were similar between the 2 groups, even though 21% of the no-treatment children eventually needed antibiotics. (LOE = 1b–)

Reference

McCormick DP, Chonmaitree T, Pittman C, et al. Nonsevere acute otitis media: a clinical trial comparing outcomes of watchful waiting versus immediate antibiotic treatment. Pediatrics 2005;115:1455–1465.

Study Design	Funding	Allocation
Randomized controlled trial (single-blinded)	Government	Uncertain

Setting

Outpatient (primary care)

Synopsis

Several studies have shown that not treating children initially with antibiotics for acute otitis media results in fewer eventual prescriptions and fewer adverse effects. This study again evaluated watchful waiting versus immediate antibiotic treatment, and also surveyed parents regarding their satisfaction with care. The researchers enrolled 223 infants and children with symptoms and otoscopic evidence of acute otitis media rated as not severe. Approximately 30% of the children were younger than 1 year, 25% were between the ages of 1 year and 2 years, and the rest were between the ages of 2 years and 13 years. The children were randomized (allocation concealment uncertain) to receive either high-dose amoxicillin, 90 mg per kg per day for 10 days, or no treatment. Children were concurrently treated with ibuprofen, a decongestant, and saline nose drops. They were also given an antihistamine, although this class of drugs was shown to be ineffective more than 20 years ago and were recently shown to extend the duration of middle ear effusion. Parents were instructed to return to the clinic if symptoms failed to improve or worsened, which occurred in 5% of antibiotic-treated children and 21% of no-antibiotic children ($P = .001$; number needed to treat with antibiotic to prevent one failure = 7). Treatment failure occurred significantly more often in children who had received antibiotics in the previous 30 days. On a questionnaire of satisfaction, which included questions regarding the parents' feelings toward medication side effects, extra time spent receiving care for the infection, difficulty giving the antibiotic, work absences, and overall satisfaction, the average score was not significantly different between the 2 groups of parents when measured on day 12 and day 30 of the study, with scores in both groups averaging about 44 of a possible 48. The study has many limitations: there is no mention whether the parent questionnaires were written in Spanish, which is important since the study was conducted in a predominantly Spanish-speaking area of the United States; the questionnaire was not validated; and there was unblinding of the investigators in a number of instances. Parents were also not given a delayed prescription to fill if symptoms didn't resolve, but were asked to return to the clinic for further evaluation.

Essential Evidence: Medicine that Matters, Edited by David Slawson, Allen Shaughnessy, Mark Ebell, and Henry Barry.

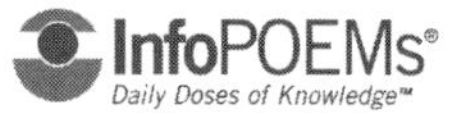

Parents prefer shared decision-making for AOM

Clinical question

Do parents with children with acute otitis media prefer to share in the decision to use antibiotics?

Bottom line

Presenting information about the pros and cons of antibiotic treatment for acute otitis media and letting parents decide whether and when to start treatment increases parents' satisfaction with their visit and could decrease antibiotic use. These results were found in wealthy, white, older parents and may not apply to other socioeconomic groups. (LOE = 2c)

Reference

Merenstein D, Diener-West M, Krist A, Pinneger M, Cooper LA. An assessment of the shared-decision model in parents of children with acute otitis media. Pediatrics 2005;116:1267–1275.

Study Design

Cross-sectional

Funding

Foundation

Setting

Outpatient (primary care)

Synopsis

The researchers conducting this study wished to determine to what extent parents would like to participate in the decision-making regarding the treatment of their child, given a scenario in which their child had acute otitis media. The parents in this study were not typical; they were older with an average age of 46 years), wealthy (76% had a family income >$75,000), well educated (87% attended college), mostly non-Hispanic white, and almost all had health insurance. During a visit to a family practice, 466 parents were asked to imagine their reaction to 1 of 3 clinical vignettes. All vignettes presented a mother taking her 2 1/2-year-old son to the doctor with a fever. The child is diagnosed with acute otitis media. In each vignette the doctor explains a desire to decrease antibiotic use and the lack of need for antibiotic use in most instances. In the "paternalistic" vignette the doctor clearly recommends antibiotics. In the "shared decision-making" vignettes the doctor makes no specific recommendation but gives a prescription for an antibiotic to be started in 2 days if the child is not better; in 1 of these vignettes acetaminophen is also recommended as treatment. Before reading the vignettes, 93% of parents reported that they felt that antibiotics were needed if an ear infection is present. After reading the vignettes, 82% reported being willing to wait 48 hours before starting treatment. However, 27% of the parents receiving the paternalistic vignette would start antibiotics immediately; only 7% receiving the shared decision-making vignettes would do so ($P < .001$). All reported similar degrees of satisfaction with the amount of information they received. Significantly more patients reported being satisfied with the shared decision-making approaches than with the paternalistic approach (76% satisfied in the paternalistic group vs 84% and 93% in the shared decision-making groups; $P < .001$).

Essential Evidence: Medicine that Matters, Edited by David Slawson, Allen Shaughnessy, Mark Ebell, and Henry Barry.

Intensive insulin only helpful if MICU stay 3 days or longer

Clinical question

Does intensive insulin therapy reduce mortality for patients in the medical intensive care unit?

Bottom line

Intensive insulin treatment of patients in the medical intensive care unit (ICU) is helpful if patients spend at least 3 days in the unit. Unfortunately, those with a shorter stay may be harmed, and physicians were unable to accurately predict who would actually stay 3 or more days (36% of those predicted to stay at least 3 days were discharged sooner in this study). (LOE = 1b)

Reference

Van den Berghe G, Wilmer A, Hermans G, et al. Intensive insulin therapy in the medical ICU. N Engl J Med 2006;354:449–461.

Study Design

Randomized controlled trial (single-blinded)

Funding

Government

Allocation

Concealed

Setting

Inpatient (ICU only)

Synopsis

Studies in the surgical ICU have demonstrated reduced mortality among patients receiving strict blood sugar control, especially if they had a longer stay in the ICU. In this study, 1200 patients admitted to a Belgian medical ICU expected to have a stay of at least 3 days were randomized with concealed allocation to intensive insulin treatment (target blood glucose 80 to 110 mg/dL, 4.4 to 6.1 mmol/L) or conventional insulin treatment (target blood glucose 180 to 200 mg/dL, 10 to 11 mmol/L) using an insulin pump. Groups were balanced at the start of the study and analysis was by intention to treat. The intention was to enroll only patients who would be in the ICU for 3 or more days, but only 767 of the 1200 patients actually stayed that long. Although there was no difference in in-hospital mortality rates between the 2 treatment groups as a whole, there were morbidity benefits: less new renal injury (5.9% vs 8.9%); earlier weaning from mechanical ventilation; and earlier discharge from the ICU and hospital. In the subgroup of 767 patients who actually spent at least 3 days in the ICU, in-hospital mortality was lower in the intensive treatment group (43% vs 52.5%; P = .009; number needed to treat [NNT] = 10). On the other hand, among patients staying in the ICU less than 3 days, there were more deaths in the intensive treatment group (26.8% vs 18.7%; P = .05; number needed to treat to harm = 12). Post-hoc analysis suggests that the higher rate of death in patients in the intensive-treatment group who stayed less than 3 days could be due to the higher number in whom care was limited or withdrawn for reasons of futility within 72 hours of admission. Morbidity was also reduced by intensive treatment in the group staying in the ICU less than 3 days.

Essential Evidence: Medicine that Matters, Edited by David Slawson, Allen Shaughnessy, Mark Ebell, and Henry Barry.

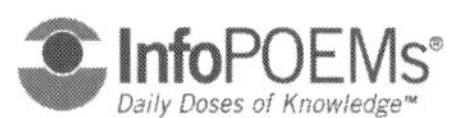

Normal saline similar to 4% albumin in ICU fluid resuscitation

Clinical question

What is the best intravenous fluid for patients in the intensive care unit?

Bottom line

Crystalloids and colloids are equally effective for fluid resuscitation in patients admitted to the intensive care unit, with the possible exception of the patients admitted with trauma and an associated brain injury (saline better) or severe sepsis (colloid better). (LOE = 1b)

Reference

The SAFE Study Investigators. A comparison of albumin and saline for fluid resuscitation in the intensive care unit. N Engl J Med 2004;350:2247–2256.

Study Design

Randomized controlled trial (double-blinded)

Allocation

Concealed

Setting

Inpatient (ICU only)

Synopsis

One meta-analysis of 1419 patients suggested that mortality is higher when colloid fluids are used instead of crystalloids for fluid resuscitation in patients admitted to the intensive care unit, while a larger meta-analysis in less severely ill patients did not find such an effect. This large, well-designed randomized trial of 7000 adults in the intensive care unit was designed to settle the issue. The patients' mean age was 59 years, 40% were female, 64% were mechanically ventilated, and slightly more than 10% had failure of 2 or more organs. Patients were excluded if they were admitted after liver transplant, for cardiac surgery, or for burn therapy. The groups were well balanced at the start of the study. Allocation was appropriately concealed, and blinding of participants, physicians, and outcome assessors was effective. Patients were randomly assigned to receive either 4% albumin or 0.9% normal saline. The primary outcome was mortality at 28 days, which was nearly identical between groups (20.9% for albumin vs 21.1% for normal saline). There was a trend toward greater mortality for patients admitted because of trauma who were given albumin (n = 1186; 13.6% vs 10.0%; P = .06), but only if they had an associated brain injury (n = 492; 24.5% vs 15.1%; P = .009). There was also a trend toward greater mortality for patients admitted with severe sepsis who were given normal saline (n = 1218; 35.3% vs 30.7%; P = .09). All other outcomes were similar between groups.

Essential Evidence: Medicine that Matters, Edited by David Slawson, Allen Shaughnessy, Mark Ebell, and Henry Barry.

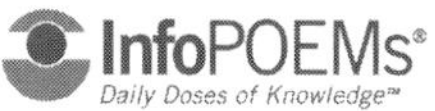

No benefit from pulmonary artery catheters for critically ill patients

Clinical question

Are pulmonary artery catheters useful in the management of critically ill patients?

Bottom line

Evidence is lacking to show benefit or harm of the pulmonary artery catheter (PAC) in the management of critically ill patients. Patients managed with the PAC are more likely to receive inotropic medications and vasodilators. There are few data showing that either class of medication improves outcomes in critically ill patients. Individual patients may benefit from use of the PAC, so clinical judgment should guide optimal management. The PAC should not be a standard of care or be used routinely in the intensive care unit for all patients. (LOE = 1a)

Reference

Shah MR, Hasselblad V, Stevenson LW, et al. Impact of the pulmonary artery catheter in critically ill patients. Meta-analysis of randomized clinical trials. JAMA 2005;294:1664–1670.

Study Design

Meta-analysis (randomized controlled trials)

Funding

Foundation

Setting

Various (meta-analysis)

Synopsis

Although the PAC is widely used in the management of critically ill patients, data regarding the utility of this device are conflicting. The investigators thoroughly searched MEDLINE, the Cochrane Controlled Trials Registry, bibliographies of identified articles, and government databases for English language randomized trials evaluating the effectiveness of PAC in various clinical settings. Two independent reviewers assessed the eligibility of individual trials and abstracted data in an unblinded manner. Disagreements were resolved by consensus. A total of 13 randomized trials involving 5051 patients met inclusion criteria for both methodology and quality. The meta-analysis also included a trial published in the same journal issue (The ESCAPE Trial. Evaluation study of congestive heart failure and pulmonary artery catheterization effectiveness. JAMA 2005;294:1625–33). Compared with clinical management alone, PAC use did not significantly affect mortality. Furthermore, the PAC did not significantly reduce days of hospitalization. The PAC is associated with an increased use of inotropic medications and vasodilators. The investigators did not perform a formal analysis for publication bias. The overall findings of all trials were homogeneous (ie, the results were similar among the individual trials).

Essential Evidence: Medicine that Matters, Edited by David Slawson, Allen Shaughnessy, Mark Ebell, and Henry Barry.

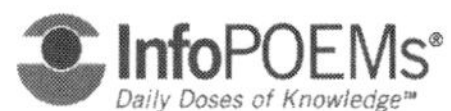

Pulmonary artery catheters: no harm, no benefit (PAC-Man)

Clinical question

Do patients in the intensive care unit benefit from being monitored by pulmonary artery catheters?

Bottom line

In this randomized trial, patients in the intensive care unit (ICU) do not benefit – nor are they harmed – by pulmonary artery catheters (PACs). (LOE = 1b–)

Reference

Harvey S, Harrison DA, Singer M, et al, for the PAC-Man study collaboration. Assessment of the clinical effectiveness of pulmonary artery catheters in management of patients in intensive care (PAC-Man): a randomised controlled trial. Lancet 2005;366:472–477.

Study Design

Randomized controlled trial (nonblinded)

Funding

Government

Allocation

Concealed

Setting

Inpatient (ICU only)

Synopsis

In a previous study, the use of PACs in critically ill postoperative patients did not provide any advantage (New Engl J Med 2003; 348:5–14). In this multicenter British study, patients older than 16 years admitted to the ICU were randomly assigned (masked allocation) to receive invasive monitoring with PACs (n = 506) or to a control group managed without PACs (n = 508). The study began with more patients in each group, but the authors excluded those who didn't consent or who withdrew consent for participation; the same number of patients were excluded from each group. Clinicians or nurses caring for the patients collected data for the acute physiology and chronic health evaluation (APACHE II) severity scoring system and the sequential organ failure assessment (SOFA) score. These are all measures of severity of illness. The main outcome, assessed by intention to treat, was hospital mortality from any cause. To have 90% power to detect a 10% absolute mortality difference, the authors needed a total of 1281 patients, more than the 1014 they were able to enroll. The hospital mortality was the same in PAC group and the control group (68% and 66%, respectively; P = 0.4). Additionally, ICU mortality was the same in each group, as was total length of stay and ICU length of stay. Approximately 10% of the patients with PACs had complications, none fatal.

Essential Evidence: Medicine that Matters, Edited by David Slawson, Allen Shaughnessy, Mark Ebell, and Henry Barry.

Door-to-balloon time important in STEMI

Clinical question

Does time to reperfusion using coronary angioplasty ("door-to-balloon time") affect mortality rates?

Bottom line

Mortality resulting from ST-segment elevation myocardial infarction (STEMI) is independently related to the time it takes to administer percutaneous coronary intervention (PCI) following presentation to the emergency department. The relationship is still seen in patients who present several hours after symptoms begin. If you have a choice of hospitals, find out their door-to-balloon times and send patients to the faster one. (LOE = 2b)

Reference

McNamara RL, Wang Y, Herrin J, et al, for the NRMI Investigators. Effect of door-to-balloon time on mortality in patients with ST-segment elevation myocardial infarction. J Am Coll Cardiol 2006;47:2180–2186.

Study Design

Cohort (retrospective)

Funding

Government

Setting

Emergency department

Synopsis

Faster use of thrombolytic therapy in the treatment of STEMI is associated with better outcomes, though this relationship is not as solid for PCI. The investigators conducting this study evaluated the role of speed of reperfusion therapy in a US registry. The registry contained data on 29,222 patients treated at 395 hospitals with PCI within 6 hours of presentation. The investigators excluded data from hospitals performing fewer than 20 PCIs over the 4 years of data collection. In-hospital mortality was associated with delays in treatment in a linear fashion with rates of 3.0%, 4.2%, 5.7%, and 7.4% at less than 91 minutes, 91 to 120 minutes, 121 to 150 minutes, and greater than 150 minutes, respectively ($P < .01$). In other words, 1 additional death is avoided for every 23 patients treated within 90 minutes rather than after 150 minutes. This trend was seen regardless of the time between symptom onset and presentation to the hospital. Faster administration of PCI was associated with improved outcomes in patients with at least one risk factor for STEMI, but not for patients with no risk factors.

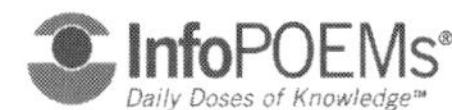

Pharmaceutical ads are often inaccurate

Clinical question

How accurate are pharmaceutical advertisements?

Bottom line

Inaccurate statements occur in one third to one half of pharmaceutical advertisements in Spanish medical journals. The findings are likely comparable with other countries, but this paper can't address that. (LOE = 4)

Reference

Villaneuva P, Peiro S, Librero J, Pereiro I. Accuracy of pharmaceutical advertisements in medical journals. Lancet 2003;361:27–32.

Study Design

Cross-sectional

Setting

Other

Synopsis

These authors reviewed 6 Spanish medical journals and extracted ads for antihypertensive and lipid-lowering medications. Using a procedure that was established a priori and was previously tested on ads not included in this study, two pairs of investigators independently reviewed the ads, obtained references cited within the ads and compared the data with those actually published. Disagreements were reviewed by a third pair of investigators. Among the 264 ads for antihypertensive medications, only 31 (12%) had references. Among the 23 ads for lipid-lowering agents, 7 (30%) had references. Many of the references couldn't be retrieved. Of those retrieved, 63% came from journals ranked in the top 20 impact journals by the Science Citations Index and 82% were randomized controlled trials. The authors report that the bibliographic references didn't support many of the promotional statement claims (45 of 102 [44.1%]; 95% CI, 34.3–54.3). Although the ads evaluated were published in 1997, the results are likely to be representative of current practice.

Essential Evidence: Medicine that Matters, Edited by David Slawson, Allen Shaughnessy, Mark Ebell, and Henry Barry.

Prescribing antibiotics does not save time

Clinical question

Does prescribing antibiotics for viral infections save time?

Bottom line

Prescribing antibiotics for respiratory infections in children does not improve patient satisfaction and, as shown in this study, doesn't save time. Of course, as you know, antibiotic prescribing also doesn?t affect the duration or severity of these viral illnesses. (LOE = 2c)

Reference

Coco A, Mainous AG. Relation of time spent in an encounter with the use of antibiotics in pediatric office visits for viral respiratory infections. Arch Pediatr Adolesc Med 2005;159:1145–1149.

Study Design

Cross-sectional

Funding

Foundation

Setting

Outpatient (primary care)

Synopsis

"If I don't give antibiotics, they won't be satisfied." "If I don't give antibiotics, they will change doctors." "If I don't give antibiotics, I will have to waste time explaining why." These are only a smattering of the excuses physicians use to justify bad practice. In this study, the authors used the National Ambulatory Medical Care Survey to evaluate the duration of visits for children presenting with colds or bronchitis. The survey, completed by physicians and office staff, includes an item labeled "time spent with a physician." The mean duration of the visits during which antibiotics were prescribed was 14.24 minutes; the mean duration of the visits when antibiotics were not prescribed was 14.18. Other studies have demonstrated that patient demand, patient satisfaction, and the likelihood of switching physicians are not affected by the receipt of an antibiotic. About the only thing prescribing antibiotics does is increase the likelihood of subsequent drug-seeking behaviors.

Essential Evidence: Medicine that Matters, Edited by David Slawson, Allen Shaughnessy, Mark Ebell, and Henry Barry.

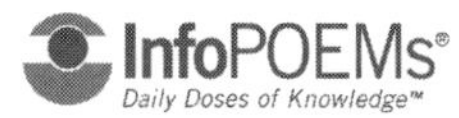

Delayed prescription for AOM reduces unnecessary antibiotics

Clinical question

Will asking parents to delay filling a prescription for the treatment of acute otitis media reduce unnecessary antibiotic use?

Bottom line

A wait-and-see approach of asking parents of children given a diagnosis of acute otitis media (AOM) in the emergency department to delay filling a prescription significantly reduces unnecessary antibiotic use. Parents of children in the delayed group reported otalgia slightly, if any, more often than the parents of children in the standard group. All parents received explicit instructions to provide both ibuprofen and otic analgesic drops to their children. Children in the standard treatment group were more likely to have diarrhea. (LOE = 1b)

Reference

Spiro DM, Tay KY, Arnold DH, Dziura JD, Baker MD, Shapiro ED. Wait-and-see prescription for the treatment of acute otitis media: a randomized controlled trial. JAMA 2006;296:1235–1241.

Study Design	Funding	Allocation
Randomized controlled trial (single-blinded)	Foundation	Concealed

Setting

Emergency department

Synopsis

Previous studies evaluating the effects of asking parents to delay filling antibiotic prescriptions for children with AOM excluded children with high fever. These investigators enrolled 283 consecutive children, aged 6 months to 12 years, seen in an emergency department who were given a diagnosis of AOM. Exclusion criteria included: another bacterial infection, such as pneumonia; "toxic" appearance; immunocompromization; myringotomy tubes or perforated tympanic membrane; or antibiotic use within 7 days. Parents of children with AOM randomly received (concealed allocation assignment) verbal and written instructions "not to fill the antibiotic prescription unless your child either is not better or is worse 48 hours (2 days) after today's visit" (intervention group) or to "fill the antibiotic prescription and give the antibiotic to your child after today's visit" (standard group). Amoxicillin was prescribed for most patients. All subjects also received ibuprofen and otic analgesic drops (containing antipyrene and benzocaine) in standard doses. Individuals blinded to treatment group assignment assessed outcomes at 4 to 6 days, 11 to 14 days, and 30 to 40 days after enrollment. In addition, a research assistant called pharmacies 4 days after enrollment to confirm whether prescriptions were filled. Follow-up occurred for more than 94% of participants. Using intention-to-treat analysis, prescriptions were filled significantly less often for children in the wait-and-see group versus the standard group (62% vs 13%). The difference was also significant in the subgroup of children younger than 2 years of age (47% wait-and-see vs 5% standard). Verification of whether prescriptions were actually filled was assessed for 28% of the study population; the pharmacy confirmed parental report in almost all instances. Otalgia occurred for a slightly greater period (0.4 days) in the wait-and-see group, but the overall rate of otalgia after 4 days was similar in both groups. Unscheduled follow-up visits were similar in both groups. No serious adverse events occurred in either treatment group, but parents in the standard group reported significantly more diarrhea in their children (23% vs 8%; number needed to treat to harm = 7).

Essential Evidence: Medicine that Matters, Edited by David Slawson, Allen Shaughnessy, Mark Ebell, and Henry Barry.

Delayed prescriptions for URIs reduce antibiotic use

Clinical question

Do delayed prescriptions reduce antibiotic use in upper respiratory tract infections?

Bottom line

Delayed prescriptions for upper respiratory tract infections reduces the use of antibiotics; patient satisfaction, however, may be worse. (LOE = 1a–)

Reference

Arroll B, Kenealy T, Kerse N. Do delayed prescriptions reduce antibiotic use in respiratory tract infections? A systematic review. Br J Gen Pract 2003;53:871–877.

Study Design

Systematic review

Setting

Outpatient (primary care)

Synopsis

For this systematic review, the authors included controlled trials of studies in which the intervention was a delayed prescription compared with an immediate prescription for patients with upper respiratory tract infections. They searched several databases (MEDLINE, Embase, Cochrane) and searched for unpublished studies. Two of the authors independently assessed the quality of the trials (randomization, concealment of allocation, co-interventions, losses to follow-up, and so forth). Disagreements among the reviewers were resolved by discussion and consensus. The authors were only able to find 5 controlled trials, 4 of which were randomized. All the randomized controlled trials had Jadad scores above 3, indicating reasonable to good quality. Since the authors found significant heterogeneity among the studies, they refrained from pooling the data. However, each study demonstrated significant reduction in the rate of antibiotic use. In 2 of the studies, however, patient satisfaction was significantly worse, and in 3 studies the symptoms were worse among those receiving a delayed prescription.

Quality of care not related to spending

Clinical question

With regional variation in Medicare spending, do increased costs reflect better quality of care?

Bottom line

Medical spending varies widely across the country. Medicare enrollees in higher-spending regions of the country receive more care but do not live as long, function better, or report more satisfaction with their care. If we could spend the same amount of money across the country as we do in the lowest cost regions, Medicare costs would decrease 30% and the Medicare Trust Fund would become solvent again. Is anyone listening? (LOE = 2b)

Reference

Fisher ES, Wennberg DE, Stukel TA, Gottlieb DJ, Lucas FL, Pinder EL. The implications of regional variations in Medicare spending, part 1: the content, quality, and accessibility of care. Ann Intern Med 2003;138:273–287. Fisher ES, Wennberg DE, Stukel TA, Gottlieb DJ, Lucas FL, Pinder EL. The implications of regional variations in Medicare spending, part 2: health outcomes and satisfaction with care. Ann Intern Med 2003;138:288–299.

Study Design

Cohort (retrospective)

Setting

Population-based

Synopsis

We know from previous research, that, after adjusting for age, sex, and race, Medicare spending in Miami, Florida, was $8414 per person, but only $3341 in Minneapolis, Minnesota. The sunshine state must be providing better care, right? Not necessarily. This national study of Medicare beneficiaries evaluated the care of patients hospitalized for hip fracture, colorectal cancer, or acute myocardial infarction (almost 1 million patients). Although not a randomized study, this type of approach has been called "natural randomization," since the geographic area assignment eliminates links between patients' initial health status and regional expenditures. Hospital referral regions, and the patients within them, were assigned to different exposure levels on the basis of the End-of-Life Expenditure Index; differences between regions in end-of-life spending are not related to underlying illness levels. They measured content of care (frequency and type of service), quality of care, and access to care. Although the average baseline health status of patients was similar across regions, patients in higher-spending regions received approximately 60% more care, mainly as more physician visits, more tests, and a higher use of specialists. The quality of care associated with this higher spending was no better in most cases and was worse with regard to preventive care measures (influenza, pneumonia vaccines, Pap smears, mammography). Patients with acute myocardial infarction were no more likely to receive acute reperfusion therapy, and were less likely to receive aspirin or angiotnesin-converting enzyme inhibitors. Access to primary care was slightly lower in the high expenditure areas, with fewer patients reporting a usual source of care. What about outcomes? For the colon cancer and acute myocardial infarction groups, adjusted mortality rates increased – yes, increased – with increased spending. Increased spending was not related to mortality in the hip fracture and general population samples. Functional status of patients did not vary by the amount of money spent on their care. There was no difference in satisfaction of care across spending categories, although there was variation across geographic regions.

Essential Evidence: Medicine that Matters, Edited by David Slawson, Allen Shaughnessy, Mark Ebell, and Henry Barry.

Disclosure of errors preferred by patients

Clinical question

How do patients report they will respond when doctors disclose errors?

Bottom line

Given a hypothetical situation in which harm occurred as the result of a medical error, patients overwhelmingly report that they would want to be told of the error. Full disclosure increases patient satisfaction, trust, and positive emotional responses. Although this disclosure may make them feel better, it may not decrease their desire to sue. Most patients (83%) would want financial compensation for an injury that occurs because an error, and 13% expressed a desire for compensation even if harm didn't occur. A questionnaire of this type does not evaluate the role of bedside manner during the process of disclosure. (LOE = 2c)

Reference

Mazor KM, Simon SR, Yood RA, et al. Health plan members' views about disclosure of medical errors. Ann Intern Med 2004;140:409–418.

Study Design

Cross-sectional

Setting

Population-based

Synopsis

This study used a self-administered questionnaire to gauge patients' responses to several types of errors and their disclosure by physicians. The questionnaires were sent to a sample of 1500 patients of a New England-based health maintenance organization (the response rate was 66%, which is high for this type of study, but less than the 70% often cited as being satisfactory). Eight versions of the questionnaire were used, which varied by type of error, clincal outcome of the error, and level of physician disclosure. The respondents were an average 2 years older and more likely to be female than nonrespondents, and more than 90% of the responding group was white. Most (90%) graduated from high school and, interestingly, 1 in 8 reported they had been injured by a medical error. Almost all patients (99%) wanted to be told of a medical error and most (83%) wanted financial compensation for harm caused by an error. Interestingly, 13% of respondents wanted compensation even if no harm occurred. Full disclosure of the error reduced the reported likelihood of changing physicians and increased patients satisfaction, trust, and positive emotional response, but for the most part did not decrease reported likelihood of seeking legal advice. This study is limited by its design; that is, by asking patients what they would think in a hypothetical situation rather than studying patients for whom the situation has occurred. This approach tends to make responses more logical and doesn't take into account the positive or negative effects that emotions play during an actual situation. Our interpretation is that how the error is communicated matters just as much as the communication itself.

Essential Evidence: Medicine that Matters, Edited by David Slawson, Allen Shaughnessy, Mark Ebell, and Henry Barry.

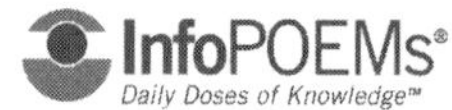

Hypertension follow-up: 3 months = 6 months

Clinical question

Can patients with hypertension be seen every 6 months without loss of control, changes in patient satisfaction, or declines in adherence to treatment?

Bottom line

Seeing patients with controlled hypertension every 6 months, rather than every 3 months, resulted in similar blood pressure measurements both in the office and at home, with no changes in patients satisfaction or adherence to therapy. (LOE = 1b)

Reference

Birtwhistle RV, Godwin MS, Delva MD, et al. Randomised equivalence trial comparing three and six months of follow-up of patients with hypertension by family practitioners. BMJ 2004;328:204–206.

Study Design

Randomized controlled trial (nonblinded)

Setting

Outpatient (primary care)

Synopsis

Canadian, British, and American guidelines regarding the management of hypertension suggest an interval of 3 to 6 months for follow-up in patients with controlled hypertension. This study explored the difference between 3-month and 6-month follow-up in 609 patients with hypertension controlled for at least 3 months by at least 1 drug. Patients were randomized (allocation assignment concealed) to return every 3 or 6 months, with earlier follow-up if blood pressure was out of control or if drug therapy was changed. Analysis was by intention to treat. As one might expect, the 6-month group had significantly fewer office visits over the 3 years of the study (average = 16.2 vs 18.8), although they still were seen much more frequently than scheduled (they should have been seen an average of 6 and 12 times). Blood pressures measured at the end of each year in the office were not different among the 2 groups. Blood pressure measurements taken at home were similar to the doctors' measurements. At each period a similar percentage of patients (~20%) in each group were deemed by their doctor to have out-of-control blood pressure. Satisfaction with their care and self-reported adherence to therapy was similar in both groups. The study had the ability to find a true difference in blood pressure of <10% at a power of 0.8.

Essential Evidence: Medicine that Matters, Edited by David Slawson, Allen Shaughnessy, Mark Ebell, and Henry Barry.

Watchful waiting acceptable option for inguinal hernia

Clinical question

Is it safe to defer surgical repair (called watchful waiting) in asymptomatic or minimally symptomatic men with inguinal hernias?

Bottom line

Watchful waiting is a safe and acceptable option for men with asymptomatic or minimally symptomatic inguinal hernias. Acute complications rarely occur, and patients who delay surgery are not at an increased risk of operative or postoperative complications. (LOE = 1b)

Reference

Fitzgibbons RJ Jr, Giobbie-Hurder A, Gibbs JO, et al. Watchful waiting vs repair of inguinal hernia in minimally symptomatic men. A randomized clinical trial. JAMA 2006;295:285–292.

Study Design

Randomized controlled trial (single-blinded)

Funding

Government

Allocation

Concealed

Setting

Outpatient (any)

Synopsis

Although many men with inguinal hernia are asymptomatic or minimally symptomatic, surgical repair is usually recommended to prevent complications, such as acute bowel incarceration. The investigators enrolled 720 men, aged 18 years or older, with asymptomatic or minimally symptomatic inguinal hernias. Subjects were randomized (concealed allocation assignment) to watchful waiting or to standard inguinal hernia repair. Complete follow-up occurred for 2 years to 4.5 years for 90% of enrollees. Patients aware of treatment group assignment self-reported outcomes. Primary outcomes included pain and discomfort interfering with usual activities and overall quality of life. Secondary outcomes included complications. Twenty-three percent of patients assigned to watchful waiting crossed over to received surgical repair and 17% of subjects assigned to surgical repair crossed over to watchful waiting. Using intention-to-treat analysis, there were no significant differences reported between the 2 groups in pain-limiting activities or overall quality of life. Postoperative complications occurred similarly in patients initially assigned to surgical repair and in those who crossed over from watchful waiting. One watchful waiting patient experienced acute hernia incarceration without strangulation within 2 years, and one patient had acute incarceration with bowel obstruction at 4 years, with an overall complication rate of watchful waiting of 1.8/1000 patient years. The sample size of 720 patients had a 90% power to detect a 10% difference for each of the primary outcomes.

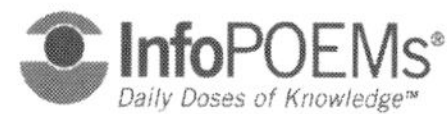

Self-monitoring of anticoagulation safe, effective

Clinical question

Can patients taking warfarin monitor and adjust their doses safely and effectively?

Bottom line

Although many patients will not wish to do so, home monitoring of anticoagulation status and subsequent self-adjustment of dosing is safe and effective. Self-monitoring of anticoagulation is a bit trickier than home blood glucose monitoring, and approximately 30% of patients dropped out during the training period. The testing equipment is expensive ($1300 US), a cost-effectiveness analysis has not been done, and there is no evidence that it leads to better clinical outcomes (ie, less bleeding and less recurrent embolic events). (LOE = 2b)

Reference

Fitzmaurice DA, Murray ET, McCahon D, et al. Self management of oral anticoagulation: randomised trial. BMJ 2005;331:1057–1062.

Study Design

Randomized controlled trial (nonblinded)

Funding

Government

Allocation

Concealed

Setting

Outpatient (primary care)

Synopsis

The marketing of simple point-of-care tools for determining anticoagulation opens up the possibility of patients self-monitoring and adjusting their own warfarin doses. These UK researchers tested this possibility in patients taking warfarin chronically for a variety of reasons. Starting by identifying 2530 patients who might be eligible, they ended up recruiting 617 adults (25%) with a long-term indication for anticoagulation who had taken warfarin for at least 6 months. All patients were considered capable of self management. Using concealed allocation, the researchers randomly assigned patients to continue either routine care or to self-monitoring. Following 2 training sessions, the patients were given testing equipment (Coaguchek S) and a dose-adjustment algorithm. The patients checked their coagulation status every 2 weeks, or weekly following a dosing change. The percentage of time the international normalized ratio (INR) was in the therapeutic range was similar between the patients who continued self-management (~70%) and the patients in routine care (72% vs 68%). Patients with a target INR of 2.5 were in the therapeutic range 74% of the time. Of patients with a higher target INR of 3.5, they were in their therapeutic range only 55% of the 12-month study period, but this percentage was significantly higher than before the study was started (45%). The rate of adverse effects was low in the routine care and self-management groups: 2.8 vs. 2.7 events per 100 patients per year. Serious bleeding rates and serious thrombosis rates were similar in both groups. These results are slightly better than a recent study conducted in Italy (Ann Intern Med 2005;142:1–10).

Essential Evidence: Medicine that Matters, Edited by David Slawson, Allen Shaughnessy, Mark Ebell, and Henry Barry.

Self-monitoring anticoagulation superior at preventing venous thromboembolic events

Clinical question

Do patients monitor and manage their oral anticoagulation at least as well as professionals?

Bottom line

Patients who self-monitor oral anticoagulation had fewer thromboembolic events than those using standard approaches to monitoring. However, self-monitoring should only be offered to literate and motivated patients. Additionally, the machines are costly and not universally covered by insurance. (LOE = 1a)

Reference

Heneghan C, Alonso-Coello P, Garcia-Alamino JM, Perera R, Meats E, Glasziou P. Self-monitoring of oral anticoagulation: a systematic review and meta-analysis. Lancet 2006;367:404–411.

Study Design

Meta-analysis (randomized controlled trials)

Funding

Self-funded or unfunded

Setting

Outpatient (any)

Synopsis

These investigators searched multiple databases for randomized controlled trials comparing self-monitoring of oral anticoagulation with standard monitoring. Additionally, they sought ongoing trials and data from equipment manufacturers in an attempt to find unpublished data. Three reviewers independently assessed each study for inclusion with discrepancies resolved by consensus. Additionally, they assessed each study's methodologic quality. Ultimately, the authors identified 14 studies including 1309 patients. These were generally small studies with an average of 94 patients. In all studies, the self-monitored patients maintained their international normalization ratio within target at least as well as those with standard monitoring. More important, only 2.2% of self-monitored patients had thromboembolic events compared with 4.6% receiving standard care (number needed to treat = 43; 95% CI, 27–92). In the studies that directly measured them, outcomes of major hemorrhage and overall death were also significantly better in the self-monitoring groups. A word of caution: A high proportion of patients (31%–88%) didn't enroll or dropped out because of the complexity of self-management.

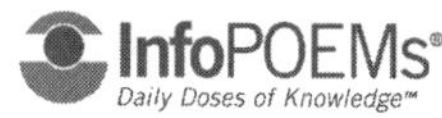

Immediate- and extended-release ciprofloxacin similar for UTI

Clinical question

Does a single dose of extended-release ciprofloxacin improve outcomes for women with uncomplicated urinary tract infection?

Bottom line

A single dose of an extended-release version of ciprofloxacin (Cipro XR) is as effective as the immediate-release version taken twice daily for 3 days. The tiny reduction in the likelihood of gastrointestinal adverse effects (number needed to treat (NNT) = 60–80) is likely to be heavily promoted, and must be balanced against the higher cost of this formulation. As we are given more such options, it is important to remember the key elements in choosing a drug: its safety, tolerability, efficacy, price, and simplicity. Although extended-release ciprofloxacin is simpler, it is no more effective and will almost certainly cost more. (LOE = 1b)

Reference

Fourcroy JL, Berner B, Chiang YK, Cramer M, Rowe L, Shore N. Efficacy and safety of a novel once-daily extended-release ciprofloxacin tablet formulation for treatment of uncomplicated urinary tract infection in women. Antimicrob Agents Chemother 2005;49:4137–4143.

Study Design

Randomized controlled trial (double-blinded)

Funding

Industry

Allocation

Concealed

Setting

Outpatient (any)

Synopsis

Although 3 days of trimethoprim-sulfamethoxazole is the recommended first-line therapy for uncomplicated urinary tract infection (UTI), ciprofloxacin is a treatment option when resistance to trimethoprim-sulfamethoxazole is greater than 20%. The critical problem with ciprofloxacin is that it is available in generic form, so manufacturers are working hard to create innovative delivery systems that can be sold under patent. In this study, the authors compared an extended-release version of ciprofloxacin 500 mg (Proquin XR) given once with the immediate-release formulation of ciprofloxacin 250 mg given twice a day for 3 days. Of 1027 nonpregnant adult women with an uncomplicated UTI, only the 540 with a positive urine culture for an organism susceptible to ciprofloxacin were included in the modified intention-to-treat analysis. Most UTIs (81%) were caused by E. coli. There was no difference between groups regarding microbiologic or clinical cure rates (86% for both groups). There was a slight reduction in the likelihood of nausea or diarrhea (NNT = 60 for nausea; NNT = 80 for diarrhea).

Essential Evidence: Medicine that Matters, Edited by David Slawson, Allen Shaughnessy, Mark Ebell, and Henry Barry.

Treating negative dipstick dysuria decreases symptoms

Clinical question

In women with dysuria and frequency but a negative dipstick test result for nitrites and leukocytes, do antibiotics decrease symptoms?

Bottom line

No infection, no antibiotic, right? Maybe not. In women with dysuria and frequency but a negative urine dipstick result for nitrites and leukocytes, 3 of 4 women will respond to antibiotic treatment as compared with 1 of 4 taking placebo. The negative dipstick result correlated with culture 92% of the time. These results imply that some women have microbial infections that are not identified by dipstick or culture. Or, perhaps, the antibiotic is doing something other than killing bacteria. (LOE = 1b)

Reference

Richards D, Toop L, Chambers S, Fletcher L. Response to antibiotics of women with symptoms of urinary tract infection but negative dipstick urine test results: double blind randomised controlled trial. BMJ 2005;331:143–146.

Study Design

Randomized controlled trial (double-blinded)

Funding

Government

Allocation

Concealed

Setting

Outpatient (primary care)

Synopsis

The authors invited women between the ages of 16 years and 50 years to participate in this study if they presented to their New Zealand general practitioner with a history of dysuria and frequency but with a midstream urine specimen that was negative for nitrites and leukocytes using a standard urine dipstick. As a check on the validity of the dipstick, urine specimens were also cultured, though the results were not known until after the treatment and assessment had been completed. The 59 participants were randomized to receive, using concealed allocation, either placebo or trimethoprim 300 mg daily for 3 days. At the end of treatment, 76% of the women treated with antibiotic had resolution of dysuria, as compared with 26% of women who were treated with placebo (P = .0005). By 7 days, 90% of treated women had resolution of dysuria as compared with 59% of women receiving placebo (P = .02). One additional patient had resolution of symptoms by 7 days for every 4 women who received treatment instead of placebo (number needed to treat = 4; 95% CI, 1.9–14.1). Urinary frequency was unaffected by treatment. It's not that the dipstick failed to diagnose infection: Culture of dipstick-negative urine grew organisms in only 5 of 59 women; therefore, the negative predictive value of the dipstick was 92%.

Essential Evidence: Medicine that Matters, Edited by David Slawson, Allen Shaughnessy, Mark Ebell, and Henry Barry.

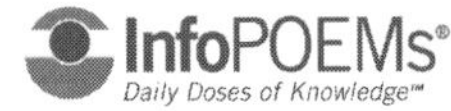

Urinary incontinence diagnosis with 3 questions

Clinical question

Can a questionnaire be used to differentiate between urge and stress incontinence?

Bottom line

A simple 3-item questionnaire – 1 question, in particular – can identify incontinence as being either stress predominant or urge predominant in 3 of 4 women. The written questionnaire is self-administered by the patient and takes approximately 30 seconds. (LOE = 2b)

Reference

Brown JS, Bradley CS, Subak LL, et al, for the Diagnostic Aspects of Incontinence Study (DAISy) Research Group. The sensitivity and specificity of a simple test to distinguish between urge and stress urinary incontinence. Ann Intern Med 2006;144:715–723.

Study Design

Diagnostic test evaluation

Funding

Industry

Setting

Population-based

Synopsis

The authors of this study tested a 3-item questionnaire to see if it could accurately differentiate urge incontinence and stress incontinence in women. They recruited through advertisements women who were at least 40 years of age and had untreated incontinence (average = 7 years) of a broad range of severity. All 301 women in the study completed the written questionnaire and then were extensively evaluated by a urologist or urogynecologist unaware of the responses to the questions. The gold standard was blinded review of the extended evaluation by a second specialist unaware of the questionnaire results or the conclusion of the first specialist. Stress incontinence was diagnosed in 44% of the patients, urge incontinence in 40%, mixed in 14%, and other causes in 3%. As compared with the gold standard, the questionnaire had a sensitivity of 0.75 and a specificity of 0.77 for urge incontinence and a sensitivity of 0.86 and a specificity of 0.60 for stress incontinence. Given a similar distribution of types of incontinence, the questions will have a positive predictive value of 73% for stress incontinence and 75% for urge incontinence. The 3-item questionnaire follows; only question #3 was used to determine diagnosis.1. Have you leaked urine (even a small amount) in the last 3 months?2. In the last 3 months, did you leak urine: A. when performing some physical activity such as coughing, sneezing, lifting, or exercise? B. when you had the urge or feeling that you needed to empty your bladder? C. without physical activity or a sense of urgency?3. During the last 3 months, did you leak urine most often: A. when you were performing some physical activity such as coughing, sneezing, lifting, or exercise? (diagnosis: stress) B. when you had the urge or the feeling that you needed to empty your bladder, but you could not get to the toilet fast enough? (diagnosis: urge) C. without physical activity and without a sense of urgency? (diagnosis: other cause) D. about equally as often with physical activity as with a sense of urgency? (diagnosis: mixed)

Essential Evidence: Medicine that Matters, Edited by David Slawson, Allen Shaughnessy, Mark Ebell, and Henry Barry.

HRT increases risk of stress, urge urinary incontinence

Clinical question

Can hormone replacement therapy decrease the risk of urinary incontinence in postmenopausal women?

Bottom line

Despite what we learned about the beneficial effects of menopausal hormone therapy on reversing urethral and bladder mucosal atrophy, postmenopausal women using either estrogen alone or estrogen plus progestin are at an increased risk of both stress and urge urinary incontinence. (LOE = 1b)

Reference

Hendrix SL, Cochrane BB, Nygaard IE, et al. Effects of estrogen with and without progestin on urinary incontinence. JAMA 2005;293:935–948.

Study Design

Randomized controlled trial (double-blinded)

Funding

Government

Allocation

Concealed

Setting

Outpatient (any)

Synopsis

As predicted, more spin-off studies are coming from the Women's Health Initiative (WHI) multicenter clinical trial of hormone therapy in postmenopausal women. These investigators randomized 27,347 postmenopausal women aged 50 to 79 years to active treatment (estrogen alone or estrogen plus progestin) or placebo. The randomization (concealed allocation assignment) was based on hysterectomy status. Outcomes were assessed by individuals blinded to treatment group assignment. Follow-up was available at 1 year for 96% of the women. Using intention-to-treat analysis, menopausal hormone replacement therapy with estrogen alone or estrogen plus progestin increased the risk for both urge urinary incontinence (14% vs 13%; number needed to treat to harm [NNTH] = 100) and stress urinary incontinence (17% vs 9%; NNTH = 13; 95% CI, 10–15) compared with placebo, respectively.

Essential Evidence: Medicine that Matters, Edited by David Slawson, Allen Shaughnessy, Mark Ebell, and Henry Barry.

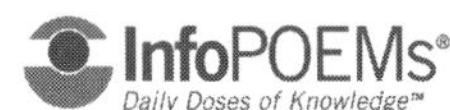

PT cures postpartum stress incontinence

Clinical question

Can physical therapy cure stress urinary incontinence in women with symptoms persisting longer than 3 months postpartum?

Bottom line

Eight weekly sessions of pelvic floor muscle physiotherapy, including electrical stimulation and biofeedback exercises, cured stress incontinence in 70% of the treated women. None of the control patients, who received massage only, were cured. Instructions for a home exercise program alone is usual care and would have been a better control intervention. (LOE = 1b)

Reference

Dumoulin C, Lemieux MC, Broubonnais D, Gravel D, Bravo G, Morin M. Physiotherapy for persistent postnatal stress urinary incontinence: a randomized controlled trial. Obstet Gynecol 2004;104:504–10.

Study Design

Randomized controlled trial (single-blinded)

Funding

Industry + govt

Allocation

Concealed

Setting

Outpatient (specialty)

Synopsis

Urinary incontinence is a common complaint among postpartum women. These authors enrolled 52 women who had persistent stress urinary incontinence at least 3 months after delivery. The diagnosis was made with a standardized test that used 20 minutes of exercises such as jumping jacks and measuring the difference in weight of a perineal pad to determine urine leakage. The women were stratified into 4 groups according to the amount of incontinence at baseline and parity. Women were then randomized into 3 groups that each had 8 weekly physiotherapy sessions. Women were aware of group assignment, but asked not to reveal it to providers and outcome assessors. One intervention group had sessions including electrical stimulation of the pelvic floor muscles for 15 minutes and exercises with biofeedback for 25 minutes. They were also instructed to do exercises at home 5 days per week. A second group got the same intervention, plus 30 minutes of deep abdominal muscle training. The control group had weekly massages of back and extremities and were asked not to do pelvic floor exercises during the study. Analysis was by treatment, and the authors reported that the intention-to-treat analysis was virtually identical. Only 2 subjects dropped out of the study. At study conclusion the pad test was repeated with a standardized volume in the bladder. To be considered cured, the woman's leakage could not exceed 2 g. Leakage did not occur in 56% of women receiving electrical sitmulation/biofeedback and 74% of women also receiving abdominal muscle training, but all of the women in the control group had leakage. The difference between the 2 active treatment groups was not significant. Improvement was not predicted by pelvic floor muscle dynamometer measurements.

Essential Evidence: Medicine that Matters, Edited by David Slawson, Allen Shaughnessy, Mark Ebell, and Henry Barry.

No long-term continence with pelvic floor muscle training

Clinical question
Do women maintain continence after intensive pelvic muscle floor exercise training?

Bottom line
Long-term urinary continence remains poor after intensive pelvic floor exercise training. Most women do not continue to do pelvic floor exercises. Unfortunately, surgical interventions for stress urinary incontinence did not provide long-term relief in this cohort of women, either. (LOE = 1b)

Reference
Bo K, Kvarstein B, Nygaard I. Lower urinary tract symptoms and pelvic floor muscle exercise adherence after 15 years. Obstet Gynecol 2005;105:999–1005.

Study Design
Randomized controlled trial (nonblinded)

Funding
Unknown/not stated

Allocation
Uncertain

Setting
Outpatient (any)

Synopsis
Pelvic floor muscle training is a successful intervention for the management of stress urinary incontinence in the short term. These authors surveyed 52 Norwegian women 15 years after participation in a successful intervention study comparing intensive pelvic floor training to a home exercise program for 6 months. A severity index was calculated based on multiplying the numerical responses to 2 questions, range 0–12. The questions were: (1) How often are you incontinent? (scored as 0 = never, 1 = less than once a month, 2 = a few times a month, 3 = a few times a week, and 4 = daily) and (2) How much urine leaked? (scored as 0 = none, 1 = drops, 2 = small splashes, and 3 = more). Women also rated how much incontinence interfered with their lives on a scale from 0 (not at all) to 10 (a great deal). The response rate was 90%, and approximately equal between the original intervention groups. There were no differences between groups on the severity index, in how much incontinence interfered with their lives, in pad use, or in other variables included. Approximately half the women in each group underwent surgical intervention to treat their incontinence during the 15-year follow-up period. However, more women in the original home exercise group than in the intensive training group had surgery within the first 5 years after the intervention study (9/13 vs 3/11). Comparisons between women who had surgery and women who didn't showed that those who underwent surgery were more likely to report severe leakage and interference with their lives ($P < .01$). Few women were performing pelvic floor exercises at the time of the survey.

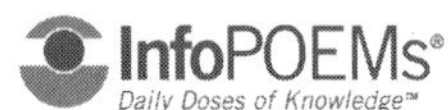

Fewer complications with condom than Foley catheters

Clinical question

Do condom catheters cause fewer complications than Foley catheters?

Bottom line

After adjusting for other factors, using condom catheters in men older than 40 is associated with fewer complications (bacteriuria, symptomatic urinary tract infection, death) than using indwelling catheters. Since more than 40% of men in each group had complications, I wonder if any kind of catheter is really necessary in most patients. (LOE = 2b)

Reference

Saint S, Kaufman SR, Rogers MA, Baker PD, Ossenkop K, Lipsky BA. Condom versus indwelling urinary catheters: a randomized trial. J Am Geriatr Soc 2006;54:1055–1061.

Study Design

Randomized controlled trial (nonblinded)

Funding

Foundation

Allocation

Concealed

Setting

Inpatient (any location) with outpatient follow-up

Synopsis

Male veterans older than 40 years admitted to a Veterans Administration (VA) nursing home or an acute medicine, neurology, or rehabilitation ward within a single VA hospital who required a urine collection device were randomly assigned to receive either a condom catheter (n = 34) or an indwelling (Foley) catheter (n = 41). The authors don't specify how this "requirement" was determined. Other studies have found that indwelling catheters are overused, typically for the convenience of the staff, and rarely have true medical indications. The main outcomes – bacteriuria, symptomatic urinary tract infection (UTI), and death – were all assessed by intention to treat for the 30-day period following enrollment. The primary outcome, bacteriuria, was assessed by staff unaware of group assignment. By chance, a significantly larger proportion of men with dementia were assigned to the condom catheter group (61% vs 20%). There was no significant difference in the overall rate of bacteriuria (38.2% with condom catheters compared with 42% with Foleys). Additionally, the composite end point of bacteriuria, symptomatic UTI, and death was similar in each group (44.1% vs 48.8%). Since the randomization resulted in baseline differences, the authors tried to take into account the effects of age, Mini-Mental State Score, prior UTI, and prior urethral catheterization. After adjusting for these factors, bacteriuria was 5 times as likely in the men with Foley catheters who did not have dementia.

Essential Evidence: Medicine that Matters, Edited by David Slawson, Allen Shaughnessy, Mark Ebell, and Henry Barry.

Tamsulosin effective for renal colic

Clinical question

Is tamsulosin (Flomax) useful in the treatment of renal colic?

Bottom line

Even though this study is fraught with methdological shortcomings, it appears highly likely that tamsulosin (Flomax) is effective in hastening the passage of juxtavesical ureteral stones and decreasing both the severity and duration of renal colic. (LOE = 2b–)

Reference

Dellabella M, Milanese G, Muzzonigro G. Efficacy of tamsulosin in the medical management of juxtavesical ureteral stones. J Urology 2003;170:2202–2205.

Study Design

Randomized controlled trial (nonblinded)

Setting

Emergency department

Synopsis

The medical management of renal colic secondary to stone retention includes the reduction of ureteral edema and spasm and the prevention of co-infection. Alpha1-adrenergic antagonists reduce ureteral contractions and spasm and may hasten the passage of retained stones. A total of 163 patients presenting to an emergency room in Italy with renal colic were identified; of these, 70 were found on imaging studies to have unilateral, juxtavesical ureteral stones. Ten subjects were excluded for various reasons, including renal colic for more than 1 day. The remaining 60 patients were randomized (nonconcealed allocation assignment) to 2 groups. Group 1 received 30 mg deflazacort (a corticosteroid to control edema) daily, cotrimoxazole (a prophylactic antibiotic) 2 times daily, 75 mg injectable diclofenac (Voltaren) on demand, and floroglucine-trimetossibenzene (a local spasmolytic drug) 3 times daily. Group 2 received similar treatment with the substitution of 0.4 mg once daily of tamsulosin (Flomax) as the spasmolytic drug. All patients were instructed to drink a lot of water. The patients, their treating clinicians, and individuals assessing outcomes were not blinded to treatment group assignment (a big methodological no-no). The mean stone size was 5.8 mm (range = 4 mm to 11 mm). Although the mean stone size was statistically larger in Group 2, the expulsion rate was greater than in Group 1 (100% vs 70%; P = .001; number needed to treat = 3). In addition, the mean hours to expulsion, the mean number of diclofenac injections, the rate of hospitalization, and the need for endoscopic stone removal were all less in the tamsulosin group. Although not specifically stated, it appears that analysis was by intention to treat.

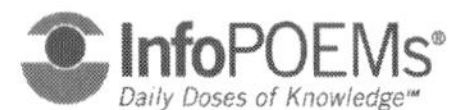

Renal colic: NSAIDs more effective, less noxious than opioid analgesics

Clinical question

Are intravenous nonsteroidal anti-inflammatory drugs more effective than narcotics in the treatment of patients with acute renal colic?

Bottom line

Nonsteroidal anti-inflammatory drugs (NSAIDs) produce equivalent or better analgesia than opioid narcotics, reduce the need for additional analgesia, and result in less vomiting in patients with renal colic. Not studied was a potential benefit of NSAIDs on the duration of colic; their ability to cause ureteral dilation may hasten stone passage. (LOE = 1a)

Reference

Holdgate A, Pollock T. Systematic review of the relative efficacy of non-steroidal anti-inflammatory drugs and opioids in the treatment of acute renal colic. BMJ 2004;328:1401–1404.

Study Design

Meta-analysis (randomized controlled trials)

Setting

Various (meta-analysis)

Synopsis

The authors of this study scoured nephrology textbooks, review articles, study bibliographies, conference proceedings, and 4 databases to find the 20 trials that compared (usually) intravenous nonsteroidal anti-inflammatory drugs (NSAIDs) with opioids in a total of 1613 patients with acute renal colic. The authors didn't describe how this search was performed or how articles were selected for inclusion. Of the 9 trials that evaluated pain at a fixed time after therapy was given, pain reports were slightly but significantly lower in the NSAID group. Studies with ketorolac (Toradol) produced heterogeneous results, but other NSAIDs produced scores that were lower, on average, by 4.6 mm on a 100 mm visual analog scale (a difference of 13 mm to 15 mm is considered clinically relevant). The number of patients with complete pain relief at 30 or 60 minutes was similar in the 2 groups. However, the risk of patients requiring rescue (ie, additional) analgesia was significantly less in the NSAID group (relative risk = 0.75; 95% CI, .61–.93). Approximately 16 patients treated with a NSAID instead of a narcotic (9 of 10 trials used meperidine [Demerol]) would need to be treated for 1 additional patient to avoid the need for additional analgesia (number needed to treat = 16; 95% CI, 10–57). Vomiting occurred less often with NSAIDs than with narcotic treatment (relative risk = 0.35; 95% CI, 0.23–0.53), with 1 fewer patient vomiting for every 8 patients treated with a NSAID instead of an opioid (95% CI, 7–11). Vomiting risk was highest with meperidine. The effect of the type of analgesia on the duration of colic was not evaluated in these studies, although their pharmacology would suggest NSAIDs, by causing relaxation of the ureters, would produce more rapid resolution.

Essential Evidence: Medicine that Matters, Edited by David Slawson, Allen Shaughnessy, Mark Ebell, and Henry Barry.

Medications help passage of kidney stones

Clinical question

Do medications help the passage of kidney stones?

Bottom line

The limited amount of available data suggest that alpha blockers and calcium channel blockers appear to speed the passage of kidney stones. Furthermore, it appears that combining these medications with steroids provides additional benefit. (LOE = 1a−)

Reference

Hollingsworth JM, Rogers MA, Kaufman SR, et al. Medical therapy to facilitate urinary stone passage: a meta-analysis. Lancet 2006;368:1171–1179.

Study Design

Meta-analysis (randomized controlled trials)

Funding

Unknown/not stated

Setting

Various (meta-analysis)

Synopsis

These authors searched multiple databases looking for randomized controlled trials of the effect of calcium channel blockers and alpha blockers on the passage of kidney stones. They also searched for unpublished studies. Two authors independently reviewed each study, assessed their quality, and extracted the data. Discrepancies were reconciled by consensus. The authors included 9 trials with a total of 693 patients in this study. Unfortunately, the authors don't report the doses of the drugs used in the included studies. In the 6 studies reporting time to stone passage, the range was as short as 6 days in several treatment groups to as long as 20 days in a control group. In 5 of those 6 trials, the treatment group had a shorter time to stone passage. The authors report that patients receiving active treatment had a 65% relative increased rate of stone passage compared with control patients. Based on the authors' estimates, we would need to treat 4 patients to facilitate the passage of 1 stone. A few studies also used steroids and the results suggest an additional benefit. Finally, the researchers report that most of the variability among the studies was attributable to variable inclusion criteria. Although they found no statistical evidence of publication bias, the authors are cautious about its potential.

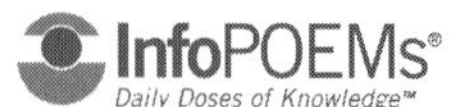

Finasteride of mixed benefit in preventing prostate cancer

Clinical question

Does finasteride reduce the risk of prostate cancer?

Bottom line

Finasteride 5 mg daily reduces the overall risk of prostate cancer from 24.4% to 18.4%, but increases the risk of high-grade disease from 5.1% to 6.4%. Since the latter is the cancer that matters in terms of mortality, and because the drug is associated with significant cost and adverse effects, it is not recommended for the prevention of prostate cancer. Patients starting finasteride for the prevention of urinary retention should be informed of these risks. (LOE = 1b)

Reference

Thompson IM, Goodman PJ, Tangen CM, et al. The influence of finasteride on the development of prostate cancer. N Engl J Med 2003;349:215–224.

Study Design

Randomized controlled trial (double-blinded)

Setting

Outpatient (any)

Synopsis

Finasteride (Proscar) inhibits the conversion of testosterone to dihydrotestosterone; it is thought that having less of this potent androgen may reduce the risk of prostate cancer. However, this theory has never been tested. In the current trial, men older than 55 years with, at most, moderate symptoms of benign prostatic hypertrophy (BPH), a normal digital rectal examination (DRE) result, and a prostate specific antigen (PSA) level of less than or equal to 3.0 ng/mL were recruited from 221 sites and randomized to oral finasteride 5 mg each day or placebo. We aren't told whether they were recruited from primary care or specialty clinics (although I suspect the latter), and 20% had a first-degree relative with prostate cancer. The allocation method was not described, but groups were balanced at baseline. Although the analysis is described as intention to treat, only men with a tissue biopsy at the end of the study were actually included. The participants had annual DRE and PSA testing, and underwent prostate biopsy if they had an abnormal DRE result or a PSA level greater than 4.0 ng/mL. All patients were supposed to undergo prostate biopsy at the end of the study, although approximately 1 in 4 refused in each group. The plan was to follow each man for 7 years, but it was stopped early by the monitoring committee, meaning that approximately 20% were followed up for less than 7 years. The overall likelihood of prostate cancer was lower in the finasteride group (18.4% vs 24.4%; $P < .001$; number needed to treat [NNT] = 16). However, there were more high-grade cancers (Gleason score 7 to 10) in the finasteride group (6.4% vs 5.1%; $P = .005$; number needed to treat to harm [NNTH] = 77). There was no difference in overall mortality over the 7-year follow-up period, although the study was too small and too short to be able to detect such a difference if it did exist. Patients taking finasteride had a greater risk of erectile dysfunction (NNTH = 16), loss of libido (NNTH = 17), and reduced volume of ejaculate (NNTH = 8), and a lower risk of benign prostatic hypertrophy (NNT = 29), incontinence (NNT = 333), and urinary retention (NNT = 48). It is interesting that more than 40% of patients had a prostate biopsy during the follow-up period because of symptoms, abnormal DRE result, or elevated PSA level. That illustrates part of the harm associated with prostate cancer screening, which must be balanced against any potential benefits.

Essential Evidence: Medicine that Matters, Edited by David Slawson, Allen Shaughnessy, Mark Ebell, and Henry Barry.

Prostate cancer screening every 4 years as good as annually

Clinical question

Is a 4-year screening interval as effective as annual screening for prostate cancer?

Bottom line

The 4-year rate of developing prostate cancer in screened men between the ages of 55 years and 75 years is pretty low. Although this study can't tell us whether men are better or worse off as a result of screening, it suggests that for those men who choose to be screened, annual screening isn't necessary. Other, smaller studies have similarly found that men with low prostate-specific antigen (PSA) levels don't need annual screening. (LOE = 2b)

Reference

van der Cruijsen-Koeter IW, van der Kwast TH, Schröder FH. Interval carcinomas in the European Randomized Study of Screening for Prostate Cancer (ERSPC)-Rotterdam. J Natl Cancer Inst 2003;95:1462–1466.

Study Design

Randomized controlled trial (nonblinded)

Setting

Population-based

Synopsis

This team studied more than 17,000 men between the ages of 55 years and 74 years randomized to screening or no screening. This study reports on the cohort of men being screened with rectal examinations, PSA, and ultrasound (n = 8350). After the first 4 years of follow-up, they report on the incidence of prostate cancer as confirmed by a review of the cancer registry. This could underestimate the true incidence of cancer. During the first screening, 412 men were given a diagnosis of prostate cancer; only 25 more cases were detected after enrollment. This translates to an incidence of 21 cases per 1000 person-years among men in the screened arm. Since the intervention group had ultrasound, these data may not reflect what one might find if PSA were used alone.

Essential Evidence: Medicine that Matters, Edited by David Slawson, Allen Shaughnessy, Mark Ebell, and Henry Barry.

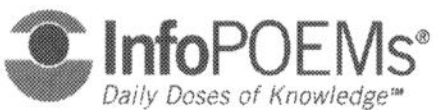

False-positive PSA associated with increased worry, fears

Clinical question

Do men who receive a positive prostate specific antigen (PSA) test result subsequently shown to be wrong worry more about prostate cancer than men who receive a negative result?

Bottom line

False positive results of screening tests are not benign but carry with them a psychological cost. As with women receiving false-positive mammogram results, men receiving false-positive prostate specific antigen (PSA) test results report having thought and worried more about prostate cancer despite receiving a negative follow-up test (prostate biopsy) result. They also think, like women, that the false-positive result makes them more likely to develop prostate cancer. Screening can be bad for our patients' mental health. (LOE = 1b)

Reference

McNaughton -Collins M, Fowler FJ, Caubet JF, et al. Psychological effects of a suspicious prostate cancer screening test followed by a benign biopsy result. Am J Med 2004;117:719–725.

Study Design

Cohort (prospective)

Funding

Foundation

Setting

Outpatient (primary care)

Synopsis

The investigators identified 167 men from a group of consecutive men who had a negative biopsy following a suspicious PSA test. In other words, these men had a false positive PSA result. For comparison, they also identified 233 men who had a normal PSA test. The men were mailed a brief questionnaire about 6 weeks after their biopsy or normal PSA test result. Overall, 85% of the men responded by returning the survey, which is a very good response for a survey. Of the men who had a false positive PSA, 49% reported having thought about prostate cancer either "a lot" or "some of the time" compared with 18% of controls ($P < .001$). As compared with 8% in the control group, 40% of the men in the false positive group also worried "a lot" (7%) or "some of the time" (33%) about the possibility of developing prostate cancer. The false positive group did not worry more than the control group about dying soon. Sixty-two percent of the men with a negative biopsy reported being "a lot" reassured by the result, despite the 10% false negative rate associated with biopsy. As with women undergoing mammogram, instead of being angry at the erroneous PSA, men with a false positive PSA but a normal biopsy felt they "dodged a bullet": Significantly more men in this group reported their lives changed for the better (31% vs. 13%, $P < .001$). And, similar to women experiencing a false positive mammogram, the men in the false positive group were more likely to think their chance of getting prostate cancer was "much more" or "a little more than average" (36% vs. 18% in the control group, $P < .001$).

Elevated PSA should be confirmed before biopsy

Clinical question

How often does an elevated PSA level return to normal?

Bottom line

Isolated elevations of serum prostate-specific antigen (PSA) frequently return to normal. Clinicians and their patients with an elevated PSA have 3 choices: (1) immediate referral for biopsy; (2) immediate repeat of the PSA test; or (3) wait 4 to 6 weeks and repeat the test. The repeat testing interval of 4 to 6 weeks is based on studies reporting the time needed for an elevated PSA to return to normal after biopsy or surgery for noncancerous conditions. Studies of prostate cancer progression conclude that a delay of several months from diagnosis to surgery does not affect outcomes. Thus, choice #3 is likely the best one for most patients before proceeding with further testing or referral. (LOE = 2b)

Reference

Eastham JA, Riedel E, Scardino PT, et al. Variation of serum prostate-specific antigen levels. An evaluation of year-to-year fluctuations. JAMA 2003:289:2695–2700.

Study Design

Cohort (prospective)

Setting

Outpatient (specialty)

Synopsis

Routine use of the PSA as a screening tool has been questioned because of its lack of specificity – meaning that many men with elevated levels do not have prostate cancer and thus undergo unnecessary and potentially harmful treatment or further testing. A variety of different methods have been studied to improve the specificity of the PSA, including age-specific reference levels, PSA velocity of change, and percentage-free PSA. Given that natural biological variations in PSA levels occur, the authors used blood samples obtained during the Polyp Prevention Trial from 1351 men aged 35 years or older with 1 or more colonic adenomas. Samples were obtained at least yearly for up to 4 years and were stored between 1 and 9 years prior to their analysis. Participants with a history of prostate cancer, those developing prostate cancer during the study period, and those with fewer than 2 blood samples were excluded from the final analysis. Most of the participants (n = 972; 79%) had PSA measurements at baseline and yearly for 4 years. Using any of the PSA thresholds, 37% of the men would have met at least 1 of the criteria for an abnormal test result. Nearly half these men subsequently had a normal PSA level on 1 or more subsequent follow-ups, including 44% with a PSA level greater than 4 ng/mL; 40% with a level greater than 2.5 ng/mL; 55% with a level above the age-specific cutoff; and 53% with level 4 ng/mL to 10 ng/mL and a free-to-total ratio of less than 0.25 ng/mL.

Essential Evidence: Medicine that Matters, Edited by David Slawson, Allen Shaughnessy, Mark Ebell, and Henry Barry.

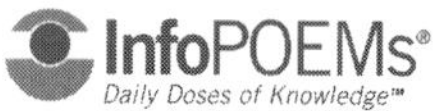

Glossary: Statistics Definitions

Blinding Also called "masking," blinding prevents people – researchers, assistants, patients, even statisticians involved in the study from knowing the treatment a subject is receiving. "Double-blinding" means that neither the researcher nor the subject knew what treatment was used. There are up to seven levels of blinding, ranging from the person enrolling patients (see "concealed allocation") to blinding of the researcher interpreting the results.

Clinical vs. Statistical Significance In most cases, statistical significance is a necessary but not the only requirement for clinical significance. Differences cannot be clinically important if they could have occurred by chance (i.e., the p-value is greater than 0.05 or so). Once statistical significance has been determined, then the reader must determine whether the difference is big enough to be relevant in practice.

Concealed Allocation: When subjects begin a study, they are allocated to a group, for example, the treatment or placebo group. There is a risk that researchers performing the study enroll some patients into the study based on what group they will be in. Concealing allocation from the investigator will prevent this from happening. It is not the same as blinding in the usual sense, which occurs after the study is started. Blinding can occur in a study even though allocation was not concealed.

For example, in many of the studies evaluating the effectiveness of breast cancer screening, researchers knew whether an individual patient would be allocated to the screening (with mammography) or no-screening group before enrolling them. If they didn't want the particular patient in the group to which they would be assigned, they simply didn't enroll them into the study. As a result, the patients in these studies who received mammography were an average 6 months older, better educated, and economically better off, three factors that are associated with decreased mortality.

Confidence Interval Sort of a statistic of a statistic. Values calculated in studies (means, etc) are estimates of the "truth." A confidence interval gives you the range of likely possibilities with a given degree of certainty. A 95% confidence interval tells us that we can be fairly (95%) certain that the true value will fall within this range.

For example, in a study looking at the BP drugs taken by people who died suddenly, beta-blockers were found to **increase** the risk of sudden death by 40% (relative risk = 1.4). However, the confidence intervals said that the risk could be as high as 3 times those not taking beta-blockers (relative risk = 3.0). The lower end of the confidence interval showed that betă blockers could have **decreased** the risk of sudden death by 40% (relative risk = 0.6). The confidence interval tells us that we really have no idea if beta-blockers are linked to sudden death.

Evidence-based Medicine The classic EBM approach consists of a 5 step process of developing a question using the populations-intervention-comparison-outcome (PICO) format, finding research that may answer the question, evaluating the research for validity, impact, and applicability, applying the information to clinical decision-making, and periodically evaluating one's effectiveness at performing the previous 4 steps

Information Mastery Information management focuses on using currently available information tools to remain up to date with new valid information that is relevant to the care of patients and is accessible while taking care of patients.

Number Needed to Treat (NNT) The number of patients that need to be treated for one to receive benefit. The NNT also can represent the number of patients that need to be treated to prevent one additional outcome event. It offers an advantage over the relative risk (see below), in that it takes into account the baseline risk as well.

p-value: P stands for "probability" – the likelihood that the difference observed between two groups could have arisen by chance. The usual p value is arbitrarily set at 0.05; it means that there is a 5% probability that the difference is actually due to chance. It does not tell you the importance of the difference. (See clinical vs. statistical significance, above).

In the phrase, "51.7% of warfarin recipients developed a DVT as compared with 36.9% of enoxaparin recipients (p = 0.003)", the probability of this difference being due to chance (and not the beneficial effect of enoxaparin over warfarin) is 0.003, or 0.3%. It does not tell us whether a 36.9% incidence represents an important therapeutic gain over the 51.7% reported with warfarin.

Relative Risk The risk of *harm* with one drug as compared with another. Conversely, it also can be the risk of *benefit* with one drug as compared with another. If RR = 1, then there is no difference between the two treatments.

Statistical Power The power of a study is the ability for that study to find a difference between two treatments if the difference *really exists*. Power depends on the number of patients in the study and the magnitude of the difference. A power of 0.80 is the standard. For example, a study of only 30 patients might not find a small difference between two drugs, whereas a study of 300 patients might find a difference.

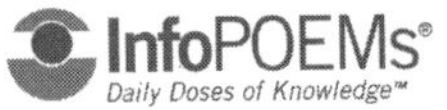

Index

Essential Evidence: Medicine that Matters, Edited by David Slawson, Allen Shaughnessy, Mark Ebell, and Henry Barry.

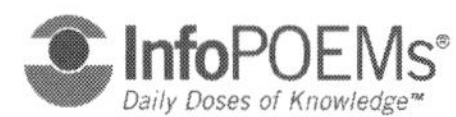
InfoPOEMs®
Daily Doses of Knowledge™

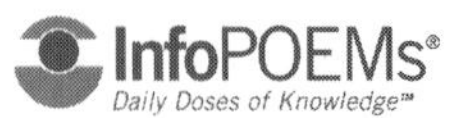

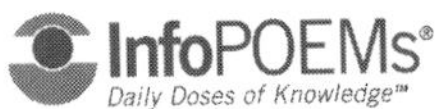
InfoPOEMs®
Daily Doses of Knowledge™

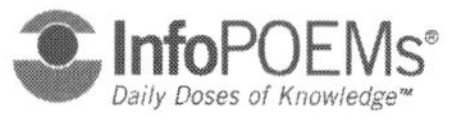
InfoPOEMs®
Daily Doses of Knowledge™

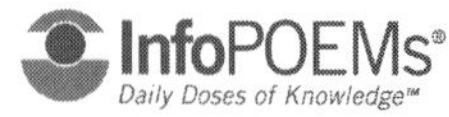
InfoPOEMs
Daily Doses of Knowledge

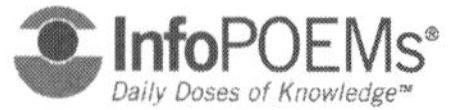
InfoPOEMs®
Daily Doses of Knowledge™